Brinda

W9-CHO-698

Davis's Guide to IV Medications

Third Edition

April Hazard Vallerand, Ph.D., R.N.
School of Nursing
University of Pennsylvania
Philadelphia, Pennsylvania

Judith Hopfer Deglin, Pharm.D.
Consultant Pharmacist
Hospice of Southeastern Connecticut
Norwich, Connecticut

 F. A. DAVIS COMPANY • **Philadelphia**

F. A. Davis Company
1915 Arch Street
Philadelphia, PA 19103

Printed in the United States of America

Last digit indicates print number: 10 9 8 7 6 5 4 3

Nursing Publisher: Robert G. Martone
Nursing Editor: Joanne Patzek DaCunha, R.N., M.S.N.
Production Editor: Jessica Howie Martin
Cover Designer: Steven R. Morrone

Library of Congress Cataloging-in-Publication Data

Vallerand, April Hazard.
  Davis's guide to IV medications / April Hazard Vallerand, Judith
Hopfer Deglin.—3rd ed.
    p.   cm.
  Includes bibliographical references and index.
  ISBN 0-8036-0092-5 (pbk.)
  1. Intravenous therapy—Handbooks, manuals, etc.   I. Vallerand,
April Hazard.   II. Title.
  [DNLM: 1. Drugs—handbooks.   2. Drugs—nurses' instruction.
3. Infusions, Intravenous—handbooks.   4. Infusions, Intravenous—
nurses' instruction.   QV 39 V184d 1996]
RM170.V35   1996
615.5'8—dc20
DNLM/DLC
for Library of Congress   95-21035
                                                              CIP

To Ben and Kate for bringing me smiles and cuddles and reminding me of what is important.
To Warren, my soulmate, colleague, husband, and friend for encouraging me, supporting me, and believing in me.

AHV

To my parents, Kurt and Charlotte Hopfer, for their unfailing love, understanding, and support.

JHD

Acknowledgments

We offer gratitude to our families, whose support and patience made possible the completion of this manuscript. We also thank those at F. A. Davis, especially Bob Martone, Ruth De George, Joanne DaCunha, and Pete Faber, who have seen our projects through to completion. We are especially grateful to the nurses, physicians, allied health workers, and students whose desire for information on the safe use of intravenous medications inspired us to create the most comprehensive and usable reference possible.

April Hazard Vallerand
Judith Hopfer Deglin

Table of Contents

Key to Commonly Used Abbreviations

ABGs	arterial blood gases
ACE	angiotensin converting enzyme
AIDS	acquired immunodeficiency syndrome
bid	two times a day
bpm	beats per minute
°C	degrees Celsius
CBC	complete blood count
CCr	creatinine clearance
CHF	congestive heart failure
CNS	central nervous system
CPK	creatine phosphokinase
CV	cardiovascular
CVP	central venous pressure
D5/LR	5% dextrose and lactated Ringer's injection
D5/0.9%	5% dextrose and 0.9% NaCl, 5% dextrose and normal saline
D5/0.25%	5% dextrose and 0.25% NaCl, 5% dextrose and quarter normal saline
D5/0.45%	5% dextrose and 0.45% NaCl, 5% dextrose and half normal saline
D5W	5% dextrose in water
D10W	10% dextrose in water
Derm	dermatologic
dl	deciliter (100 ml)
DNA	deoxyribonucleic acid
ECG	electrocardiogram
EENT	eye, ear, nose, and throat
Endo	endocrine
°F	degrees Fahrenheit
F and E	fluid and electrolyte
GI	gastrointestinal
g or Gm	gram(s)
gtt	drop(s)
GU	genitourinary
h or hr	hour(s)
Hemat	hematologic
HIV	human immunodeficiency virus
IM	intramuscular

IT . . . . intrathecal
IU . . . . international units
IV . . . . intravenous
K . . . . potassium
kg . . . . kilogram
L . . . . liter
LR . . . . lactated Ringer's solution
m^2 . . . . square meter
MAO . . . . monoamine oxidase
Metab . . . . metabolic
mcg . . . . microgram(s)
mg . . . . milligram(s)
min . . . . minute
Misc . . . . miscellaneous
ml . . . . milliliter(s)
mm^3 . . . . cubic millimeter
MS . . . . musculoskeletal
Na . . . . sodium
NaCl . . . . sodium chloride
Neuro . . . . neurologic
ng . . . . nanogram(s)
NS . . . . sodium chloride, normal saline (0.9% NaCl)
NSAIA (or NSAID)   nonsteroidal anti-inflammatory agent (drug)
Ophth . . . . ophthalmic
OTC . . . . over-the-counter (nonprescription)
PCA . . . . patient-controlled analgesia
prn . . . . when required
q . . . . every
qid . . . . four times a day
RBC . . . . red blood cell count
REM . . . . rapid eye movement
Resp . . . . respiratory
RNA . . . . ribonucleic acid
SC . . . . subcutaneous
tid . . . . three times a day
UK . . . . unknown
WBC . . . . white blood cell count
wk . . . . week(s)

How to Use Davis's Guide to IV Medications

The purpose of *Davis's Guide to IV Medications* is to provide readily accessible, concise drug information about the most commonly prescribed drugs for intravenous use. The sections below describe the organization of the monograph for each drug.

GENERIC NAME: The generic name is the accepted nonproprietary or official name of the drug and includes the name of the salt form where appropriate (sodium, potassium, hydrochloride, etc.). If the user does not know the generic name, the index includes entries for both trade names and generic names.

CLASSIFICATION: The most common classification is listed first followed by other classification(s) according to the use(s) of the drug. For example, phenytoin (Dilantin) is classified first as an anticonvulsant, but is also used as an antiarrhythmic. Subclassifications appear in parentheses.

TRADE NAMES: Trade names used by manufacturers are listed next. The index is cross-referenced by trade names. Drug monographs may also be found by looking up the trade name in the index. Common names, abbreviations, and selected foreign names are also included. Brand names available in Canada only appear in braces ({ }).

pH: The pH of the drug is listed if this information is available. For powders, the pH is listed for reconstituted solutions. For some drugs which are dispersed in unusual vehicles (i.e., castor oil derivatives), pH is not able to be determined. Drugs which are strongly acidic or alkaline are generally irritating to tissues and should be diluted appropriately or infused slowly to prevent damage to veins and surrounding tissues.

CONTROLLED SUBSTANCE SCHEDULE: If a drug is a controlled substance, its legal status or schedule in the United States will be listed. This information alerts the reader to observe the necessary regulations when handling these drugs and should help instruct the patient regarding refill allotments (see Appendix A for a description of the Schedule of Controlled Substances and a list of controlled substances included in *Davis's Guide to IV Medications*).

SODIUM (Na)/POTASSIUM (K) CONTENT: If a drug contains a significant amount of sodium (Na) or potassium (K), that information is included. For patients with severe cardiovascular or renal disease, this may be an important consideration.

ADMINISTRATION CONSIDERATIONS
Usual Dose: Usual recommended dosages are listed for adults, children, geriatric, and other more specific age/weight groups if available. In situations where dosage or interval is different from that commonly encountered, these indications will be listed separately for clarification, including unlabeled uses. Dosage units are given in the terms in which they will most likely be prescribed. (Example: Penicillin G dosage is given in units rather than milligrams.) Dosing intervals are also mentioned in the manner in which they are most likely to be ordered. If special patient characteristics exist such as renal or hepatic impairment, the text of the monograph should be consulted to see if modifications in usual doses are recommended.

Dilution: This section provides details for reconstitution and dilution. The headings **Direct IV** (IV Push), **Intermittent Infusion**, and **Continuous Infusion** specify amount and type of further dilution. Information about the color and stability of the solution is also provided.

Compatibility/Incompatibility: These sections provide information regarding the administration of the drug with other drugs when mixed in a syringe, via Y-site, as an admixture in solution with other drugs, and in solution with other infusion solutions. **Syringe Compatibility/Incompatibility** identifies the medications each drug is compatible or incompatible with when mixed in a syringe. This type of compatibility is usually limited to 15 minutes after mixing. **Y-Site Compatibility/Incompatibility** identifies those medications that are compatible or incompatible with each drug when administered via Y-injection site or 3-way stopcock in IV tubing. **Additive Compatibility/Incompatibility** identifies those medications that are compatible or incompatible when admixed in solution. This type of compatibility is usually limited to 24 hours. **Solution Compatibility/Incompatibility** identifies the compatibility of the drug in various infusion solutions.

Rate of Administration: This section provides the infusion time for each type of administration (**Direct IV or IV Push, Intermittent Infusion, Continuous Infusion**).

CLINICAL PRECAUTIONS

The Clinical Precautions section addresses information required to administer the drug safely and effectively. Guidelines are presented in a prioritized fashion so that parameters and precautions needed before the drug is administered are presented first, while other requirements follow in a logical sequence. Upon reading this section, the clinician will be able to assess for the desired response to drug therapy as well as side effects and adverse reactions to the drug. Recommendations for preventing and managing these undesired drug actions are also presented. Disease states or clinical situations where drug use involves particular risks or where dosage modification may be necessary are described in this section. A new feature designed to prevent medication error involving drugs whose names sound similar is introduced by the statement, "Do not confuse *(drug being described)* with *(drug with similar-sounding name)*." For patients receiving numerous medications, the likelihood of experiencing a drug-drug interaction increases with the number of drugs being given. The most important drug-drug interactions and their results are included here as well. Pregnancy, lactation, pediatric, and geriatric cautions have also been included. Further explanation of the FDA Pregnancy Categories is given in Appendix D. These categories allow for assessment of risk to the fetus when used in the pregnant patient or the patient who may be trying to conceive while receiving the drug.

Toxicity and Overdose Alert: Therapeutic and toxic serum drug levels and signs and symptoms of toxicity are presented in this section. The antidote and management of toxicity or overdose of medications are also included.

Lab Test Considerations: This section provides the information regarding which laboratory tests to monitor in the patient taking the drug and which lab test results may be altered by the medication.

Patient/Family Teaching: Material which should be taught to patients and/or families of patients taking each medication is provided in this section. Side effects which should be reported, information on how to minimize side effects, details on administration, and follow-up requirements are presented. The reader should also refer to the "Adverse Reactions and Side Effects" section for additional information to complete the patient/family teaching plan. A subsection, **Home Care Issues,** has been included for drugs likely to be administered in the home setting and includes information pertinent to home administration and monitoring.

PHARMACOLOGIC PROFILE

Indications: The most common clinical uses of the drug are listed. Unless otherwise noted these indications are approved by the Food and Drug Administration (FDA). Significant unlabeled uses are also noted.

Action: This section contains a concise description of how a drug is known or believed to act in producing the desired therapeutic effect. A tabular **Time/Action Profile** is presented in this section to allow the clinician to anticipate when the onset, peak, and duration of action may be expected. For many drugs, knowing the duration of action provides information for planning an effective dosing regimen. Durations of action of anti-infective agents have generally not been included. Most regimens for these agents are designed to avoid toxicity while ensuring tissue levels necessary for anti-infective action. Because of this, duration of action and blood level information are not necessarily comparable for anti-infectives.

Pharmacokinetics: The information in this section describes what happens to a drug following administration and includes an analysis of distribution, metabolism, excretion, and half-life (amount of time for blood level to decrease by 50%). **Distribution**: Following IV administration, drugs are distributed, sometimes selectively to various body tissues and fluids. These factors become important in choosing one drug over another; as in selecting antibiotics which may need to penetrate the CNS in the treatment of meningitis, or avoiding drugs which cross the placenta in pregnancy or concentrate in breast milk during lactation. During distribution many drugs interact with specific receptors and exert their pharmacologic effect. **Metabolism and Excretion**: Following their intended action, drugs leave the body by either being converted to inactive compounds by the liver (metabolism or biotransformation), which are then excreted by the kidneys, or by renal elimination of unchanged drug. In addition, some drugs may be eliminated by other pathways such as biliary excretion, sweat, feces, and breath. If drugs are extensively liver-metabolized, then patients with severe liver disease may require dosage reduction. If the kidney is the major organ of elimination, then dosage adjustment may be necessary in the face of renal impairment. The very young (premature infants and neonates) and the elderly (patients over 55–60 years) have diminished renal excretory and hepatic metabolic capacity. These patients may require dosage reduction, increased dosing intervals, or both. **Half-life:** Knowing the half-life of a drug is useful in planning effective regimens, since this parameter correlates roughly with the duration of action. Half-lives are given for patients with normal renal or hepatic function. Conditions which may alter the half-life are identified.

Contraindications: Situations where use of a specific drug should be avoided or alternative drugs strongly considered are listed as contraindications. Contraindications may be absolute; that is, the drug in question should be avoided completely; or relative, where certain clinical situations may allow cautious use of the drug.

Adverse Reactions and Side Effects: In order to simplify long lists of possible reactions, a systems approach to side effects and adverse reactions has been taken. The order is such that these reactions have been listed in head-to-toe order for systems amenable to noting in this manner (CNS, EENT, RESP, CV, GI, GU). Other systems follow in alphabetical order (DERM, ENDO, F and E, HEMAT, LOCAL, METAB, MS, NEURO), ending with a miscellaneous section. While it is not possible to include all reported reactions, an effort has been made to include major side effects. Life-threatening adverse reactions or side effects are CAPITALIZED, while the most commonly encountered problems are underlined. The following abbreviations are used for body systems: **CNS:** central nervous system; **EENT:** eye, ear, nose and throat; **Resp:** respiratory; **CV:** cardiovascular; **GI:** gastrointestinal; **GU:** genitourinary; **Derm:** dermatologic; **Endo:** endocrinologic; **F and E:** fluid and electrolyte; **Hemat:** hematologic; **Local:** local (at the injection site); **Metab:** metabolic; **MS:** musculoskeletal; **Neuro:** neurologic; **Misc:** miscellaneous.

Acetazolamide Sodium

*Antiglaucoma,
Anticonvulsant,
Carbonic anhydrase
inhibitor*

Diamox   **pH 9.2**

≋ ADMINISTRATION CONSIDERATIONS

Usual Dose

Antiglaucoma

ADULTS: *Short-term therapy*—250 mg q 4 hr or 250 mg twice
   daily. *Acute therapy*—500 mg initially followed by 125–
   250 mg q 4 hr.
CHILDREN: 5–10 mg/kg q 6 hr.

Anticonvulsant

ADULTS AND CHILDREN: 10 mg/kg/day (range 8–30 mg/kg/day)
   in 4 divided doses. If given with other anticonvulsants, 250
   mg once daily.

Dilution

• **Direct IV: Dilute** 500 mg in at least 5 ml of sterile water
for injection. Use reconstituted solutions within 24 hours.
• **Intermittent Infusion: Further dilute** in D5W, D10W,
0.45% NaCl, 0.9% NaCl, Ringer's or lactated Ringer's solutions, or combinations of dextrose and saline or dextrose and
Ringer's solution.

Compatibility

• **Additive:** cimetidine • ranitidine.

Incompatibility

• **Additive:** multiple vitamins.

Rate of Administration

• **Direct IV:** Administer over at least 1 minute. • **Intermittent Infusion:** Infuse over 4–8 hours.

1

≋ CLINICAL PRECAUTIONS

- Monitor intake and output, and fluid and electrolyte status. Observe patient for signs of hypokalemia (muscle weakness, malaise, fatigue, ECG changes, vomiting). Hypokalemia increases the risk of cardiac glycoside toxicity. Because acetazolamide diuresis is self-limiting, use as a diuretic should be intermittent.
- Assess for allergy to sulfonamides. Cross-sensitivity may occur.
- Assess for eye discomfort or decrease in visual acuity.
- Encourage fluids to 2000–3000 ml/day, unless contraindicated, to prevent crystalluria and stone formation. Acetazolamide should be used cautiously in patients with electrolyte imbalance, renal or hepatic disease, or a history of kidney stones.
- Alters the effects of drugs whose excretion is pH dependent. Excretion of barbiturates, aspirin, lithium, and primidone is accelerated. Observe for decreased clinical effectiveness of these agents. Excretion of amphetamines, cyclosporine, quinidine, flecainide, mexiletine, and tricyclic antidepressants is decreased. Observe patients for toxic effects of these drugs. Acetazolamide may increase CNS toxicity in salicylate overdose. Salicylates may increase the toxic effects of acetazolamide.
- Monitor neurological status in patients receiving acetazolamide for seizures. Initiate seizure precautions.
- Acetazolamide should be avoided in pregnant patients, especially during the first trimester. Use cautiously in patients with childbearing potential (Pregnancy Category C).

Lab Test Considerations

- Serum electrolytes, complete blood counts, and platelet counts should be evaluated initially and periodically throughout prolonged therapy. Acetazolamide may cause decreased potassium, bicarbonate, WBCs, and RBCs. May cause increased serum chloride. • Acetazolamide may cause increase in serum glucose. Monitor serum and urine glucose carefully in diabetic patients. • May cause false-positive results for urine protein and 17-hydroxysteroid tests. • Acetazolamide may cause increased blood ammonia, bilirubin, uric acid, and increased urine urobilinogen and calcium. May decrease urine citrate.

Patient/Family Teaching

• Advise patient to report numbness, tingling, or tremors of extremities, weakness, rash, sore throat, unusual bleeding or bruising, flank pain, or fever to the physician. • Advise patients with glaucoma of the need for periodic ophthalmologic exams as loss of vision may be gradual and painless.

 PHARMACOLOGIC PROFILE

Indications

• Acetazolamide is used to lower intraocular pressure in patients with glaucoma. • It is also used as an adjunct in treating drug-induced edema and edema due to CHF and as an adjunct in treating epilepsy.

Action

• Acetazolamide inhibits carbonic anhydrase in the eye, which decreases the secretion of aqueous humor and subsequently lowers intraocular pressure. • Acetazolamide also inhibits renal carbonic anhydrase, resulting in self-limiting urinary excretion of sodium, potassium, bicarbonate, and water.

Time/Action Profile (effect on intraocular pressure)

Onset	Peak	Duration
2 min	15 min	4–5 hr

Pharmacokinetics

• **Distribution:** Acetazolamide is widely distributed to body tissues and crosses the placenta. • **Metabolism and Excretion:** Excretion of acetazolamide occurs primarily in the urine as unchanged drug. • **Half-life:** 2.4–5.8 hours.

Contraindications

• Acetazolamide is contraindicated in patients with hypersensitivity to it. Cross-sensitivity with sulfonamides may occur.

Adverse Reactions and Side Effects*

• **CNS:** drowsiness • **EENT:** transient myopia • **GI:** nausea, vomiting, anorexia • **GU:** crystalluria, renal calculi • **Derm:** rash • **Endo:** hyperglycemia • **F and E:** <u>hyperchloremic acidosis</u>, hypokalemia • **Hemat:** APLASTIC ANEMIA, HEMOLYTIC ANEMIA, LEUKOPENIA • **Metab:** hyperuricemia • **Neuro:** paresthesias • **Misc:** allergic reactions.

Acyclovir Sodium   *Antiviral*
{Avirax}, Zovirax   pH 10.5–11.6

 ADMINISTRATION CONSIDERATIONS

Usual Dose

Initial Genital Herpes
ADULTS: 5 mg/kg q 8 hr for 5 days.
INFANTS AND CHILDREN UP TO 12 yr: 250 mg/m² q 8 hr for 5 days.

Mucocutaneous Herpes Simplex Infections in Immunosuppressed Patients
ADULTS AND CHILDREN >12 yr: 5–10 mg/kg q 8 hr for 7–10 days.
CHILDREN <12 yr: 250 mg/m² q 8 hr for 7 days.

Herpes Simplex Encephalitis
ADULTS: 10 mg/kg q 8 hr for 10 days.
CHILDREN <12 yr: 10 mg/kg or 500 mg/m² q 8 hr for 10 days.

Varicella Zoster Infections in Immunosuppressed Patients
ADULTS: 10 mg/kg q 8 hr for 7 days.
CHILDREN <12 yr: 500 mg/m² q 8 hr for 7 days.

---

*<u>Underlines</u> indicate most frequent; CAPITALS indicate life-threatening.

{} = Available in Canada only.

Dilution

• **Intermittent Infusion: Reconstitute** 500 mg with 10 ml or 1000 mg with 20 ml of sterile water for injection for a concentration of 50 mg/ml. Do not reconstitute with bacteriostatic water with benzyl alcohol or parabens; may result in precipitation. Shake well to dissolve completely. • **Dilute** in D5W, D5/0.25% NaCl, D5/0.45% NaCl, D5/0.9% NaCl, 0.9% NaCl, or lactated Ringer's solution for a concentration not to exceed 7 mg/ml. • Use reconstituted solutions within 12 hours. Once diluted for infusion, should be used within 24 hours. Refrigeration results in precipitation, which dissolves at room temperature.

Compatibility

• **Y-site:** allopurinol sodium • amikacin • ampicillin • cefamandole • cefazolin • cefonicid • cefoperazone • ceforanide • cefotaxime • cefoxitin • ceftazidime • ceftizoxime • ceftriaxone • cefuroxime • cephapirin • chloramphenicol • cimetidine • clindamycin • dexamethasone sodium phosphate • dimenhydrinate • diphenhydramine • doxycycline • erythromycin lactobionate • filgrastim • fluconazole • gallium nitrate • gentamicin • heparin • hydrocortisone sodium succinate • hydromorphone • imipenem/cilastatin • lorazepam • magnesium sulfate • melphalan • methylprednisolone sodium succinate • metoclopramide • metronidazole • multivitamin infusion • nafcillin • oxacillin • paclitaxel • penicillin G potassium • pentobarbital • perphenazine • piperacillin • potassium chloride • ranitidine • sodium bicarbonate • tacrolimus • theophylline • ticarcillin • tobramycin • trimethoprim/sulfamethoxazole • vancomycin • zidovudine.

• **Additive:** fluconazole.

Incompatibility

• **Y-site:** dobutamine • dopamine • fludarabine • foscarnet • idarubicin • ondansetron • piperacillin/tazobactam • sargramostim • vinorelbine.

• **Additive:** blood products or protein-containing solutions • dobutamine • dopamine.

Rate of Administration

• **Intermittent Infusion:** Administer slowly, via infusion pump, over at least 1 hour to minimize renal tubular damage.

≋ CLINICAL PRECAUTIONS

- Assess lesions prior to and daily during therapy. Acyclovir treatment should be started as soon as possible after herpes symptoms appear.
- Assess for history of seizures. Risk of seizures may be increased by concurrent intrathecal methotrexate. Neuropsychiatric adverse effects are more common in geriatric or immunosuppressed patients. Concurrent use with zidovudine may result in drowsiness.
- Assess fluid and electrolyte status and renal function. Maintain adequate hydration (2000–3000 ml/day in adults), especially during first 2 hours following IV infusion, to prevent crystalluria. Renal failure is more likely to occur following bolus injections with concurrent nephrotoxic medications in dehydrated patients or patients with pre-existing renal impairment. Dosage reduction and/or increased dosing interval is recommended if creatinine clearance is less than 50 ml/min.
- Assess IV site frequently for signs of inflammation or phlebitis. Rotate infusion site to prevent phlebitis.
- Toxicity may also be increased by concurrent probenecid, which decreases renal excretion and increases blood levels.
- Dosing of acyclovir in obese patients should be based on ideal body weight.
- Safe use during pregnancy has not been established (Pregnancy Category C). Enters breast milk in lactating patients, although toxicity has not been noted in infants.

Lab Test Considerations

- Monitor BUN, serum creatinine, and creatinine clearance prior to and during therapy. Increased BUN and serum creatinine levels or decreased creatinine clearance may indicate renal failure.

Patient/Family Teaching

- Advise patients with genital herpes that condoms should be used during sexual contact and that no sexual contact should be made while lesions are present. • Instruct women with genital herpes to have yearly Pap smears because they may be more likely to develop cervical cancer. • If IV acyclovir is to be followed by chronic oral therapy, instruct patient on the importance of maintaining good dental hygiene and seeing a dentist for teeth cleaning regularly to prevent tenderness, bleeding, and gingival hyperplasia.

PHARMACOLOGIC PROFILE

Indications

• Acyclovir is used in the treatment of severe initial episodes of genital herpes in nonimmunosuppressed patients and in the management of initial or recurrent mucosal or cutaneous herpes simplex infections in immunosuppressed patients. • It is also used in the treatment of herpes simplex encephalitis in patients older than 6 months and in the treatment of varicella zoster infections (chickenpox) in immunosuppressed patients.

Action

• Acyclovir interferes with viral DNA synthesis, resulting in inhibition of viral replication, decreased viral shedding, and reduced time to healing of lesions.

Time/Action Profile (blood levels)

Onset	Peak
prompt	end of infusion

Pharmacokinetics

• **Distribution:** Acyclovir is widely distributed; crosses the placenta, and enters breast milk. CSF concentrations are 50% of plasma levels. • **Metabolism and Excretion:** More than 90% of acyclovir is excreted by the kidneys. • **Half-life:** 2.5 hours (increased in renal impairment).

Contraindications

• Acyclovir is contraindicated in patients with hypersensitivity to the drug. • Cross-sensitivity with ganciclovir or famciclovir may occur.

Adverse Reactions and Side Effects*

• **CNS:** <u>dizziness</u>, <u>headache</u>, hallucinations, trembling, SEIZURES • **EENT:** gingival hyperplasia • **GI:** diarrhea, nausea, vomiting, anorexia, abdominal pain • **GU:** RENAL FAILURE, hematuria, crystalluria • **Derm:** acne, unusual sweating, skin rashes, hives • **Endo:** changes in menstrual cycle • **Local:** <u>pain</u>, <u>phlebitis</u> • **MS:** joint pain • **Misc:** polydipsia.

Adenosine	Antiarrhythmic
Adenocard	pH 5.5–7.5

ADMINISTRATION CONSIDERATIONS

Usual Dose

ADULTS: 6 mg by rapid IV bolus; if no results repeat 1–2 min later as 12-mg rapid bolus. This dose may be repeated. (Single dose not to exceed 12 mg.)

CHILDREN: *Unlabeled*—37.5–50 mcg/kg q 1–2 min up to a total of three doses.

Dilution

• **Direct IV:** Administer undiluted directly into vein or via proximal IV line. • Crystals may occur if adenosine is refrigerated. Warm to room temperature to dissolve crystals. Solution must be clear before use. Discard unused portions.

Incompatibility

• **Additive:** Do not admix with any other drug or solution.

Rate of Administration

• **Direct IV:** Administer over 1–2 seconds. Follow with rapid saline flush to ensure injection reaches systemic circulation. Slow administration may cause increased heart rate in response to vasodilation.

---

*<u>Underlines</u> indicate most frequent; CAPITALS indicate life-threatening.

≋ CLINICAL PRECAUTIONS

- Monitor heart rate frequently (every 15–30 seconds) and ECG continuously throughout therapy. Response should be rapid (within seconds), but is short lived (1–2 minutes). Once conversion to normal sinus rhythm is achieved, transient arrhythmias (premature ventricular contractions, atrial premature contractions, sinus tachycardia, sinus bradycardia, skipped beats, AV nodal block) may occur but generally last only a few seconds. Carbamazepine may increase the likelihood of progressive heart block. Dipyridamole potentiates the effects of adenosine (dosage reduction of adenosine recommended). Effects of adenosine may be decreased by theophylline or caffeine (larger doses of adenosine may be required). Nicotine (in cigarette smoke, nicotine transdermal patches, or gum) may increase risk of adverse cardiovascular reactions.
- Monitor blood pressure during therapy. Dose-related hypotension may occur.
- Assess respiratory status (breath sounds, rate) following administration. Shortness of breath and facial flushing are common effects of the drug.
- Use cautiously in patients with asthma. Bronchospasm may occur.
- Do not confuse adenosine with adenosine phosphate.
- Safe use in pregnancy, lactation, or children has not been established (Pregnancy Category C).

Patient/Family Teaching

- Caution patient to make position changes slowly to minimize orthostatic hypotension. Doses greater than 12 mg decrease blood pressure by decreasing peripheral vascular resistance. • Instruct patient to report facial flushing, shortness of breath, or dizziness.

≋ PHARMACOLOGIC PROFILE

Indications

- Adenosine is used in the conversion of paroxysmal supraventricular tachycardia to normal sinus rhythm when vagal maneuvers have been unsuccessful.

Action
• Adenosine restores normal sinus rhythm by interrupting re-entrant pathways in the AV node. • It also slows conduction time through the AV node.

Time/Action Profile

Onset	Peak	Duration
3–4 sec	UK	1–2 min

Pharmacokinetics
• **Distribution:** Adenosine is taken up by reticulocytes and vascular endothelium. • **Metabolism and Excretion:** Adenosine is rapidly cleared by conversion of inosine and adenosine monophosphate. • **Half-life:** Less than 10 seconds.

Contraindications
• Hypersensitivity • Avoid using in patients with second- or third-degree AV block or sick sinus syndrome, unless a functional artificial pacemaker is present.

Adverse Reactions and Side Effects*
• **CNS:** headache, light-headedness, dizziness, apprehension, head pressure • **EENT:** blurred vision, throat tightness • **Resp:** shortness of breath, chest pressure, hyperventilation • **CV:** facial flushing, transient arrhythmias, palpitations, chest pain, hypotension • **GI:** nausea, metallic taste • **Derm:** sweating, burning sensation • **MS:** neck and back pain • **Neuro:** tingling, numbness • **Misc:** pressure sensation in groin, heaviness in arms.

Albumin, Human	*Volume expander*
Albuminar, Albutein, Buminate, normal serum albumin, Plasbumin	pH 6.4–7.4

≋ ADMINISTRATION CONSIDERATIONS
Usual Dose

Hypovolemia
ADULTS: 25 g; an additional dose may be given 15–30 min later.

---

*Underlines indicate most frequent; CAPITALS indicate life-threatening.

CHILDREN: 2.5–12.5 g (0.5–1 g/kg); an additional dose may be given 15–30 min later.

Hypoproteinemia

ADULTS: 50–75 g.

CHILDREN: 2.5–12.5 g (0.5–1 g/kg); an additional dose may be given 15–30 min later.

Burns

ADULTS AND CHILDREN: 24 hr following initial administration of appropriate crystalloid, 25 g; additional amounts may be given to maintain serum albumin and protein.

Nephrotic Syndrome

ADULTS: 25 g/day with diuretic therapy for 7–10 days.

Neonatal Hyperbilirubinemia

NEONATES: 1 g/kg concurrent with or 1–2 hr prior to exchange transfusion.

Dilution

• Administer 5% normal serum albumin **undiluted.** • 25% normal serum albumin may be administered **undiluted** or **diluted** in 0.9% NaCl, D5W, D5/0.9% NaCl, D5/0.45% NaCl, D5/LR, lactated Ringer's solution. • Do not use if solution is turbid or contains a precipitate. Use vial within 4 hours of opening.

Compatibility

• **Y-site:** diltiazem.

Incompatibility

• **Y-site:** vancomycin ✦ verapamil.

• **Additive:** alcohol-containing solutions ✦ amino acid solutions ✦ fat emulsions ✦ Ionosol D-CM ✦ Ionosol G with 10% dextrose ✦ protein hydrolysates ✦ verapamil.

Rate of Administration

• Rate of administration is determined by concentration of solution, blood volume, indication, and patient response. In patients with normal blood volume, 5% normal serum albumin should be administered at 2–4 ml/min and 25% normal serum albumin at a rate of 1 ml/min. The rate for children is usually one quarter to one half the adult rate. • Infusion must be completed within 4 hours. • **Shock with Associated Hypovolemia:** 5% or 25% normal serum albumin may be administered as rapidly as tolerated and repeated in 15–30 minutes if necessary. • **Burns:** Rate after the first 24 hours should be set to maintain a plasma albumin level of 2.5 g/100 ml or a total serum protein level of 5.2 g/100 ml. • **Hypoproteinemia:** Normal serum albumin 25% is the preferred solution due to the increased concentration of protein. The rate should not exceed 3 ml/min of 25% or 5–10 ml/min of 5% solution to prevent circulatory overload and pulmonary edema. This treatment provides a temporary rise in plasma protein until the cause of the hypoproteinemia is corrected.

☰ CLINICAL PRECAUTIONS

- Monitor vital signs, intake and output, and hemodynamic parameters throughout therapy. Vascular overload may occur. Assess for rales/crackles, dyspnea, hypertension, elevated CVP or jugular venous distention. Due to high sodium content (130–160 mEq Na/L), avoid use in patients with congestive heart failure.
- Additional fluids may be required in dehydrated patients.
- If hypersensitivity or pyrogenic reactions occur manifesting as fever, tachycardia, or hypotension, therapy should be discontinued. Antihistamines may be required.
- Hypotension may also result from rapid administration.
- Use cautiously in patients with severe hepatic or renal disease. Protein content may be excessive for these patients.
- Following administration, assess surgical patients for increased bleeding caused by increased blood pressure and circulating blood volume. Albumin does not contain clotting factors.
- Follow manufacturer's recommendations for administration and use set provided. Administer through a large-gauge (at least 20 g) needle or catheter.
- Solutions should be clear amber; do not administer cloudy solutions or those containing a precipitate. Store at room temperature.
- There is no danger of serum hepatitis or HIV infection from normal serum albumin. Crossmatching is not required.
- Twenty-five grams of normal serum albumin are osmoti-

cally equivalent to 2 units of fresh frozen plasma; 100 ml of normal serum albumin 25% provides the plasma protein of 500 ml plasma or 2 pints of whole blood. Normal serum albumin 5% is isotonic and osmotically equivalent to an equal amount of plasma. The 25% albumin solution is equal to 5 times the osmotic value of plasma.

- Administration of large quantities of normal serum albumin may need to be supplemented with whole blood to prevent anemia. If more than 1000 ml of 5% normal serum albumin are given or if hemorrhage has occurred, the administration of whole blood or packed red blood cells may be needed.
- Safe use in pregnancy has not been established. Use only if necessary (Pregnancy Category C).

Lab Test Considerations

- Serum protein levels should increase with albumin therapy. • Monitor serum sodium; may cause increased concentrations. • Infusions of normal serum albumin may cause false elevation of alkaline phosphatase levels. • **Hemorrhage:** Monitor hemoglobin and hematocrit. These values may decrease due to hemodilution.

Patient/Family Teaching

- Explain the purpose of this solution to the patient.
- Instruct patient to report signs and symptoms of hypersensitivity reaction.

≋ PHARMACOLOGIC PROFILE

Indications

- Albumin is used to attain expansion of plasma volume and maintenance of cardiac output in situations associated with fluid volume deficit including shock, hemorrhage, or burns. • It temporarily replaces albumin in diseases associated with edema secondary to hypoproteinemia such as the nephrotic syndrome or end-stage liver disease.

Action

- Albumin provides colloidal oncotic pressure, which serves to mobilize fluid from extravascular tissues back into intravascular space. • Temporarily replaces albumin in hypo-proteinemic states.

Time/Action Profile (oncotic effect)

Onset	Peak	Duration
15–30 min	UK	UK

Pharmacokinetics

• **Distribution:** Albumin is confined to the vascular space, unless capillary permeability is increased. • **Metabolism and Excretion:** Albumin is normally produced by the liver and is probably degraded by the liver as well. • **Half-life:** UK.

Contraindications

• Previous allergic reactions to albumin. • Avoid using in patients with severe anemia, congestive heart failure, or increased intravascular volume.

Adverse Reactions and Side Effects*

• **CNS:** headache • **CV:** hypertension, hypotension, fluid overload, PULMONARY EDEMA, tachycardia • **GI:** nausea, vomiting, increased salivation • **Derm:** urticaria, rash, flushing • **MS:** back pain • **Misc:** fever, chills.

Aldesleukin	*Antineoplastic (modified recombinant interleukin)*
interleukin-2, IL-2, Proleukin	pH 7.5

 ADMINISTRATION CONSIDERATIONS

Usual Dose

ADULTS: 600,000 IU/kg (0.037 mg/kg) q 8 hr for 14 doses. Cycle is repeated once after a 9-day rest period to a total of 28 doses. After a rest period of 7 weeks, patients who have

---

*Underlines indicate most frequent; CAPITALS indicate life-threatening.

had a beneficial response may be evaluated for additional courses.

Dilution
  • **Intermittent Infusion: Reconstitute** each vial with 1.2 ml of sterile water for injection for a concentration of 18 million IU (1.1 mg)/ml. Direct the sterile water during reconstitution at the side of the vial and swirl contents gently to prevent excess foaming. Do not shake. • Solution should be clear and colorless to slightly yellow. Administer within 48 hours of reconstitution. Discard unused portion. • **Dilute** reconstituted dose in 50 ml of D5W. • Do not reconstitute or dilute with bacteriostatic water for injection, 0.9% NaCl, or albumin.

Compatibility
  • **Y-site:** amikacin ◆ fat emulsion ◆ gentamycin ◆ morphine ◆ piperacillin ◆ ticarcillin ◆ tobramycin.

Incompatibility
  • **Additive:** Do not admix with other drugs.

Rate of Administration
  • **Intermittent Infusion:** Infuse each dose over 15 minutes.

≋ CLINICAL PRECAUTIONS

  • Aldesleukin should be administered only in a hospital setting with intensive care facilities available.
  • Use with caution in any patient with a history of cardiovascular, hepatic, or renal disease. Baseline thallium cardiac stress testing, pulmonary function testing, and arterial blood gases should be performed and evaluated prior to therapy and periodically during continued courses. Concurrent cardiotoxic, hepatotoxic, nephrotoxic, or neurotoxic drug therapy increases the risk of toxicity in these organ systems. Continuous monitoring of ECG should be performed during infusion. Monitor respiratory status frequently.
  • Monitor vital signs and weight daily. Assess patient for the development of capillary leak syndrome (hypotension, hypovolemia, edema, ascites, pleural effusions). This initially manifests as a drop in arterial blood pres-

sure beginning 2–12 hours from start of administration. Concurrent antihypertensive therapy increases the risk of hypotension. Maintenance of normovolemia with IV fluids and dopamine may help maintain organ perfusion.

• Use cautiously in patients with a history of seizures or suspected CNS metastases. Symptoms may be exaggerated and seizures may occur. Monitor for changes in mental status. Hold administration if patient develops moderate to severe lethargy or somnolence. This may progress to coma.

• Monitor for bone marrow depression. Assess frequently for signs of infection, particularly sepsis and bacterial endocarditis. Antibiotic prophylaxis directed against *Staphylococcus aureus* is recommended for all patients with central lines. Any infections occurring during therapy should be managed aggressively. Aldesleukin impairs the function of white blood cells. Assess for signs of anemia (increased fatigue, dyspnea, orthostatic hypotension). Assess for bleeding (bleeding gums, bruising, petechiae, guaiac stools, urine, and emesis). Avoid IM injections and rectal temperatures. Apply pressure to venipuncture sites for 10 minutes. Transfusions of red blood cells and/or platelets are usually required.

• Glucocorticoids decrease the antitumor effect of aldesleukin. Concurrent use should be avoided. Acetaminophen and a nonsteroidal anti-inflammatory drug should be administered prior to therapy to decrease fever. Meperidine may be given to control the rigors (chills), which commonly accompany aldesleukin therapy.

• Safe use in pregnancy, lactation, or children less than 18 years old has not been established (Pregnancy Category C). Use cautiously in patients with childbearing potential.

Lab Test Considerations

• Monitor CBC, differential, platelet count, blood chemistries including electrolytes, and renal and hepatic function prior to and daily throughout therapy. • May cause elevated bilirubin, BUN, serum creatinine, AST (SGOT), ALT (SGPT), LDH, and alkaline phosphatase. • May cause hypomagnesemia, acidosis, hypocalcemia, hypophosphatemia, hypokalemia, hyperuricemia, hypoalbuminemia, and hypoproteinemia. • Monitor thyroid function periodically during therapy.

Patient/Family Teaching

• Advise patient to use a nonhormonal method of contraception throughout therapy. • Instruct patient to notify physician promptly if fever; sore throat; signs of infection; bleeding gums; bruising; petechiae; blood in stools, urine, or emesis; increased fatigue; dyspnea; or orthostatic hypotension occurs. Caution patient to avoid crowds and persons with known infections. Instruct patient to use a soft toothbrush and an electric razor, and to avoid falls. Patient should be cautioned not to drink alcoholic beverages or to take medication containing aspirin, ibuprofen, or naproxen because these may precipitate gastric bleeding.

PHARMACOLOGIC PROFILE

Indications

• Aldesleukin is used in the management of metastatic renal cell carcinoma.

Action

• Aldesleukin increases cellular immunity (as seen by lymphocytosis and eosinophilia), increases the production of cytokines (including tumor necrosis factor, interleukin-1, and gamma interferon), and inhibits tumor growth.

Time/Action Profile (tumor regression after completion of first course)

Onset	Peak	Duration
4 wk	UK	12 mo

Pharmacokinetics

• **Distribution:** Aldesleukin rapidly distributes to extravascular, extracellular space. 70% is taken up by the liver, kidneys, and lungs. • **Metabolism and Excretion:** Aldesleukin is metabolized by cells in the kidneys to amino acids. • **Half-life:** 85 minutes.

Contraindications

• Aldesleukin should not be used in patients with previous hypersensitivity to it or mannitol. • Patients with any history of cardiac or pulmonary disease as assessed by abnormal thallium stress testing or abnormal pulmonary function testing should not receive aldesleukin. • If patients have experienced any of the following toxicities during previous courses of aldesleukin, they should not be given additional courses— sustained ventricular tachycardia (5 bpm or more), angina pectoris or myocardial infarction as indicated by ECG changes, respiratory problems requiring more than 72 hours of intubation, pericardial tamponade, renal toxicity requiring more than 72 hours of dialysis, CNS dysfunction consisting of more than 48 hours of coma or psychosis, intractable seizures, bowel perforation or ischemia, or GI bleeding requiring surgical intervention. • Patients who have had allograft organ transplantation should not receive aldesleukin because of increased risk of rejection.

Adverse Reactions and Side Effects*

• **CNS:** COMA, <u>mental status changes</u>, lethargy, somnolence, confusion, agitation • **Resp:** <u>pulmonary congestion</u>, <u>dyspnea</u>, <u>pulmonary edema</u>, RESPIRATORY FAILURE, APNEA, tachypnea, pleural effusion, wheezing, pneumothorax, hemoptysis • **CV:** MYOCARDIAL INFARCTION, CARDIAC ARREST, CONGESTIVE HEART FAILURE, STROKE, MYOCARDITIS, <u>hypotension</u>, <u>tachycardia</u>, <u>arrhythmias</u>, myocardial ischemia, pericardial effusion, thrombosis • **GI:** BOWEL PERFORATION, GI BLEEDING, <u>jaundice</u>, ascites, hepatomegaly • **GU:** <u>renal dysfunction</u>, oliguria, anuria • **Derm:** <u>pruritus</u> • **Hemat:** <u>anemia</u>, <u>leukopenia</u>, <u>thrombocytopenia</u>, <u>coagulation disorders</u>, leukocytosis, eosinophilia • **Misc:** CAPILLARY LEAK SYNDROME, <u>fever</u>, <u>chills</u>, gangrene, SEPSIS.

---

*<u>Underlines</u> indicate most frequent; CAPITALS indicate life-threatening.

Alfentanil Hydrochloride	*Opioid analgesic (agonist)*
Alfenta	pH 4.0–6.0

Schedule II

≋ ADMINISTRATION CONSIDERATIONS

Usual Dose

Incremental Injection (Duration of anesthesia ≤30 min)

Adults: Induction—8–20 mcg (0.008–0.020 mg)/kg; followed by **maintenance** of 3–5 mcg (0.003–0.005 mg)/kg increments or 0.5–1.0 mcg (0.0005–0.001 mg)/kg/min infusion (total dose 8–40 mcg/kg).

Incremental Injection (Duration of anesthesia 30–60 min)

Adults: Induction—20–50 mcg (0.02–0.05 mg)/kg; followed by **maintenance** of 5–15 mcg/kg increments [up to total dose of 75 mcg (0.075 mg)/kg].

Continuous Infusion (Duration of anesthesia >45 min)

Adults: Induction—50–75 mcg/kg; followed by **maintenance** of 0.5–3.0 mcg/kg/min (average infusion rate 1–1.5 mcg/kg/min). Infusion rate should be decreased by 30–50% after first hour of maintenance. If lightening occurs, infusion rate may be increased up to 4 mcg/kg/min or boluses of 7 mcg/kg may be administered.

Anesthetic Induction (Duration of anesthesia >45 min)

Adults: 130–245 mcg (0.13–0.245 mg)/kg followed by 0.5–1.5 mcg (0.0005–0.0015 mg)/kg/min or general anesthesia.

Dilution

• **Direct IV:** Use **undiluted** solution. • **Continuous Infusion: Dilute** to a concentration of 25–80 mcg/ml (20 ml of alfentanil in 230 ml of diluent provides a 40 mcg/ml solution) with 0.9% NaCl, D5W, D5/0.9% NaCl, or lactated Ringer's solution.

Incompatibility

- Information unavailable. Do not admix with other drugs or solutions.

Rate of Administration

- **Direct IV:** Injections should be administered slowly over 90 seconds–3 minutes. Slow IV administration may reduce the incidence and severity of muscle rigidity, bradycardia, or hypotension. Neuromuscular blocking agents may be administered concurrently to decrease muscle rigidity.

≋ CLINICAL PRECAUTIONS

- Assess vital signs, especially respiratory status and ECG, following and frequently throughout administration. Notify physician of significant changes immediately. Monitor drug effect continuously. Postoperative pain may require treatment relatively early in the recovery period due to short duration of alfentanil.
- Benzodiazepines may be administered prior to administration of alfentanil to reduce the induction dose requirements and decrease the time to loss of consciousness. This combination may also increase the risk of hypotension. Monitor blood pressure.
- Administer small volumes for direct IV use via tuberculin syringe for accuracy.
- IV infusion should be discontinued at least 10–15 minutes prior to the end of surgery.
- Elderly, severely ill, or debilitated patients are very sensitive to the effects of opioid analgesics. Smaller doses may be necessary.
- Because of respiratory depressant effects, use with caution in patients with severe pulmonary disease. Muscle rigidity from alfentanil may hinder mechanical ventilation.
- Assess for history of cardiovascular disease, as arrhythmias may occur.
- Patients with hepatic disease, adrenal insufficiency, or hypothyroidism are more prone to adverse reactions.
- Avoid using in patients with undiagnosed abdominal pain, as symptoms may be masked.
- May increase intracranial pressure and therefore should

be used cautiously in patients with CNS tumors, increased intracranial pressure, or head trauma.
- Concurrent use with alcohol, antihistamines, antidepressants, and other sedatives results in additive CNS depression. Observe for increased drug effect. During induction, the concentration of inhalation agents should be decreased by 30–50%.
- Duration of recovery may be prolonged by concurrent administration of cimetidine or erythromycin.
- Avoid use of MAO inhibitors for 14 days prior to use to avoid serious and unpredictable adverse reactions.
- Safe use in pregnancy has not been established (Pregnancy Category C). Should not be used during labor. Avoid use in patients who are breast-feeding because alfentanil enters breast milk.

Toxicity and Overdose Alert

- Symptoms of toxicity include respiratory depression, hypotension, arrhythmias, bradycardia, and asystole. Opioid antagonist, oxygen, and resuscitative equipment should be readily available during the administration of alfentanil. • Atropine may be used to treat bradycardia. Use of a neuromuscular blocking agent with vagolytic activity, such as pancuronium or gallamine, may prevent bradycardia caused by alfentanil. • If respiratory depression persists following surgery, prolonged mechanical ventilation may be necessary. If an opioid antagonist is required to reverse respiratory depression or coma, naloxone (Narcan) is the antidote. Dilute the 0.4-mg ampule of naloxone in 10 ml of 0.9% NaCl and administer 0.5 ml (0.02 mg) by direct IV push every 2 minutes. For children and patients weighing <40 kg, dilute 0.1 mg of naloxone in 10 ml of 0.9% NaCl for a concentration of 10 mcg/ml and administer 0.5 mcg every 1–2 minutes. Titrate the dose to avoid withdrawal, seizures, and severe pain. Administration of naloxone in these circumstances, especially in cardiac patients, has resulted in hypertension and tachycardia, occasionally causing left ventricular failure and pulmonary edema. Monitor respiratory status continuously; the duration of respiratory depression may exceed the duration of a dose of naloxone. Continuous infusion of naloxone may be required (see *naloxone hydrochloride* monograph on page 690). • If hypotension occurs, administer parenteral fluids, position patient to improve venous return to the heart when surgical conditions permit, and administer a vasopressor as necessary. • If muscle rigidity occurs during surgery, a neuromuscular blocking agent and mechanical ventilation should be used. Muscle rigidity occurring upon emergence may be treated with naloxone.

Lab Test Considerations

• May cause elevated serum amylase and lipase concentrations.

Patient/Family Teaching

• Discuss the use of anesthetic agents and the sensations to expect with the patient prior to surgery. • Alfentanil may cause drowsiness and dizziness. Advise patient to call for assistance when ambulating or smoking. • Advise patient to make position changes slowly to minimize orthostatic hypotension. • Following outpatient surgery, instruct patient to avoid alcohol or CNS depressants for 24 hours after the administration of alfentanil.

≋ PHARMACOLOGIC PROFILE

Indications

• Alfentanil is an analgesic adjunct in the maintenance of anesthesia with barbiturate/nitrous oxide/oxygen. • It is used as an analgesic with nitrous oxide/oxygen while maintaining general anesthesia. • It is also used in primary induction of general anesthesia when intubation and ventilation are required.

Action

• Alfentanil binds to opiate receptors in the CNS, altering the response to and perception of pain and causing generalized CNS depression.

Time/Action Profile (analgesia and respiratory depression)

Onset	Peak	Duration
immediate	1–1.5 min	5–10 min

Pharmacokinetics

• **Distribution:** Alfentanil does not readily penetrate adipose tissue. It crosses the placenta and enters breast milk.
• **Metabolism and Excretion:** More than 95% of alfentanil is metabolized by the liver. • **Half-life:** 60–130 minutes.

Contraindications

• Do not use in patients with known hypersensitivity or intolerance. • Safe use in pediatric patients (<12 years) has not been established.

Adverse Reactions and Side Effects*

• **CNS:** dizziness, sleepiness • **EENT:** blurred vision • **CV:** bradycardia, tachycardia, hypotension, hypertension, arrhythmias • **Resp:** apnea • **GI:** nausea, vomiting • **MS:** thoracic muscle rigidity, skeletal muscle rigidity.

Alglucerase	Enzyme replacement
Ceredase	pH 5.5–6

≋ ADMINISTRATION CONSIDERATIONS

Usual Dose

ADULTS AND CHILDREN: 60 units/kg once every 2 weeks (frequency may be adjusted from once every other day up to once every 4 weeks based on disease severity and patient convenience). Dose may be reduced every 3–6 months while monitoring response. Doses as low as 1 unit/kg may be effective.

Dilution

• **Intermittent Infusion: Dilute** each dose with preservative-free 0.9% NaCl to a final volume not to exceed 100 ml. • Do not shake; may denature the glycoprotein and render it inactive. • Do not use solutions that are discolored or contain particulate matter. • Small dosage adjustments can be made

---

*Underlines indicate most frequent; CAPITALS indicate life-threatening.

to avoid discarding partially used bottles, as long as monthly dose remains unaltered. • Stable for up to 18 hours if refrigerated. Discard unused vials after opening; contains no preservative.

Incompatibility

• Information unavailable. Do not admix with other drugs or solutions.

Rate of Administration

• **Intermittent Infusion:** Administer over 1–2 hours. Use an in-line filter during administration.

≋ CLINICAL PRECAUTIONS

• Monitor for an improvement in symptoms including hepatomegaly, splenomegaly, anemia, thrombocytopenia, bone demineralization, and increased appetite and energy level. In pediatric patients, cachexia and wasting should diminish.

• Safe use in pregnancy or lactation has not been established (Pregnancy Category C).

Lab Test Considerations

• Decreasing serum acid phosphatase levels and increasing hemoglobin and platelet counts indicate response to therapy. Monitor serum acid phosphatase every 2 months and hemoglobin and platelet counts monthly during therapy. If hemoglobin falls below 7 grams/dl and platelet count is less than 50,000/mm^3, levels may be monitored every 2 weeks. • Chemistry panels may be monitored every 6 months.

Patient/Family Teaching

• Inform patient of the purpose of this medication and importance of treatment at least every 4 weeks. Alglucerase helps control the symptoms, but does not cure Gaucher's disease. Lifelong therapy may be required. • Advise the patient that precautions have been taken to prevent transmission of HIV and hepatitis B virus; risk of transmission is slight. • Emphasize the importance of follow-up examinations and lab tests.

PHARMACOLOGIC PROFILE

Indications

• Alglucerase is used in the symptomatic treatment of type I Gaucher's disease associated with splenomegaly, hepatomegaly, hematologic abnormalities, and bone demineralization.

Action

• Alglucerase replaces the naturally occurring enzyme glucocerebrosidase, which is deficient in type I Gaucher's disease. Lack of the enzyme results in accumulation of lipid glucocerebroside in macrophages.

Time/Action Profile (improvement in hepatomegaly/splenomegaly)

Onset	Peak	Duration
within 6 mo	UK	UK

Pharmacokinetics

• **Distribution:** The distribution of alglucerase is not known. • **Metabolism and Excretion:** Metabolism and excretion of alglucerase are not known. • **Half-life:** 3.6–11 minutes.

Contraindications

• Alglucerase should not be used in patients who exhibit hypersensitivity to it.

Adverse Reactions and Side Effects*

• **GI:** abdominal pain • **Local:** burning, swelling, discomfort at injection site • **Misc:** chills, fever.

Allopurinol Sodium	*Antigout agent (xanthine oxidase inhibitor)*
Zyloprim	pH UK

• IV allopurinol is not approved by the FDA. It is available on a compassionate-use basis from the manufacturer.

---

*Underlines indicate most frequent; CAPITALS indicate life-threatening.

≋ ADMINISTRATION CONSIDERATIONS

Usual Dose
ADULTS: 200–400 mg/m^2/day (not to exceed 600 mg/day).
CHILDREN: 200 mg/m^2/day initially.

Dilution
• **Intermittent Infusion: Reconstitute** with 25 ml of sterile water for injection. • **Dilute further** with 0.9% NaCl or D5W for a concentration not to exceed 6.0 mg/ml. • Use reconstituted solution within 24 hours, then discard.

Incompatibility
• Information unavailable. Do not admix with other drugs or solutions.

Rate of Administration
• **Intermittent Infusion:** Rate will vary depending on the volume of the solution.

≋ CLINICAL PRECAUTIONS

- The patient should be switched to oral allopurinol as soon as possible.
- Monitor intake and ouput ratios. Decreased kidney function can cause drug accumulation and toxic effects. Ensure that patient maintains adequate fluid intake to produce a urinary output of at least 2000 ml/day to minimize risk of kidney stone formation. Use allopurinol cautiously in patients with renal insufficiency (dosage reduction required if creatinine clearance is <20 ml/min). Geriatric patients may require lower doses due to age-related decrease in renal function.
- Monitor for hypersensitivity reactions. If rash appears, allopurinol should be discontinued. The incidence of rash may be increased by concurrent diuretic, ampicillin, or amoxicillin therapy. Patients with pre-existing renal impairment may be more likely to develop a rash.
- Because allopurinol prevents the metabolism of mercaptopurine and azathioprine, the bone marrow depressant properties of these drugs are markedly enhanced by allopurinol. Dosages of these drugs must be reduced to ⅓–¼ of the usual dose when used concurrently with allopurinol. Allopurinol increases the risk of hypogly-

cemia in patients receiving insulin or oral hypoglycemic agents (dosage alteration may be required). The effects of warfarin may be potentiated by allopurinol.
• Safe use during pregnancy or lactation has not been established.

Lab Test Considerations

• Obtain hemoglobin, WBC, platelet count, serum uric acid, AST (SGOT), ALT (SGPT), and serum creatinine prior to initiating therapy. • Serum and urine uric acid levels usually begin to decrease 2–3 days after initiation of therapy. • Allopurinol may cause elevation of serum alkaline phosphatase, AST (SGOT), and ALT (SGPT) levels. Decreased CBC and platelets may indicate bone marrow depression. Elevated BUN, serum creatinine, and creatinine clearance may indicate nephrotoxicity. These are usually reversed with discontinuation of therapy. • Monitor blood glucose in patients receiving oral hypoglycemic agents or insulin as allopurinol may cause hypoglycemia. • Monitor prothrombin time closely in patients receiving concurrent warfarin and allopurinol therapy.

Patient/Family Teaching

• Alkaline diet may be ordered. Advise patient that urinary acidification with large doses of vitamin C or other acidic compounds may increase kidney stone formation (see Appendix H). Advise patient of need for increased fluid intake. • Allopurinol may occasionally cause drowsiness. Caution patient to avoid activities requiring alertness until response to drug is known. • Instruct patient to report itching, skin rash, chills, fever, nausea, or vomiting promptly. • Advise patient that large amounts of alcohol increase uric acid concentrations and may decrease the effectiveness of allopurinol. • Emphasize the importance of follow-up examinations to monitor effectiveness and side effects.

≋ PHARMACOLOGIC PROFILE

Indications

• IV allopurinol is used in the treatment of secondary hyperuricemia, which may occur during treatment of tumors or leukemias in patients who are unable to take or tolerate oral allopurinol. Lowering of serum uric acid levels in this situation prevents uric acid nephropathy.

Action

• Allopurinol inhibits the production of uric acid by inhibiting the enzyme xanthine oxidase.

Time/Action Profile (hypouricemic effect)

Onset	Peak	Duration
2–3 days	1–3 wk	1–2 wk†

†Duration after discontinuation of allopurinol.

Pharmacokinetics

• **Distribution:** Allopurinol is widely distributed in tissue water. • **Metabolism and Excretion:** Allopurinol is metabolized to oxypurinol, an active compound with a long half-life. Both allopurinol and oxypurinol are excreted mainly by the kidneys. • **Half-life:** allopurinol 2–3 hours; oxypurinol 24 hours.

Contraindications

• Allopurinol should not be used in patients with hypersensitivity to it or to oxypurinol. Pregnant or lactating patients should not receive allopurinol. Injection contains alcohol and should be avoided in patients with known intolerance.

Adverse Reactions and Side Effects*

• **CNS:** drowsiness • **GI:** nausea, vomiting, diarrhea, hepatitis • **GU:** renal failure • **Derm:** rash, urticaria • **Hemat:** bone marrow depression • **Misc:** hypersensitivity reactions.

Alpha₁-Proteinase Inhibitor	Enzyme inhibitor
alpha₁-antitrypsin, Prolastin	pH 6.6–7.4

≋ ADMINISTRATION CONSIDERATIONS

Usual Dose

ADULTS: 60 mg/kg once weekly.

---

*Underlines indicate most frequent; CAPITALS indicate life-threatening.

Dilution

• **Direct IV:** Bring bottles to room temperature. • **Reconstitute** with sterile water for injection provided by manufacturer to yield a concentration of 20 mg/ml. Follow manufacturer's instructions for vacuum transfer using filter needle. Swirl to mix; do not shake. • May be **diluted** in 0.9% NaCl if necessary. • Do not refrigerate after reconstitution. • Use within 3 hours.

Incompatibility

• Administer alone. Do not mix with other drugs or diluents.

Rate of Administration

• **Direct IV:** Administer direct IV at rate of 0.08 ml/kg/min or greater.

≋ CLINICAL PRECAUTIONS

- Monitor respiratory status (rate, lung sounds, dyspnea) prior to and weekly throughout therapy.
- Monitor for signs of fluid overload. Fever may occur up to 12 hours after infusion and resolve by 24 hours. Treat symptomatically.
- Observe for dizziness and light-headedness.
- Safe use in pregnancy, lactation, or children has not been established (Pregnancy Category C).

Lab Test Considerations

• Monitor serum alpha₁-proteinase inhibitor levels to determine response to therapy. Minimum serum concentration should be 80 mg/100 ml. • May cause transient mild increase in leukocytes.

Patient/Family Teaching

• Explain to patient and family the purpose of the medication and the need for chronic weekly therapy. The patient should avoid smoking and notify physician of any changes in breathing pattern or sputum production. • Advise patient that fever may occur up to 12 hours after infusion and resolves by 24 hours. Fever may be treated symptomatically. • Advise patient of need for periodic pulmonary function tests to determine progression of disease and response to therapy. • Explain purpose of vaccination with hepatitis B vaccine prior to beginning therapy. A small risk of hepatitis is caused by the manufacturing process, and vaccination is recommended to prevent hepatitis.

 PHARMACOLOGIC PROFILE

Indications

• Alpha₁-proteinase inhibitor is used as replacement therapy in patients with demonstrated panacinar emphysema associated with congenital alpha₁-antitrypsin deficiency. This agent is not useful in patients with irreversible destruction of lung tissue secondary to alpha₁-antitrypsin deficiency.

Action

• Alpha₁-proteinase inhibitor prevents the destructive action of elastase on pulmonary alveolar tissue in patients who have alpha₁-antitrypsin deficiency.

Time/Action Profile (Increased levels of alpha₁-proteinase inhibitor)

Onset	Peak	Duration
within a few weeks	several weeks	UK

Pharmacokinetics

• **Distribution:** Alpha₁-proteinase inhibitor achieves high concentration in lung tissue. • **Metabolism and Excretion:** This agent is broken down in the intravascular space. • **Half-life:** 4.5–5.2 days.

Contraindications

• Do not use in patients with known hypersensitivity to polyethylene glycol. • Avoid using in patients whose emphysema is associated with alpha₁-antitrypsin deficiency where risk of panacinar emphysema is small (PiMZ and PiMS phenotype). • Patients with IgA deficiency who have antibodies against IgA should not receive alpha₁-proteinase inhibitor due to the increased risk of severe hypersensitivity reactions.

Adverse Reactions and Side Effects*

• **CNS:** light-headedness, dizziness • **Hemat:** transient leukocytosis • **Misc:** delayed fever.

Alprostadil	Prostaglandin
prostaglandin E$_1$, PGE$_1$, Prostin VR Pediatric	pH UK

☰ ADMINISTRATION CONSIDERATIONS

Usual Dose

NEONATES: 0.05–0.1 mcg/kg/min initially until satisfactory response is obtained, then decrease to a rate that maintains desired response. (Initial dose may be increased up to 0.4 mcg/kg/min if no response is obtained.) Some infants may respond to maintenance doses as low as 0.002 mcg/kg/min.

Dilution

• **Intermittent Infusion:** Available in solution at concentration of 500 mcg/ml. • **Dilute further** in 0.9% NaCl or D5W. Diluting 1 ml (500 mcg) of alprostadil in 250 ml of IV fluid will yield a final concentration of 2 mcg/ml; in 100 ml of IV fluid, will yield 5 mcg/ml; in 50 ml of IV fluid, will yield 10 mcg/ml; in 25 ml of IV fluid, will yield 20 mcg/ml. • Do not use solutions containing benzyl alcohol as a diluent. • Stable for 24 hours at room temperature.

Incompatibility

• Information unavailable. Do not mix with any other drugs.

Rate of Administration

• Once desired response is obtained, use lowest rate and shortest time possible to achieve therapeutic effect. This may be accomplished by progressively decreasing the infusion rate by 50%. • Infusion must be administered via infusion pump

---

*Underlines indicate most frequent; CAPITALS indicate life-threatening.

to ensure precise dose delivered. • For dose of 0.1 mcg/kg/min use 2 mcg/ml solution at infusion rate of 0.05 ml/kg/min or use 20 mcg/ml solution at infusion rate of 0.005 ml/kg/min.

≋ CLINICAL PRECAUTIONS

- Monitor rectal temperature, respiratory rate, pulse, blood pressure, ECG continuously during therapy. In neonates with aortic arch anomalies, also monitor pulmonary artery and descending aorta pressures, and urinary output. Palpate femoral pulse frequently to assess circulation to lower extremities. Blood pressure may be monitored in a lower and upper extremity simultaneously. Neonates with cyanotic congenital heart defects respond more rapidly (onset 15–30 minutes) than neonates with acynotic congenital heart defects (onset 1.5–3 hours). Monitor for appearance of congestive heart failure. Fever or hypotension may be resolved by slowing infusion rate.
- Monitor respiratory status and blood gases frequently. Low-birth-weight neonates (<2 kg) are more prone to respiratory (apnea, wheezing), cardiovascular (bradycardia, hypotension), and neurological (seizures, lethargy, cerebral bleeding) side effects. A ventilator should be readily available.
- Monitor for signs of bleeding. Use cautiously in neonates with bleeding tendencies due to effects on platelet function.
- May also be administered intra-arterially through an umbilical artery catheter or pulmonary artery catheter, or by intra-aortic infusion. During intra-aortic and intra-arterial administration, assess frequently for facial or arm flushing, which may indicate catheter displacement and necessitate repositioning of the catheter.
- Duration of therapy is usually limited to 24–48 hours. Closure of the ductus arteriosus usually begins within 1 or 2 hours after discontinuation of therapy.

Toxicity and Overdose Alert

- Symptoms of overdose include flushing, hypotension, bradycardia, fever, and decreased respiratory rate or apnea.

Infusion should be discontinued if apnea or bradycardia occurs.

Lab Test Considerations

• Monitor arterial blood gases prior to and periodically throughout therapy. In cyanotic defects, PaO$_2$ should increase within 30 minutes. In noncyanotic defects, correction of metabolic acidosis should occur within 4–11 hours.
• May rarely cause decreased serum glucose or increased serum bilirubin levels. May increase or decrease serum potassium levels.

Patient/Family Teaching

• Explain to the parents the purpose of alprostadil and the need for continuous monitoring.

≋ PHARMACOLOGIC PROFILE

Indications

• Alprostadil is used in the temporary maintenance of patent ductus arteriosus in neonates who depend on patency to maintain blood oxygenation and perfusion of the lower body until surgery can be performed.

Action

• Alprostadil directly relaxes smooth muscle of the ductus arteriosus. Other effects include vasodilation, inhibition of platelet aggregation, and stimulation of intestinal smooth muscle.

Time/Action Profile (improvement in blood gases and pulmonary blood flow)

	Onset	Peak	Duration
achd	UK	1.5–3 hr	duration of infusion
cchd	UK	30 min	duration of infusion

achd = acyanotic congenital heart disease.
cchd = cyanotic congenital heart disease.

Pharmacokinetics

• **Distribution:** UK • **Metabolism and Excretion:** Up to 80% of alprostadil is rapidly metabolized in the lungs. • **Half-life:** 5–10 minutes.

Contraindications

• Alprostadil is contraindicated in neonates with respiratory distress syndrome. • Product contains dehydrated alcohol. Avoid using in patients with known intolerance.

Adverse Reactions and Side Effects*

• **CNS:** SEIZURES, cerebral bleeding, irritability, jitteriness, lethargy • **CV:** bradycardia, hypotension • **Resp:** APNEA, wheezing, hypercapnia, respiratory depression, altered respiratory rate (slow and fast) • **GI:** diarrhea, gastric regurgitation, hyperbilirubinemia • **GU:** anuria, hematuria • **Derm:** flushing • **F and E:** hypokalemia • **Hemat:** disseminated intravascular coagulation, anemia, thrombocytopenia, bleeding • **Metab:** hypoglycemia • **MS:** neck hyperextension, stiffness • **Misc:** fever, hypothermia, sepsis, peritonitis.

Alteplase, Recombinant	*Thrombolytic*
Activase, tissue plasminogen activator, recombinant, rt-PA, t-PA	pH 7.3

≋ ADMINISTRATION CONSIDERATIONS

Usual Dose

Myocardial Infarction (Standard Regimen)

ADULTS ≥**65 kg:** 60 mg over the first hr (6–10 mg of this given as a bolus over the first 1–2 min), 20 mg over the second hr, and 20 mg over the third hr for a total of 100 mg.

ADULTS <**65 kg:** 1.25 mg/kg total dose over 3 hr given as 0.75 mg/kg over the first hr (0.045–0.075 mg/kg of this given as a bolus over the first 1–2 min), 0.25 mg/kg over the second hr, and 0.25 mg/kg over the third hr.

Myocardial Infarction (Accelerated Regimen)

ADULTS: 15 mg initially, then 0.75 mg/kg (up to 50 mg) over 30 min, then 0.75 mg/kg (up to 35 mg) over the next 60 min.

*Underlines indicate most frequent; CAPITALS indicate life-threatening.

Pulmonary Embolism

ADULTS: 100 mg over 2 hr. Follow with heparin therapy.

Dilution

• **Intermittent Infusion:** Vials are packaged with sterile water for injection (without preservatives) to be used as diluent. Do not use bacteriostatic water for injection. • **Reconstitute** 20-mg vials with 20 ml and 50-mg vials with 50 ml using 18-g needle. Avoid excess agitation during dilution; swirl or invert gently to mix. Solution may foam upon reconstitution. Bubbles will resolve upon standing a few minutes. Solution will be clear to pale yellow. Stable for 8 hours at room temperature. • May be administered as reconstituted (1 mg/ml) or may be **further diluted** immediately prior to use in equal amount of 0.9% NaCl or D5W.

Compatibility

• **Y-site:** lidocaine • metoprolol • propranolol.

Incompatibility

• **Y-site:** dobutamine • dopamine • heparin • nitroglycerin.

• **Additive:** Do not admix.

Rate of Administration

• **Intermittent Infusion:** Standard dose for *myocardial infarction* is given over 3 hours. See infusion rate table below. Flush line with 25–30 ml saline at completion of infusion to ensure entire dose is received. For *pulmonary embolism* administer dose over 2 hours.

ALTEPLASE INFUSION RATES (STANDARD REGIMEN)

Dilution: 20-mg vial with 20 ml diluent or 50-mg vial with 50 ml diluent = 1 mg/ml

Patient Weight	DOSE		
	1st hr†	2nd hr	3rd hr
>65 kg	60 mg	20 mg	20 mg
	DOSE (mg/kg)		
	1st hr‡	2nd hr	3rd hr
<65 kg	0.75 mg/kg	0.25 mg/kg	0.25 mg/kg

†Give 6–10 mg (6–10 ml) as a bolus over first 1–2 min.
‡Give 0.045–0.075 mg/kg as a bolus over the first 1–2 min.

≋ CLINICAL PRECAUTIONS

- Starting two IV lines is recommended, one for alteplase, the other for any additional IV infusions, prior to therapy.
- Assess patient for signs of bleeding and hemorrhage. Avoid IM injections prior to and throughout period of anticoagulation. Avoid unnecessary venipunctures. Apply pressure to all arterial and venous punctures for at least 30 minutes. Avoid venipunctures at all noncompressible sites (e.g., jugular and subclavian sites). Monitor all previous puncture sites every 15 minutes. May cause internal bleeding including intracranial hemorrhage. Guaiac test all body fluids and stools. Monitor neurological status. Assess peripheral pulses. If uncontrolled bleeding occurs, stop medication immediately. Patients at greatest risk of bleeding are those who have had recent (within 10 days) surgery, trauma, GI or GU bleeding, pre-existing hepatic or renal disease, or uncontrolled hypertension.
- Monitor vital signs until stable, then every 4 hours during therapy. Do not use lower extremities to monitor blood pressure. Alteplase should not be given if hypertension is uncontrolled. Hypotension may result from the drug, hemorrhage, or cardiogenic shock.
- Monitor ECG continuously in patients with coronary thrombosis for significant arrhythmias. Accelerated idioventricular rhythm, bradycardia, asystole, and ventricular arrhythmias due to reperfusion have been reported. Prophylactic, short-term antiarrhythmic therapy may be ordered concurrently and following alteplase administration. Arrhythmias are usually self-limiting. Coronary angiography or radionuclide myocardial scanning may be used to assess effectiveness of therapy.
- Assess intensity, character, location, and radiation of chest pain. Note presence of associated symptoms (nausea, vomiting, diaphoresis). Administer analgesics as ordered by physician. Notify physician if chest pain is unrelieved or recurs.
- Monitor heart sounds and breath sounds frequently. Inform physician if signs of congestive heart failure occur (rales/crackles, dyspnea, S3 heart sound, jugular venous distention, elevated CVP).

- Concurrent use of aspirin, oral anticoagulants, heparin, or dipyridamole may increase the risk of bleeding, although these agents are frequently used together or in sequence. Nonsteroidal anti-inflammatory agents, some cephalosporins, plicamycin, and valproic acid may also increase the risk of bleeding. Heparin may be started when the APTT or thrombin time has dropped to twice normal or less.
- Assess neurological status throughout therapy. Altered sensorium or mental changes may be indicative of intracranial bleeding. Cerebral or peripheral embolization may occur in patients with left heart thrombus. Geriatric patients (older than 75 years) are at increased risk of cerebrovascular bleeding, especially when doses greater than 150 mg are used.
- Assess patient for development of urticaria, which may indicate hypersensitivity reaction. Inform physician promptly if this occurs.
- Assess IV sites and other sites of potential phlebitis frequently. Septic embolization may occur if septic phlebitis is present.
- *Extreme caution* should be used during the early (10 days) postpartum period in order to avoid serious bleeding complications (Pregnancy Category C).

Toxicity and Overdose Alert

- Alteplase is rapidly cleared from the body; discontinue immediately if serious bleeding occurs.

Lab Test Considerations

- Monitor prothrombin time, partial thromboplastin time, fibrinogen, fibrin degradation products, CBC and platelets, and CPK-MB to assess effectiveness of therapy and prevent hemorrhage. CPK-MB may rise from washout of reperfused area. Confer with physician about type and crossmatch of blood in the event of hemorrhage. • Stools should be tested for occult blood loss and urine tested for hematuria periodically during therapy.

Patient/Family Teaching

- Advise patient to remain on bed rest. • Avoid all unnecessary procedures such as shaving and vigorous toothbrushing for 24 hours. • Explain purpose of alteplase and the need for close monitoring to patient and family. • Instruct patient to report signs of hypersensitivity and bleeding promptly.

 PHARMACOLOGIC PROFILE

Indications
• Alteplase is used in the acute (within 4–6 hours from onset of chest pain) management of myocardial infarction. • It is also used in management of acute massive pulmonary embolism associated with obstructed pulmonary blood flow or unstable hemodynamics.

Action
• Alteplase stimulates the conversion of plasminogen trapped in thrombi to plasmin by binding to fibrin. • It lyses thrombi and subsequently limits infarct size in myocardial infarction. • Alteplase lyses life-threatening emboli in pulmonary embolism.

Time/Action Profile (reperfusion of occluded coronary arteries)

Onset	Peak†	Duration‡
UK	20 min–2 hr (average 45 min)	4 hr

†Lysis of pulmonary emboli occurs within 2–6 hr.
‡Thrombin time returns to less than twice normal.

Pharmacokinetics
• **Distribution:** UK. • **Metabolism and Excretion:** More than 80% of alteplase is rapidly metabolized by the liver. • **Half-life:** 35 minutes.

Contraindications
• Active internal bleeding • History of cerebrovascular accident • Recent (within 2 months) intracranial or intraspinal trauma or surgery • Intracranial neoplasm • Severe uncontrolled hypertension • Arteriovenous malformation • Known bleeding tendencies.

Adverse Reactions and Side Effects*

• **CNS:** INTRACRANIAL BLEEDING, headache • **CV:** <u>arrhythmias</u> (due to reperfusion), hypotension • **EENT:** epistaxis, gingival bleeding • **GI:** GASTROINTESTINAL BLEEDING, RETROPERITONEAL BLEEDING, nausea, vomiting • **GU:** GENITOURINARY TRACT BLEEDING • **Derm:** ecchymoses, urticaria, itching, flushing • **Hemat:** <u>BLEEDING</u> • **MS:** musculoskeletal pain • **Misc:** fever.

Amikacin Sulfate	*Anti-infective* *(aminoglycoside)*
Amikin	pH 3.5–5.5

≋ ADMINISTRATION CONSIDERATIONS

Usual Dose

ADULTS, CHILDREN, AND OLDER INFANTS: 5 mg/kg q 8 hr or 7.5 mg/kg q 12 hr. 250 mg q 12 hr has been used for urinary tract infections.

YOUNGER INFANTS AND NEONATES: 10 mg/kg initially, 7.5 mg/kg q 12 hr.

PREMATURE NEONATES: 10 mg/kg initially, then 7.5 mg/kg q 18–24 hr.

Dilution

• **Intermittent Infusion:** Dilute 500 mg of amikacin in 100–200 ml of D5W, D10W, 0.9% NaCl, D5/0.9% NaCl, D5/0.45% NaCl, D5/0.25% NaCl, or lactated Ringer's solution. • Solution may be pale yellow without decreased potency. Stable for 24 hours at room temperature.

Compatibility

• **Y-site:** acyclovir ◆ cyclophosphamide ◆ diltiazem ◆ enalaprilat ◆ esmolol ◆ filgrastim ◆ fluconazole ◆ fludarabine ◆ foscarnet ◆ furosemide ◆ idarubicin ◆ labetalol ◆ magnesium sulfate ◆ melphalan ◆ morphine ◆ ondansetron ◆ paclitaxel ◆ perphenazine ◆ sargramostim ◆ vinorelbine ◆ zidovudine.

---

*<u>Underlines</u> indicate most frequent; CAPITALS indicate life-threatening.

- **Additive:** ascorbic acid ✦ bleomycin ✦ calcium chloride ✦ calcium gluconate ✦ chloramphenicol ✦ chlorpheniramine ✦ cimetidine ✦ ciprofloxacin ✦ clindamycin ✦ diphenhydramine ✦ epinephrine ✦ fluconazole ✦ furosemide ✦ hyaluronidase ✦ hydrocortisone ✦ metronidazole ✦ phytonadione ✦ polymyxin B ✦ ranitidine ✦ sodium bicarbonate ✦ succinylcholine ✦ vancomycin. However, manufacturer recommends administering separately.

Incompatibility

- **Syringe:** allopurinol sodium ✦ heparin.
- **Y-site:** hetastarch. If aminoglycosides and penicillins or cephalosporins must be administered concurrently, administer in separate sites at least 1 hour apart.
- **Additive:** heparin. Manufacturer does not recommend admixing.

Rate of Administration

- Infuse over 30–60 minutes (1–2 hours for infants). Flush IV line with D5W or 0.9% NaCl following administration.

≋ CLINICAL PRECAUTIONS

- Assess patient for infection (vital signs; wound appearance, sputum, urine, and stool; WBC) at beginning and throughout course of therapy.
- Obtain culture and sensitivity specimens. First dose may be administered prior to receiving results.
- Monitor intake and output, daily weight, and renal function tests. Renal failure may be related to excess peak and trough blood levels. Risk is also increased by dehydration, concurrent loop diuretic therapy, advanced age, or nephrotoxic drugs. Any degree of renal impairment requires dosage adjustment. Keep patient well hydrated (1500–2000 ml/day) during therapy.
- Evaluate eighth cranial nerve function by audiometry prior to and throughout course of therapy. Hearing loss is usually in the high-frequency range. Prompt recognition and intervention is essential in preventing permanent damage. Also monitor for vestibular dysfunction (vertigo, ataxia, nausea, vomiting). Eighth cranial nerve

dysfunction is associated with persistently elevated peak amikacin levels. Assessment of hearing may be difficult in very young or geriatric patients.

- Use with caution in patients with neuromuscular diseases such as myasthenia gravis. Amikacin has neuromuscular blocking properties. This property is accentuated by neuromuscular blocking agents (tubocurarine, succinylcholine). Respiratory paralysis may occur with inhalation anesthetics (ether, cyclopropane, halothane, or nitrous oxide).
- Amikacin may be inactivated by penicillins when coadministered to patients with renal insufficiency.
- Dosing in obese patients should be based on ideal body weight.
- Safe use in pregnancy and lactation has not been established (Pregnancy Category D).

Toxicity and Overdose Alert

- Therapeutic blood levels should be monitored periodically during therapy. Timing of blood levels is important in interpreting results. Draw blood for peak levels 15–30 minutes after IV infusion is completed. Trough levels should be drawn just prior to next dose. Acceptable peak level is 30–35 mcg/ml; trough level should not exceed 5–10 mcg/ml.

Lab Test Considerations

- Monitor renal function by urinalysis, specific gravity, BUN, creatinine, and creatinine clearance prior to and throughout therapy. • May cause increased BUN, AST (SGOT), ALT (SGPT), serum alkaline phosphatase, bilirubin, creatinine, and LDH concentrations. • May cause decreased serum calcium, magnesium, potassium, and sodium concentrations.

Patient/Family Teaching

- Instruct patient to report signs of hypersensitivity, tinnitus, vertigo, or hearing loss. • Advise patient to report signs of superinfection (fever, upper respiratory infection, vaginal itching or discharge, increasing malaise, diarrhea).

≋ PHARMACOLOGIC PROFILE

Indications
- Amikacin is used in the treatment of serious Gram-negative bacillary infections and infections due to staphylococci when penicillins or other less toxic drugs are contraindicated.

Action
- Amikacin inhibits bacterial protein synthesis at the level of the 30S ribosome, resulting in death of susceptible organisms. • Spectrum notable for activity against *Pseudomonas aeruginosa, Klebsiella pneumoniae, Escherichia coli, Proteus, Serratia, Acinetobacter* (where resistance to gentamicin or tobramycin has occurred), and *Staphylococcus aureus.* • In the treatment of enterococcal infections, synergy with a penicillin is required.

Time/Action Profile (blood levels)

Onset	Peak
rapid	end of infusion

Pharmacokinetics
- **Distribution:** Amikacin is widely distributed throughout extracellular fluids. Penetration into CSF is poor. • **Metabolism and Excretion:** Excretion of amikacin is mainly renal (>90%). Small amounts are metabolized by the liver. • **Half-life:** 2–3 hours (increased in renal impairment, decreased in burn patients).

Contraindications
- Hypersensitivity to amikacin or bisulfites. • Cross-sensitivity with other aminoglycosides may occur.

Adverse Reactions and Side Effects*
- **EENT:** ototoxicity (vestibular and cochlear) • **GU:** nephrotoxicity • **Neuro:** enhanced neuromuscular blockade • **Misc:** hypersensitivity reactions.

---

*Underlines indicate most frequent; CAPITALS indicate life-threatening.

Amino Acids	*Caloric agent (protein source)*
Aminess, Aminosyn, BranchAmin, FreAmine, HepatAmine, NeprAmine, Novamine, ProcalAmine, RenAmin, Travasol, Trophamine	pH 5–8

≋ ADMINISTRATION CONSIDERATIONS

Usual Dose

NOTE: Doses must be carefully individualized and titrated to meet metabolic needs. If amino acids are part of total parenteral nutrition (hyperalimentation), then additional calories and fluid (as dextrose and lipid emulsions) must be provided along with electrolytes, vitamins, trace minerals, and other necessary micronutrients.

ADULTS: 0.9–2 g protein/kg/day.
CHILDREN: 1–4 g protein/kg/day.
NEONATES: 2–4 g protein/kg/day.

Dilution

• **Continuous Infusion:** Parenteral amino acids are a component of total parenteral nutrition. They are usually given in conjunction with hypertonic dextrose. Trace elements, vitamins, electrolytes, and insulin are usually incorporated into formulation. • Special formulas are available for patients with hepatic or renal dysfunction, patients under extreme stress (trauma, sepsis), and children. Amino acids are also available as a component of total nutrient admixtures (TNA), known as multicomponent admixtures, all-in-one, 3-in-1, or triple mix, which combine amino acids, dextrose, and lipids in one container. • Solution should be clear. Do not administer if precipitates have formed. Addition of multivitamins will result in bright yellow color.

Compatibility

• **Y-site:** cefamandole • cefazolin • cefoperazone • cefotaxime • cefoxitin • ceftazidime • cephalothin • cephapirin • chloramphenicol • ciprofloxacin • clindamycin • digoxin • dobutamine • dopamine • doxycycline • erythromycin lactobionate • fluconazole • foscarnet • furosemide • gentamicin • idarubicin • isoproterenol • kanamycin • lidocaine • meperidine • methicillin • mezlocillin • miconazole • morphine

• nafcillin • netilmicin • norepinephrine • oxacillin • penicillin G potassium • piperacillin • sargramostim • ticarcillin • tobramycin • urokinase • vancomycin.

Incompatibility

• **Y-site:** cephradine • indomethacin.

• **Additive:** Do not add anything to solution without conferring with pharmacist. Total parenteral nutrition solutions should be prepared aseptically in a biologic cabinet.

Rate of Administration

• **Continuous Infusion:** Infuse through 0.22-micron filter unless mixed with dextrose and fat emulsion in a total nutrient admixture. Control infusion rate with pump or controller.

≋ CLINICAL PRECAUTIONS

• Nutritional status must be assessed prior to and periodically throughout therapy. Parameters to assess include height, weight, skinfold thickness, arm circumference, total protein, serum albumin, CBC, electrolytes, nitrogen balance, function of gastrointestinal tract, and caloric need. **Treatment must be individualized for each patient and requires facilities and personnel skilled in its use.** Patients with advanced cardiac, renal, and hepatic disease may require specific formulations.

• Monitor intake and output; assess for fluid overload (rales/crackles, dyspnea, peripheral edema).

• Monitor for infection (fever, chills, diaphoresis). If sepsis occurs, physician may order changing site, culturing catheter tip, hanging new solution and tubing, and obtaining blood cultures. Due to the risk of infection associated with amino acids, patients with uncontrolled sepsis should be treated before therapy is initiated.

• Monitor vital signs, fluid and electrolyte status, glucose, weight, and nitrogen balance. Patients on long-term therapy require monitoring of trace elements. Glucocorticoids, diuretics, or tetracyclines may exaggerate negative nitrogen balance.

• If administered peripherally, change peripheral site every 48–72 hours or according to institutional policy. Monitor for thrombophlebitis. Avoid infiltration; may cause tissue necrosis.

• Peripheral line may be used to administer protein-sparing regimen using dilute amino acid solution (3.5%) with or without D5W or D10W and fat emulsion. Central line must be used to administer more concentrated solutions when mixed with hypertonic glucose.

- Fat emulsion may be piggybacked with amino acids. Fat emulsion container should be hung at a higher level than amino acid container.
- Use aseptic technique when handling central line. Change dressing every 48 hours or according to institutional policy. Auscultate breath sounds and assess site for erythema, edema, and leakage.
- Use cautiously in pregnant or lactating patients. Safe use during pregnancy and lactation has not been established (Pregnancy Category C).

Lab Test Considerations

- May cause increased BUN. A 10–15% increase for 3 consecutive days may necessitate discontinuing therapy or altering formulation. • May cause increased ammonia and ketone levels.

Patient/Family Teaching

- If amino acids are used as a component of total parenteral nutrition, assure the patient and family that the solution is capable of fulfilling all nutritional needs. • Instruct patient to report fever, chills, or swelling, pain, and leakage at infusion site immediately.
- **Home Care Issues:** Patients receiving total parenteral nutrition at home may receive infusion only at night.
- Prior to discharge, the patient and family must understand rationale for therapy, procedure, and symptoms to report to physician. Patients must correctly demonstrate aseptic technique in caring for site, spiking bag, priming tubing, and regulating infusion pump. • Discharge planning should be coordinated with home care agency that will provide equipment, solutions, and professional support to the patient and family.

☰ PHARMACOLOGIC PROFILE

Indications

- Amino acids provide protein to patients who are unable to ingest enough protein by mouth to maintain positive nitrogen balance. They are used perioperatively in patients who are unable to ingest protein as in GI disorders or to provide an extra source of protein in patients with large requirements who are unable to ingest necessary quantities, as seen in extensive burns, severe trauma, or overwhelming sepsis.

Action
• Amino acids promote protein synthesis by acting as a protein calorie source, decreasing the rate of protein breakdown (catabolism), and maintaining positive nitrogen balance.

Pharmacokinetics
• **Distribution:** Amino acids are widely distributed.
• **Metabolism and Excretion:** Amino acids are metabolized as part of anabolic processes, then excreted in urine as urea nitrogen. • **Half-life:** UK.

Contraindications
• There are no known contraindications to amino acid therapy.

Adverse Reactions and Side Effects*
• **CNS:** headache, confusion • **CV:** congestive heart failure, hypotension, hypertension • **GI:** nausea, vomiting • **F and E:** hypervolemia, hypovolemia, electrolyte disturbances • **Metab:** hyperglycemia, hypoglycemia, azotemia, fatty acid deficiency, hyperammonemia • **Misc:** INFECTION.

Aminocaproic Acid	*Hemostatic agent*
epsilon aminocaproic acid, Amicar	pH 6–7.6

≋ ADMINISTRATION CONSIDERATIONS
Usual Dose
Acute Bleeding Syndromes Due to Elevated Fibrinolytic Activity
ADULTS: 4–5 g over first hr, followed by 1 g/hr for 8 hr or until hemorrhage is controlled (not to exceed 30 g/day). Lower doses may be used following prostatic surgery.

---

*Underlines indicate most frequent; CAPITALS indicate life-threatening.

CHILDREN: 100 mg/kg or 3 g/m^2 over first hr, followed by continuous infusion of 33.3 mg/kg/hr or 1 g/m^2/hr (total dosage not to exceed 18 g/m^2/24 hr).

Dilution

- **Continuous Infusion:** Do not administer undiluted. Dilute 4–5 g in 250 ml of sterile water, 0.9% NaCl, D5W, or lactated Ringer's solution. Do not dilute with sterile water in patients with subarachnoid hemorrhage.

Incompatibility

- **Additive:** Do not admix with other medications.

Rate of Administration

- **Continuous Infusion:** Administer initial 4–5 g over the first hour. • Initial dose may be followed by a continuous infusion of 1 g/hr in 50–100 ml diluent. Administer IV solutions using infusion pump to ensure accurate dose. Rapid infusion rate may cause hypotension, bradycardia, or other arrhythmias.

≋ CLINICAL PRECAUTIONS

- Monitor blood pressure, pulse, and respiratory status as indicated by severity of bleeding. Monitor for signs of bleeding every 15–30 minutes. Use cautiously in patients with hematuria originating in the upper urinary tract.
- Stabilize intravenous catheter to minimize thrombophlebitis. Monitor site closely.
- Monitor neurological status (pupils, level of consciousness, motor activity) in patients with subarachnoid hemorrhage.
- Monitor intake and output ratios frequently; notify physician if significant discrepancies occur.
- Assess for thromboembolic complications (especially in patients with previous history). Notify physician if positive Homans' sign, leg pain and edema, hemoptysis, dyspnea, or chest pain occurs.
- Patients being treated for disseminated intravascular coagulation (DIC) must be treated concurrently with heparin to avoid potentially fatal thrombus formation.

- Patients with cardiac, renal, or liver disease may require reduced dosage.
- Safe use in pregnancy or lactation has not been established.

Lab Test Considerations

- Monitor platelet count and clotting factors prior to and periodically throughout therapy in patients with systemic fibrinolysis. • Increased CPK may indicate myopathy.

Patient/Family Teaching

- Instruct patient to notify the nurse immediately if bleeding recurs, or if thromboembolic symptoms develop. • Caution patient to make position changes slowly to avoid orthostatic hypotension.

≋ PHARMACOLOGIC PROFILE

Indications

- Aminocaproic acid is used in the management of acute, life-threatening hemorrhage due to systemic hyperfibrinolysis or urinary fibrinolysis.

Action

- Aminocaproic acid inhibits activation of plasminogen. This results in inhibition of fibrinolysis and stabilization of clot.

Time/Action Profile (blood levels)

Onset	Peak	Duration
UK	2 hr	UK

Pharmacokinetics

- **Distribution:** Aminocaproic acid is widely distributed.
- **Metabolism:** The kidneys are the major organ of elimination for aminocaproic acid. • **Half-life:** UK.

Contraindications

- Do not use in patients with active intravascular clotting.
- Some products contain benzyl alcohol and should be avoided in patients with known intolerance.

Adverse Reactions and Side Effects*

• **CNS:** dizziness, malaise • **EENT:** tinnitus, nasal stuffiness • **CV:** arrhythmias, hypotension • **GI:** nausea, cramping, diarrhea, anorexia, bloating • **GU:** diuresis, renal failure • **MS:** myopathy.

Aminophylline	*Bronchodilator* *(phosphodiesterase inhibitor)*
theophylline ethylenediamine	pH 8.6–9

ADMINISTRATION CONSIDERATIONS

Aminophylline Dosing

It is necessary to know if aminophylline or theophylline products have been taken in the past 24 hours before initiating therapy. Serum level monitoring is useful in determining the need for partial or full loading doses in these patients.

Usual Dose

Bronchodilator

ADULTS: 6 mg/kg initially over 20–30 min, then in *otherwise healthy nonsmoking adults*—0.5 mg/kg/hr; *young adult smokers*—0.9 mg/kg/hr; *patients >60 yr or patients with cor pulmonale*—0.3 mg/kg/hr; *patients with congestive heart failure or liver disease*—0.2 mg/kg/hr. Maintenance infusion rates may be decreased after 12 hr.

CHILDREN 12–16 yr: 6 mg/kg initially, then in *nonsmokers*—0.6 mg/kg/hr; *smokers*—0.9 mg/kg/hr.

CHILDREN 9–12 yr: 6 mg/kg initially, then 0.9 mg/kg/hr.

CHILDREN 1–9 yr: 6 mg/kg initially, then 1 mg/kg/hr.

CHILDREN UP TO 1 yr: 6 mg/kg initially, then dose in mg/kg/hr = 0.01 (age in weeks) + 0.25.

Respiratory Stimulant

NEONATES: 6 mg/kg initially, then 1.2–1.8 mg/kg q 12 hr.

---

*Underlines indicate most frequent; CAPITALS indicate life-threatening.

Dilution

• **Intermittent Infusion: Dilute** in 100–200 ml of D5W, D10W, D20W, 0.9% NaCl, 0.45% NaCl, D5/0.9% NaCl, D5/0.45% NaCl, D5/0.25% NaCl, or lactated Ringer's solution. Mixture is stable for 24 hours if refrigerated. • Do not administer discolored or precipitated solutions. • Flush main IV line prior to administration. • **Continuous Infusion:** Usually given as a loading dose in a small volume followed by continuous infusion in a larger volume.

Compatibility

• **Syringe:** heparin ✦ metoclopramide ✦ pentobarbital ✦ thiopental.

• **Y-site:** allopurinol sodium ✦ amrinone ✦ atracurium ✦ cimetidine ✦ enalaprilat ✦ esmolol ✦ famotidine ✦ filgrastim ✦ fluconazole ✦ fludarabine ✦ foscarnet ✦ gallium nitrate ✦ labetalol ✦ melphalan ✦ morphine ✦ netilmicin ✦ paclitaxel ✦ pancuronium ✦ piperacillin/tazobactam ✦ potassium chloride ✦ ranitidine ✦ sargramostim ✦ tacrolimus ✦ tolazoline ✦ vecuronium ✦ vitamin B complex with C.

• **Additive:** calcium gluconate ✦ cimetidine ✦ dexamethasone sodium phosphate ✦ diphenhydramine ✦ erythromycin lactobionate ✦ esmolol ✦ furosemide ✦ heparin ✦ hydrocortisone sodium succinate ✦ potassium chloride ✦ ranitidine ✦ sodium bicarbonate ✦ terbutaline.

Incompatibility

• **Syringe:** doxapram.

• **Y-site:** ciprofloxacin ✦ dobutamine ✦ hydralazine ✦ ondansetron ✦ vinorelbine.

• **Additive:** ascorbic acid ✦ bleomycin ✦ ciprofloxacin ✦ clindamycin ✦ dobutamine ✦ doxorubicin ✦ epinephrine ✦ erythromycin gluceptate ✦ hydralazine ✦ insulin ✦ isoproterenol ✦ meperidine ✦ morphine ✦ penicillin G potassium ✦ vitamin B complex with C.

Rate of Administration

• **Direct IV:** Administer loading dose over 20–30 minutes. Do not administer at a rate faster than 25 mg/min. If acute adverse reactions occur during administration of the loading dose, the infusion may be stopped for 5–10 minutes or administered at a slower rate. • **Intermittent/Continuous**

Infusion: Do not exceed 25 mg/min in adults. Administer via infusion pump to ensure accurate dosage. Rapid administration may cause hypotension, arrhythmias, syncope, and death.

AMINOPHYLLINE INFUSION RATES (ml/hr)
Concentration = 1 mg/ml

Dilution: 250 mg in 250 ml or 500 mg in 500 ml or 1000 mg in 1000 ml = 1 mg/ml.

Loading dose in patients who have not received aminophylline in preceding 24 hr = 6 mg/kg (6 ml/kg of above dilution) administered over 20–30 min.

PATIENT WEIGHT

Dose	50 kg	60 kg	70 kg	80 kg	90 kg	100 kg
Loading dose (mg)*	280 mg	336 mg	392 mg	448 mg	504 mg	560 mg

INFUSION RATES						
1.0 mg/kg	50 ml/hr	60 ml/hr	70 ml/hr	80 ml/hr	90 ml/hr	100 ml/hr
0.9 mg/kg/hr	45 ml/hr	54 ml/hr	63 ml/hr	72 ml/hr	81 ml/hr	90 ml/hr
0.8 mg/kg/hr	40 ml/hr	48 ml/hr	56 ml/hr	64 ml/hr	72 ml/hr	80 ml/hr
0.7 mg/kg/hr	35 ml/hr	42 ml/hr	49 ml/hr	56 ml/hr	63 ml/hr	70 ml/hr
0.6 mg/kg/hr	30 ml/hr	36 ml/hr	42 ml/hr	48 ml/hr	54 ml/hr	60 ml/hr
0.5 mg/kg/hr	25 ml/hr	30 ml/hr	35 ml/hr	40 ml/hr	45 ml/hr	50 ml/hr
0.4 mg/kg/hr	20 ml/hr	24 ml/hr	28 ml/hr	32 ml/hr	36 ml/hr	40 ml/hr
0.3 mg/kg/hr	15 ml/hr	18 ml/hr	21 ml/hr	24 ml/hr	27 ml/hr	30 ml/hr
0.2 mg/kg/hr	10 ml/hr	12 ml/hr	14 ml/hr	16 ml/hr	18 ml/hr	20 ml/hr
0.1 mg/kg/hr	5 ml/hr	6 ml/hr	7 ml/hr	8 ml/hr	9 ml/hr	10 ml/hr

*Loading dose administered over 20–30 min.

≋ CLINICAL PRECAUTIONS

- Dosage should be determined by theophylline serum level monitoring. Determine previous use of theophylline-containing products. Loading dose should be decreased or eliminated if theophylline preparation has been used in preceding 24 hours. Aminophylline releases free theophylline upon administration (aminophylline = 85% theophylline). Wait at least 4 hours after discontinuing IV therapy to begin immediate release oral dosage; for extended-release oral dosage form, administer first oral dose at time of IV discontinuation.

- Assess blood pressure, pulse, respiration, and lung sounds before administering medication and throughout therapy. Patients with a history of cardiovascular problems should be monitored for chest pain and ECG changes (PACs, supraventricular tachycardia, PVCs, ventricular tachycardia). Resuscitative equipment should be readily available.

- If extravasation occurs, local injection of 1% procaine and application of heat may relieve pain and promote vasodilation.

- Use cautiously in patients older than 60 years of age and patients with liver disease or congestive heart failure. These patients metabolize aminophylline more slowly and have an increased risk for developing toxicity. Dosage reduction in these populations is required, and blood level monitoring is valuable in assessing therapy. Erythromycin, beta blockers, cimetidine, ranitidine, influenza vaccination, oral contraceptives, glucocorticoids, disulfiram, interferon, mexiletine, thiabendazole, fluoroquinolones, and large doses of allopurinol also decrease metabolism. Monitor these patients for CNS, GI, and cardiovascular toxicity.

- Cigarette smokers and children metabolize theophylline more rapidly and may require larger doses or more frequent administration. A similar effect is seen with concurrent use of adrenergic agents, barbiturates, phenytoin, ketoconazole, rifampin, and excessive intake of charcoal-broiled foods. Monitor for decreased drug effect in these patients.

- Monitor intake and output ratios for an increase in diuresis.

- Excessive intake of xanthine-containing foods or beverages (colas, coffee, chocolate) may increase the risk of CV and CNS side effects.

- Monitor neonates for apnea, bradycardia, and cyanosis. Neonatal patients may accumulate caffeine, a by-product of aminophylline metabolism.

- Additive CV and CNS side effects may occur with concurrent adrenergic (sympathomimetic) agents. Cardiovascular side effects may be accentuated by halothane.

- Theophylline may decrease the effects of lithium.

- Isoniazid, carbamazepine, and loop diuretics have variable effects on theophylline levels. Monitor patients for altered response.
- Aminophylline crosses the placenta and enters breast milk in concentrations 70% of plasma levels. Although it has been used safely during pregnancy, irritability, tachycardia, and insomnia may occur in the newborn (Pregnancy Category C).

Toxicity and Overdose Alert

• Monitor drug levels routinely. Therapeutic plasma levels range from 10 to 20 mcg/ml. Drug levels in excess of 20 mcg/ml are associated with toxicity. • Observe patient closely for symptoms of progressive drug toxicity (anorexia, nausea, vomiting, restlessness, insomnia, tachycardia, arrhythmias, seizures). Notify physician immediately if any of these occur.

Patient/Family Teaching

• Encourage the patient to drink adequate liquids (2000 ml/day minimum) to decrease the viscosity of the airway secretions. • Encourage patients not to smoke. A change in smoking habits may necessitate a change in dosage.
• **Home Care Issues:** Instruct family or care-giver on dilution, rate, and administration of drug and proper care of IV equipment. • Advise patient to minimize intake of xanthine-containing foods or beverages (colas, coffee, chocolate) and not to eat charcoal-broiled foods daily. • Advise patient to contact physician promptly if the usual dose of medication fails to produce the desired results, symptoms worsen after treatment, or toxic effects occur. • Emphasize the importance of having serum levels routinely tested every 6–12 months during chronic therapy or more often during dosage adjustment.

≋ PHARMACOLOGIC PROFILE

Indications

• Aminophylline produces bronchodilation in patients with reversible airway obstruction due to asthma or COPD.

• **Unlabeled Use:** Respiratory and myocardial stimulant in apnea of infancy.

Action

• Aminophylline inhibits phosphodiesterase, producing increased tissue concentrations of cyclic adenosine monophosphate (cAMP). Increased levels of cAMP result in bronchodilation, CNS stimulation, positive inotropic and chronotropic effects, diuresis, and gastric acid secretion. Aminophylline is a salt of theophylline and releases free theophylline following administration.

Time/Action Profile (therapeutic blood levels)

Onset	Peak	Duration
rapid	end of infusion	6–8 hr

Pharmacokinetics

• **Distribution:** Aminophylline is widely distributed as theophylline. Theophylline crosses the placenta and enters breast milk. • **Metabolism and Excretion:** Theophylline is metabolized by the liver to caffeine, which may accumulate in neonates. Metabolites are renally excreted. • **Half-life:** 3–13 hours. Half-life is longer in elderly (>60 years) patients, neonates, and in patients with congestive heart failure or liver disease, but is shorter in cigarette smokers and children.

Contraindications

• Aminophylline should not be used in patients with uncontrolled arrhythmias or hyperthyroidism.

Adverse Reactions and Side Effects*

• **CNS:** <u>nervousness</u>, <u>anxiety</u>, headache, insomnia, SEIZURES
• **CV:** <u>tachycardia</u>, palpitations, arrhythmias, angina pectoris
• **GI:** <u>nausea</u>, <u>vomiting</u>, anorexia, cramps • **Neuro:** tremor.

---

*<u>Underlines</u> indicate most frequent; CAPITALS indicate life-threatening.

Amobarbital Sodium	*Sedative/hypnotic, Anticonvulsant (barbiturate)*
Amytal	**pH 9.6–10.5 (as 5% solution)**

Schedule II

 ADMINISTRATION CONSIDERATIONS

Usual Dose

Anticonvulsant
ADULTS AND CHILDREN >6 yr: 65–500 mg (not to exceed 1 g).
CHILDREN <6 yr: 3–5 mg/kg or 125 mg/m² per dose.

Hypnotic
ADULTS: 65–200 mg.
CHILDREN >6 yr: 65–500 mg/dose.

Sedative
ADULTS: 30–50 mg 2–3 times daily.
CHILDREN: 65–500 mg (3–5 mg/kg/dose) as a preoperative sedative.

Dilution
• **Direct IV: Reconstitute** with sterile water for a concentration of 100 mg/ml. Rotate vial to mix; do not shake. • May be **further diluted** in D5W, D10W, D20W, D5/0.9% NaCl, D5/LR, 0.9% NaCl, 3% NaCl, and lactated Ringer's injection. • Solution should be used within 30 minutes of reconstitution. Do not use if solution does not become absolutely clear within 5 minutes following reconstitution or if precipitate forms after solution clears.

Incompatibility
• **Additive:** cimetidine ◆ chlorpromazine ◆ droperidol ◆ insulin ◆ levorphanol ◆ meperidine ◆ morphine ◆ pentazocine ◆ propiomazine ◆ pancuronium ◆ streptomycin ◆ vancomycin.

Rate of Administration
• **Direct IV:** Administer at a rate of 50 mg over at least 1 minute for adults or 60 mg/m²/min for children. Titrate slowly for desired response. Rapid administration may result

in respiratory depression, apnea, laryngospasm, broncho-spasm, or hypotension.

≋ CLINICAL PRECAUTIONS

- Assess location, duration, and characteristics of seizure activity. Institute seizure precautions.
- Sedation lasts for 6–8 hours after a dose. Remove cigarettes and monitor ambulation following administration.
- May cause hypotension and bradycardia. Monitor blood pressure and heart rate. Respiratory status may be compromised by rapid administration. Equipment for resuscitation and artificial ventilation should be readily available.
- Use largest vein possible to prevent thrombosis.
- Solution is highly alkaline; avoid extravasation, which may cause tissue damage and necrosis. If extravasation occurs, infiltration of 5% procaine solution into affected area and application of moist heat may be ordered.
- Use cautiously in patients with hepatic dysfunction or renal impairment. These patients may have exaggerated responses and be at increased risk of adverse reactions.
- Geriatric or debilitated patients may be more sensitive to drug effects. Dosage should be reduced. Excitement and confusion may also occur.
- The following drugs will potentiate the CNS depressant effects of amobarbital: alcohol, antidepressants, antihistamines, opioid analgesics, and other sedative/hypnotics. MAO inhibitors may prolong sedation.
- Barbiturates induce hepatic enzymes that metabolize other drugs, thereby decreasing their effectiveness; included are oral contraceptives, chloramphenicol, acebutolol, propranolol, metoprolol, timolol, doxycycline, glucocorticoids, tricyclic antidepressants, phenothiazines, and quinidine.
- This drug crosses the placenta and enters breast milk. Avoid using in pregnant or lactating patients (Pregnancy Category D).

Patient/Family Teaching

- Caution patient to request assistance with ambulation and transfer to prevent injury due to drowsiness.

≋ PHARMACOLOGIC PROFILE

Indications
• Amobarbital is used as an anticonvulsant in the management of seizures of diverse causes. • It is also used as a sedative/hypnotic.

Action
• Amobarbital produces all levels of CNS depression. It depresses sensory cortex, decreases motor activity, and alters cerebral function. • Amobarbital inhibits transmission in the CNS and raises the seizure threshold.

Time/Action Profile (sedation)

Onset	Peak	Duration
several minutes	UK	6–8 hr

Pharmacokinetics
• **Distribution:** Amobarbital is rapidly and widely distributed, with high concentrations occurring in the brain, liver, and kidneys. Amobarbital readily crosses the placenta, and small amounts enter breast milk. • **Metabolism and Excretion:** Amobarbital is mostly metabolized by the liver. • **Half-life:** 16–40 hours.

Contraindications
• Hypersensitivity to amobarbital. • Cross-sensitivity with other barbiturates may occur. • Amobarbital should not be used in patients with any degree of CNS depression, including comatose patients. • Do not use in patients with severe uncontrolled pain; amobarbital has no analgesic properties.

Adverse Reactions and Side Effects*
• **CNS:** <u>drowsiness</u>, lethargy, vertigo, depression, <u>hangover</u>, excitation, delirium, syncope • **CV:** hypotension, bradycardia • **Resp:** respiratory depression, LARYNGOSPASM, BRONCHOSPASM • **GI:** nausea, vomiting, diarrhea, constipation • **Derm:** rashes, urticaria, photosensitivity, exfoliative dermatitis • **MS:** myalgia, arthralgia • **Neuro:** neuralgia • **Local:** phlebitis at IV site, pain at IM site • **Misc:** hypersensitivity reactions including STEVENS-JOHNSON SYNDROME.

---

*<u>Underlines</u> indicate most frequent; CAPITALS indicate life-threatening.

Amphotericin B   *Antifungal*
Fungizone Intravenous   **pH 5.7–8.0**

≋ ADMINISTRATION CONSIDERATIONS

Usual Dose

ADULTS: Give test dose of 1 mg, then initial dose of 0.25 mg/ kg, slowly over 6 hr, increase daily doses slowly by 5–10 mg to 0.5 mg/kg (can give up to 1 mg/kg/day or 1.5 mg/kg every other day, not to exceed 50 mg/day). Escalation depends on patient's condition. In severely ill patients, therapy may be started at full dose.

CHILDREN: 0.25 mg/kg infused over 6 hr initially, increase by 0.125–0.25 mg/kg every day or every other day to maximum of 1 mg/kg/day or 30 mg/m^2/day.

Dilution

• **Test Dose:** Dilute 1 mg in 20 ml of D5W. • **Intermittent Infusion:** Reconstitute 50-mg vial with 10 ml of sterile water without a bacteriostatic agent. Concentration equals 5 mg/ml. Shake until clear. • **Further dilute** each 1 mg with at least 10 ml of D5W (pH >4.2) for a concentration of 0.1 mg/ml. Do not use other diluents. Avoid use of precipitated solutions. • Use 20-gauge needle; change for each step of dilution. Wear gloves while handling. • If an in-line filter is used, the mean pore diameter should be no less than 1 micron. • Agitate hanging solution every half hour to mix. Short-term exposure to light (8–24 hours) does not appreciably alter potency. If administered via heparin lock containing 0.9% NaCl, flush heparin lock with D5W before and after administration of amphotericin. • Store in a dark area. Reconstituted solution is stable for 24 hours at room temperature and 1 week if refrigerated.

Compatibility

• **Syringe:** heparin.
• **Y-site:** diltiazem ◆ tacrolimus ◆ zidovudine.
• **Additive:** fluconazole ◆ heparin ◆ hydrocortisone ◆ methylprednisolone ◆ sodium bicarbonate.

Incompatibility

• **Y-site:** allopurinol sodium ◆ enalaprilat ◆ filgrastim ◆ fluconazole ◆ fludarabine ◆ foscarnet ◆ melphalan ◆ ondansetron ◆ piperacillin/tazobactam ◆ vinorelbine.

* **Additive:** calcium chloride ✦ calcium gluconate ✦ cimetidine ✦ diphenhydramine ✦ magnesium sulfate ✦ potassium chloride ✦ ranitidine ✦ saline solutions.

Rate of Administration
* **Test Dose:** Administer 1 mg in 20 ml of D5W over 10–30 minutes to determine the patient's tolerance. If the medication is held for 7 days, restart at the lowest dose level.
* **Intermittent Infusion:** Administer slowly via infusion pump over 6 hours.

≋ CLINICAL PRECAUTIONS

* This drug should be administered intravenously only under close medical supervision. Diagnosis should be confirmed with cultures prior to administration.
* Monitor patient closely during test dose and the first 1–2 hours of each dose for fever, chills, headache, anorexia, nausea, vomiting. Premedication with aspirin, glucocorticoid (25 mg or less of hydrocortisone), antihistamines, and antiemetics and maintaining sodium balance may decrease these reactions. Febrile reaction usually subsides within 4 hours after the infusion is completed.
* Assess injection site frequently for thrombophlebitis or leakage. Drug is extremely irritating to tissues. The addition of heparin to IV solution may decrease the likelihood of thrombophlebitis. Administration through a central line is preferred. If peripheral site is used, change site with each dose to prevent phlebitis.
* Monitor pulse and blood pressure every 15–30 minutes during test dose and initial therapy. Assess respiratory status (lung sounds, dyspnea) daily. Notify physician of any changes.
* Monitor intake and output and weigh patient daily. Use cautiously in patients with renal impairment or pre-existing electrolyte abnormalities. Adequate hydration (2000–3000 ml/day) may minimize nephrotoxicity. Nephrotoxicity is usually heralded by hypokalemia.
* Cumulative doses greater than 4 g increase the risk of adverse renal reactions.
* Diuretics, glucocorticoids, mezlocillin, piperacillin, or ticarcillin may potentiate hypokalemia. Risk of nephrotoxicity is increased by concurrent aminoglycosides and

other nephrotoxic agents. Hypokalemia increases the risk of cardiac glycoside (digoxin) toxicity.
• Although safe use during pregnancy and lactation has not been established, amphotericin has been used without ill effects on mother or fetus (Pregnancy Category B).

Lab Test Considerations

• Monitor weekly hemoglobin and hematocrit, magnesium, BUN, and serum creatinine, and biweekly potassium levels. Life-threatening hypokalemia may occur following each dose. If BUN exceeds 40 mg/100 ml or serum creatinine exceeds 3 mg/100 ml, dosage should be decreased or discontinued until renal function improves. May cause decreased hemoglobin, hematocrit, and magnesium levels. • Liver function tests should be monitored periodically throughout therapy. Elevated alkaline phosphatase and bilirubin may require discontinuation of therapy.

Patient/Family Teaching

• Explain need for long duration of IV therapy. • Inform patient of potential side effects and discomfort at IV site.
• **Home Care Issues:** Instruct family or care-giver on dilution, rate, and administration of drug and proper care of IV equipment.

≋ PHARMACOLOGIC PROFILE

Indications

• Amphotericin B is used in the treatment of active, progressive, potentially fatal fungal infections.

Action

• Amphotericin B binds to fungal cell membrane, allowing leakage of cellular contents. • Antifungal spectrum includes activity against aspergillosis, blastomycosis, disseminated candidiasis, coccidioidomycosis, histoplasmosis, and mucormycosis.

Time/Action Profile (blood levels)

Onset	Peak
rapid	end of infusion

Pharmacokinetics

• **Distribution:** Amphotericin B distributes to body tissues and fluids. Penetration into the CSF is poor. • **Metabolism and Execretion:** The elimination of amphotericin B is very prolonged, being detectable in urine up to 7 weeks after discontinuation.

Contraindications

• Hypersensitivity.

Adverse Reactions and Side Effects*

• **CNS:** <u>headache</u> • **CV:** <u>hypotension</u>, arrhythmias • **Resp:** dyspnea, wheezing • **GI:** <u>nausea</u>, <u>vomiting</u>, <u>diarrhea</u> • **GU:** <u>nephrotoxicity</u>, hematuria • **F and E:** <u>hypokalemia</u> • **Hemat:** anemia, dyscrasias • **Local:** phlebitis • **MS:** myalgia, arthralgia • **Neuro:** peripheral neuropathy • **Misc:** <u>fever</u>, <u>chills</u>, HYPERSENSITIVITY REACTIONS.

Ampicillin Sodium	*Anti-infective (penicillin)*
{Ampicin}, Ampilean, Omnipen-N, {Penbritin}, Polycillin-N, Totacillin-N	pH 8–10

≋ ADMINISTRATION CONSIDERATIONS

Usual Dose

ADULTS AND CHILDREN ≥**20 kg:** 250–500 mg q 6 hr (up to 2 g q 3 hr for meningitis).

INFANTS AND CHILDREN <**20 kg:** *Most indications*— 12.5 mg/kg q 6 hr (up to 200 mg/kg/day for meningitis).

NEONATES ≥**2 kg:** *Meningitis*— 50 mg/kg q 8 hr for first week of life, then 50 mg/kg q 6 hr.

NEONATES <**2 kg:** *Meningitis*— 25–50 mg/kg for the first week of life, then 50 mg/kg q 8 hr.

---

*<u>Underlines</u> indicate most frequent; CAPITALS indicate life-threatening.

{} = Available in Canada only.

Dilution

• **Reconstitute** with sterile water 0.9–1.2 ml to the 125-mg vial; 0.9–1.9 ml to the 250-mg vial; 1.2–1.8 ml to the 500-mg vial; 2.4–7.4 ml to the 1-g vial, and 6.8 ml to the 2-g vial. Administer within 4 hours of reconstitution. • **Direct IV:** Administer **undiluted.** • **Intermittent Infusion: Dilute further** in 50 ml or more of 0.9% NaCl, D5W, D5/0.45% NaCl, or lactated Ringer's solution for a concentration of no more than 30 mg/ml.

Compatibility

• **Syringe:** chloramphenicol ✦ heparin ✦ procaine.
• **Y-site:** acyclovir ✦ allopurinol sodium ✦ cyclophospha-mide ✦ enalaprilat ✦ esmolol ✦ famotidine ✦ filgrastim ✦ flu-darabine ✦ foscarnet ✦ insulin ✦ labetalol ✦ magnesium sulfate ✦ melphalan ✦ meperidine ✦ morphine ✦ perphenazine ✦ phy-tonadione ✦ potassium chloride ✦ tacrolimus ✦ tolazidine ✦ vitamin B complex with C.
• **Additive:** clindamycin ✦ verapamil.

Incompatibility

• **Syringe:** erythromycin lactobionate ✦ gentamicin ✦ kan-amycin ✦ metoclopramide ✦ streptomycin.
• **Y-site:** epinephrine ✦ fluconazole ✦ hydralazine ✦ on-dansetron ✦ sargramostim ✦ verapamil ✦ vinorelbine. If ami-noglycosides and penicillins must be administered concur-rently, administer in separate sites at least 1 hour apart.
• **Additive:** amikacin ✦ gentamicin ✦ kanamycin.

Rate of Administration

• **Direct IV:** May be administered over 3–5 minutes (125–500 mg) or over 10–15 minutes (1–2 g) within 1 hour of reconstitution. More rapid administration may cause sei-zures. • **Intermittent Infusion:** Administer over a period of up to 4 hours.

≋ CLINICAL PRECAUTIONS

• Assess patient for infection (vital signs, wound appear-ance, sputum, urine, and stool; WBC) at beginning and throughout therapy.
• Obtain specimens for culture and sensitivity prior to ini-

tiating therapy. First dose may be given prior to receiving results.

- Obtain a history before initiating therapy to determine use and reactions to penicillins or cephalosporins. Persons with a negative history of penicillin sensitivity may still have an allergic response. Observe patient for signs and symptoms of anaphylaxis (rash, pruritus, laryngeal edema, wheezing). Discontinue the drug and notify the physician immediately if these occur. Keep epinephrine, an antihistamine, and resuscitation equipment close by in the event of an anaphylactic reaction.
- Assess skin daily for ampicillin rash—a nonallergic, dull red, macular or maculopapular, and mildly pruritic rash. Incidence of rash is greatly increased with concurrent allopurinol therapy or in the presence of infectious mononucleosis.
- Probenecid decreases renal excretion and increases blood levels of ampicillin. Therapy may be combined for this purpose. Observe for seizures with large doses of ampicillin.
- Observe for signs of bleeding in patients taking oral anticoagulants, as ampicillin may increase the risk of bleeding.
- Increased dosing interval is recommended if creatinine clearance <30 ml/min.
- Has been used safely during pregnancy and lactation (Pregnancy Category B).

Lab Test Considerations

• May cause false-positive copper sulfate urine glucose tests (Clinitest); test urine with glucose enzymatic tests (Ketodiastix or Tes-Tape). • May cause increased AST (SGOT) and ALT (SGPT).

Patient/Family Teaching

• Advise patient to report the signs of superinfection (furry overgrowth on the tongue, vaginal itching or discharge, loose or foul-smelling stools) and allergy. • Determine if patient is taking oral contraceptives, and advise patient to use a nonhormonal method of contraception while taking ampicillin and for the remainder of the contraceptive cycle because the effectiveness of oral contraceptives is decreased and breakthrough bleeding or pregnancy may result. • Instruct the patient to notify the physician if symptoms do not improve.

• **Home Care Issues:** Instruct family or care-giver on dilution, rate, and administration of drug and proper care of IV equipment.

PHARMACOLOGIC PROFILE

Indications

• Ampicillin is used in the treatment of a variety of skin and skin structure infections, soft tissue infections including otitis media, sinusitis, respiratory tract infections, genitourinary tract infections, meningitis, and septicemia.

Action

• Ampicillin binds to the bacterial cell wall, resulting in cell death. • It resists action of beta-lactamase, an enzyme produced by bacteria, which is capable of inactivating some penicillins. • Ampicillin is active against streptococci, pneumococci, enterococci, *Haemophilus influenzae, Escherichia coli, Proteus mirabilis, Neisseria meningitidis, N. gonorrhoeae, Shigella,* and *Salmonella.*

Time/Action Profile (blood levels)

Onset	Peak
rapid	end of infusion

Pharmacokinetics

• **Distribution:** Ampicillin diffuses readily into most body tissues and fluids. CSF penetration is increased in the presence of inflamed meninges. Ampicillin crosses the placenta and enters breast milk. • **Metabolism and Excretion:** Ampicillin is variably metabolized by the liver (12–50%). Renal excretion of unchanged drug is also variable. • **Half-life:** 1–1.5 hours.

Contraindications

• Ampicillin should not be used in patients with previous hypersensitivity to penicillins or cephalosporins.

Adverse Reactions and Side Effects*

- **CNS:** SEIZURES (high doses) • **GI:** nausea, vomiting, <u>diarrhea</u> • **Hemat:** blood dyscrasias • **Derm:** <u>rashes</u>, urticaria • **Misc:** superinfection, allergic reactions including ANAPHYLAXIS and serum sickness.

Ampicillin Sodium/ Sulbactam Sodium	Anti-infective
Unasyn	pH 8–10
	5 mEq Na/1.5 g

ADMINISTRATION CONSIDERATIONS

Usual Dose

1.5 g ampicillin/sulbactam = 1 g ampicillin plus 0.5 g sulbactam.

ADULTS: 1.5–3 g (1 g ampicillin plus 0.5 g sulbactam—2 g ampicillin plus 1 g sulbactam) q 6 hr (not to exceed 4 g sulbactam/day).

Dilution

- **Reconstitute** each 1.5 g with at least 4 ml of sterile water for a concentration of 375 mg/ml (250 mg ampicillin/125 mg sulbactam). Foaming should dissipate upon standing. Administer only clear solutions. • **Dilute** immediately for infusion in 50–100 ml of 0.9% NaCl, D5W, D5/0.45% NaCl, or lactated Ringer's solution. • Stability of solution varies from 2–8 hours at room temperature or 3–72 hours if refrigerated, depending on concentration and diluent.

Compatibility

- **Y-site:** enalaprilat • famotidine • filgrastim • fluconazole • fludarabine • gallium nitrate • insulin • meperidine • morphine • paclitaxel • tacrolimus.

---

*<u>Underlines</u> indicate most frequent; CAPITALS indicate life-threatening.

Incompatibility

• **Y-site:** idarubicin ◆ ondansetron ◆ sargramostim. If aminoglycosides and penicillins must be administered concurrently, administer in separate sites.

Rate of Administration

• **Direct IV:** May be administered over 10–15 minutes (1–2 g) within 1 hour of reconstitution. More rapid administration may cause seizures. • **Intermittent Infusion:** Infuse over 15–30 minutes.

≋ CLINICAL PRECAUTIONS

- Assess patient for infection (vital signs, wound appearance, sputum, urine, and stool; WBC) at beginning and throughout course of therapy.
- Obtain specimens for culture and sensitivity prior to initiating therapy. First dose may be given before receiving results.
- Obtain a history before initiating therapy to determine previous use and reactions to penicillins or cephalosporins. Persons with a negative history of penicillin sensitivity may still have an allergic response. Observe patient for signs and symptoms of anaphylaxis (rash, pruritus, laryngeal edema, wheezing). Discontinue the drug and notify the physician immediately if these occur. Keep epinephrine, an antihistamine, and resuscitation equipment close by in the event of an anaphylactic reaction.
- Assess skin daily for ampicillin rash—a nonallergic, dull red, macular or maculopapular, and mildly pruritic rash. Incidence of rash is greatly increased with concurrent allopurinol therapy or in the presence of infectious mononucleosis.
- Probenecid decreases renal excretion and increases blood levels of ampicillin. Therapy may be combined for this purpose.
- Observe for signs of bleeding in patients taking oral anticoagulants.
- Increased dosing interval is recommended if creatinine clearance is less than 30 ml/min.
- Diarrhea is common during therapy. If fever and bloody diarrhea occur, notify physician.

- Ampicillin has been used safely during pregnancy and lactation. It crosses the placenta and enters breast milk in small amounts (ampicillin/sulbactam has the Pregnancy Category B). Safety of ampicillin/sulbactam in children younger than 12 years of age has not been established.

Lab Test Considerations

- May cause false-positive copper sulfate urine glucose tests (Clinitest); test urine with glucose enzymatic tests (Ketodiastix or Tes-Tape). • May cause increased AST (SGOT), ALT (SGPT), LDH, alkaline phosphatase, monocytes, basophils, eosinophils, BUN, and creatinine. May also cause presence of RBCs and hyaline casts in the urine. • May cause decreased hemoglobin, hematocrit, RBC, WBC, neutrophils, lymphocytes, platelets, serum albumin, and total proteins.

Patient/Family Teaching

- Advise patient to report the signs of superinfection (furry overgrowth on the tongue, vaginal itching or discharge, loose or foul-smelling stools) and allergy. • Determine if patient is taking oral contraceptives, and advise patient to use a nonhormonal method of contraception while taking ampicillin/sulbactam, because the effectiveness of oral contraceptives is decreased and breakthrough bleeding or pregnancy may result. • Instruct the patient to notify the physician if symptoms do not improve.

- **Home Care Issues:** Instruct family or care-giver on dilution, rate, and administration of drug and proper care of IV equipment.

≋ PHARMACOLOGIC PROFILE

Indications

- Ampicillin/sulbactam is used in the treatment of a variety of skin and skin structure infections and soft tissue infections including otitis media, sinusitis, respiratory tract infections, genitourinary tract infections, meningitis, and septicemia.

Action

- Ampicillin binds to the bacterial cell wall, resulting in cell death. Addition of sulbactam increases resistance to beta-lactamases, enzymes produced by bacteria that may inactivate ampicillin. • The combination displays activity against the following pathogens: streptococci, pneumococci, enterococci, *Haemophilus influenzae, Escherichia coli, Proteus mirabilis, Neisseria meningitidis, N. gonorrhoeae, Shigella,* and *Salmonella.* Therapy with ampicillin/sulbactam should be reserved for infections caused by beta-lactamase-producing strains.

Time/Action Profile (blood levels)

Onset	Peak
immediate	end of infusion

Pharmacokinetics

• **Distribution:** Ampicillin diffuses readily into most body tissues and fluids. CSF penetration is increased in the presence of inflamed meninges. Ampicillin crosses the placenta and enters breast milk. • **Metabolism and Excretion:** Ampicillin is variably metabolized by the liver (12–50%). Renal excretion of unchanged drug is also variable. • **Half-life:** 1–1.5 hours (ampicillin).

Contraindications

• Ampicillin/sulbactam should not be used in patients with previous hypersensitivity to penicillins/cephalosporins or sulbactam.

Adverse Reactions and Side Effects*

• **CNS:** SEIZURES (high doses) • **GI:** nausea, vomiting, diarrhea • **Derm:** rashes, urticaria • **Hemat:** blood dyscrasias • **Local:** pain at IV site • **Misc:** superinfection, allergic reactions including ANAPHYLAXIS and serum sickness.

---

*Underlines indicate most frequent; CAPITALS indicate life-threatening.

Amrinone Lactate   *Inotropic agent*

Inocor   **pH 3.2–4**

≋ ADMINISTRATION CONSIDERATIONS

Usual Dose

ADULTS: 750 mcg (0.75 mg)/kg loading dose may be repeated in 30 min if necessary, then 5–10 mcg/kg/min infusion (total daily dose should not exceed 10 mg/kg).

CHILDREN: 0.75–3 mg/kg initially, then 5–10 mcg/kg/min infusion (unlabeled).

NEONATES: 0.75–3 mg/kg initially, then 3–5 mcg/kg/min infusion (unlabeled).

Dilution

• **Direct IV**: Administer **undiluted** or **dilute** with 0.9% NaCl or 0.45% NaCl only, for a concentration of 1–3 mg/ml. Dilution with dextrose products may lead to decomposition of amrinone, but amrinone may be administered through Y-tubing or directly into tubing of a running dextrose solution. • Change tubing whenever concentration of solution is changed. • Solution should be clear yellow. Use reconstituted solutions within 24 hours of preparation.

Compatibility

• **Syringe:** propranolol ✦ verapamil.

• **Y-site:** aminophylline ✦ atropine ✦ bretylium ✦ calcium chloride ✦ cimetidine ✦ digoxin ✦ dobutamine ✦ dopamine ✦ epinephrine ✦ famotidine ✦ hydrocortisone sodium succinate ✦ isoproterenol ✦ lidocaine ✦ metaraminol ✦ methylprednisolone sodium succinate ✦ nitroglycerin ✦ nitroprusside ✦ norepinephrine ✦ phenylephrine ✦ potassium chloride ✦ propranolol ✦ verapamil.

Incompatibility

• **Y-site:** furosemide ✦ sodium bicarbonate.

Rate of Administration

• **Direct IV:** Loading dose should be administered over 2–3 minutes. Loading doses greater than 0.75 mg/kg should be divided into 2–3 smaller doses. An additional loading dose may be given in 30 minutes.

• **Continuous Infusion:** Rate is titrated according to patient response. See infusion rate table below. Administer via infusion pump to ensure accurate dosage.

AMRINONE (Inocor) INFUSION RATES

Loading dose: 0.75 mg/kg (0.75 ml/kg) over 2–3 min.
To calculate infusion rate (ml/min), multiply patient's weight (kg) by dose in ml/kg/min.
To calculate infusion rate (ml/hr), multiply patient's weight (kg) by dose in mg/kg/min × 60.

AMRINONE INFUSION RATES (ml/hr)

CONCENTRATION = 1 mg/ml

PATIENT WEIGHT

Dose	50 kg	60 kg	70 kg	80 kg	90 kg	100 kg
loading dose (mg)*	37.5 mg	45 mg	52.5 mg	60 mg	67.5 mg	75 mg
5 mcg/kg/min	15 ml/hr	18 ml/hr	21 ml/hr	24 ml/hr	27 ml/hr	30 ml/hr
6 mcg/kg/min	18 ml/hr	21.6 ml/hr	25.5 ml/hr	28.8 ml/hr	32.4 ml/hr	36 ml/hr
7 mcg/kg/min	21 ml/hr	25.2 ml/hr	29.4 ml/hr	33.6 ml/hr	37.8 ml/hr	42 ml/hr
8 mcg/kg/min	24 ml/hr	28.8 ml/hr	33.6 ml/hr	38.4 ml/hr	43.2 ml/hr	48 ml/hr
9 mcg/kg/min	27 ml/hr	32.4 ml/hr	37.8 ml/hr	43.2 ml/hr	48.6 ml/hr	54 ml/hr
10 mcg/kg/min	30 ml/hr	36 ml/hr	42 ml/hr	48 ml/hr	54 ml/hr	60 ml/hr

* Given over 2–3 min.

≋ CLINICAL PRECAUTIONS

• Monitor blood pressure, pulse, ECG, respiratory rate, cardiac index, pulmonary capillary wedge pressure, and central venous pressure frequently during the administration of this medication. Notify physician promptly if drug-induced hypotension occurs. Hypotension may be exaggerated by disopyramide. Inotropic effects may be additive with cardiac glycosides (digoxin).

• Use cautiously in patients with atrial fibrillation or flutter. Amrinone may increase ventricular response; pretreatment with cardiac glycosides may be necessary. Amrinone may cause hypokalemia, which could increase the risk of cardiac glycoside toxicity. Hypokalemia should be corrected prior to administration of amrinone.

- Monitor intake and output and weigh patient daily. Assess patient for resolution of signs and symptoms of congestive heart failure (peripheral edema, dyspnea, rales/crackles, weight gain). Fluid intake may need to be increased cautiously to ensure adequate cardiac filling pressure.
- Observe the patient for the appearance of hypersensitivity reactions (pleuritis, pericarditis, ascites). Withhold drug and notify physician immediately if a reaction occurs.
- Safe use in children <18 years of age has not been established.
- Safety in pregnancy, lactation, or children under 18 years has not been established (Pregnancy Category C).

Lab Test Considerations

• Platelet counts, CBC, serum electrolytes, liver enzymes, and renal function should be evaluated periodically throughout the course of therapy. Reversible thrombocytopenia is common. If platelet count is less than 150,000/mm^3, notify physician promptly. Increased liver enzymes may indicate hepatotoxicity. May cause decreased potassium levels.

Patient/Family Teaching

• Advise patient to report an increase in dyspnea or chest pain, or the onset of hypersensitivity reactions promptly. • Advise patient to make position changes slowly to minimize any drug-induced postural hypotension.

 PHARMACOLOGIC PROFILE

Indications

• Amrinone lactate is used in the short-term treatment of congestive heart failure unresponsive to conventional therapy with cardiac glycosides, diuretics, and vasodilators.

Action

• Amrinone lactate increases myocardial contractility. • It decreases preload and afterload by a direct dilating effect on vascular smooth muscle. The net hemodynamic effect is increased cardiac output (inotropic effect).

Time/Action Profile (blood levels)

Onset	Peak	Duration
2–5 min	10 min	0.5–2 hr

Pharmacokinetics

• **Distribution:** UK • **Metabolism and Excretion:** 50% of amrinone is excreted by the liver; 10–40% is excreted unchanged by the kidneys. • **Half-life:** 3.6–5.8 hours (increased in congestive heart failure).

Contraindications

• Hypersensitivity to amrinone or bisulfites • Idiopathic hypertrophic subaortic stenosis.

Adverse Reactions and Side Effects*

• **CV:** <u>arrhythmias</u>, <u>hypotension</u> • **Resp:** dyspnea • **GI:** nausea, vomiting, diarrhea, hepatotoxicity • **F and E:** hypokalemia • **Hemat:** <u>thrombocytopenia</u> • **Misc:** hypersensitivity reactions, fever.

Anistreplase *Thrombolytic agent*

anisoylated plasminogen-streptokinase
activator complex, APSAC, Eminase   pH 3.2–4.0

 ADMINISTRATION CONSIDERATIONS

Usual Dose

ADULTS: 30 units over 2–5 min.

Dilution

• **Reconstitute** with 5 ml of sterile water (direct to sides of vial) and swirl gently; do not shake to minimize foaming. **Do not dilute further.** Solution is colorless to transparent pale yellow. Use reconstituted solution within 30 minutes of preparation.

---

*<u>Underlines</u> indicate most frequent; CAPITALS indicate life-threatening.

Incompatibility

• **Y-site/Additive:** Do not admix or administer via **Y-site** injection with any other medication.

Rate of Administration

• Administer via IV line or vein over 2–5 minutes.

≋ CLINICAL PRECAUTIONS

• Therapy should be administered as soon as possible after the onset of symptoms.

• Assess patient for signs of bleeding and hemorrhage. Avoid IM injections prior to and throughout period of anticoagulation. Avoid unnecessary venipunctures. Apply pressure to all arterial and venous puncture sites for at least 30 minutes. Avoid venipunctures at all noncompressible sites (e.g., jugular and subclavian sites). Monitor all previous puncture sites every 15 minutes. May cause internal bleeding including intracranial hemorrhage. Guaiac test all body fluids and stools. If uncontrolled bleeding occurs, stop medication immediately. Monitor neurological status. Assess peripheral pulses. Patients at greatest risk of bleeding are those who have had recent (within 10 days) surgery, trauma, GI or GU bleeding, pre-existing hepatic or renal disease, or uncontrolled hypertension.

• Monitor vital signs, including temperature, continuously until stable, then every 4 hours. Do not use lower extremities to measure blood pressure. Anistreplase should not be given if hypertension is uncontrolled. Hypotension may result from the drug, hemorrhage, or cardiogenic shock. Acetaminophen may be ordered to control fever.

• Monitor ECG continuously in patients with coronary thrombosis for significant arrhythmias. Document changes in ST segment. Accelerated idioventricular rhythm, bradycardia, asystole, and ventricular arrhythmias due to reperfusion have been reported. Short-term, prophylactic antiarrhythmic therapy may be ordered concurrently and following anistreplase administration. Arrhythmias are usually self-limiting. Peak effect on reperfusion occurs in 20 minutes–2 hours (average 45 minutes). Coronary angiography or radionuclide myocardial scanning may be used to assess effectiveness of therapy.

- Assess intensity, character, location, and radiation of chest pain. Note presence of associated symptoms (nausea, vomiting, diaphoresis). Administer analgesics as ordered. Notify physician if chest pain is unrelieved or recurs. Monitor cardiac enzymes. Radionuclide myocardial scanning and/or coronary angiography may be ordered ≥10 days following therapy.

- Monitor heart sounds and breath sounds frequently. Inform physician if signs of congestive heart failure occur (rales/crackles, dyspnea, S3 heart sound, jugular venous distention, elevated CVP).

- Concurrent use of aspirin, oral anticoagulants, heparin, or dipyridamole may increase the risk of bleeding, although these agents are frequently used together or in sequence. Most nonsteroidal anti-inflammatory agents, some cephalosporins, plicamycin, and valproic acid may also increase the risk of bleeding.

- Assess neurological status throughout therapy. Altered sensorium or mental changes may be indicative of intracranial bleeding. Cerebral or peripheral embolization may occur in patients with left heart thrombus. Geriatric patients (>75 years) are at increased risk of cerebrovascular bleeding.

- Inquire about previous reaction to anistreplase or streptokinase therapy. Assess patient for hypersensitivity reaction (changes in facial skin color, rash, dyspnea, swelling around eyes, wheezing). If these occur, inform physician promptly. Keep epinephrine, an antihistamine, and resuscitation equipment close by in the event of an anaphylactic reaction.

- Assess IV sites and other sites of potential phlebitis frequently. Septic embolization may occur if septic phlebitis is present.

- Assess patient for recent streptococcal infection or previous therapy with anistreplase or streptokinase (from 5 days–6 months), which may produce resistance due to antibody formation. Increased dosage requirements may be encountered.

- *Extreme caution* should be used during the early (10 days) postpartum period in order to avoid serious bleeding complications (Pregnancy Category C).

Toxicity and Overdose Alert

• If local bleeding occurs, apply pressure to site. If severe or internal bleeding occurs, clotting factors and/or blood volume may be restored through infusions of whole blood, packed red blood cells, fresh frozen plasma, cryoprecipitate, platelets, and/or desmopressin. Do not administer dextran, because it has an antiplatelet activity. If heparin is being administered, discontinue and consider administration of protamine. Aminocaproic acid (Amicar) may be used as an antidote (see *aminocaproic acid* monograph on page 46).

Lab Test Considerations

• Hematocrit, hemoglobin, platelet count, prothrombin time, thrombin time, bleeding time, activated partial thromboplastin time, and fibrinolytic activity should be evaluated prior to and frequently throughout course of therapy. • Obtain type and crossmatch and have blood available at all times in case of hemorrhage. • Stools should be tested for occult blood loss and urine for hematuria periodically during therapy.

Patient/Family Teaching

• Explain purpose of the medication. Instruct patient to report hypersensitivity reactions (rash, dyspnea), bleeding, or bruising. • Explain need for bed rest and minimal handling during therapy to avoid injury.

≋ PHARMACOLOGIC PROFILE

Indications

• Anistreplase is used in the acute management of myocardial infarction, in order to lyse thrombi in coronary arteries and thereby preserve ventricular function.

Action

• Anistreplase consists of an inactive complex of plasminogen and streptokinase. Following administration, controlled activation of the complex occurs, allowing the conversion of plasminogen to plasmin and subsequent fibrinolysis.

Time/Action Profile (fibrinolysis)

Onset	Peak	Duration
UK	45 min	6 hr†

†Systemic hyperfibrinolytic state may persist for 2 days.

Pharmacokinetics

• **Distribution:** Minimal amounts cross the placenta.
• **Metabolism and Excretion:** Anistreplase is inactivated by binding to plasmin inactivators. • **Half-life:** 70–120 minutes.

Contraindications

• Active internal bleeding • History of cerebrovascular accident • Recent (within 2 months) intracranial or intraspinal trauma • Intracranial neoplasm • Severe uncontrolled hypertension • Arteriovenous malformation • Known bleeding tendencies • Hypersensitivity to anistreplase or streptokinase.

Adverse Reactions and Side Effects*

• **CNS:** INTRACRANIAL HEMORRHAGE • **EENT:** epistaxis, gingival bleeding • **Resp:** hemoptysis • **CV:** arrhythmias, hypotension • **GI:** GASTROINTESTINAL BLEEDING, RETROPERITONEAL BLEEDING • **GU:** GENITOURINARY TRACT BLEEDING • **Hemat:** BLEEDING • **Misc:** allergic reactions, including ANAPHYLAXIS, fever.

Antihemophilic Factor	*Hemostatic agent*
AHF, Hemofil M, Humate-P, Hyate:C, Koate-HP, Kogenate, MelATE, Monoclate-P, Profilate OSD, Recombinate	pH UK

〰 ADMINISTRATION CONSIDERATIONS

Usual Dose

Consult individual product information for specific dosing information. Dosage may be calculated using either of the following formulas:
Desired AHF increase (% normal) = [dose AHF (units)/body weight (kg)] × 2

---

*<u>Underlines</u> indicate most frequent; CAPITALS indicate life-threatening.

Dose AHF (units) = body weight (kg) × desired AHF increase × 0.5

ANTIHEMOPHILIC FACTOR (HUMAN)

Hemofil M, Humate-P, Koate-HP, MelATE, Monoclate-P, Profilate OSD

ANTIHEMOPHILIC FACTOR (RECOMBINANT)

Kogenate, Recombinate

Prevention of Spontaneous Hemorrhage

ADULTS AND CHILDREN: 25–40 units/kg three times weekly.

Treatment of Minor Hemorrhage

ADULTS AND CHILDREN: 8–15 units/kg (or amount required to increase plasma Factor VIII levels to 20–40% of normal). If required, may be repeated q 8–10 hr for 1–3 days.

Treatment of Moderate Hemorrhage

ADULTS AND CHILDREN: 15–25 units/kg (or amount required to increase plasma Factor VIII levels to 30–50% of normal) initially, then 10–25 units/kg q 8–12 hr as needed.

Treatment of Severe Hemorrhage or Hemorrhage into or near Vital Organs

ADULTS AND CHILDREN: 30–50 units/kg (or amount required to increase plasma Factor VIII levels to 60–100% of normal) initially, then 20–25 units/kg q 8–12 hr as needed.

Management of Perioperative Hemostasis— Tooth Extraction

ADULTS AND CHILDREN: Amount necessary to raise plasma Factor VIII levels to 30–50% of normal given 1 hr prior to surgery. May be repeated if required.

Management of Perioperative Hemostasis— Minor Procedures

ADULTS AND CHILDREN: 15–20 units/kg (or amount necessary to raise plasma Factor VIII levels to 30–50% of normal) initially, then 10–15 units/kg q 8–12 hr as required.

Management of Perioperative Hemostasis— Major Procedures

ADULTS AND CHILDREN: Amount necessary to raise plasma Factor VIII levels to 50–100% of normal) given 1 hr prior to procedure. Administer a second dose of half the initial dose 5 hr later. May be repeated as required q 6–14 hr or maintain plasma Factor VIII levels of at least 30% of normal for 10–14 days postoperatively.

ANTIHEMOPHILIC FACTOR (PORCINE)

Hyate:C

Prevention of Bleeding in Patients with Antibodies to Factor VIII

ADULTS AND CHILDREN: 100–150 porcine units/kg (may be increased as needed).

Dilution

• Refrigerate concentrate until just prior to reconstitution. Warm concentrate and diluent (provided by manufacturer) to room temperature before reconstituting. Use plastic syringe for preparation and administration. Use an additional needle as an air vent to the vial when reconstituting. After adding diluent, rotate vial gently until completely dissolved. • Solution may vary in color from light yellow to clear with a bluish tint. Do not refrigerate after reconstitution; use within 3 hours. • Preparations should be filtered prior to administration.

Incompatibility

• **Y-site/Additive:** Do not admix or administer in the same line with any other medication or solution.

Rate of Administration

• **Direct IV:** May be administered by slow IV push (see Intermittent Infusion for rates). • **Intermittent Infusion:** Administration rate is based on the patient's comfort. *Hemofil M, Profilate OSD,* and *Recombinate* may be administered at a rate not to exceed 10 ml/min. *Monoclate-P* should be administered at a rate of 2 ml/min; *Humate-P* at a rate of 4 ml/min; and *Hyate:C* at a rate of 2–5 ml/min. The entire dose of *Koate-HP* or *Kogenate* can be administered over 5–10 minutes.

≋ CLINICAL PRECAUTIONS

• Monitor for bleeding from any site. Assess blood loss. Inform all personnel of bleeding tendency to prevent further trauma. Apply pressure to all venipuncture sites for at least 5 minutes; avoid all IM injections.

- Monitor blood pressure, pulse, and respirations. If tachycardia occurs, slow or stop infusion rate and notify physician.
- Obtain history of current trauma; estimate amount of blood loss. Obtain type and crossmatch of blood in case a transfusion is necessary.
- Monitor for renewed bleeding every 15–30 minutes. Immobilize and apply ice to affected joints.
- Monitor intake and output ratios; note color of urine. Notify physician if significant discrepancy occurs or if urine becomes red or orange. Patients with type A, B, or AB blood are particularly at risk for hemolytic reaction.
- Assess for allergic reaction (wheezing, tachycardia, urticaria, hives, chest tightness, stinging at IV site, nausea and vomiting, lethargy). Premedication with diphenhydramine (Benadryl) or a similar antihistamine to prevent acute reactions may be ordered. Stop infusion; notify physician if signs of an acute reaction occur.
- For major surgical procedures, the first dose of antihemophilic factor is given 1 hour before surgery. The second dose (half of the first dose) is given 5–8 hours postoperatively. Factor VIII level must be maintained at 30% of the normal level for 10–14 days postoperatively.
- Cryoprecipitated antihemophilic factor is only available from blood banks.
- Safe use in pregnancy not established (Pregnancy Category C).

Lab Test Considerations

- Monitor plasma Factor VIII levels. To prevent spontaneous bleeding, at least 5% of the normal Factor VIII level must be present. To control moderate bleeding or prior to minor surgery, 30–50% must be present. For severe bleeding associated with trauma, or patient undergoing major surgery, 80–100% of the normal Factor VIII level must be present.
- Obtain baseline and periodic CBC, platelet count, direct Coombs', urinalysis, partial thromboplastin time (PTT), thromboplastin generation test, and prothrombin generation test. Decreased hematocrit and increased Coombs' test may indicate hemolytic anemia. • Monitor coagulation studies before, during, and after therapy to assess

effectiveness of therapy. • Patients with increased inhibitor levels may not respond or may require increased doses.

Patient/Family Teaching

• Instruct patient to notify nurse immediately if bleeding recurs. Advise patient to observe for bleeding of gums, skin, or blood in urine, stool, or emesis. • Advise patient to carry identification describing disease process at all times. • Caution patient to consult a physician or pharmacist prior to using products containing aspirin, ibuprofen, or naproxen because they may further impair clotting. • Review methods of preventing bleeding with patient and family (use of soft toothbrush, avoid IM and SC injections, avoid potentially traumatic activities). • Inform newly diagnosed hemophilia patients of the need for hepatitis B vaccine. Advise patient that the risk of hepatitis or AIDS transmission may be diminished by the use of heat-treated, pasteurized, solvent/detergent treated or monoclonal antibody preparations. Screening programs currently used should also decrease the risk.

• **Home Care Issues:** Instruct family or care giver on dilution, rate, storage, and administration of drug and proper care of IV equipment.

≋ PHARMACOLOGIC PROFILE

Indications

• Antihemophilic factor is used in the management of hemophilia A associated with a deficiency of Factor VIII. Antihemophilic factor (porcine) is used in patients who have antibodies to Factor VIII.

Action

• Antihemophilic factor is an essential clotting factor required for the conversion of prothrombin to thrombin. Administration of antihemophilic factor controls excessive bleeding in deficiency states.

Time/Action Profile (hemostatic effect)

Onset	Peak	Duration
rapid	1–2 hr	8–12 hr

Pharmacokinetics

• **Distribution:** Antihemophilic factor is rapidly cleared from plasma. It does not cross the placenta. • **Metabolism and Excretion:** Antihemophilic factor is used up in the clotting process. • **Half-life:** 4–24 hours (12-hour average).

Contraindications

• Hypersensitivity to mouse protein (monoclonal antibody–derived product–Monoclate only).

Adverse Reactions and Side Effects*

• **CNS:** headache, somnolence, lethargy, loss of consciousness • **EENT:** visual disturbances • **CV:** tachycardia, hypotension, chest tightness • **GI:** nausea, vomiting • **Hemat:** intravascular hemolysis • **Derm:** flushing, urticaria • **MS:** back pain • **Neuro:** paresthesia • **Misc:** rigor, jaundice, allergic reactions, Hepatitis B or HIV infection (small risk from frequent use of large amounts).

Aprotinin	Hemostatic agent (protease inhibitor)
Trasylol	pH 4.5–6.5

ADMINISTRATION CONSIDERATIONS

Usual Dose

ADULTS: 1 ml (1.4 mg or 10,000 kallikrein inhibitor units [KIU]) test dose is given 10 min prior to loading dose. If no allergic reaction occurs, loading dose is 200 ml (280 mg or 2 million KIU) followed by constant infusion of 50 ml/hr (70 mg/hr) or 500,000 KIU/hr. In addition, 200 ml (280 mg or 2 million KIU) may be added to the priming fluid ("pump prime" dose) of the cardiopulmonary bypass circuit. Other regimens have been used.

---

*Underlines indicate most frequent; CAPITALS indicate life-threatening.

Dilution

• **Intermittent/Continuous Infusion:** Administer **undiluted**.

Incompatibility

• **Y-site:** Do not administer any other drug in the same venous line or catheter.

• **Additive:** corticosteroids • heparin • tetracyclines • nutrient solutions containing amino acids or fat emulsion.

Rate of Administration

• **Intermittent Infusion:** Administer loading dose over
20–30 minutes. Rapid administration may cause transient fall
in blood pressure. • **Continuous Infusion:** Administer at a
rate of 50 ml/hr.

≋ CLINICAL PRECAUTIONS

• Administer with patient in a supine position. The loading dose is administered after induction of anesthesia but
  prior to sternotomy. Follow the loading dose with a continuous infusion until the surgery is completed and the
  patient leaves the operating room.

• Monitor for the development of allergic reactions (skin
  eruptions, dyspnea, nausea, tachycardia, circulatory failure). If any of these reactions occur, discontinue the
  use of aprotinin immediately. Treatment with antihistamines, epinephrine, glucocorticoids, vasopressors, and
  fluids may be required. Resuscitation equipment should
  be readily available. Use cautiously in patients with a
  prior history of allergic reactions to drugs or other
  agents, as they may be at increased risk for allergic reactions to aprotinin. The risk of hypersensitivity reactions,
  including anaphylaxis, is greatly increased in patients
  who have been previously exposed to aprotinin. If there
  is a history of prior exposure, an antihistamine should be
  administered shortly before the loading dose. If an allergic reaction occurs following the test dose, do not administer further aprotinin. Even with a negative response
  to the test dose, anaphylaxis may occur with the full
  therapeutic dose.

• Aprotinin may decrease the effectiveness of fibrinolytic
  agents.

• Safe use of aprotinin in pregnancy, lactation, or children has not been established (Pregnancy Category B).

Lab Test Considerations

• Laboratory assessment of concurrent heparin therapy is altered by aprotinin. Aprotinin prolongs the whole blood clotting time of heparinized blood. Standard loading doses of heparin should be used, with subsequent doses determined by either using a fixed-dose regimen based on the patient's weight and duration of cardiopulmonary bypass, giving a loading dose of heparin prior to cannulation followed by a second dose 90 minutes after cardiopulmonary bypass, or determining the heparin dose by a method not affected by aprotinin, such as protamine titration. • May cause elevated serum creatinine, glucose, serum transaminases, and creatine kinase levels. • Usually causes elevations in partial thromboplastin time (PTT) and activated clotting time (ACT).

Patient/Family Teaching

• Instruct the patient on the importance of notifying the physician if the patient has previously received aprotinin.

≋ PHARMACOLOGIC PROFILE

Indications

• Aprotinin is used to reduce the incidence of bleeding in patients undergoing repeat coronary artery bypass graft (CABG) surgery and in high-risk patients (impaired hemostasis, presence of aspirin, or other coagulopathy) undergoing such surgery for the first time, or in patients in whom transfusion is unavailable or unacceptable. Aprotinin decreases bleeding and the need for transfusions.

Action

• Aprotinin acts as a protease inhibitor and has the following effects on coagulation: inhibition of plasmin and kallikrein, inhibition of contact phase activation of coagulation, and maintenance of the integrity of the platelet membrane. Its overall effect is inhibition of fibrinolysis and decreased turnover of coagulation factors with a decrease in bleeding.

Time/Action Profile (effects on bleeding)

Onset	Peak	Duration
rapid	UK	UK

Pharmacokinetics
   • **Distribution:** Aprotinin rapidly distributes into the to-tal extracellular space. • **Metabolism and Excretion:** Small amounts of aprotinin (9%) are excreted unchanged by the kidneys. Most aprotinin is slowly degraded by lysosomal enzymes. • **Half-life:** 150 minutes (postdistribution); 10 hours (terminal elimination).

Contraindications
   • Aprotinin is contraindicated in patients with known hypersensitivity.

Adverse Reactions and Side Effects*
   • **GU:** renal tubular necrosis • **Local:** phlebitis • **Misc:** hypersensitivity reactions, including ANAPHYLAXIS.

Ascorbic Acid	Vitamin (water soluble)
Cee-500, Cetane 500, Cevalin	pH 5.5–7

≋ ADMINISTRATION CONSIDERATIONS

Usual Dose
ADULTS: 100–250 mg 1–3 times daily.
CHILDREN: 100–300 mg/day in divided doses.

Dilution
   • **Direct IV:** Ascorbic acid may be administered IV undiluted. • **Intermittent Infusion:** Dilute with D5W, D10W, 0.9% NaCl, 0.45% NaCl, lactated Ringer's or Ringer's solution, dextrose and saline, or dextrose and Ringer's combinations. At room temperature, pressure in ampules may increase; wrap with protective cover before breaking.

---

   *Underlines indicate most frequent; CAPITALS indicate life-threatening.

Compatibility
- **Syringe:** metoclopramide.
- **Additive:** amikacin • calcium chloride • calcium gluceptate • calcium gluconate • cephalothin • chloramphenicol • cyanocobalamin • diphenhydramine • heparin • kanamycin • methicillin • methyldopa • penicillin G potassium • prednisolone.

Incompatibility
- **Syringe:** cefazolin • doxapram.
- **Additive:** bleomycin • cephapirin • nafcillin • sodium bicarbonate.

Rate of Administration
- **Direct IV:** Administer at a rate of 100 mg over at least 1 minute. Rapid IV administration may result in temporary dizziness and fainting.

≋ CLINICAL PRECAUTIONS

- Assess patient for signs of vitamin C deficiency (faulty bone and tooth development, gingivitis, bleeding gums, and loosened teeth) prior to and throughout therapy. Vitamin C deficiency is also called scurvy.
- Use cautiously in patients with recurrent kidney stones. Vitamin C produces acidic urine, which may aggravate stone formation. Patients receiving doses over 1 g/day who have underlying renal disease are at increased risk for stone formation. If urinary acidification occurs, excretion of mexiletine, amphetamines, or tricyclic antidepressants may be increased.
- Large doses may decrease the response to oral anticoagulants.
- Requirements for ascorbic acid are increased by smoking, salicylates, and primidone.
- Ascorbic acid increases iron toxicity when given concurrently with deferoxamine.
- Vitamin C crosses the placenta and enters breast milk and has been used safely during pregnancy and lactation (Pregnancy Category C).

Lab Test Considerations

- Megadoses of ascorbic acid (>10 times the RDA requirement) may cause false-negative results for occult blood in the stool, false-positive urine glucose test results with the copper sulfate method (Clinitest), and false-negative urine glucose test results with the glucose enzymatic tests (Tes-Tape). • May cause decreased serum bilirubin and increased urine oxalate, urate, and cysteine levels.

Patient/Family Teaching

• Encourage patient to comply with physician's diet recommendations. Explain that the best source of vitamins is a well-balanced diet with foods from the basic food groups. • Foods high in ascorbic acid include citrus fruits, tomatoes, strawberries, cantaloupe, and raw peppers. Gradual loss of ascorbic acid occurs when fresh food is stored, but not when frozen. Rapid loss is caused by drying, salting, and cooking.

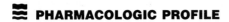 **PHARMACOLOGIC PROFILE**

Indications

• Ascorbic acid is used in the treatment and prevention of vitamin C deficiency (scurvy) in conjunction with dietary supplementation. • It is also used as supplemental therapy in some GI diseases and during long-term parenteral nutrition or chronic hemodialysis. • Supplemental ascorbic acid is also used in states of increased requirements, such as pregnancy, lactation, stress, hyperthyroidism, trauma, burns, or infancy.

Action

• Ascorbic acid is necessary for collagen formation and tissue repair. • It is involved in oxidation–reduction reactions; tyrosine, folic acid, iron, and carbohydrate metabolism; lipid and protein synthesis; cellular respiration; and resisting infection.

Time/Action Profile (response to skeletal and hemorrhagic changes in scurvy)

Onset	Peak	Duration
2 days–3 wk	UK	UK

Pharmacokinetics

• **Distribution:** Ascorbic acid is widely distributed, crosses the placenta, and enters breast milk. • **Metabolism and Excretion:** Ascorbic acid is oxidized to inactive compounds that are excreted by the kidneys. When serum levels are high, unchanged ascorbic acid is excreted by the kidneys. • **Half-life:** UK.

Contraindications

• Chronic use of large doses should be avoided during pregnancy.

Adverse Reactions and Side Effects*

• **CNS:** fatigue, headache, insomnia, drowsiness, dizziness, faintness • **GI:** nausea, vomiting, heartburn, cramps, diarrhea • **GU:** kidney stones • **Derm:** flushing • **Hemat:** deep vein thrombosis, sickle cell crisis, hemolysis (in G6-PD deficiency).

Asparaginase	Antineoplastic agent (enzyme)
Elspar, {Kidrolase}	pH 7.4

ADMINISTRATION CONSIDERATIONS

Usual Dose

Various other regimens may be used. Dose and regimen must be individualized. IU = international units.

As a Component of *Multiple-Agent* Induction Regimens in Children with Acute Lymphocytic Leukemia (in Combination with Vincristine and Prednisone)

CHILDREN: 1000 IU/kg/day for 10 successive days beginning on day 22 of regimen (in combination with prednisone and vincristine).

---

*Underlines indicate most frequent; CAPITALS indicate life-threatening.

{} = Available in Canada only.

Single-Agent Therapy for Acute Lymphocytic Leukemia

ADULTS: 200 IU/kg daily for 28 days.

Desensitization Regimen

ADULTS AND CHILDREN: Administer 1 IU, then double dose every 10 min until total dose for that day has been given or reaction occurs.

Dilution

• Solutions should be prepared in a biologic cabinet. Wear gloves, gown, and mask while handling medication. Discard equipment in specially designated containers (see Appendix F). • **Test Dose:** Intradermal test dose must be performed prior to initial dose and doses separated by more than 1 week. • **Reconstitute** vial with 5 ml of sterile water or 0.9% NaCl for injection (without preservatives). Add 0.1 ml of this 2000-IU/ml solution to 9.9 ml of additional diluent to yield a 20-IU/ml solution. Inject 0.1 ml (2 IU) intradermally. Observe site for 1 hour for formation of wheal. Wheal is indicative of a positive reaction; physician may order desensitization therapy. • **Direct IV:** Prepare IV dose by **diluting** 10,000-IU vial with 5 ml of sterile water or 0.9% NaCl (without preservatives) for *Elspar* or with 4 ml of sterile water for *Kidrolase*. If gelatinous fibers are present, administration through a 5-micron filter will not alter potency. Administration through a 0.2-micron filter may cause loss of potency. Solution should be clear after reconstitution. Discard if cloudy. Stable for 8 hours if refrigerated.

Incompatibility

• Information unavailable. Do not mix with other drugs.

Rate of Administration

• Administer through Y-site of rapidly flowing IV of D5W or 0.9% NaCl over at least 30 minutes. Maintain IV infusion for 2 hours after dose.

≋ CLINICAL PRECAUTIONS

• Monitor for hypersensitivity reaction (urticaria, diaphoresis, facial swelling, joint pain, hypotension, bronchospasm). Epinephrine and resuscitation equipment should be readily available. Reaction may occur up to

2 hours after administration. Use cautiously in patients with previous hypersensitivity reactions to other drugs or agents. An intradermal test dose of 2 IU may be used to determine reactions. If reaction is positive or previous reactions have occurred, desensitization may be undertaken.

- Monitor vital signs prior to and frequently during therapy. Inform physician if fever or chills occur.
- Monitor intake and output. Notify physician if significant discrepancies occur. Encourage patient to drink 2000–3000 ml/day to promote excretion of uric acid. Allopurinol and alkalinization of the urine may be ordered to help prevent urate stone formation.
- Assess nausea, vomiting, and appetite. Weigh patient weekly. Confer with physician regarding an antiemetic prior to administration.
- Monitor blood sugar. Hyperglycemia is more likely to occur in patients receiving glucocorticoids.
- Monitor affect and neurological status. Notify physician if depression, drowsiness, or hallucinations occur. Symptoms usually resolve 2–3 days after drug is discontinued. Use with care in patients with severe liver disease, renal disease, pancreatic disease, or CNS depression. These patients may be more prone to adverse CNS and hepatotoxic effects. Neurotoxicity may be additive with vincristine.
- Risk of hepatotoxicity is increased by concurrent use of hepatotoxic agents.
- Concurrent IV use with or immediately preceding vincristine and prednisone may result in increased toxicity.
- Clotting abnormalities may be exaggerated in patients receiving asparaginase. If coagulopathy develops, apply pressure to venipuncture sites; avoid intramuscular injections.
- Patients with chronic debilitating illnesses may not tolerate usual doses. Dosage reduction may be necessary.
- Asparaginase may negate the antineoplastic activity of methotrexate.
- Do not confuse asparaginase with pegaspargase (Oncaspar). Their doses and toxicities are different (see *pegaspargase* monograph on page 755).
- Use asparaginase cautiously in patients with childbearing potential. Safe use in pregnancy has not been estab-

lished; use only if required (Category C). Avoid using during lactation.

Lab Test Considerations

• Monitor CBC prior to and periodically throughout therapy. May alter coagulation studies. Platelets, PT, PTT, and thrombin time may be increased. • May cause elevated BUN. • Hepatotoxicity may be manifested by increased AST (SGOT), ALT (SGPT), alkaline phosphatase, bilirubin, or cholesterol. Liver function tests usually return to normal after therapy. May cause pancreatitis; monitor for elevated amylase or glucose. • May cause decreased serum calcium. • May cause elevated serum and urine uric acid. • May interfere with thyroid function tests.

Patient/Family Teaching

• Instruct patient to notify physician if abdominal pain, severe nausea and vomiting, jaundice, fever, chills, sore throat, bleeding or bruising, excess thirst or urination, or mouth sores occur. Caution patient to avoid crowds and persons with known infections. Instruct patient to use a soft toothbrush and electric razor, and to be especially careful to avoid falls. Patients should also be cautioned not to drink alcoholic beverages or take medication containing aspirin, ibuprofen, or naproxen because these may precipitate gastric bleeding. • Due to teratogenic effects of asparaginase, advise patient of the need for contraception. • Instruct patient not to receive any vaccinations without advice of physician. Advise parents that this may alter child's immunization schedule. • Emphasize need for periodic lab test to monitor for side effects.

☰ PHARMACOLOGIC PROFILE

Indications

• Asparaginase is part of single or combination chemotherapy in the treatment of acute lymphocytic leukemia (ALL) unresponsive to first-line agents.

Action

• Asparaginase acts as a catalyst in the conversion of asparagine (an amino acid) to aspartic acid and ammonia. This results in depletion of asparagine in leukemic cells and their subsequent death.

Time/Action Profile (depletion of asparagine)

Onset	Peak	Duration
within 14–24 hr	UK	23–33 days

Pharmacokinetics

• **Distribution:** Asparaginase remains mostly in the intravascular space. Penetration into the CSF is poor. • **Metabolism and Excretion:** Asparaginase is slowly sequestered in the reticuloendothelial system. • **Half-life:** 8–30 hours.

Contraindications

• Previous hypersensitivity to asparaginase.

Adverse Reactions and Side Effects*

• **CNS:** depression, somnolence, fatigue, SEIZURES, coma, headache, confusion, irritability, agitation, dizziness, hallucinations • **GI:** nausea, vomiting, anorexia, cramps, weight loss, pancreatitis, hepatotoxicity • **Derm:** rashes, urticaria • **Endo:** hyperglycemia • **Hemat:** coagulation abnormalities, transient bone marrow depression • **Metab:** hyperuricemia, hyperammonemia • **Misc:** hypersensitivity reactions including ANAPHYLAXIS.

Atenolol *Beta-adrenergic blocker (selective)*

Tenormin pH 5.5–6.5

≋ ADMINISTRATION CONSIDERATIONS

Usual Dose

ADULTS: 5 mg over 5 min initially, wait 10 min, then give another 5 mg.

Dilution

• May be **diluted** in D5W, 0.9% NaCl, or D5/0.9% NaCl.
• Stable for 48 hours.

---

*Underlines indicate most frequent; CAPITALS indicate life-threatening.

Compatibility
- **Y-site:** meperidine • morphine.

Rate of Administration
- **Direct IV:** Administer 5 mg over 5 minutes, followed by another 5 mg 10 minutes later. • If patient tolerates 10-mg IV dose, administer 50 mg PO 10 minutes after last IV dose and give another 50-mg PO dose 12 hours later.

≋ CLINICAL PRECAUTIONS

- Monitor heart rate, blood pressure, and ECG during therapy. If heart rate is less than 50 bpm, hold medication and notify physician. Excessive slowing of the heart rate and hypotension may occur. Atenolol may exacerbate congestive heart failure or precipitate pulmonary edema. Monitor intake and output ratios, and weigh patient daily. Assess patient routinely for signs and symptoms of fluid overload (peripheral edema, dyspnea, rales/crackles, weight gain, jugular venous distention). General anesthesia, IV phenytoin, and verapamil may cause additive myocardial depression. Additive bradycardia may occur with concurrent use of cardiac glycosides. Additive hypotension may occur with antihypertensive agents or nitrates.
- Use with epinephrine may result in unopposed alpha-adrenergic stimulation and hypertension.
- Concurrent thyroid administration may decrease clinical effectiveness.
- Use cautiously in patients with renal impairment or elderly patients. Decrease maintenance dose or increase dosing interval if creatinine clearance is 35 ml/min or less.
- Geriatric patients may exhibit altered (increased or decreased) sensitivity to beta-adrenergic blockers. Dosage adjustment may be necessary.
- Use with caution during pregnancy. Atenolol crosses the placenta and may cause apnea, bradycardia, or hypoglycemia in the newborn (Pregnancy Category C).

Lab Test Considerations
- May cause elevated serum uric acid, BUN, lipoproteins, and triglyceride concentrations.

Patient/Family Teaching

• Advise patients to make position changes slowly to minimize orthostatic hypotension.

PHARMACOLOGIC PROFILE

Indications
• Prevention of myocardial reinfarction.

Action
• Atenolol blocks stimulation of beta$_1$ (myocardial) adrenergic receptors. In therapeutic doses, it does not usually affect beta$_2$ (pulmonary, vascular, or uterine) receptor sites.

Time/Action Profile (cardiovascular effects)

Onset	Peak	Duration
rapid	within 5 min	12 hr

Pharmacokinetics
• **Distribution:** Atenolol does not significantly cross the blood–brain barrier. However, it does cross the placenta and enter breast milk. • **Metabolism and Excretion:** 40–50% of atenolol is excreted unchanged by the kidneys. • **Half-life:** 6–7 hours (increases in renal impairment to 16–27 hours; if impairment is severe, half-life may be up to 144 hours).

Contraindications
• Beta blockers should be avoided in uncompensated congestive heart failure or patients experiencing pulmonary edema, cardiogenic shock, bradycardia, or heart block. Because atenolol enters breast milk, its use should be avoided in patients who are breast-feeding.

Adverse Reactions and Side Effects*
• **CNS:** fatigue, weakness, dizziness, depression, memory loss, mental changes, nightmares, drowsiness • **EENT:** dry eyes, blurred vision • **Resp:** bronchospasm, wheezing • **CV:** BRADYCARDIA, CONGESTIVE HEART FAILURE, PULMONARY EDEMA, peripheral vasoconstriction, hypotension • **Endo:** hyperglycemia • **GI:** impotence, diminished libido.

---

*Underlines indicate most frequent; CAPITALS indicate life-threatening.

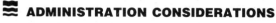

Atracurium Besylate	*Neuromuscular blocking agent (nondepolarizing)*
Tracrium	pH 3.25–3.65

≋ ADMINISTRATION CONSIDERATIONS

Usual Dose

ADULTS AND CHILDREN >**2 yr:** 400–500 mcg (0.4–0.5 mg)/kg initially; *if following steady-state anesthesia with isoflurane or enflurane,* 250–350 mcg (0.25–0.35 mg)/kg; *if following succinylcholine or in patients for whom histamine release is dangerous,* 300–400 mcg (0.3–0.4 mg)/kg. This may be followed by 80–100 mcg (0.08–0.1 mg)/kg as needed or 5–9 mcg/kg/min by continuous infusion (range 2–15 mcg/kg/min). Maintenance doses should be decreased by 1/3 in patients undergoing isoflurane or enflurane anesthesia and by 50% in patients undergoing hypothermic cardiopulmonary bypass.

CHILDREN 1 mo–**2 yr:** 300–400 mcg (0.3–0.4 mg)/kg initially (while under halothane anesthesia). Maintenance doses may be required more frequently than in adults. Continuous infusion is not recommended in children.

Dilution

• **Direct IV:** Initial dose may be given undiluted as a bolus. • **Intermittent Infusion:** Maintenance dose is usually required 20–45 minutes following initial dose and must be **further diluted** in D5W, 0.9% NaCl, or D5/0.9% NaCl. • Store in refrigerator.

Compatibility

• **Syringe:** alfentanil ◆ fentanyl ◆ midazolam ◆ sufentanil. • **Y-site:** aminophylline ◆ cefazolin ◆ cefuroxime ◆ cimetidine ◆ dobutamine ◆ dopamine ◆ epinephrine ◆ esmolol ◆ fentanyl ◆ gentamicin ◆ heparin ◆ hydrocortisone sodium succinate ◆ isoproterenol ◆ lorazepam ◆ midazolam ◆ morphine ◆ nitroglycerin ◆ ranitidine ◆ sodium nitroprusside ◆ trimethoprim/sulfamethoxazole ◆ vancomycin.

Incompatibility

- **Syringe:** Incompatible with most barbiturates and sodium bicarbonate; do not administer in the same syringe or through the same needle during infusion.
- **Y-site:** diazepam.

Rate of Administration

- **Direct IV:** Administer initial IV dose as a bolus over 1 minute. • **Intermittent/Continuous Infusion:** Maintenance dose is administered every 15–25 minutes or by continuous infusion. Titrate according to patient response.

≋ CLINICAL PRECAUTIONS

- Assess respiratory status continuously throughout atracurium therapy. Atracurium should be used only by individuals experienced in endotracheal intubation, and equipment for this procedure should be readily available.
- Neuromuscular response to atracurium should be monitored with a peripheral nerve stimulator. Paralysis is initially selective and usually occurs sequentially in the following muscles: levator muscles of eyelids, muscles of mastication, limb muscles, abdominal muscles, muscles of the glottis, intercostal muscles, and the diaphragm. Recovery of muscle function usually occurs in reverse order. Observe the patient for residual muscle weakness and respiratory distress during the recovery period.
- Atracurium has *no* effect on consciousness or the pain threshold. Adequate anesthesia should *always* be used when atracurium is used as an adjunct to surgical procedures.
- Use cautiously in patients with a history of pulmonary disease, renal or liver impairment, or in elderly or debilitated patients; these patients may be very sensitive to drug effects. Smaller doses may be used. Patients who are sensitive to the effects of histamine, including those with a history of cardiovascular disease, should receive lower doses.
- Patients with electrolyte disturbances or who are receiving cardiac glycosides may experience more arrhythmias.

- Using atracurium in patients with myasthenia gravis or myasthenic syndromes should be undertaken with extreme caution, because prolonged respiratory paralysis may occur. The intensity and duration of paralysis may also be prolonged by pretreatment with succinylcholine, general anesthesia, aminoglycoside antibiotics, polymyxin, colistin, clindamycin, lidocaine, quinidine, procainamide, beta-adrenergic blocking agents, potassium-losing diuretics, and magnesium.
- Atracurium crosses the placenta but has been used safely in pregnant women undergoing cesarean section (Pregnancy Category C).

Toxicity and Overdose Alert

- If overdose occurs, use peripheral nerve stimulator to determine the degree of neuromuscular blockade. Maintain airway patency and ventilation until recovery of normal respiration occurs. • Administration of anticholinesterase agents (edrophonium, neostigmine, pyridostigmine) may be used to antagonize the action of atracurium. Atropine is usually administered prior to or concurrently with anticholinesterase agents to counteract the muscarinic effects. • Administration of fluids and vasopressors may be necessary to treat severe hypotension or shock.

Patient/Family Teaching

- Explain all procedures to patient receiving atracurium therapy without anesthesia, as consciousness is not affected by atracurium alone. • Reassure patient that communication abilities will return as the medication wears off.

≋ PHARMACOLOGIC PROFILE

Indications

- Atracurium is used to produce skeletal paralysis, after induction of anesthesia.

Action

- Atracurium prevents neuromuscular transmission by blocking the effect of acetylcholine at the myoneural junction. It has no anxiolytic or analgesic properties.

Time/Action Profile (neuromuscular blockade)

Onset	Peak	Duration
2–2.5 min	5 min	30–40 min

Pharmacokinetics

• **Distribution:** Atracurium distributes into the extracellular space. It also crosses the placenta. • **Metabolism and Excretion:** Metabolism of atracurium occurs in plasma. • **Half-life:** 20 minutes.

Contraindications

• Hypersensitivity to atracurium or benzyl alcohol.

Adverse Reactions and Side Effects*

• **CV:** bradycardia, hypotension • **Resp:** wheezing, increased bronchial secretions • **Derm:** skin flush, erythema, pruritus, urticaria • **Misc:** allergic reactions, including ANAPHYLAXIS.

Atropine Sulfate	Anticholinergic
	pH 3–6.5

≋ ADMINISTRATION CONSIDERATIONS

Usual Dose

Bradycardia

ADULTS: 0.4–1.0 mg; may repeat as needed q 3–5 min until desired heart rate is achieved. The total dose should not exceed 3 mg or 0.04 mg/kg (total vagolytic dose). Once the heart rate is lowered, the dose may be repeated less frequently, as needed.

CHILDREN: 10–30 mcg/kg (0.01–0.03 mg/kg) (maximum dose 0.5 mg in pediatric patients or 1 mg in adolescents); may repeat q 5 min (total dose not to exceed 1 mg in pediatric patients or 2 mg in adolescents).

---

*Underlines indicate most frequent; CAPITALS indicate life-threatening.

Reversal of Adverse Muscarinic Effects of Anticholinesterases

ADULTS: 0.6–1.2 mg for each 0.5–2.5 mg of neostigmine methylsulfate or 10–20 mg of pyridostigmine bromide concurrently with anticholinesterase.

Organophosphate Poisoning Antidote

ADULTS: 1–2 mg initially, then 2 mg q 5–60 min as needed. In severe cases, 2–6 mg may be used initially and repeated every 5–60 min as needed.

CHILDREN: 0.01 mg/kg test dose, then 50 mcg/kg (0.05 mg/kg) q 10–30 min as needed.

Dilution

• **Direct IV:** Give IV **undiluted** or **dilute** in 10 ml of sterile water.

Compatibility

• **Syringe:** benzquinamide • butorphanol • chlorpromazine • cimetidine • dimenhydrinate • diphenhydramine • droperidol • fentanyl • glycopyrrolate • heparin • hydromorphone • hydroxyzine • meperidine • metoclopramide • midazolam • milrinone • morphine • nalbuphine • pentazocine • perphenazine • prochlorperazine • promazine • promethazine • propiomazine • ranitidine • scopolamine.

• **Y-site:** amrinone • famotidine • heparin • hydrocortisone sodium succinate • nafcillin • potassium chloride • vitamin B complex with C.

Incompatibility

• **Additive:** metaraminol • methohexital • norepinephrine • sodium bicarbonate.

Rate of Administration

• Administer at a rate of 0.6 mg over 1 minute. Inject through Y-tubing or 3-way stopcock. When given IV in doses less than 0.5 mg or over more than 1 minute, atropine may cause paradoxical bradycardia, which usually resolves in approximately 2 minutes.

≋ CLINICAL PRECAUTIONS

• Assess vital signs and ECG tracings frequently during the course of IV drug therapy. Note any significant changes in heart rate or blood pressure, or increased ventricular ectopy or angina.

- Use cautiously in patients with intra-abdominal infections (may cause ileus); prostatic hypertrophy (may produce urinary retention); or chronic renal, hepatic, pulmonary, or cardiac disease (increased risk of adverse reactions).
- Geriatric patients may exhibit increased sensitivity to atropine. Dosage adjustment may be required.
- Atropine readily crosses the blood–brain barrier, which accounts for common CNS side effects. Monitor for drowsiness and confusion. Elderly patients and the very young display increased susceptibility to CNS adverse reactions. Atropine also crosses the placenta and enters breast milk. Safe use in pregacy has not been established (Pregnancy Category C).

Toxicity and Overdose Alert

- If overdose occurs, physostigmine is the antidote.

Patient/Family Teaching

- Instruct patient that oral rinses, sugarless gum or candy, and frequent oral hygiene may help relieve dry mouth. • Inform men with benign prostatic hypertrophy that atropine may cause urinary hesitancy and retention. Changes in urinary stream should be reported to the physician.

PHARMACOLOGIC PROFILE

Indications

- Atropine is used in the acute management of sinus bradycardia. • It reverses adverse muscarinic effects of anticholinesterase agents (neostigmine, physostigmine, or pyridostigmine). • It is also used in the treatment of anticholinesterase (organophosphate pesticide) poisoning.

Action

- Atropine inhibits the action of acetylcholine at postganglionic sites located in smooth muscle, secretory glands, and the CNS (antimuscarinic activity). • Low doses of atropine decrease sweating, salivation, and respiratory secretions, whereas intermediate doses result in mydriasis (pupillary dilation), cycloplegia (loss of visual accommodation), and increased heart rate. • GI and GU tract motility are decreased at larger doses.

Time/Action Profile (inhibition of salivation)

Onset	Peak	Duration
immediate	2–4 min	4–6 hr

Pharmacokinetics

• **Distribution:** Atropine is widely distributed, crossing the blood–brain barrier and placenta and entering breast milk. • **Metabolism and Excretion:** Metabolism of atropine occurs mostly in the liver, with 30–50% excreted unchanged by the kidneys. • **Half-life:** 13–38 hours.

Contraindications

• Hypersensitivity to atropine. Do not use in patients with narrow-angle glaucoma, acute hemorrhage, or tachycardia secondary to cardiac insufficiency or thyrotoxicosis.

Adverse Reactions and Side Effects*

• **CNS:** <u>drowsiness</u>, confusion • **EENT:** dry eyes, <u>blurred vision</u>, mydriasis, cycloplegia • **CV:** palpitations, <u>tachycardia</u> • **GI:** <u>dry mouth</u>, constipation • **GU:** <u>urinary hesitancy</u>, retention • **Misc:** decreased sweating.

Azathioprine	*Immunosuppressant*
Imuran	**pH 9.6**

≋ ADMINISTRATION CONSIDERATIONS

Usual Dose

ADULTS AND CHILDREN: 3–5 mg/kg/day initially; maintenance dose 1–2 mg/kg/day.

Dilution

• **Direct IV: Reconstitute** each 100 mg with 10 ml of sterile water for injection. Swirl the vial gently until com-

---

*<u>Underlines</u> indicate most frequent; CAPITALS indicate life-threatening.

pletely dissolved. Reconstituted solutions may be administered for up to 24 hours after preparation. • **Intermittent Infusion:** Solution may be **further diluted** in 50 ml of 0.9% NaCl, 0.45% NaCl, D5/0.9% NaCl, or D5W.

Incompatibility

• **Additive:** Do not **admix** with other drugs.

Rate of Administration

• **Direct IV:** Administer over at least 5 minutes. • **Intermittent Infusion:** Infuse over 30–60 minutes. Has been infused up to 8 hours.

≋ CLINICAL PRECAUTIONS

- Use with caution in patients with active infections, decreased bone marrow reserve, or history of recent radiation therapy. Azathioprine lowers WBC count, increasing the risk of infection. Monitor blood counts and assess for infection (vital signs, sputum, urine, stool) throughout therapy. Myelosuppression caused by azathioprine is additive with other antineoplastics, myelosuppressive agents, and radiation therapy. Protect transplant patients from staff and visitors who may carry infection. Maintain protective isolation as indicated.
- Monitor intake and output and daily weight. Decreased urine output may lead to toxicity with this medication.
- Monitor patient's nutritional status. Azathioprine commonly causes GI adverse reactions.
- Allopurinol inhibits the metabolism of azathioprine, increasing toxicity. Decrease azathioprine dose by 25–33% in patients taking allopurinol concurrently.
- Patients with other chronic debilitating illnesses may not tolerate the usual doses of azathioprine. Dosage reduction may be necessary in these patients and in those with renal impairment.
- Azathioprine is not recommended during pregnancy or lactation. Use cautiously in patients with childbearing potential (Pregnancy Category D).

Lab Test Considerations

• Renal, hepatic, and hematologic functions should be monitored prior to beginning the course of therapy, weekly during the first 2 months, and monthly thereafter during the course of therapy. If leukocyte count is less than 3000/mm³ or if platelets are less than 100,000/mm³ a reduction in dosage may be necessary. • A decrease in hemoglobin may indicate bone marrow suppression. • Hepatotoxicity may be manifested by increased alkaline phosphatase, bilirubin, AST (SGOT), ALT (SGPT), and amylase. Doses greater than 2.5 mg/kg/day are associated with increased risk of hepatotoxicity, which is usually reversible if azathioprine is discontinued. • May decrease serum and urine uric acid and plasma albumin.

Patient/Family Teaching

• Advise patient to report the onset of infection, bleeding gums, bruising, signs and symptoms of hepatic dysfunction (abdominal pain, pruritus, clay-colored stools), or transplant rejection to the physician immediately. • Reinforce the need for lifelong therapy to prevent transplant rejection. • Instruct the patient to consult with physician or pharmacist before taking any over-the-counter medications or receiving any vaccinations while taking this medication. • Advise patient to avoid persons with known contagious illnesses and those who have recently taken oral poliovirus vaccine. • This drug may have teratogenic properties. Advise patient to use a nonhormonal method of contraception during therapy and for at least 4 months after therapy has been completed. • Emphasize the importance of follow-up examinations and lab tests.

≋ PHARMACOLOGIC PROFILE

Indications

• Azathioprine is used as an adjunct with glucocorticoids, local radiation, or other cytotoxic agents in the prevention of renal transplant rejection. It has also been used to prevent rejection following cardiac, hepatic, and pancreatic transplants (unlabeled use).

Action

• Azathioprine antagonizes purine metabolism, with subsequent inhibition of DNA and RNA synthesis. This results in suppression of cell-mediated immunity and altered antibody formation. The body converts azathioprine to mercaptopurine, which is the active form of the drug.

Time/Action Profile (immunosuppression)

Onset	Peak	Duration
days–weeks	UK	days–weeks

Pharmacokinetics

• **Distribution:** Azathioprine is rapidly cleared from the body and also crosses the placenta. Small amounts enter breast milk. • **Metabolism and Excretion:** Azathioprine is metabolized to mercaptopurine, which is then further metabolized. There is minimal excretion of unchanged drug. • **Half-life:** 3 hours.

Contraindications

• Hypersensitivity to azathioprine. • Azathioprine crosses the placenta and should not be used during pregnancy or lactation.

Adverse Reactions and Side Effects*

• **EENT:** retinopathy • **Resp:** pulmonary edema • **Misc:** fever, chills, serum • **GI:** nausea, vomiting, diarrhea, anorexia, mucositis, hepatotoxicity, pancreatitis • **Derm:** rash, alopecia • **Hemat:** leukopenia, anemia, pancytopenia, thrombocytopenia • **MS:** arthralgia • **Misc:** serum sickness, retinopathy, Raynaud's phenomenon, increased risk of neoplasia.

Aztreonam	*Anti-infective*
Azactam	**pH 4.5–7.5**

ADMINISTRATION CONSIDERATIONS

Usual Dose

ADULTS: 0.5–2.0 g q 6–12 hr (not to exceed 8 g/day).

---

*Underlines indicate most frequent; CAPITALS indicate life-threatening.

Dilution

• **Direct IV:** **Add** 6–10 ml of sterile water for injection to each 15-ml vial. • **Intermittent Infusion:** **Dilute** each 15-ml vial with at least 3 ml of sterile water for injection for each g of aztreonam. **Further dilute** with 50–100 ml of 0.9% NaCl, Ringer's or lactated Ringer's solution, D5W, D10W, D5/0.9% NaCl, D5/0.45% NaCl, D5/0.25% NaCl, sodium lactate, 5% or 10% mannitol. Shake vigorously. Final concentration should not exceed 20 mg/ml. Solutions range from colorless to light straw yellow or may develop a pink tint upon standing; this does not alter potency. • Solution is stable for 48 hours at room temperature or 7 days if refrigerated.

Compatibility

• **Y-site:** allopurinol sodium ◆ ciprofloxacin ◆ diltiazem ◆ enalaprilat ◆ filgrastim ◆ fluconazole ◆ fludarabine ◆ foscarnet ◆ insulin ◆ melphalan ◆ meperidine ◆ morphine ◆ ondansetron ◆ piperacillin/tazobactam ◆ ranitidine ◆ sargramostim ◆ vinorelbine ◆ zidovudine.

• **Additive:** ampicillin/sulbactam ◆ cefazolin ◆ ciprofloxacin ◆ clindamycin ◆ gentamicin ◆ tobramycin.

Incompatibility

• **Y-site:** vancomycin.
• **Additive:** cephradine ◆ metronidazole ◆ nafcillin.

Rate of Administration

• **Direct IV:** Administer slowly over 3–5 minutes by direct IV or into tubing of a compatible solution. • **Intermittent Infusion:** Infuse over 20–60 minutes.

☰ CLINICAL PRECAUTIONS

• Assess patient for infection (vital signs; wound appearance; sputum, urine, and stool; WBC) at beginning and throughout therapy.
• Obtain a history before initiating therapy to determine previous use of and reactions to penicillins or cephalosporins. Patients allergic to these drugs may exhibit hypersensitivity reactions to aztreonam.
• Obtain specimens for culture and sensitivity to aztreonam. First dose may be given before results are available.
• Observe IV site for phlebitis/irritation.

- Use cautiously in patients with renal impairment. Dosage reduction is recommended in patients with creatinine clearance of less than 30 ml/min. Patients with severe impairment of liver function receiving high-dose, long-term therapy may also require dosage reduction.
- Aztreonam may have a synergistic or antagonistic effect when combined with other anti-infectives. Observe for possible decreased response or re-emergence of infection.
- Aztreonam crosses the placenta (Pregnancy Category B). Although aztreonam enters breast milk in low concentrations, it is not absorbed from the GI tract. Safe use in children has not been established.

Lab Test Considerations

• May cause elevations in AST (SGOT), ALT (SGPT), alkaline phosphatase, LDH, and serum creatinine. • May cause increased prothrombin and partial thromboplastin times, eosinophilia, and positive Coombs' test.

Patient/Family Teaching

• Inform patient that IV infusion may cause a mild taste alteration. • Advise patient to report the signs and symptoms of superinfection (furry overgrowth on the tongue, vaginal itching or discharge, loose or foul-smelling stools) and allergy.

☰ PHARMACOLOGIC PROFILE

Indications

• Aztreonam is used in the treatment of serious Gram-negative infections including bone and joint infections, septicemia, skin and skin structure infections, intra-abdominal infections, gynecologic infections, respiratory tract infections, and urinary tract infections.

Action

• Aztreonam binds to the bacterial cell wall membrane, causing cell death. Anti-infective spectrum is significant only against Gram-negative aerobic organisms: *Escherichia coli, Serratia, Klebsiella, Enterobacter, Shigella, Providencia, Salmonella, Neisseria gonorrhoeae, Haemophilus influenzae,* and *Pseudomo-*

nas aeruginosa, including strains resistant to other drugs.
• Aztreonam is not active against *Staphylococcus aureus,* enterococci, or *Bacteroides fragilis.*

Time/Action Profile (blood levels)

Onset	Peak
rapid	end of infusion

Pharmacokinetics

• **Distribution:** Aztreonam is widely distributed, crosses the placenta, and enters breast milk in low concentrations.
• **Metabolism and Excretion:** 65–75% of aztreonam is excreted unchanged by the kidneys. Small amounts are metabolized by the liver. • **Half-life:** 1.5–2.5 hours (increased in renal impairment).

Contraindications

• Hypersensitivity to aztreonam, although possible cross-sensitivity with penicillins or cephalosporins may occur.

Adverse Reactions and Side Effects*

• **CNS:** SEIZURES • **GI:** diarrhea, nausea, vomiting • **Derm:** rashes • **Local:** phlebitis at IV site • **Misc:** superinfection, allergic reactions including ANAPHYLAXIS.

Benzquinamide Hydrochloride	*Antiemetic*
Emete-Con	pH 3–4

≋ ADMINISTRATION CONSIDERATIONS

Usual Dose

ADULTS: 25 mg (0.2–0.4 mg/kg).

Dilution

• **Direct IV: Reconstitute** with 2.2 ml of sterile or bacteriostatic water for injection. Results in 2 ml of solution with a

---

*Underlines indicate most frequent; CAPITALS indicate life-threatening.

concentration of 25 mg/ml. Do not use 0.9% NaCl for reconstitution, because solution may form a precipitate. • Reconstituted solution is stable at room temperature for 14 days if protected from light. Do not refrigerate.

Compatibility

- **Syringe:** atropine ◆ droperidol/fentanyl ◆ glycopyrrolate ◆ hydroxyzine ◆ ketamine ◆ meperidine ◆ midazolam ◆ morphine ◆ naloxone ◆ pentazocine ◆ propranolol ◆ scopolamine.
- **Y-site:** foscarnet.

Incompatibility

- **Syringe:** chlordiazepoxide ◆ diazepam ◆ pentobarbital ◆ phenobarbital ◆ secobarbital ◆ sodium chloride ◆ thiopental.
- **Y-site:** Do not administer through an IV line containing saline.

Rate of Administration

- **Direct IV:** Administer slowly, 1 ml (25 mg) over 30–60 seconds through Y-tubing or 3-way stopcock.

≋ CLINICAL PRECAUTIONS

- Assess nausea, vomiting, bowel sounds, and abdominal pain prior to and following administration. Benzquinamide may mask the signs of an acute abdomen.
- Monitor intake and output and nutritional status. Patients with severe nausea and vomiting may require IV fluids in addition to antiemetics.
- This drug may be administered prophylactically at least 15 minutes prior to emergence from anesthesia.
- Although the initial dose may be given intravenously, the IM route is preferred.
- CNS depression is more likely to occur with concurrent use of other CNS depressants including alcohol, antihistamines, opioid analgesics, and sedative/hypnotics.
- Monitor patient for arrhythmias and changes in blood pressure. Use cautiously in patients with a history of cardiovascular disease. Patients receiving vasopressors should receive benzquinamide in fractions of the usual dose.

• Safe use during lactation or in children less than 12 has not been established.

Patient/Family Teaching

• Advise patient to call for assistance when ambulating, because this drug may cause drowsiness. • Instruct patient to make position changes slowly to minimize orthostatic hypotension. • Inform patient that this drug may cause dry mouth. Frequent oral rinses, good oral hygiene, and sugarless gum or candy may minimize this effect. • Advise patient and family to use general measures to decrease nausea (begin with sips of liquids, small nongreasy meals; provide oral hygiene; remove noxious stimuli from the environment).

PHARMACOLOGIC PROFILE

Indications

• Benzquinamide is used in the prevention and treatment of nausea and vomiting associated with anesthesia and surgery.

Action

• Benzquinamide depresses the chemoreceptor trigger zone in the CNS.

Time/Action Profile (antiemetic effect)

Onset	Peak	Duration
15 min	UK	3–4 hr

Pharmacokinetics

• **Distribution:** Benzquinamide is widely distributed. • **Metabolism and Excretion:** Metabolism of benzquinamide occurs mainly in the liver. Minimal amounts are excreted unchanged by the kidneys. • **Half-life:** 30–40 minutes.

Contraindications

• Hypersensitivity to benzquinamide. • This agent is not recommended for use during pregnancy.

Adverse Reactions and Side Effects*

- **CNS:** <u>drowsiness</u>, insomnia, restlessness, tremor
- **EENT:** blurred vision, increased salivation, dry mouth
- **CV:** hypotension, hypertension, arrhythmias • **GI:** nausea, vomiting, cramps.

Benztropine Mesylate	Antiparkinson (anticholinergic)
Cogentin	pH 5–8

ADMINISTRATION CONSIDERATIONS

Usual Dose
ADULTS: 1–4 mg 1–2 times daily (not to exceed 6 mg/day).
GERIATRIC PATIENTS: 0.5 mg 1–2 times daily initially.

Dilution
- **Direct IV:** May be administered **undiluted**.

Compatibility
- **Syringe:** metoclopramide.
- **Y-site:** fluconazole • tacrolimus.

Rate of Administration
- **Direct IV:** Administer at a rate of 1 mg over 1 minute.

CLINICAL PRECAUTIONS

- Monitor pulse and blood pressure closely and maintain bed rest for 1 hour after administration.
- Parenteral doses of benztropine are only used in acute situations. IV route is rarely used because onset is same as with IM route.
- Assess parkinsonian and extrapyramidal symptoms (akinesia, rigidity, tremors, pill rolling, mask facies, shuffling gait, muscle spasms, twisting motions, drooling).

*<u>Underlines</u> indicate most frequent; CAPITALS indicate life-threatening.

- Use with caution in geriatric patients due to increased risk of confusion and hallucinations.
- Anticholinergic effects (dry eyes, dry mouth, blurred vision) will be additive with drugs sharing anticholinergic properties such as antihistamines, phenothiazines, quinidine, disopyramide, and tricyclic antidepressants.
- Benztropine counteracts the cholinergic effects of bethanecol.
- Safe use in pregnancy or lactation has not been established (Pregnancy Category C).

Patient/Family Teaching

• Advise patient to make position changes slowly to minimize orthostatic hypotension. • May cause drowsiness or dizziness. Caution patient to call for assistance with ambulation or transfer. • Instruct patient that frequent oral rinses, good oral hygiene, and sugarless candy or gum may minimize dry mouth. • Instruct patient to notify physician or nurse if difficulty with urination, constipation, or abdominal discomfort occurs.

PHARMACOLOGIC PROFILE

Indications

• Benztropine is used in the adjunctive treatment of acute drug-induced extrapyramidal effects and dystonic reactions.

Action

• Benztropine blocks cholinergic activity in the CNS that is partially responsible for the symptoms of Parkinson's disease and drug-induced extrapyramidal and dystonic reactions. • It restores the natural balance of neurotransmitters in the CNS.

Time/Action Profile (antidyskinetic effect)

Onset	Peak	Duration
within 15 min	UK	24 hr

Pharmacokinetics

• **Distribution:** UK. • **Metabolism and Excretion:** UK.
• **Half-life:** UK.

Contraindications
• Hypersensitivity to benztropine. • Benztropine is not to be used in children less than 3 years of age. • Patients with narrow-angle glaucoma should not receive benztropine.

Adverse Reactions and Side Effects*
• **CNS:** confusion, weakness, hallucinations, headache, sedation, depression, dizziness • **EENT:** <u>dry eyes</u>, <u>blurred vision</u>, mydriasis • **CV:** tachycardia, arrhythmias, palpitations • **GI:** <u>constipation</u>, <u>dry mouth</u>, nausea, ileus • **GU:** urinary retention, hesitancy • **Misc:** decreased sweating.

Betamethasone Sodium Phosphate	*Glucocorticoid anti-inflammatory*
Celestone Phosphate, Cel-U-Jec, Selestoject	pH 8.5

 ADMINISTRATION CONSIDERATIONS

Usual Dose
Adults: Up to 9 mg/day.

Dilution
• **Direct IV:** May be administered **undiluted**. • **Intermittent Infusion:** May be **diluted** in D5W, 0.9% NaCl, Ringer's solution, D5/Ringer's solution, or D5/LR.

Compatibility
• **Y-site:** heparin • hydrocortisone sodium succinate • potassium chloride • vitamin B complex with C.

Rate of Administration
• **Direct IV:** Administer over at least 1 minute.

---

*<u>Underlines</u> indicate most frequent; CAPITALS indicate life-threatening.

≋ CLINICAL PRECAUTIONS

- Potency of 0.6 mg betamethasone is equivalent to 20 mg of hydrocortisone. Note that the suspension dosage form (betamethasone sodium phosphate combined with betamethasone acetate) is for intramuscular use only.
- Monitor blood/urine glucose. Because glucocorticoids may produce hyperglycemia, diabetic patients may display an increased need for insulin or hypoglycemic agents.
- Monitor blood pressure. Hypertensive patients may require additional drug therapy during glucocorticoid treatment.
- Assess for signs of infection. Chronic treatment decreases host defense systems and increases the risk of infection.
- Assess skin during chronic therapy. Petechiae, increased fragility, acne, and other changes may occur. Patient's appearance may change dramatically during long-term therapy. Moon face, buffalo hump, and other cushingoid features may lead to altered body image.
- Monitor intake and output, and daily weight. Assess for fluid overload (edema, steady weight gain, rales/crackles, dyspnea).
- Assess mental status. A variety of changes may occur, ranging from excitement to depression.
- Hypokalemia produced by glucocorticoids is increased by concurrent diuretics, amphotericin B, mezlocillin, or ticarcillin. Hypokalemia may increase the risk of cardiac glycoside (digoxin) toxicity.
- Barbiturates, phenytoin, and rifampin increase metabolism of betamethasone and may decrease effectiveness.
- Chronic treatment (doses >0.6 mg/day for more than 2 weeks) causes adrenal suppression. Supplemental doses may be necessary during periods of stress, trauma, or surgery. Use lowest dose for shortest period of time.
- Patients with glaucoma may experience increased intraocular pressures.
- Geriatric patients are more likely to develop hypertension, osteoporosis, and mental status changes during chronic therapy.
- Chronic therapy in children should be undertaken with caution. Decreased growth may result; use of short- or intermediate-acting glucocorticoids is recommended.

- Glucocorticoids should not be abruptly discontinued during chronic use due to adrenal suppression.
- Betamethasone crosses the placenta in small amounts. Safe use in pregnancy has not been established.

Lab Test Considerations

• Monitor serum electrolytes and glucose. May cause hyperglycemia, especially in persons with diabetes. • May cause hypokalemia. • Guaiac test stools. Promptly report presence of guaiac-positive stools. • Periodic adrenal function tests may be ordered to assess degree of hypothalamic–pituitary–adrenal axis suppression during chronic therapy.

Patient/Family Teaching

• Advise patient to notify physician immediately if signs of adrenal suppression (anorexia, nausea, weakness, fatigue, hypotension, hypoglycemia) occur. • This drug causes immunosuppression and may mask symptoms of infection. Instruct patient to avoid persons with known contagious illnesses and to notify physician if infection occurs. • Caution patient to avoid vaccinations without first consulting with physician. • Instruct patient to notify physician if severe abdominal pain, tarry stools, unusual pain, swelling, weight gain, tiredness, bone pain, bruising, non-healing sores, visual disturbances, or behavioral changes occur. • Explain the need for continued medical follow-up to assess effectiveness and possible side effects of medication. Physician may order periodic lab tests and eye examinations. • Instruct patient to inform physician if symptoms of underlying disease return or worsen. • Advise patient to carry identification describing disease process and medication regimen in the event of emergency in which patient cannot relate medical history. • Encourage patients receiving long-term therapy to eat a diet high in protein, calcium, and potassium, and low in sodium and carbohydrates (see Appendix H). Alcohol should be avoided during therapy.

≋ PHARMACOLOGIC PROFILE

Indications

• Betamethasone sodium phosphate is used in a wide variety of chronic inflammatory, allergic, hematologic, neoplastic, and autoimmune diseases. This is a long-acting glucocorticoid and is therefore not suitable for alternate-day therapy.

Action

• Glucocorticoids suppress inflammation and normal immune response, while displaying numerous intense metabolic effects (see Adverse Reactions and Side Effects). Therapeutic results include suppression of inflammation and modification of normal immune response. Adrenal function is suppressed at chronic doses of 0.6 mg/day.

Time/Action Profile (anti-inflammatory effect)

Onset	Peak	Duration
rapid	UK	UK

Pharmacokinetics

• **Distribution:** Betamethasone crosses the placenta, and small amounts enter breast milk. The remainder of distribution is not known. • **Metabolism and Excretion:** Metabolism of betamethasone occurs primarily in the liver. • **Half-life:** 3–5 hours (plasma); 36–54 hours (tissue).

Contraindications

• Glucocorticoids should be avoided during acute untreated infections except for some forms of meningitis. • Because small amounts enter breast milk, patient should avoid chronic use during lactation. • Some products contain bisulfites (Celestone, Cel-U-Jec) and should be avoided in patients with hypersensitivity.

Adverse Reactions and Side Effects*

Adverse reactions and side effects occur mostly in patients on high-dose chronic therapy.

• **CNS:** headache, restlessness, psychoses, depression, euphoria, personality changes, increased intracranial pressure (children only) • **EENT:** increased intraocular pressure • **CV:** hypertension • **GI:** nausea, vomiting, anorexia, peptic ulceration, increased appetite • **Derm:** impaired wound healing, petechiae, ecchymoses, skin fragility, hirsutism, acne • **Endo:** adrenal suppression, hyperglycemia • **F and E:** hypokalemia,

---

*Underlines indicate most frequent; CAPITALS indicate life-threatening.

hypokalemic alkalosis, fluid retention • **Hemat:** thromboembolism, thrombophlebitis • **MS:** <u>muscle wasting</u>, muscle pain, aseptic necrosis of joints, <u>osteoporosis</u> • **Misc:** <u>increased susceptibility to infection</u>, <u>cushingoid appearance (moon face, buffalo hump)</u>.

Biperiden Lactate	*Antiparkinson (anticholinergic)*
Akineton	pH 4.8–5.8

≋ ADMINISTRATION CONSIDERATIONS

Usual Dose
ADULTS: 2 mg; may repeat q 30 min (not to exceed 8 mg in 24 hr).
GERIATRIC PATIENTS: 2 mg 1–2 times daily.

Dilution
• **Direct IV:** May be administered **undiluted**.

Incompatibility
• Information unavailable. Do not admix with other drugs or solutions.

Rate of Administration
• **Direct IV:** Administer each dose over at least 1 minute.

≋ CLINICAL PRECAUTIONS

• Monitor pulse and blood pressure closely and maintain bed rest for 1 hour after administration.
• IV use of biperiden is reserved only for acute situations.
• Assess parkinsonian and extrapyramidal symptoms (akinesia, rigidity, tremors, pill rolling, mask facies, shuffling gait, muscle spasms, twisting motions, drooling).
• Use with caution in elderly patients due to increased risk of CNS adverse reactions.
• Anticholinergic effects (dry eyes, dry mouth, blurred vision) will be additive with drugs sharing anticholiner-

gic properties, such as antihistamines, phenothiazines, quinidine, disopyramide, and tricyclic antidepressants.
- Biperiden counteracts the cholinergic effects of bethanechol.
- Use with caution in patients with a history of seizure disorders or cardiac arrhythmias, because of risk of CNS and cardiac adverse reactions. Geriatric patients are at increased risk for confusion and hallucinations.
- Safe use in pregnancy or lactation has not been established (Pregnancy Category C). The intravenous route is not recommended in children.

Patient/Family Teaching

- Advise patient to make position changes slowly to minimize orthostatic hypotension. • May cause drowsiness or dizziness. Caution patient to call for assistance with ambulation or transfer. • Instruct patient that frequent oral rinses, good oral hygiene, and sugarless candy or gum may minimize dry mouth. • Instruct patient to notify physician or nurse if difficulty with urination, constipation, or abdominal discomfort occurs.

PHARMACOLOGIC PROFILE

Indications

- Biperiden is used in the adjunctive treatment of acute drug-induced extrapyramidal effects and dystonic reactions.

Action

- Biperiden blocks cholinergic activity in the CNS, which is partially responsible for the symptoms of Parkinson's disease. • It restores the natural balance of neurotransmitters in the CNS.

Time/Action Profile (antidyskinetic effect)

Onset	Peak	Duration
UK	UK	UK

Pharmacokinetics

- **Distribution:** UK. • **Metabolism and Excretion:** UK. • **Half-life:** UK.

Contraindications

• Biperiden is contraindicated in patients with hypersensitivity to it. It should not be used in patients less than 3 years old, or patients with narrow-angle glaucoma, bowel obstruction, or megacolon.

Adverse Reactions and Side Effects*

• **CNS:** confusion, weakness, hallucinations, headache, sedation, depression, dizziness • **EENT:** <u>dry eyes</u>, <u>blurred vision</u>, mydriasis • **CV:** tachycardia, arrhythmias, palpitations • **GI:** <u>constipation</u>, <u>dry mouth</u>, nausea, ileus • **GU:** urinary retention, hesitancy • **Misc:** decreased sweating.

Bleomycin Sulfate	*Antineoplastic (antitumor antibiotic)*
Blenoxane	**pH 4.5–6** (depends on diluent)

≋ ADMINISTRATION CONSIDERATIONS

Usual Dose

Lymphoma patients should receive initial test doses of 1–2 units 2–4 hr prior to treatment.

ADULTS: 0.25–0.5 units/kg (10–20 units/m²) weekly or twice weekly initially. If favorable response occurs, lower maintenance doses are employed (1 unit/day or 5 units/wk). May also be given as a 24-hr infusion of 0.25 units/kg (15 units/m²) for 4–5 days.

Dilution

• **Direct IV:** Reconstitute IV and intra-arterial doses by diluting 15-unit vial with 5 ml of D5W or 0.9% NaCl. • **Intermittent Infusion:** May be **further diluted** in 50–100 ml of D5W or 0.9% NaCl. • Solutions should be prepared in a biologic cabinet. Wear gloves, gown, and mask while handling medication. Discard equipment in specially designated containers. • Reconstituted solution is stable for 24 hours at room

---

*<u>Underlines</u> indicate most frequent; CAPITALS indicate life-threatening.

temperature or 14 days if refrigerated but use within 24 hours is recommended due to lack of preservatives.

Compatibility

- **Syringe:** cisplatin ✦ cyclophosphamide ✦ doxorubicin ✦ droperidol ✦ fluorouracil ✦ furosemide ✦ heparin ✦ leucovorin calcium ✦ methotrexate ✦ metoclopramide ✦ mitomycin ✦ vinblastine ✦ vincristine.

- **Y-site:** allopurinol sodium ✦ cisplatin ✦ cyclophosphamide ✦ doxorubicin ✦ droperidol ✦ filgrastim ✦ fludarabine ✦ fluorouracil ✦ heparin ✦ leucovorin ✦ melphalan ✦ methotrexate ✦ metoclopramide ✦ mitomycin ✦ ondansetron ✦ paclitaxel ✦ piperacillin/tazobactam ✦ sargramostim ✦ vinblastine ✦ vincristine ✦ vinorelbine.

- **Additive:** amikacin ✦ cephapirin ✦ dexamethasone sodium phosphate ✦ diphenhydramine ✦ fluorouracil ✦ gentamicin ✦ heparin ✦ hydrocortisone sodium phosphate ✦ phenytoin ✦ streptomycin ✦ tobramycin ✦ vinblastine ✦ vincristine.

Incompatibility

- **Additive:** aminophylline ✦ ascorbic acid injection ✦ cefazolin ✦ cephalothin ✦ diazepam ✦ hydrocortisone sodium succinate ✦ methotrexate ✦ mitomycin ✦ nafcillin ✦ penicillin G sodium ✦ terbutaline.

Rate of Administration

- **Direct IV:** Administer slowly over 10 minutes.

≋ CLINICAL PRECAUTIONS

- Assess for anaphylactic reactions. Keep epinephrine, antihistamines, and resuscitative equipment nearby. These reactions are more common in patients with lymphoma. The use of small initial test doses in these patients may be helpful.
- Assess for fever and chills, which may occur within 2–4 hours of therapy. Antipyretics may diminish this reaction.
- Assess pulmonary status. Bleomycin produces dose-related pulmonary toxicity. Risk is greatly increased at cumulative doses greater than 225–400 units, in patients older than 70 years, with concurrent use of other

antineoplastic agents or thoracic radiation. Pulmonary function tests and carbon monoxide diffusion capacity may be monitored for early detection of pulmonary toxicity. Patients with renal, pulmonary, or hepatic impairment may experience pulmonary toxicity at lower total doses. Patients undergoing general anesthesia are also at increased risk of pulmonary toxicity.

- Assess for history of renal impairment. Dosage reduction is recommended if creatinine clearance is less than 25 ml/min.
- Hematologic toxicity is infrequent with bleomycin alone, but risk increases with concurrent antineoplastic therapy.
- Assess for changes in skin. A variety of lesions, including alopecia and hyperpigmentation, may be noted. Assure patient that these are not permanent changes. Skin toxicity is more common in patients receiving cumulative doses of more than 150 units. Mucocutaneous mouth lesions may be managed with supportive local measures, such as frequent rinsing and local anesthetics (viscous lidocaine).
- Presence of nonmalignant chronic debilitating illness increases the risk for adverse reactions.
- Cisplatin decreases renal elimination of bleomycin and increases the risk of toxicity.
- Assess for regression of tumor. Beneficial response occurs within 2–3 weeks.
- Safe use in pregnancy, lactation, or children has not been established. Use cautiously in patients with childbearing potential.

Lab Test Considerations

- Monitor CBC prior to and periodically throughout therapy. May cause mild thrombocytopenia and leukopenia (nadir 2 weeks). Monitor baseline and periodic renal and hepatic function.

Patient/Family Teaching

- Instruct patient to notify physician if fever, chills, wheezing, faintness, diaphoresis, shortness of breath, prolonged nausea and vomiting, or mouth sores occur. • Encourage patient not to smoke, because this may worsen pulmonary toxicity. • Explain to the patient that skin toxicity may manifest itself as skin sensitivity, hyperpigmentation (especially at skin folds and points of skin irritation), rashes, and thickening of the skin. • Instruct patient to inspect oral mucosa for erythema and ulceration. If ulceration occurs, advise patient to use sponge brush and rinse mouth with water after eating and drinking. Physician may order viscous lidocaine swishes if pain interferes with eating. • Discuss with patient the possibility of hair loss. Explore coping strategies. • Advise patient of the need for contraception. • Instruct patient not to receive any vaccinations without advice of physician. Bleomycin may decrease antibody response to vaccinations and increase the risk of adverse reactions. • Emphasize need for periodic lab tests to monitor for side effects.

PHARMACOLOGIC PROFILE

Indications

• Bleomycin is used alone or in combination with other antineoplastic agents in the treatment of lymphomas, squamous cell carcinoma, testicular embryonal cell carcinoma, choriocarcinoma, and teratocarcinoma.

Action

• Bleomycin inhibits DNA and RNA synthesis resulting in death of rapidly replicating cells, particularly malignant ones.

Time/Action Profile (tumor response)

Onset	Peak	Duration
2–3 wk	UK	UK

Pharmacokinetics

• **Distribution:** Widely distributed; concentrates mainly in skin, lungs, peritoneum, kidneys, and lymphatics. • **Metabolism and Excretion:** 60–70% excreted unchanged by the kidneys. • **Half-life:** 2 hours (increased with renal impairment).

Contraindications

• Hypersensitivity to bleomycin. • Pregnant or lactating patients should not receive bleomycin.

Adverse Reactions and Side Effects*

• **CNS:** weakness, disorientation, aggressive behavior
• **Resp:** pneumonitis, PULMONARY FIBROSIS • **CV:** hypotension, peripheral vasoconstriction • **GI:** nausea, vomiting, anorexia
• **Derm:** mucocutaneous toxicity, urticaria, erythema, hyper-pigmentation, alopecia, rashes, vesiculation • **Hemat:** thrombocytopenia, leukopenia, anemia • **Local:** pain at tumor site, phlebitis at IV site • **Metab:** weight loss • **Misc:** fever, chills, ANAPHYLACTOID REACTIONS.

Bretylium Tosylate	*Antiarrhythmic (group III)*
{Bretylate}, Bretylol	pH 4.5–7 (injection), 4 (premixed infusion)

ADMINISTRATION CONSIDERATIONS

Usual Dose

Ventricular Fibrillation

ADULTS: 5 mg/kg undiluted bolus over 15–30 sec initially; if no response, increase to 10 mg/kg; repeat as necessary q 15–30 min (not to exceed 30 mg/kg/24 hr). For maintenance: Dilute and infuse at 1–2 mg/min *or* dilute and infuse 5–10 mg/kg over more than 8 min q 6 hr.

CHILDREN: 5 mg/kg initially, then 10 mg/kg q 15–30 min up to 30 mg/kg total dose. May be followed by 5–10 mg/kg q 6 hr.

Other Ventricular Arrhythmias

ADULTS: Dilute and infuse 5–10 mg/kg over more than 8 min; may repeat in 1–2 hr if arrhythmia persists, and then q 6 hr or continuous infusion at 1–2 mg/min.

CHILDREN: 5–10 mg/kg q 6 hr.

Dilution

• **Direct IV:** Administer **undiluted**, for ventricular fibrillation. • **Intermittent Infusion:** For other arrhythmias, di-

---

*Underlines indicate most frequent; CAPITALS indicate life-threatening.

{} = Available in Canada only.

lute 500 mg in at least 50 ml of D5W, 0.9% NaCl, D5/0.45% NaCl, D5/0.9% NaCl, D5/LR, 1/6 M sodium lactate or lactated Ringer's solution. • **Continuous Infusion:** Bretylium can be diluted in any amount of solution (1 g in 1000 ml equals 1 mg/ml). Available in premixed solutions with 5% dextrose.

Compatibility

   • **Y-site:** amrinone ♦ diltiazem ♦ dobutamine ♦ famotidine ♦ isoproterenol ♦ ranitidine.
   • **Additive:** 5% sodium bicarbonate ♦ 20% mannitol ♦ aminophylline ♦ atracurium ♦ calcium chloride ♦ calcium gluconate ♦ digoxin ♦ dopamine ♦ esmolol ♦ insulin ♦ lidocaine ♦ potassium chloride ♦ quinidine ♦ verapamil.

Rate of Administration

   • **Direct IV:** For ventricular fibrillation, administer over 1 minute; arrhythmia usually resolves within minutes. Repeat in 15–30 minutes if arrhythmia persists. Do not exceed 30 mg/kg/24 hr. Employ usual resuscitative procedures, including CPR and electrical cardioversion, prior to and following injection. • **Intermittent Infusion:** Administer over more than 8 minutes. More rapid infusion in the alert patient may cause nausea and vomiting. May repeat after 1–2 hours if necessary. Ventricular tachycardia usually resolves within 20 minutes. • **Continuous Infusion:** Infuse at 1–2 mg of diluted solution/minute. Administer via infusion pump to ensure accurate dosage.

BRETYLIUM INFUSION RATES

A. FOR LIFE-THREATENING VENTRICULAR ARRHYTHMIAS

(V Fib or hemodynamically unstable V tach). Administer 5 mg/kg (0.1 ml/kg) of *undiluted* drug by rapid IV injection. *Undiluted* drug concentration = 50 mg/ml.

Rapid IV Injection of Undiluted Bretylium
(doses given in volume of undiluted bretylium injection) 50 mg/ml.

| | PATIENT WEIGHT | | | | | |
Dose	50 kg	60 kg	70 kg	80 kg	90 kg	100 kg
5 mg/kg	5 ml	6 ml	7 ml	8 ml	9 ml	10 ml

B. FOR OTHER VENTRICULAR ARRHYTHMIAS

Dilution: 2 g (40 ml) in 500 ml = 2 g/540 ml = 3.7 mg/ml
Administer as 5–10 mg/kg (1.35–2 ml/kg) IV over 10–30 min. May
be repeated q 6 hr or administered as a continuous infusion at
1–2 mg/min.

Intermittent Infusion
Volume of *diluted* bretylium to infuse over more than 8 minutes
Concentration = 3.7 mg/ml.

	PATIENT WEIGHT					
Dose	50 kg	60 kg	70 kg	80 kg	90 kg	100 kg
5 mg/kg	67.6 ml	81.1 ml	94.6 ml	108.1 ml	121.6 ml	135.1 ml
6 mg/kg	81.8 ml	97.3 ml	113.5 ml	129.7 ml	145.9 ml	162.2 ml
7 mg/kg	94.6 ml	113.5 ml	132.4 ml	151.4 ml	170.3 ml	189.2 ml
8 mg/kg	108.1 ml	129.7 ml	151.4 ml	173.0 ml	194.6 ml	216.2 ml
9 mg/kg	121.6 ml	145.9 ml	170.3 ml	194.6 ml	218.9 ml	243.2 ml
10 mg/kg	135.1 ml	162.2 ml	189.1 ml	216.2 ml	243.2 ml	270.3 ml

BRETYLIUM CONTINUOUS INFUSION RATES FOR MAINTENANCE THERAPY

DILUTION				RATE OF ADMINISTRATION	
Amount of bretylium injection (50 mg/ml)	Volume of dextrose or sodium chloride injection (ml)	Final volume (ml)	Final concentration (mg/ml)	Dose (mg/min)	ml/hr
500 mg (10 ml)	50	60	8.3	1	7
				1.5	11
				2	14
2 g (40 ml)	500	540	3.7	1	16
1 g (20 ml)	250	270	3.7	1.5	24
				2	32
1 g (20 ml)	500	520	1.9	1	32
500 mg (10 ml)	250	260	1.9	1.5	47
				2	63

≋ CLINICAL PRECAUTIONS

- Assess ECG frequently throughout administration. Fibrillation should respond within minutes. Ventricular tachycardia and PVCs respond within 20 minutes–6 hours. Initial dose may be followed in 1 hour by recurrence of arrhythmia and hypertension.

- Assess blood pressure frequently. Postural hypotension is common following an initial rise in blood pressure. Keep patient in supine position, and instruct patient to make position changes slowly.
- Nausea or vomiting may improve or be alleviated by slowing infusion rate.
- Combination use with other antiarrhythmics may result in additive or antagonistic properties.
- Assess for previous use of cardiac glycosides. If bretylium is used during suspected cardiac glycoside (digoxin, digitoxin) toxicity, arrhythmias may be aggravated.
- Assess cardiac output. Patients with fixed cardiac output may experience severe hypotension requiring supportive therapy.
- Assess renal function. Dosage reduction is required if creatinine clearance is less than 50 ml/min. Bretylium should be avoided in patients with creatinine clearance less than 10 ml/min.
- Dosage should be reduced gradually and discontinued over 3–5 days with close ECG monitoring. Maintenance with an oral antiarrhythmic may be initiated.
- Safety in pregnancy, lactation, and children is not established. Bretylium may decrease uterine blood flow (Pregnancy Category C).

Patient/Family Teaching

- Instruct patient to make position changes slowly to minimize the effects of drug-induced orthostatic hypotension.

≋ PHARMACOLOGIC PROFILE

Indications
- Bretylium is used in the treatment of ventricular tachycardia and prophylaxis against ventricular fibrillation. • It is also used in the treatment of other serious ventricular arrhythmias resistant to lidocaine.

Action
- Bretylium initially releases norepinephrine, then inhibits its release. • It suppresses ventricular tachycardia and fibrillation.

Time/Action Profile (suppression of arrhythmias)

	Onset	Peak	Duration
fibrillation	within minutes	end of infusion	6–24 hr
V Tach, PVCs	20 min–6 hr	end of infusion	6–24 hr

Pharmacokinetics

• **Distribution:** Bretylium reaches high concentrations in areas of adrenergic stimulation. • **Metabolism and Excretion:** All of bretylium is excreted unchanged by the kidneys. • **Half-life:** 5–10 hours (increased in renal impairment).

Contraindications

• No significant contraindications.

Adverse Reactions and Side Effects*

• **CNS:** syncope, faintness, vertigo, dizziness • **EENT:** nasal stuffiness • **CV:** postural hypotension, transient hypertension, bradycardia, angina • **GI:** nausea, vomiting (with rapid administration), diarrhea.

Bumetanide	Loop diuretic
Bumex	pH 6.8–7.8

≋ ADMINISTRATION CONSIDERATIONS

Usual Dose

ADULTS: 0.5–1.0 mg; may give 1–2 more doses q 2–3 hr (not to exceed 10 mg/24 hr).

Dilution

• **Direct IV:** May be administered **undiluted**. • May also be **diluted** in D5W, 0.9% NaCl, or lactated Ringer's solution, and administered through Y-tubing or a 3-way stopcock. • Use diluted solution within 24 hours.

---

*Underlines indicate most frequent; CAPITALS indicate life-threatening.

Compatibility

- **Syringe:** doxapram.
- **Y-site:** allopurinol sodium ◆ diltiazem ◆ filgrastim ◆ melphalan ◆ meperidine ◆ morphine ◆ piperacillin/tazobactam ◆ vinorelbine.

Incompatibility

- **Additive:** dobutamine ◆ milrinone.

Rate of Administration

- **Direct IV:** Administer slowly over 1–2 minutes.

≋ CLINICAL PRECAUTIONS

- One mg of bumetanide is approximately equivalent to 40 mg of furosemide.
- Assess for allergy to sulfonamides.
- Assess fluid status throughout therapy. Monitor intake and output ratios, daily weight, amount and location of edema, lung sounds, skin turgor, and mucous membranes. Notify physician if excessive thirst, dry mouth, weakness, hypotension, lethargy, or oliguria occurs.
- Monitor blood pressure and pulse throughout therapy.
- Because bumetanide causes loss of many electrolytes, correct any electrolyte depletion before administering.
- Excessive hypotension may occur with concurrent use of antihypertensive agents or nitrates.
- Bumetanide increases the risk of ototoxicity and nephrotoxicity with aminoglycosides or cisplatin. Monitor aminoglycoside serum levels and assess for hearing loss in patients receiving concurrent or prolonged therapy, and maintain adequate hydration.
- Additive hypokalemia may occur with other diuretics, piperacillin, ticarcillin, mezlocillin, amphotericin B, and glucocorticoids. Hypokalemia may increase cardiac glycoside (digoxin) toxicity.
- Use cautiously in patients with severe liver disease. Rapid diuresis may precipitate hepatic coma.
- Bumetanide decreases lithium excretion and may cause toxicity.
- Bumetanide may enhance the effect of warfarin. Nonsteroidal anti-inflammatory agents or probenecid may decrease the diuretic effect of bumetanide.

- Use with caution in patients with diabetes mellitus. Requirements for insulin or oral hypoglycemic agents may be increased.
- Safe use in pregnancy or in children younger than 18 years has not been established (Pregnancy Category C).

Lab Test Considerations

- Monitor electrolytes, renal and hepatic function, serum glucose and uric acid levels prior to and periodically throughout therapy. May cause decreased electrolyte levels (especially potassium). May cause elevated serum glucose, BUN, uric acid, and urinary phosphate levels.

Patient/Family Teaching

- Caution patient to make position changes slowly to minimize orthostatic hypotension. • Instruct patient regarding diet with adequate potassium (see Appendix H). • Advise patient to contact physician immediately if muscle weakness, cramps, nausea, dizziness, numbness, or tingling of extremities occurs.

≋ PHARMACOLOGIC PROFILE

Indications

- Bumetanide is used in the management of edema secondary to congestive heart failure, hepatic disease, or renal disease.

Action

- Loop diuretics inhibit the reabsorption of sodium and chloride from the loop of Henle and distal renal tubule. This results in increased renal excretion of water, sodium, chloride, magnesium, hydrogen, and calcium. Bumetanide may also have renal and peripheral vasodilatory effects. Unlike thiazide diuretics, its effectiveness persists despite impaired renal function.

Time/Action Profile (onset of diuresis)

Onset	Peak	Duration
within minutes	15–45 min	3–6 hr

Pharmacokinetics

• **Distribution:** The distribution of bumetanide is not known. • **Metabolism and Excretion:** Bumetanide is partially metabolized by the liver, 50% is eliminated unchanged by the kidneys, and 20% is excreted in feces. • **Half-life:** 1–1.5 hours.

Contraindications

• Hypersensitivity to bumetanide. • Cross-sensitivity with thiazides, furosemide, and sulfonamides may occur. • Ampules contain EDTA; vials contain benzyl alcohol. Avoid using in patients with known intolerance. • Avoid use of bumetanide during lactation, anuria, or increasing azotemia.

Adverse Reactions and Side Effects*

• **CNS:** dizziness, headache, encephalopathy • **CV:** hypotension • **Derm:** rashes • **EENT:** hearing loss, tinnitus • **F and E:** metabolic alkalosis, hypovolemia, dehydration, hyponatremia, hypokalemia, hypochloremia, hypomagnesemia • **GI:** nausea, vomiting, diarrhea, constipation, dry mouth • **GU:** frequency • **Metab:** hyperglycemia, hyperuricemia • **MS:** muscle cramps.

Buprenorphine	Opioid analgesic (agonist/antagonist)
Buprenex	pH 3.5–5.5

Schedule V

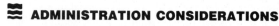 **ADMINISTRATION CONSIDERATIONS**

Usual Dose

Adults: 300 mcg q 6 hr as needed (a second dose may be given after 30–60 min). Doses up to 600 mcg IM (0.6 mg) q 4 hr have been used. May also be given as an infusion at 25–250 mcg/hr (unlabeled use).

---

*Underlines indicate most frequent; CAPITALS indicate life-threatening.

Geriatric Patients: 150 mcg (0.15 mg) q 6 hr as needed initially.
Children: 2–6 mcg (0.002–0.006 mg)/kg q 4–6 hr (unlabeled use).

Dilution

• **Direct IV:** May be given **undiluted.** • May be **further diluted** with D5W, 0.9% NaCl, D5/0.9% NaCl, Ringer's or lactated Ringer's solutions. • **Continuous Infusion:** Has been diluted in 0.9% NaCl for a concentration of 15 mcg/ml.

Compatibility

• **Syringe:** atropine ✦ diphenhydramine ✦ droperidol ✦ glycopyrrolate ✦ haloperidol ✦ hydroxyzine ✦ midazolam ✦ promethazine ✦ scopolamine.
• **Y-site:** allopurinol sodium ✦ filgrastim ✦ melphalan ✦ piperacillin/tazobactam ✦ vinorelbine.

Incompatibility

• **Syringe:** diazepam ✦ lorazepam.
• **Additive:** furosemide.

Rate of Administration

• **Direct IV:** Administer slowly over 2 minutes. Rapid administration may cause respiratory depression, hypotension, and cardiac arrest. • **Continuous Infusion:** Administer at a rate of 25–250 mcg/hr.

≋ CLINICAL PRECAUTIONS

• Assess type, location, and intensity of pain prior to and 20 minutes (peak) following administration. Buprenorphine 0.3–0.4 mg has approximately equal analgesic and respiratory depressant effects as morphine 10 mg. When titrating opioid doses, increases of 25–50% should be administered until there is either a 50% reduction in the patient's pain rating on a numerical or visual analog scale or the patient reports satisfactory pain relief. Subsequent doses may be safely administered at the time of the peak if the previous dose is ineffective and side effects are minimal. Patients requiring higher doses should be converted to an opioid agonist. Buprenorphine is not recommended for prolonged use or as first-line therapy for acute or cancer pain.

- An equianalgesic chart (Appendix B, p. 1045) should be used when changing routes or when changing from one opioid to another.
- Regularly administered doses are more effective than p.r.n. administration. Analgesic is more effective if administered before pain becomes severe. Coadministration with nonopioid analgesics may have additive effects and permit lower opioid doses.
- Assess blood pressure, pulse, and respirations prior to and periodically during administration. If respiratory rate is less than 10/minute, assess level of sedation. Physical stimulation may be sufficient to prevent significant hypoventilation. Dose may need to be decreased by 25–50%.
- Patient should remain supine during and following administration to minimize adverse effects.
- Avoid using with other opioid analgesics, as buprenorphine will decrease their analgesic properties.
- Assess prior analgesic history. Buprenorphine may precipitate withdrawal symptoms (vomiting, restlessness, abdominal cramps, increased blood pressure and temperature) in patients who are physically dependent on opioid analgesic agonists. Symptoms may occur up to 15 days after discontinuation and may persist for 1–2 weeks.
- Buprenorphine has a low potential for dependence; however, prolonged use may lead to physical and psychological dependence and tolerance although rarely to true addiction. Fear of addiction should not prevent patient from receiving adequate analgesia. Progressively higher doses may be required to relieve pain with long-term therapy.
- Assess mental status. Buprenorphine commonly produces sedation, confusion, hallucinations, and dysphoria. Initial drowsiness will diminish with continued use. Additive CNS depression is likely to occur with concurrent use of alcohol, antihistamines, antidepressants, and sedative/hypnotics.
- Elderly or debilitated patients, and patients with respiratory or CNS depression are more sensitive to the effects of opioid analgesics and may require reduced dosage. Initial dosage should be decreased by 50%.

- Exercise caution in administering buprenorphine to patients with increased intracranial pressure.
- Use cautiously in patients with severe renal, hepatic, or pulmonary disease, because of increased sensitivity to CNS adverse reactions, including respiratory depression.
- Buprenorphine may mask symptoms in patients with undiagnosed abdominal pain.
- Patients with hypothyroidism, adrenal insufficiency, or alcoholism have an increased risk of adverse reactions to opioid analgesics.
- Use with caution in patients receiving MAO inhibitors. Severe, unpredictable, and potentially fatal reactions may occur; decrease buprenorphine dose by 50%. MAO inhibitor dose may need to be decreased.
- Patients with prostatic hypertrophy may experience urinary retention.
- Buprenorphine crosses the placenta and enters breast milk. Safe use during pregnancy, labor, and lactation, or in children has not been established (Pregnancy Category C).

Toxicity and Overdose Alert

- If an opioid antagonist is required to reverse respiratory depression or coma, naloxone (Narcan) is the antidote. Dilute the 0.4-mg ampule of naloxone in 10 ml of 0.9% NaCl and administer 0.5 ml (0.02 mg) by direct IV push every 2 minutes. For children and patients weighing <40 kg, dilute 0.1 mg of naloxone in 10 ml of 0.9% NaCl for a concentration of 10 mcg/ml and administer 0.5 mcg every 1–2 minutes. Titrate the dose to avoid withdrawal, seizures, and severe pain. Doxapram may also be ordered as a respiratory stimulant.

Lab Test Considerations

- May cause elevated serum amylase and lipase levels.

Patient/Family Teaching

- Instruct patient on how and when to ask for pain medication. • To enhance the analgesic effect, explain the therapeutic value of the medication prior to administration. • Buprenorphine may cause drowsiness or dizziness.

Advise patient to call for assistance when ambulating and to avoid activities requiring alertness until response to medication is known. • Instruct patient to change positions slowly to minimize orthostatic hypotension. • Encourage patient to turn, cough, and deep-breathe every 2 hours to prevent atelectasis. • Advise patient that good oral hygiene, frequent mouth rinses, and sugarless gum or candy may decrease dry mouth. • Advise patient to avoid concurrent use of alcohol or other CNS depressants with buprenorphine.

 PHARMACOLOGIC PROFILE

Indications
• Buprenorphine is used in the management of moderate to severe pain.

Action
• Buprenorphine binds to opiate receptors in the CNS, where it alters the perception of and response to painful stimuli, while producing generalized CNS depression. • In addition, buprenorphine has partial antagonist properties, which may result in opioid withdrawal in physically dependent patients.

Time/Action Profile (pain relief)

Onset	Peak	Duration
rapid	rapid	up to 6 hr

Pharmacokinetics
• **Distribution:** Buprenorphine crosses the placenta and enters breast milk. • **Metabolism and Excretion:** Metabolism of buprenorphine occurs mainly in the liver. • **Half-life:** 2–3 hours.

Contraindications
• Hypersensitivity to buprenorphine.

Adverse Reactions and Side Effects*
• **CNS:** <u>sedation</u>, <u>confusion</u>, headache, euphoria, floating feeling, unusual dreams, <u>hallucinations</u>, <u>dysphoria</u> • **EENT:**

---

*<u>Underlines</u> indicate most frequent; CAPITALS indicate life-threatening.

miosis (high doses), blurred vision, diplopia • **Resp:** respiratory depression • **CV:** hypotension, hypertension, palpitations • **GI:** nausea, vomiting, constipation, ileus, dry mouth • **GU:** urinary retention • **Derm:** sweating, clammy feeling • **Misc:** sweating, tolerance, physical dependence, psychological dependence.

Butorphanol	Opioid analgesic (agonist/antagonist)
Stadol	pH 3–5.5

 ADMINISTRATION CONSIDERATIONS

Usual Dose
ADULTS: 1 mg q 3–4 hr as needed (range 0.5–2 mg).
GERIATRIC PATIENTS: 1 mg q 4–6 hr.

Dilution
• **Direct IV:** May be administered **undiluted**.

Compatibility
• **Syringe:** atropine ✦ chlorpromazine ✦ cimetidine ✦ diphenhydramine ✦ droperidol ✦ fentanyl ✦ hydroxyzine ✦ meperidine ✦ methotrimeprazine ✦ metoclopramide ✦ midazolam ✦ morphine ✦ pentazocine ✦ perphenazine ✦ prochlorperazine ✦ promethazine ✦ scopolamine ✦ thiethylperazine.
• **Y-site:** allopurinol sodium ✦ enalaprilat ✦ esmolol ✦ filgrastim ✦ fludarabine ✦ labetalol ✦ melphalan ✦ paclitaxel ✦ piperacillin/tazobactam ✦ sargramostim ✦ vinorelbine.

Incompatibility
• **Syringe:** dimenhydrinate ✦ pentobarbital.

Rate of Administration
• **Direct IV:** Administer over 3–5 minutes. Rapid administration may cause respiratory depression, hypotension, and cardiac arrest.

≋ CLINICAL PRECAUTIONS

- Assess type, location, and intensity of pain prior to and 4–5 minutes (peak) following administration. When titrating opioid doses, increases of 25–50% should be administered until there is either a 50% reduction in the patient's pain rating on a numerical or visual analog scale or the patient reports satisfactory pain relief. Subsequent doses may be safely administered at the time of the peak if the previous dose is ineffective and side effects are minimal. Patients requiring higher doses should be converted to an opioid agonist. Butorphanol is not recommended for prolonged use or as first-line therapy for acute or cancer pain.

- An equianalgesic chart (Appendix B, page 1045) should be used when changing routes or when changing from one opioid to another.

- Regularly administered doses are more effective than p.r.n. administration. Analgesic is more effective if administered before pain becomes severe. Coadministration with nonopioid analgesics may have additive effects and permit lower opioid doses.

- Assess mental status. Butorphanol commonly produces sedation, confusion, hallucinations, and dysphoria. Initial drowsiness will diminish with continued use. Additive CNS depression is likely to occur with concurrent use of alcohol, antihistamines, antidepressants, and sedative/hypnotics.

- Assess blood pressure, pulse, and respirations prior to and periodically during administration. Patient should remain supine during and following administration to minimize adverse effects. If respiratory rate is <10/minute, assess level of sedation. Physical stimulation may be sufficient to prevent significant hypoventilation. Dose may need to be decreased by 25–50%.

- Avoid using with other opioid analgesics, because butorphanol will decrease their analgesic properties.

- Assess prior analgesic history. Butorphanol may precipitate withdrawal symptoms (vomiting, restlessness, abdominal cramps, increased blood pressure and temperature) in patients who are physically dependent on opioid analgesics.

- Butorphanol has a low potential for dependence; however, prolonged use may lead to physical and psychological dependence and tolerance, although rarely to true addiction. Fear of addiction should not prevent patient from receiving adequate analgesia. Progressively higher doses may be required to relieve pain with long-term therapy.

- Debilitated patients are more sensitive to the effects of opioid analgesics and may require reduced dosage.
- Exercise caution in administering butorphanol to patients with increased intracranial pressure.
- Use cautiously in patients with severe renal, hepatic, or pulmonary disease, because of increased sensitivity to CNS adverse reactions including respiratory depression.
- Butorphanol may mask symptoms in patients with undiagnosed abdominal pain.
- Patients with hypothyroidism, adrenal insufficiency, or alcoholism have an increased risk of adverse reactions to opioid analgesics.
- Use with caution in patients receiving MAO inhibitors. Severe, unpredictable, and potentially fatal reactions may occur; decrease butorphanol dose by 25%. MAO inhibitor dose may also need to be decreased.
- Patients with prostatic hypertrophy may experience urinary retention.
- Butorphanol crosses the placenta, enters breast milk, and has been used safely during labor. Assess newborns for possible respiratory depression. Safe use in pregnancy, lactation, or children under 18 years has not been established (Pregnancy Category C).

Toxicity and Overdose Alert

- If an opioid antagonist is required to reverse respiratory depression or coma, naloxone (Narcan) is the antidote. Dilute the 0.4-mg ampule of naloxone in 10 ml of 0.9% NaCl and administer 0.5 ml (0.02 mg) by direct IV push every 2 minutes. For children and patients weighing <40 kg, dilute 0.1 mg of naloxone in 10 ml of 0.9% NaCl for a concentration of 10 mcg/ml and administer 0.5 mcg every 1–2 minutes. Titrate the dose to avoid withdrawal, seizures, and severe pain.

Lab Test Considerations

- May cause elevated serum amylase and lipase levels.

Patient/Family Teaching

• Instruct patient on how and when to ask for pain medication. • Butorphanol may cause drowsiness or dizziness. Advise patient to call for assistance when ambulating and to avoid activities requiring alertness until response to medication is known. • Instruct patient to change positions slowly to minimize orthostatic hypotension. • Encourage patient to turn, cough, and deep-breathe every 2 hours to prevent atelectasis. • Advise patient that good oral hygiene, frequent mouth rinses, and sugarless gum or candy may decrease dry mouth. • Advise patient to avoid concurrent use of alcohol or other CNS depressants with butorphanol.

 PHARMACOLOGIC PROFILE

Indications

• Butorphanol is used in the management of moderate to severe pain, as an analgesic during labor, as a sedative prior to surgery, and as a supplement in balanced anesthesia.

Action

• Butorphanol binds to opiate receptors in the CNS, where it alters the perception of and response to painful stimuli, while producing generalized CNS depression. • In addition, butorphanol has partial antagonist properties, which may result in opioid withdrawal in physically dependent patients.

Time/Action Profile (pain relief)

Onset	Peak	Duration
1 min	4–5 min	2–4 hr

Pharmacokinetics

• **Distribution:** Butorphanol crosses the placenta and enters breast milk. • **Metabolism and Excretion:** Most of butorphanol is metabolized by the liver; 11–14% is excreted in the feces. Minimal amounts are execreted unchanged by the kidneys.

Contraindications

• Hypersensitivity to butorphanol. • Some products contain benzethonium chloride and should be avoided in patients with known intolerance.

Adverse Reactions and Side Effects*

• **CNS:** <u>sedation</u>, <u>confusion</u>, headache, euphoria, floating feeling, unusual dreams, <u>hallucinations</u>, <u>dysphoria</u> • **EENT:** miosis (high doses), blurred vision, diplopia • **Resp:** respiratory depression • **CV:** hypotension, hypertension, palpitations • **GI:** <u>nausea</u>, vomiting, constipation, ileus, dry mouth • **GU:** urinary retention • **Derm:** sweating, clammy feeling • **Misc:** <u>sweating</u>, tolerance, physical dependence, psychological dependence.

Calcitriol	*Vitamin D analog*
Calcijex, vitamin D_3	pH 7

 ADMINISTRATION CONSIDERATIONS

Usual Dose

Adults: 0.5 mcg (0.01 mcg/kg) 3 times weekly initially. May be increased by 0.25–0.5 mcg/dose at 2–4 wk intervals. Maintenance dose is 0.5–3 mcg (0.01–0.05 mcg/kg) 3 times weekly.

Dilution

• **Direct IV:** May be administered **undiluted**.

Compatibility

• **Solution:** D5W • 0.9% NaCl • sterile water for injection.

Rate of Administration

• **Direct IV:** Administer by rapid IV injection through a catheter at the end of a period of hemodialysis.

---

*<u>Underlines</u> indicate most frequent; CAPITALS indicate life-threatening.

≋ CLINICAL PRECAUTIONS

- Calcitriol should be used cautiously in patients with sarcoidosis or hyperparathyroidism due to increased risk of hypercalcemia. Assess frequently for signs of hypocalcemia or hypercalcemia.
- Use calcitriol with caution in patients receiving cardiac glycosides, magnesium-containing antacids, or thiazide diuretics. The effects of calcitriol may be antagonized by glucocorticoids. Concurrent ingestion of foods high in calcium content may lead to hypercalcemia.
- Safe use in children or during pregnancy and lactation has not been established (Pregnancy Category C).

Lab Test Considerations

- Monitor serum calcium and ionized calcium concentrations at least weekly during early treatment. Therapeutic range is narrow; serum calcium concentrations should be maintained at 8.8–10.3 mg/100 ml. • Monitor BUN and serum creatinine periodically during therapy. • Monitor serum alkaline phosphatase and phosphorus concentrations, 24-hour urinary calcium concentrations, and urinary calcium/creatinine ratio every 1–3 months during therapy as long as the patient remains stable. Serum alkaline phosphatase concentrations may be decreased prior to the development of hypercalcemia in patients receiving excessive doses. Serum calcium, cholesterol, and phosphorus concentrations may be increased with high doses. Urinary calcium and phosphorus concentrations may be increased with therapeutic doses, even when serum concentrations are still low.

Patient/Family Teaching

- Emphasize the importance of regular laboratory tests to monitor progress. • Instruct the patient to avoid over-the-counter medications or dietary supplements containing calcium, phosphorus, or vitamin D unless directed by the physician. • Advise the patient to avoid the concurrent use of antacids containing magnesium.

≋ PHARMACOLOGIC PROFILE

Indications
- Calcitriol is used in the management of hypocalcemia in chronic renal failure patients.

Action
- Calcitriol is a synthetic form of active vitamin D. It promotes absorption of calcium from the GI tract and helps to regulate calcium homeostasis in conjunction with parathyroid hormone and calcitonin.

Time/Action Profile (effect on serum calcium†)

Onset	Peak	Duration
2–6 hr	UK	3–5 days

†Following oral administration.

Pharmacokinetics
- **Distribution:** Calcitriol crosses the placenta. Very small amounts enter breast milk. It is stored in the liver. • **Metabolism and Excretion:** Calcitriol is metabolized by the liver and excreted in bile. • **Half-life:** 3–8 hours.

Contraindications
- Calcitriol is contraindicated in hypercalcemic patients or patients exhibiting any other signs of vitamin D toxicity.

Adverse Reactions and Side Effects*
Seen primarily as manifestations of toxicity (hypercalcemia).
- **CNS:** weakness, headache, somnolence • **EENT:** photophobia, conjunctivitis, rhinorrhea • **GI:** nausea, vomiting, dry mouth, constipation, metallic taste, polydipsia, anorexia, weight loss • **GU:** polyuria, nocturia, decreased libido, albuminuria • **Derm:** pruritus • **F and E:** hypercalcemia • **Metab:** hyperthermia • **MS:** muscle pain, bone pain.

---

*Underlines indicate most frequent; CAPITALS indicate life-threatening.

Calcium Chloride	*Electrolyte*
{Calciject}	**pH 5.5–7.5**

≋ ADMINISTRATION CONSIDERATIONS

Usual Dose
Calcium chloride contains 27% calcium by weight or 13.6 mEq/g. Doses are expressed in g or mEq of elemental calcium.

Emergency Treatment of Hypocalcemia
ADULTS: 7–14 mEq.
CHILDREN: 1–7 mEq.
INFANTS: <1 mEq.

Hypocalcemic Tetany
ADULTS: 4.5–16 mEq; repeat until symptoms are controlled.
CHILDREN: 0.5–0.7 mEq/kg 3–4 times daily.
NEONATES: 2.4 mEq/kg/day in divided doses.

Hyperkalemia with Cardiac Toxicity
ADULTS: 2.25–14 mEq; may repeat in 1–2 min.

Magnesium Intoxication
ADULTS: 7 mEq.

Exchange Transfusions in Neonates
NEONATES: 0.45 mEq after each 100 ml of citrated blood exchanged.

Citrated Blood Transfusions in Adults
ADULTS: 1.35 mEq with each 100 ml of blood.

Dilution
• **Direct IV:** May be administered **undiluted.** • **Intermittent/Continuous Infusion:** May be **diluted** with D5W, D10W, 0.9% NaCl, D5/0.25% NaCl, D5/0.45% NaCl, D5/0.9% NaCl, or D5/LR.

Compatibility
• **Syringe:** milrinone.
• **Y-site:** amrinone ✦ dobutamine ✦ epinephrine ✦ esmolol ✦ morphine ✦ paclitaxel.
• **Additive:** amikacin ✦ ascorbic acid ✦ bretylium ✦ cepha-

---

{} = Available in Canada only.

pirin • chloramphenicol • dopamine • hydrocortisone sodium succinate • isoproterenol • lidocaine • methicillin • norepinephrine • penicillin G • pentobarbital • phenobarbital • verapamil • vitamin B complex with C.

Incompatibility
- **Y-site:** sodium bicarbonate.
- **Additive:** amphotericin B • cephalothin • chlorpheniramine.

Rate of Administration
- **Direct IV/Intermittent/Continuous Infusion:** Maximum rate should not exceed 0.7–1.5 mEq/min (0.5–1 ml of 10% solution); for children, 0.5 ml/min.

≋ CLINICAL PRECAUTIONS

- Milligram doses of calcium chloride, calcium gluconate, and calcium gluceptate are not equal. Doses should be expressed in mEq of calcium. Calcium chloride 10% injection contains 1 g calcium chloride/10 ml (13.6 m/Eq of calcium).
- In arrest situations, calcium use is now limited to patients with hyperkalemia, hypocalcemia, and calcium channel blocker toxicity. Physician should specify form of calcium desired.
- Warm solution to body temperature and administer through a small-bore needle in a large vein to minimize phlebitis. Do not use scalp vein. If cutaneous burning occurs, discontinue administration. Calcium chloride is rarely used in children because of vein irritation. Assess site for patency. Extravasation may cause cellulitis, sloughing, and necrosis.
- Patient should remain recumbent for 30 minutes to 1 hour following administration.
- Observe patient carefully for evidence of hypocalcemia (paresthesia, muscle twitching, laryngospasm, colic, cardiac arrhythmias, and Chvostek's or Trousseau's sign). Protect symptomatic patients by raising and padding side rails; keep bed in low position.
- Monitor blood pressure, pulse, and ECG frequently throughout therapy. May cause vasodilation resulting in hypotension, bradycardia, arrhythmias, and cardiac arrest.

- Use calcium supplements carefully in patients with cardiac disease or patients receiving cardiac glycosides (digoxin), because of increased risk of arrhythmias. Administration of calcium may decrease the effectiveness or reverse the toxic effects of verapamil.
- Patients with renal calculi should receive calcium supplements cautiously due to increased risk of stone formation.
- Calcium crosses the placenta and enters breast milk and may be used during pregnancy or lactation (supplements may be recommended; Pregnancy Category C).

Toxicity and Overdose Alert

- Observe patient for appearance of symptoms of hypercalcemia (nausea, vomiting, anorexia, excessive thirst, weakness, constipation, paralytic ileus, bradycardia).

Lab Test Considerations

- Monitor electrolytes (especially calcium) and albumin concentrations prior to and periodically throughout therapy. May cause false decrease in serum and urine magnesium levels. • Hypercalcemia increases the risk of cardiac glycoside (digoxin) toxicity. Monitor serum calcium and digoxin levels.

Patient/Family Teaching

- Instruct patient to remain recumbent for 30 minutes to 1 hour following IV administration. • With physician's order, encourage patient to maintain a diet adequate in vitamin D (fish liver oils, fortified milk, breads, and cereals) and calcium (milk, leafy green vegetables, sardines, oysters, clams); see Appendix H. • Instruct patient to contact physician immediately if the signs of hypocalcemia or hypercalcemia occur.

≋ PHARMACOLOGIC PROFILE

Indications

- Calcium chloride is used in the treatment and prevention of calcium depletion in diseases associated with hypocalcemia, which include hypoparathyroidism, achlorhydria, chronic diarrhea, pancreatitis, vitamin D deficiency, and hyperphosphatemia. • Calcium chloride may also be used in the management of hyperkalemia with cardiac toxicity and magnesium toxicity.

Action

• Calcium is essential for nervous, muscular, and skeletal systems. • It maintains cell-membrane and capillary permeability and acts as an activator in the transmission of nerve impulses and the contraction of cardiac, skeletal, and smooth muscle. • Calcium is essential for bone formation and blood coagulation.

Time/Action Profile (effect on serum calcium)

Onset	Peak	Duration
immediate	immediate	0.5–2 hr

Pharmacokinetics

• **Distribution:** Calcium readily enters extracellular fluids, crosses the placenta, and enters breast milk. • **Metabolism and Excretion:** Calcium is excreted mainly in the feces, with 20% excreted unchanged by the kidneys. • **Half-life:** UK.

Contraindications

• Do not administer calcium supplements to patients with hypercalcemia, renal calculi, or ventricular fibrillation.

Adverse Reactions and Side Effects*

• **CNS:** tingling, syncope • **CV:** bradycardia, <u>arrhythmias</u>, CARDIAC ARREST • **GI:** nausea, vomiting, <u>constipation</u> • **GU:** hypercalciuria, calculi • **Local:** <u>phlebitis</u> at IV site.

Calcium Gluceptate	Electrolyte
	pH 5.6–7

☰ ADMINISTRATION CONSIDERATIONS

Usual Dose

Contains 8.2% calcium by weight or 4.1 mEq/g. Doses are expressed in g or mEq of elemental calcium.

---

*<u>Underlines</u> indicate most frequent; CAPITALS indicate life-threatening.

Emergency Treatment of Hypocalcemia
ADULTS: 7–14 mEq.
CHILDREN: 1–7 mEq.
INFANTS: <1 mEq.

Hypocalcemic Tetany
ADULTS: 4.5–16 mEq; repeat until symptoms are controlled.
CHILDREN: 0.5–0.7 mEq/kg 3–4 times daily.
NEONATES: 2.4 mEq/kg/day in divided doses.

Hyperkalemia with Cardiac Toxicity
ADULTS: 2.25–14 mEq, may repeat in 1–2 min.

Magnesium Intoxication
ADULTS: 7 mEq.

Exchange Transfusions in Neonates
NEONATES: 0.45 mEq after each 100 ml of citrated blood exchanged.

Citrated Blood Transfusions in Adults
ADULTS: 1.35 mEq with each 100 ml of blood.

Dilution
• **Direct IV:** May be administered **undiluted**. • **Intermittent/Continuous Infusion:** May be **diluted** with D5W, D10W, 0.9% NaCl, 0.45% NaCl, D5/LR, or lactated Ringer's solution.

Compatibility
• **Additive:** ascorbic acid • isoproterenol • lidocaine • norepinephrine • phytonadione.

Incompatibility
• **Additive:** cefamandole • cephalothin • magnesium sulfate • prednisolone sodium phosphate • prochlorperazine.

Rate of Administration
• **Direct IV/Intermittent/Continuous Infusion:** Administer at a rate not to exceed 2 ml (1.8 mEq)/min for adults; 0.5 ml (0.45 mEq)/min for children. In exchange transfusion in neonates, 0.5 ml (0.45 mEq) is given after each 100 ml of citrated blood.

≋ CLINICAL PRECAUTIONS

- Milligram doses of calcium chloride, calcium gluconate, and calcium gluceptate are not equal. Doses should be expressed in mEq of calcium. Calcium gluceptate injection contains 1.1 g calcium gluceptate/5 ml (4.5 mEq of calcium).

- Warm solution to body temperature and administer through a small-bore needle in a large vein to minimize phlebitis. Do not use scalp vein. If cutaneous burning occurs, discontinue administration. Assess site for patency. Extravasation may cause cellulitis, sloughing, and necrosis.

- Patient should remain recumbent for 30 minutes–1 hour following administration.

- Observe patient carefully for evidence of hypocalcemia (paresthesia, muscle twitching, laryngospasm, colic, cardiac arrhythmias, and Chvostek's or Trousseau's sign). Protect symptomatic patients by raising and padding side rails; keep bed in low position.

- Monitor blood pressure, pulse, and ECG frequently throughout therapy. May cause vasodilation resulting in hypotension, bradycardia, arrhythmias, and cardiac arrest.

- Use calcium supplements carefully in patients with cardiac disease or patients receiving cardiac glycosides (digoxin), because of increased risk of arrhythmias. Administration of calcium may decrease the effectiveness or reverse the toxic effects of verapamil.

- Patients with renal calculi should receive calcium supplements cautiously due to increased risk of stone formation.

- Calcium crosses the placenta and enters breast milk and may be used during pregnancy or lactation (supplements may be recommended; Pregnancy Category C).

Toxicity and Overdose Alert

- Observe patient for appearance of symptoms of hypercalcemia (nausea, vomiting, anorexia, excessive thirst, weakness, constipation, paralytic ileus, bradycardia).

Lab Test Considerations

• Monitor electrolytes (especially calcium) and albumin concentrations prior to and periodically throughout therapy. May cause false decrease in serum and urine magnesium levels. • Hypercalcemia increases the risk of cardiac glycoside (digoxin) toxicity. Monitor serum calcium and digoxin levels.

Patient/Family Teaching

• Instruct patient to remain recumbent for 30 minutes– 1 hour following IV administration. • With physician's order, encourage patient to maintain a diet adequate in vitamin D (fish liver oils, fortified milk, breads, and cereals) and calcium (milk, leafy green vegetables, sardines, oysters, clams); see Appendix H. • Instruct patient to contact physician immediately if the signs of hypocalcemia or hypercalcemia occur.

 PHARMACOLOGIC PROFILE

Indications

• Calcium gluceptate is used in the treatment and prevention of calcium depletion in diseases associated with hypocalcemia, which include hypoparathyroidism, achlorhydria, chronic diarrhea, pancreatitis, vitamin D deficiency, and hyperphosphatemia. • Calcium gluceptate may also be used in the management of hyperkalemia with cardiac toxicity and magnesium toxicity.

Action

• Calcium is essential for nervous, muscular, and skeletal systems. • It maintains cell-membrane and capillary permeability and acts as an activator in the transmission of nerve impulses and contraction of cardiac, skeletal, and smooth muscle. • Calcium is essential for bone formation and blood coagulation.

Time/Action Profile (effect on serum calcium)

Onset	Peak	Duration
immediate	immediate	0.5–2 hr

Pharmacokinetics

• **Distribution:** Calcium readily enters extracellular fluids, crosses the placenta, and enters breast milk. • **Metabolism and Excretion:** Elimination of calcium occurs mainly in the feces; 20% is eliminated by the kidneys. • **Half-life:** UK.

Contraindications

• Do not administer calcium supplements to patients with hypercalcemia, renal calculi, or ventricular fibrillation.

Adverse Reactions and Side Effects*

• **CNS:** tingling, syncope • **CV:** bradycardia, <u>arrhythmias</u>, CARDIAC ARREST • **GI:** nausea, vomiting, <u>constipation</u> • **GU:** hypercalciuria, calculi • **Local:** <u>phlebitis</u> at IV site.

Calcium Gluconate	Electrolyte
Kalcinate	pH 6–8.2

ADMINISTRATION CONSIDERATIONS

Usual Dose

Contains 9% calcium by weight or 4.5 mEq/g. Doses are expressed in g or mEq of elemental calcium.

Emergency Treatment of Hypocalcemia
ADULT: 7–14 mEq.
CHILDREN: 1–7 mEq.
NEONATES: <1 mEq.

Hypocalcemic Tetany
ADULT: 4.5–16 mEq; repeat until symptoms are controlled.
CHILDREN: 0.5–0.7 mEq/kg 3–4 times daily.
NEONATES: 2.4 mEq/kg/day in divided doses.

Hyperkalemia with Cardiac Toxicity
ADULTS: 2.25–14 mEq; may repeat in 1–2 min.

Magnesium Intoxication
ADULTS: 7 mEq.

---

*<u>Underlines</u> indicate most frequent; CAPITALS indicate life-threatening.

Exchange Transfusions in Neonates

NEONATES: 0.45 mEq after each 100 ml of citrated blood exchanged.

Citrated Blood Transfusions in Adults

ADULTS: 1.35 mEq with each 100 ml of blood.

Dilution

• **Direct IV:** May be administered **undiluted** as a 10% solution. • **Intermittent/Continuous Infusion:** May also be **diluted** in 1000 ml of D5W, D10W, D20W, D5/0.9% NaCl, 0.9% NaCl, D5/LR, or lactated Ringer's solution. • Solution should be clear. Do not use if crystals are present.

Compatibility

• **Y-site:** allopurinol sodium ⬩ cefazolin ⬩ ciprofloxacin ⬩ dobutamine ⬩ enalaprilat ⬩ epinephrine ⬩ famotidine ⬩ filgrastim ⬩ labetalol ⬩ melphalan ⬩ netilmicin ⬩ piperacillin/tazobactam ⬩ potassium chloride ⬩ sargramostim ⬩ tacrolimus ⬩ tolazoline ⬩ vinorelbine ⬩ vitamin B complex with C.

• **Additive:** amikacin ⬩ aminophylline ⬩ ascorbic acid ⬩ bretylium ⬩ cephapirin ⬩ chloramphenicol ⬩ corticotropin ⬩ dimenhydrinate ⬩ erythromycin glucceptate ⬩ furosemide ⬩ heparin ⬩ hydrocortisone sodium succinate ⬩ lidocaine ⬩ magnesium sulfate ⬩ methicillin ⬩ norepinephrine ⬩ penicillin G ⬩ phenobarbital ⬩ potassium ⬩ tobramycin ⬩ vancomycin ⬩ verapamil ⬩ vitamin B complex with C.

Incompatibility

• **Syringe:** metoclopramide.
• **Y-site:** fluconazole.
• **Additive:** amphotericin B ⬩ cefamandole ⬩ cephalothin ⬩ dobutamine ⬩ methylprednisolone sodium succinate.

Rate of Administration

• **Direct IV:** Administer slowly at a rate not to exceed 0.5–2 ml/min. • **Intermittent/Continuous Infusion:** Do not exceed 200 mg/minute.

≋ CLINICAL PRECAUTIONS

• Milligram doses of calcium chloride, calcium gluconate, and calcium glucceptate are not equal. Doses should be expressed in mEq of calcium. Calcium gluconate 10%

injection contains 1 g calcium gluconate/10 ml (4.5 mEq of calcium).

- In arrest situations, calcium use is now limited to patients with hyperkalemia, hypocalcemia, and calcium channel blocker toxicity. Physician should specify form of calcium desired.
- Warm solution to body temperature and administer through a small-bore needle in a large vein to minimize phlebitis. Do not use scalp vein. If cutaneous burning occurs, discontinue administration. Assess site for patency. Extravasation may cause cellulitis, sloughing, and necrosis.
- Patient should remain recumbent for 30 minutes–1 hour following administration.
- Observe patient carefully for evidence of hypocalcemia (paresthesia, muscle twitching, laryngospasm, colic, cardiac arrhythmias, and Chvostek's or Trousseau's sign). Protect symptomatic patients by raising and padding side rails; keep bed in low position.
- Monitor blood pressure, pulse, and ECG frequently throughout therapy. May cause vasodilation resulting in hypotension, bradycardia, arrhythmias, and cardiac arrest.
- Use calcium supplements carefully in patients with cardiac disease or patients receiving cardiac glycosides (digoxin), because of increased risk of arrhythmias. Administration of calcium may decrease the effectiveness or reverse the toxic effects of verapamil.
- Patients with renal calculi should receive calcium supplements cautiously due to increased risk of stone formation.
- Calcium crosses the placenta and enters breast milk and may be used during pregnancy or lactation (supplements may be recommended; Pregnancy Category C).

Toxicity and Overdose Alert

- Observe patient for appearance of symptoms of hypercalcemia (nausea, vomiting, anorexia, excessive thirst, weakness, constipation, paralytic ileus, bradycardia).

Lab Test Considerations

- Monitor electrolytes (especially calcium) and albumin concentrations prior to and periodically throughout therapy. May cause false decrease in serum and urine magnesium levels. • Hypercalcemia increases the risk of cardiac glycoside (digoxin) toxicity. Monitor serum calcium and digoxin levels.

Patient/Family Teaching

• Instruct patient to remain recumbent for 30 minutes–1 hour following IV administration. • With physician's order, encourage patient to maintain a diet adequate in vitamin D (fish liver oils, fortified milk, breads, and cereals) and calcium (milk, leafy green vegetables, sardines, oysters, clams); see Appendix H. • Instruct patient to contact physician immediately if the signs of hypocalcemia or hypercalcemia occur.

 PHARMACOLOGIC PROFILE

Indications

• Calcium gluconate is used in the treatment and prevention of calcium depletion in diseases associated with hypocalcemia, which include hypoparathyroidism, achlorhydria, chronic diarrhea, pancreatitis, vitamin D deficiency, and hyperphosphatemia. • Calcium gluconate may also be used in the management of hyperkalemia with cardiac toxicity and magnesium toxicity.

Action

• Calcium is essential for nervous, muscular, and skeletal systems. • It maintains cell-membrane and capillary permeability and acts as an activator in the transmission of nerve impulses and the contraction of cardiac, skeletal, and smooth muscle. • Calcium is essential for bone formation and blood coagulation.

Time/Action Profile (effect on serum calcium)

Onset	Peak	Duration
immediate	immediate	0.5–2 hr

Pharmacokinetics

• **Distribution:** Calcium readily enters extracellular fluids, crosses the placenta, and enters breast milk. • **Metabolism and Excretion:** Elimination of calcium occurs mainly

in the feces; 20% is eliminated by the kidneys. • **Half-life:**
UK.

Contraindications
• Do not administer calcium supplements to patients with
hypercalcemia, renal calculi, or ventricular fibrillation.

Adverse Reactions and Side Effects*
• **CNS:** tingling, syncope • **CV:** bradycardia, <u>arrhythmias</u>,
CARDIAC ARREST • **GI:** nausea, vomiting, <u>constipation</u> • **GU:**
hypercalciuria, calculi • **Local:** <u>phlebitis</u> at IV site.

Carboplatin	Antineoplastic (alkylating agent)
Paraplatin	pH 5–7 (1% solution)

 ADMINISTRATION CONSIDERATIONS

Usual Dose
ADULTS: 300–360 mg/m^2 as a single dose; may be repeated at
4-wk intervals depending on response. A 300 mg/m^2 dose
is used as part of combination chemotherapy. A 360 mg/m^2
dose is used for single-agent chemotherapy. Other regimens may be used.

Dilution
• **Intermittent/Continuous Infusion: Reconstitute** to a
concentration of 10 mg/ml with sterile water for injection,
D5W, or 0.9% NaCl for injection. May be **further diluted** in
D5W or 0.9% NaCl for a concentration of 0.5 mg/ml. • Solution should be prepared in a biologic cabinet. Wear gloves,
gown, and mask while handling medication. Discard equipment in specially designated containers (see Appendix F).
• Solution is stable for 8 hours at room temperature.

---

*<u>Underlines</u> indicate most frequent; CAPITALS indicate life-
threatening.

Compatibility

- **Y-site:** allopurinol sodium ✦ filgrastim ✦ fludarabine ✦ melphalan ✦ ondansetron ✦ paclitaxel ✦ piperacillin/tazobactam ✦ sargramostim ✦ vinorelbine.
- **Additive:** ifosfamide ✦ ifosfamide with etoposide.

Incompatibility

- **Additive:** fluorouracil ✦ mesna.

Rate of Administration

- **Intermittent Infusion:** Administer over 15–60 minutes.

≋ CLINICAL PRECAUTIONS

- Do not use aluminum needles or equipment during preparation or administration, because aluminum reacts with carboplatin.
- Monitor for signs of anaphylaxis (rash, urticaria, pruritus, wheezing, tachycardia, hypotension). Discontinue medication immediately if these occur. Epinephrine and resuscitation equipment should be readily available.
- Monitor fluid and electrolyte status, renal function studies, and nutrition. Adequate hydration is necessary to prevent nephrotoxic and ototoxic reactions. Nausea and vomiting may be severe, often occurring 6–12 hours after treatment and persisting for 24 hours. Pretreatment with antiemetics may be helpful. Correct underlying electrolyte abnormalities before administration. Severe electrolyte depletion may occur. Hypokalemia may increase the risk of cardiac glycoside (digoxin) toxicity.
- Monitor hearing before and during treatment. Since most of carboplatin is excreted by the kidneys, dosage reduction is recommended if creatinine clearance is less than 60 ml/min. Nephrotoxicity and ototoxicity are additive with other nephrotoxic and ototoxic drugs (aminoglycosides).
- Monitor for bone marrow depression. Observe for signs of bleeding, and avoid IM injections if platelet count is low. Assess for signs of infection during period of neutropenia. Use cautiously in patients with active infections. Additive bone marrow depression will occur with other antineoplastic agents or radiation therapy. Patients

with chronic debilitating illnesses or decreased bone marrow reserve may be more sensitive to the bone marrow–depressing properties of carboplatin. • Monitor for development of peripheral neuropathy. This usually begins with mild paresthesias.

- Do not confuse carboplatin (Paraplatin) with cisplatin (Platinol). Indications, dosage, and toxicity are different. See *cisplatin* monograph on page 230.
- Carboplatin should be avoided in pregnancy, especially the first trimester (Pregnancy Category D). Breast-feeding should also be avoided. Safe use in children has not been established.

Lab Test Considerations

• CBC, differential, and clotting studies should be monitored prior to and periodically throughout therapy. Bone marrow depression is maximum at 21 days after a dose, with recovery at 28 days after a dose. The nadir of thrombocytopenia occurs within 14–28 days. Withhold subsequent doses until neutrophil count is >2000/mm^3 and platelet count >100,000/mm^3. • Monitor renal and hepatic function prior to and periodically throughout course of therapy.

Patient/Family Teaching

• Instruct patient to notify physician promptly if fever, sore throat, signs of infection, bleeding gums, bruising, petechiae; blood in stools, urine or emesis; increased fatigue, dyspnea, or orthostatic hypotension occurs. Caution patient to avoid crowds and persons with known infections. Instruct patient to use a soft toothbrush and electric razor, and to be especially careful to avoid falls. Patients should be cautioned not to drink alcoholic beverages or take medications containing aspirin, ibuprofen, or naproxen, because these may precipitate gastric bleeding. • Instruct patient to report promptly any numbness or tingling in extremities or face, decreased coordination, difficulty with hearing or tinnitus, unusual swelling, or weight gain to physician. • Carboplatin may decrease antibody response to live virus vaccines and increase the risk of adverse reactions. Advise patient not to receive any vaccinations without advice of physician. • Patients with childbearing potential should use a nonhormonal method of contraception. • Instruct patient to inspect oral mucosa for erythema and ulceration. If ulceration occurs, advise patient to notify physician, rinse mouth with water after eating, and use sponge brush. • Discuss with patient the possibility of hair loss. Explore methods of coping. • Emphasize the need for periodic lab tests to monitor for side effects.

≋ PHARMACOLOGIC PROFILE

Indications
• Carboplatin is used in combination with other agents as initial treatment of advanced ovarian carcinoma and alone as palliative treatment of ovarian carcinoma unresponsive to other chemotherapeutic modalities.

Action
• Carboplatin inhibits DNA synthesis by producing cross-linking of parent DNA strands (cell cycle–phase nonspecific). This results in death of rapidly replicating cells, particularly malignant cells. It is converted in solution to its active form.

Time/Action Profile (effect on blood counts)

Onset	Peak	Duration
UK	21 days	28 days

Pharmacokinetics
• **Distribution:** UK • **Metabolism and Excretion:** Carboplatin is excreted mostly by the kidneys. • **Half-life:** 2.6–5.9 hours (increased in renal impairment).

Contraindications
• Hypersensitivity to carboplatin, cisplatin, or mannitol. • Carboplatin should not be used in pregnant or lactating patients (Pregnancy Category D).

Adverse Reactions and Side Effects*
• **CNS:** weakness • **EENT:** ototoxicity • **GI:** <u>vomiting</u>, <u>nausea</u>, <u>abdominal pain</u>, diarrhea, constipation, hepatitis, sto-

---

*<u>Underlines</u> indicate most frequent; CAPITALS indicate life-threatening.

matitis • **GU:** nephrotoxicity, gonadal suppression • **Derm:** rash, alopecia • **F and E:** hyponatremia, hypocalcemia, hypomagnesemia, hypokalemia • **Hemat:** leukopenia, thrombocytopenia, anemia • **Neuro:** peripheral neuropathy • **Misc:** hypersensitivity reactions including ANAPHYLAXIS.

Carmustine	Antineoplastic (alkylating agent)
BCNU, BiCNU	pH 5.6–6

 ADMINISTRATION CONSIDERATIONS

Usual Dose

ADULTS AND CHILDREN: 150–200 mg/m² given as a single dose q 6–8 wk or 75–100 mg/m² daily for 2 days q 6 wk or 40 mg/m²/day for 5 days q 6 wk.

Dilution

• **Intermittent Infusion:** **Dilute** the contents of each 100-mg vial with 3 ml of absolute ethyl alcohol provided as diluent. **Dilute** this solution with 27 ml of sterile water for injection. Solution is colorless to pale yellow. **Dilute further** with 500 ml of D5W or 0.9% NaCl in a glass container.
• Solution should be prepared in a biological cabinet. Wear gloves, gown, and mask while handling medication. Discard equipment in specially designated containers (see Appendix F). Contact with skin may cause transient hyperpigmentation.
• Do not use vials that contain an oily film, which is indicative of decomposition. • Reconstituted solution is stable for 24 hours when refrigerated and protected from light. Solution contains no preservatives and should not be used as a multidose vial.

Compatibility

• **Y-site:** filgrastim ✦ fludarabine ✦ melphalan ✦ ondansetron ✦ piperacillin/tazobactam ✦ sargramostim ✦ vinorelbine.

Incompatibility
- **Y-site:** allopurinol sodium.
- **Additive:** sodium bicarbonate.

Rate of Administration
- **Intermittent Infusion:** Administer dose over 1–2 hours. Rapid infusion rate may cause local pain, burning at site, and flushing. Facial flushing may persist for 4 hours. • IV lines may be flushed with 5–10 ml of 0.9% NaCl prior to and following carmustine infusion.

≋ CLINICAL PRECAUTIONS

- Monitor vital signs prior to and frequently during therapy.
- Monitor hydration and nutritional status. Nausea and vomiting may be severe, often occurring within 2 hours of administration and persisting for 6 hours. Pretreatment with antiemetics may be useful.
- Observe IV site closely for redness/irritation. Instruct patient to notify nurse immediately if discomfort at IV site occurs. Confer with physician about application of ice to site. May cause hyperpigmentation of skin along vein.
- Assess pulmonary status for dyspnea or cough. Pulmonary infiltrates and irreversible fibrosis are usually associated with total doses greater than 1400 mg/m^2. Smoking increases the risk of adverse pulmonary reactions.
- Monitor for bone marrow depression. Assess for signs of bleeding (bleeding gums, bruising, petechiae; guaiac test stool, urine, and emesis). Avoid IM injections, use of rectal thermometer, and products containing aspirin, ibuprofen, or naproxen. Assess for fever, chills, sore throat, and signs of infection during period of neutropenia. Use cautiously in patients with active infections. Anemia may occur. Monitor for increased fatigue, dyspnea, and orthostatic hypotension. Additive bone marrow depression will occur with other antineoplastic agents or radiation therapy.
- Patients with chronic debilitating illnesses or decreased bone marrow reserve may be more sensitive to the bone marrow–depressing properties of carmustine.

• Carmustine should be avoided in pregnancy, especially during the first trimester. Use cautiously in patients with child-bearing potential. Breast-feeding should also be avoided (Pregnancy Category D).

Lab Test Considerations

• Monitor CBC, differential, and platelet count prior to and periodically throughout therapy. The nadir of thrombocytopenia occurs 4–5 weeks after a dose and the nadir of leukopenia occurs in 5–6 weeks. Recovery usually occurs within 6–7 weeks but may take 10–12 weeks with prolonged therapy. Withhold the dose if the platelet count is <100,000/mm^3 or leukocyte count is <4000/mm^3. Anemia is usually mild. • Monitor liver function studies. May cause mild, reversible increase in AST (SGOT), alkaline phosphatase, and bilirubin. • Monitor renal studies for elevated BUN.

Patient/Family Teaching

• Instruct patient to notify physician promptly if fever, sore throat, signs of infection, bleeding gums, bruising, petechiae; blood in stools, urine, or emesis; increased fatigue, dyspnea, or orthostatic hypotension occurs. Caution patient to avoid crowds and persons with known infections. Instruct patient to use a soft toothbrush and electric razor, and to be especially careful to avoid falls. Patients should be cautioned not to drink alcoholic beverages or take medications containing aspirin, ibuprofen, or naproxen because these may precipitate gastric bleeding. • Instruct patient to notify physician if shortness of breath or increased cough occurs. Encourage patient not to smoke. • Patients with childbearing potential should use a nonhormonal method of contraception. • Carmustine may decrease antibody response to live virus vaccines and increase the risk of adverse reactions. Advise patient not to receive any vaccinations without advice of physician. • Instruct patient to inspect oral mucosa for erythema and ulceration. If ulceration occurs, advise patient to notify physician, rinse mouth with water after eating, and use sponge brush. • Discuss with patient the possibility of hair loss. Explore methods of coping. • Emphasize the need for periodic lab tests to monitor therapy.

≋ PHARMACOLOGIC PROFILE

Indications

• Carmustine is used alone or in combination with other treatment modalities (surgery, radiation) in the treatment of brain tumors, multiple myeloma, Hodgkin's disease, and other lymphomas.

Action

• Carmustine inhibits DNA and RNA synthesis (cell cycle–phase nonspecific). This results in death of rapidly replicating cells, especially malignant ones.

Time/Action Profile (effect on platelet count)

Onset	Peak	Duration
days	4–5 wk	6 wk

Pharmacokinetics

• **Distribution:** Carmustine is highly lipid soluble and readily penetrates CSF. This accounts for its effectiveness in the treatment of brain tumors. In addition, it enters breast milk. • **Metabolism and Execretion:** Metabolism is rapid, with some metabolites having antineoplastic activity. • **Half-life:** 15–30 minutes.

Contraindications

• Hypersensitivity to carmustine. • Carmustine should not be used during pregnancy or lactation.

Adverse Reactions and Side Effects*

• **Resp:** pulmonary infiltrates, pulmonary fibrosis • **GI:** nausea, vomiting, diarrhea, esophagitis, anorexia, hepatotoxicity • **GU:** renal failure • **Derm:** alopecia • **Hemat:** leukopenia, thrombocytopenia, anemia • **Local:** pain at IV site.

---

*Underlines indicate most frequent; CAPITALS indicate life-threatening.

Cefamandole Nafate	*Anti-infective* *(second generation* *cephalosporin)*
Mandol	**pH 6–8.5** **contains 3.3 mEq Na/g**

ADMINISTRATION CONSIDERATIONS

Usual Dose

ADULTS: 500–2000 mg q 4–8 hr (up to 12 g/day). *Perioperative prophylaxis:* 1–2 g 30–60 min preoperatively, then q 6 hr for up to 24 hr.

CHILDREN >1 mo: 8.3–16.7 mg/kg q 4 hr, 12.5–25 mg/kg q 6 hr, or 16.7–33.3 mg/kg q 8 hr (not to exceed 150 mg/kg/day or adult dose).

Dilution

• Powder is difficult to dissolve. **Reconstitute** by keeping powder at stopper end of the vial and adding diluent to other end of vial. Shake vigorously to dissolve. • Reconstitution causes gas to form. Vial can be vented prior to withdrawal, or use gas to facilitate withdrawal of solution by inverting the vial over the syringe needle, allowing the solution the flow into the needle. • Solution ranges in color from light yellow to amber. Do not use if solution is a different color or contains a precipitate. • **Direct IV: Dilute** each g with 10 ml of sterile water for injection, D5W, or 0.9% NaCl. • **Intermittent Infusion:** Reconstituted solution may be **further diluted** in 100 ml of 0.9% NaCl, D5W, D10W, D5/0.25% NaCl, D5/0.45% NaCl, D5/0.9% NaCl, or D5/LR. Solution is stable for 24 hours at room temperature and 96 hours if refrigerated. • **Continuous Infusion:** May be diluted in up to 1000 ml for continuous infusion.

Compatibility

• **Syringe:** heparin.

• **Y-site:** acyclovir • cyclophosphamide • hydromorphone • magnesium sulfate • meperidine • morphine • perphenazine.

• **Additive:** clindamycin.

Incompatibility

- **Syringe:** cimetidine ◆ gentamicin ◆ tobramycin.
- **Y-site:** hetastarch. Aminoglycosides should be administered at a separate site, at least 1 hour apart, if given concurrently.
- **Additive:** calcium glucceptate ◆ calcium gluconate ◆ gentamicin ◆ ranitidine ◆ tobramycin.
- **Solution:** lactated Ringer's solution ◆ Ringer's solution.

Rate of Administration

- **Direct IV:** Administer slowly over 3–5 minutes. ● **Intermittent Infusion:** Administer over 15–30 minutes.

≋ CLINICAL PRECAUTIONS

- Obtain specimens for culture and sensitivity prior to initiating therapy. First dose may be given before results are available.
- Determine past history of allergic reactions to penicillins or cephalosporins. Persons with a negative history of penicillin sensitivity may still have an allergic response. Observe patient for signs and symptoms of anaphylaxis (rash, pruritus, laryngeal edema, wheezing). Discontinue the drug immediately if these occur. Keep epinephrine, an antihistamine, and resuscitation equipment close by in the event of an anaphylactic reaction.
- Assess patient for infection (vital signs; appearance of wound, sputum, urine, and stool; WBC).
- Monitor for phlebitis. Change IV site every 48–72 hours to prevent phlebitis.
- Assess renal function. Cefamandole is excreted primarily by the kidneys. Dosage adjustment may be necessary in renal impairment and in elderly patients. Decrease dose and/or increase dosing interval if creatinine clearance is 80 ml/min/1.73m^2 or less.
- Probenecid decreases excretion and increases blood levels of cefamandole.
- Cefamandole crosses the placenta and enters breast milk in low concentrations. Although safe use in pregnancy has not been established, cefamandole has been used during obstetrical surgery (Pregnancy Category B).

Lab Test Considerations

• Cefamandole may cause hypoprothrombinemia. Monitor prothrombin time and assess for bleeding (guaiac test stools; check for hematuria, bleeding gums, ecchymosis). Risk factors for this adverse reaction are hepatic or renal dysfunction, thrombocytopenia, concurrent anticoagulant or antiplatelet therapy, malnutrition, old age, or the presence of chronic debilitating illness. If bleeding occurs, it can be reversed with vitamin K, or prophylactic vitamin K 10 mg/wk may be given. • May cause transient increase in BUN, AST (SGOT), ALT (SGPT), LDH, and alkaline phosphatase. • May cause false-positive proteinuria, Coombs' test, and urine glucose when tested with copper sulfate method (Clinitest). Use glucose enzymatic tests (Clinistix or Tes-Tape) to test urine glucose.

Patient/Family Teaching

• Advise patient to report the signs of superinfection (furry overgrowth on the tongue, vaginal itching or discharge, loose or foul-smelling stools) and allergy. • Caution patient that if alcohol is ingested within 48–72 hours of cefamandole, a disulfiram-like reaction (abdominal cramps, nausea, vomiting, hypotension, palpitations, dyspnea, tachycardia, sweating, flushing) may occur. Alcohol and medications containing alcohol should be avoided during and for several days after therapy. • Instruct patient that diarrhea is a side effect, but if diarrhea becomes bloody, contains pus or mucus, or is accompanied by fever, contact physician as pseudomembranous colitis has been associated with cephalosporin use. Advise patient not to treat diarrhea without consulting physician or pharmacist.

 PHARMACOLOGIC PROFILE

Indications

• Cefamandole is used in the treatment of the following infections due to susceptible organisms: respiratory tract infections, skin and skin structure infections, bone and joint infections, urinary tract and gynecologic infections, septicemia, and intra-abdominal and biliary tract infections. • Cefamandole has also been used as a perioperative prophylactic anti-infective.

Action

• Cefamandole binds to the bacterial cell wall membrane, causing cell death. It is active against many Gram-positive cocci including *Streptococcus pneumoniae,* group A beta-hemolytic streptococci, and penicillinase-producing staphylococci. In addition, cefamandole has increased activity against several Gram-negative pathogens, including *Haemophilus influenzae, Acinetobacter, Enterobacter, Escherichia coli, Klebsiella pneumoniae, Neisseria gonorrhoeae* (including penicillinase-producing strains), *Providencia, Proteus,* and *Serratia.* • It is also active against *Bacteroides fragilis,* but has no activity against methicillin-resistant staphylococci or enterococci.

Time/Action Profile (blood levels)

Onset	Peak
rapid	end of infusion

Pharmacokinetics

• **Distribution:** Cefamandole is widely distributed, crosses the placenta, and enters breast milk in low concentrations. CSF penetration is poor. • **Metabolism and Excretion:** Excretion occurs primarily as unchanged drug eliminated by the kidneys. • **Half-life:** 0.5–1.2 hours (increased in renal impairment).

Contraindications

• Cefamandole is contraindicated in patients with a history of hypersensitivity to cephalosporins or serious hypersensitivity to penicillins.

Adverse Reactions and Side Effects*

• **GI:** <u>nausea</u>, <u>vomiting</u>, cramps, <u>diarrhea</u>, PSEUDOMEMBRANOUS COLITIS • **Derm:** <u>rashes</u>, urticaria • **Hemat:** blood dyscrasias, hemolytic anemia, bleeding • **Local:** <u>phlebitis</u> at IV site • **Misc:** superinfection, allergic reactions including ANAPHYLAXIS and serum sickness.

---

*<u>Underlines</u> indicate most frequent; CAPITALS indicate life-threatening.

Cefazolin Sodium	*Anti-infective (first generation cephalosporin)*
Ancef, Kefzol, Zolicef	pH 4.5–7 contains 2 mEq Na/g

 ADMINISTRATION CONSIDERATIONS

Usual Dose

ADULTS: 250 mg–2 g q 6–12 hr (up to 12 g/day). *Perioperative prophylaxis:* 1 g 30–60 min preoperatively, 0.5–1 g during procedure, then 0.5–1 g q 8 hr for up to 24 hr.

CHILDREN AND INFANTS >1 mo: 6.25–25 mg/kg q 6 hr or 8.3–33.3 mg/kg q 8 hr.

Dilution

• **Direct IV: Dilute** in 10 ml of sterile water for injection.
• **Intermittent Infusion:** Reconstituted 500 mg or 1 g solution may be **further diluted** with 50–100 ml of 0.9% NaCl, D5W, D10W, D5/0.25% NaCl, D5/0.45% NaCl, D5/0.9% NaCl, D5/LR, or lactated Ringer's solution for a concentration of 75–125 mg/ml. Also available as premixed solution of 500 mg or 1 g cefazolin in 50 ml of D5W. • Solution is stable for 24 hours at room temperature or 96 hours if refrigerated. Do not use a solution that is cloudy or contains a precipitate.

Compatibility

• **Syringe:** heparin • vitamin B complex.
• **Y-site:** acyclovir • allopurinol sodium • atracurium • calcium gluconate • cyclophosphamide • diltiazem • enalaprilat • esmolol • famotidine • filgrastim • fluconazole • fludarabine • foscarnet • gallium nitrate • insulin • labetalol • lidocaine • magnesium sulfate • melphalan • meperidine • morphine • multivitamins • ondansetron • pancuronium • perphenazine • sargramostim • tacrolimus • vecuronium • vitamin B complex with C.
• **Additive:** aztreonam • clindamycin • fluconazole • metronidazole.

Incompatibility

- **Syringe:** ascorbic acid ✦ cimetidine ✦ lidocaine.
- **Y-site:** idarubicin ✦ vinorelbine. Aminoglycosides should be administered at a separate site, at least 1 hour apart, if given concurrently.
- **Additive:** amikacin ✦ atracurium ✦ bleomycin.

Rate of Administration

- **Direct IV:** Administer slowly over 3–5 minutes. • **Intermittent Infusion:** Administer over 30–60 minutes.

☰ CLINICAL PRECAUTIONS

- Obtain specimens for culture and sensitivity prior to initiating therapy. First dose may be given before results are available.
- Determine past history of allergic reactions to penicillins or cephalosporins. Persons with a negative history of penicillin sensitivity may still have an allergic response. Observe patient for signs and symptoms of anaphylaxis (rash, pruritus, laryngeal edema, wheezing). Discontinue the drug immediately if these occur. Keep epinephrine, an antihistamine, and resuscitation equipment close by in the event of an anaphylactic reaction.
- Assess patient for infection (vital signs; appearance of wound, sputum, urine, and stool; WBC).
- Monitor for phlebitis. Change IV site every 48–72 hours to prevent phlebitis.
- Assess renal function; monitor intake and output, and daily weight. Cefazolin is excreted primarily by the kidneys. Dosage adjustment may be necessary in renal impairment and in elderly patients. Decrease dose and/or increase dosing interval if creatinine clearance is less than 55 ml/min in adults or 70 ml/min in children. Cefazolin may also potentiate nephrotoxicity from other nephrotoxic agents. Risk of nephrotoxicity is greater in patients over 50 years of age.
- Probenecid decreases excretion and increases blood levels of cefazolin.
- Cefazolin crosses the placenta and enters breast milk in low concentrations. Safe use in pregnancy has not been established (Pregnancy Category B).

Lab Test Considerations

• May cause transient increase in BUN, AST (SGOT), ALT (SGPT), and alkaline phosphatase. • May cause false-positive results for Coombs' test and urine glucose when tested with copper sulfate method (Clinitest). Use glucose enzymatic tests (Clinistix or Tes-Tape) to test urine glucose.

Patient/Family Teaching

• Advise patient to report the signs of superinfection (furry overgrowth on the tongue, vaginal itching or discharge, loose or foul-smelling stools) and allergy. • Inform patient that diarrhea is a side effect, but if diarrhea becomes bloody, contains pus or mucus, or is accompanied by fever, contact physician as pseudomembranous colitis has been associated with cephalosporin use. Advise patient not to treat diarrhea without consulting physician or pharmacist.

 PHARMACOLOGIC PROFILE

Indications

• Cefazolin is used in the treatment of lower respiratory tract infections, serious skin and skin structure infections, urinary tract infections, and intra-abdominal infections due to susceptible organisms. • Cefazolin has also been used as a perioperative prophylactic anti-infective.

Action

• Cefazolin binds to the bacterial cell wall membrane, causing cell death. It displays activity against many Gram-positive cocci including *Streptococcus pneumoniae,* group A beta-hemolytic streptococci, and penicillinase-producing staphylococci. • Cefazolin also has activity against some Gram-negative rods including *Klebsiella pneumoniae, Proteus mirabilis,* and *Escherichia coli,* but is not active against methicillin-resistant staphylococci, *Bacteroides fragilis,* or enterococci.

Time/Action Profile (blood levels)

Onset	Peak
rapid	end of infusion

Pharmacokinetics

• **Distribution:** Cefazolin is widely distributed, crosses the placenta, and enters breast milk in low concentrations. Penetration into CSF is minimal. • **Metabolism and Excretion:** Excreted almost entirely unchanged by the kidneys. • **Half-life:** 1.2–2.2 hours (increased in renal impairment).

Contraindications

• History of hypersensitivity to cephalosporins or serious hypersensitivity to penicillins.

Adverse Reactions and Side Effects*

• **CNS:** SEIZURES (high doses) • **GI:** <u>nausea</u>, <u>vomiting</u>, cramps, <u>diarrhea</u>, PSEUDOMEMBRANOUS COLITIS • **Derm:** <u>rashes</u>, urticaria • **Hemat:** Blood dyscrasias, hemolytic anemia • **Local:** <u>phlebitis</u> at IV site • **Misc:** superinfection, allergic reactions including ANAPHYLAXIS and serum sickness.

Cefmetazole Sodium	*Anti-infective (second generation cephalosporin)*
Zefazone	**pH 4.2–6.2** **contains 2 mEq Na/g**

 ADMINISTRATION CONSIDERATIONS

Usual Dose

ADULTS: 2 g q 6–12 hr. *Perioperative prophylaxis:* 1–2 g 30–90 min preoperatively; may be repeated q 8 hr for 2 more doses.

Dilution

• **Intermittent Infusion: Reconstitute** with sterile water, bacteriostatic water, or 0.9% NaCl for injection. Reconstituted solution may be **further diluted** to concentrations of 1–20 mg/ml in 0.9% NaCl, D5W, or lactated Ringer's solution.

---

*<u>Underlines</u> indicate most frequent; CAPITALS indicate life-threatening.

• Solution is stable for 24 hours at room temperature and 7 days if refrigerated.

Incompatibility

• **Y-site:** Aminoglycosides should be administered at a separate site, at least 1 hour apart, if given concurrently.

Rate of Administration

• **Intermittent Infusion:** Administer over 30–60 minutes.

☰ CLINICAL PRECAUTIONS

- Obtain specimens for culture and sensitivity prior to initiating therapy. First dose may be given before results are available.
- Determine history of allergic reactions to penicillins or cephalosporins. Persons with a negative history of penicillin sensitivity may still have an allergic response. Observe patient for signs and symptoms of anaphylaxis (rash, pruritus, laryngeal edema, wheezing). Discontinue the drug immediately if these occur. Keep epinephrine, an antihistamine, and resuscitation equipment close by in the event of an anaphylactic reaction.
- Assess patient for infection (vital signs; appearance of wound, sputum, urine, and stool; WBC).
- Monitor for phlebitis. Change IV site every 48–72 hours to prevent phlebitis.
- Assess renal function. Cefmetazole is excreted primarily by the kidneys. Dosage adjustment may be necessary in renal impairment and geriatric patients. If creatinine clearance is less than 40 ml/min, increased dosing interval is recommended.
- Probenecid decreases excretion and increases blood levels of cefmetazole.
- Cefmetazole crosses the placenta and enters breast milk in low concentrations. Although safety in pregnancy has not been established, cefmetazole has been used during obstetrical surgery (Pregnancy Category B).

Lab Test Considerations

• Cefmetazole may cause hypoprothrombinemia. Monitor prothrombin time and assess for bleeding (guaiac test stools; check for hematuria, bleeding gums, ecchymosis). Risk factors for this adverse reaction are hepatic or renal dysfunction, thrombocytopenia, concurrent anticoagulant or antiplatelet therapy, malnutrition, old age, or the presence of chronic debilitating illnesses. If bleeding occurs, it can be reversed with vitamin K, or prophylactic vitamin K 10 mg/wk may be given. • May cause transient increase in BUN, AST (SGOT), ALT (SGPT), LDH, and alkaline phosphatase. • May cause false-positive proteinuria, Coombs' test, and urine glucose when tested with copper sulfate method (Clinitest). Use glucose enzymatic tests (Clinistix or Tes-Tape) to test urine glucose.

Patient/Family Teaching

• Advise patient to report the signs of superinfection (furry overgrowth on the tongue, vaginal itching or discharge, loose or foul-smelling stools) and allergy. • Caution patient that if alcohol is ingested within 48–72 hours of cefmetazole, a disulfiram-like reaction (abdominal cramps, nausea, vomiting, hypotension, palpitations, dyspnea, tachycardia, sweating, flushing) may occur. Alcohol and medications containing alcohol should be avoided during therapy and for several days thereafter. • Instruct patient that diarrhea is a side effect, but if diarrhea becomes bloody, contains pus or mucus, or is accompanied by fever, contact physician as pseudomembranous colitis has been associated with cephalosporin use. Advise patient not to treat diarrhea without consulting physician or pharmacist.

≋ PHARMACOLOGIC PROFILE

Indications

• Cefmetazole is used in the treatment of the following infections due to susceptible organisms: lower repiratory tract infections, skin and skin structure infections, urinary tract infections, and intra-abdominal infections. • It has also been used as a perioperative prophylactic anti-infective.

Action

• Cefmetazole binds to the bacterial cell wall membrane, causing cell death. It is active against many Gram-positive cocci, including *Streptococcus pneumoniae,* group A beta-hemolytic streptococci, and penicillinase-producing staphylococci; while possessing increased activity against several Gram-negative pathogens, including *Haemophilus influenzae, Acinetobacter, Enterobacter, Escherichia coli, Klebsiella* sp, *Neisseria gonorrhoeae* (including penicillinase-producing strains), *Providencia, Proteus,* and *Serratia.* • It is also active against *Bacteroides fragilis,* but has no activity against methicillin-resistant staphylococci or enterococci.

Time/Action Profile (blood levels)

Onset	Peak
rapid	end of infusion

Pharmacokinetics

• **Distribution:** Cefmetazole is widely distributed, crosses the placenta, and enters breast milk in low concentrations. Penetration into CSF is minimal. • **Metabolism and Excretion:** 85% of cefmetazole is excreted unchanged by the kidneys. • **Half-life:** 0.8–1.8 hours (increased in renal impairment).

Contraindications

• Cefmetazole is contraindicated in patients with hypersensitivity to cephalosporins or serious hypersensitivity to penicillins.

Adverse Reactions and Side Effects*

• **GI:** <u>nausea</u>, <u>vomiting</u>, cramps, <u>diarrhea</u>, PSEUDOMEMBRANOUS COLITIS • **Derm:** <u>rashes</u>, urticaria • **Hemat:** blood dyscrasias, hemolytic anemia, bleeding, bruising • **Local:** <u>phlebitis</u> at IV site • **Misc:** superinfection, allergic reactions including ANAPHYLAXIS and serum sickness.

---

*<u>Underlines</u> indicate most frequent; CAPITALS indicate life-threatening.

Cefonicid Sodium	*Anti-infective (second generation cephalosporin)*
Monocid	pH 3.5–6.5 contains 3.7 mEq Na/g

≋ ADMINISTRATION CONSIDERATIONS

Usual Dose

ADULTS: 0.5–1 g/day, single dose (up to 2 g/day). *Perioperative prophylaxis:* 1 g 60 min preoperatively.

Dilution

• **Direct IV:** Reconstitute each dose with 2 ml of sterile water for injection to each 500-mg vial and 2.5 ml to each 1-g vial for concentrations of 220 and 325 mg/ml, respectively. Solution may be colorless to light amber. • **Intermittent Infusion:** Reconstituted doses may be **further diluted** with 50–100 ml of D5W, D10W, D5/LR, D5/0.25% NaCl, D5/0.45% NaCl, D5/0.9% NaCl, 0.9% NaCl, or Ringer's or lactated Ringer's solution. • Solution is stable for 24 hours at room temperature or 72 hours if refrigerated.

Compatibility

• **Y-site:** acyclovir.
• **Additive:** clindamycin.

Incompatibility

• **Y-site:** filgrastim • sargramostim. Aminoglycosides should be administered at a separate site, at least 1 hour apart, if given concurrently.

Rate of Administration

• **Direct IV:** Administer slowly over 3–5 minutes. • **Intermittent Infusion:** Administer over 30 minutes.

≋ CLINICAL PRECAUTIONS

• Obtain specimens for culture and sensitivity prior to initiating therapy. First dose may be given before results are available.

- Determine history of allergic reactions to penicillins or cephalosporins. Persons with a negative history of penicillin sensitivity may still have an allergic response. Observe patient for signs and symptoms of anaphylaxis (rash, pruritus, laryngeal edema, wheezing). Discontinue the drug immediately if these occur. Keep epinephrine, an antihistamine, and resuscitation equipment close by in the event of an anaphylactic reaction.
- Assess patient for infection (vital signs; appearance of wound, sputum, urine, and stool; WBC).
- Monitor for phlebitis. Change IV site every 48–72 hours to prevent phlebitis.
- Assess renal function; monitor intake and output, and daily weight. Cefonicid is excreted primarily by the kidneys. Dosage adjustment may be necessary in renal impairment and geriatric patients. Decreased dose and/or increased dosing interval is recommended if creatinine clearance is less than 80 ml/min.
- Probenecid decreases excretion and increases blood levels of cefonicid.
- Cefonicid crosses the placenta and enters breast milk in low concentrations. Safe use in pregnancy has not been established (Pregnancy Category B).

Lab Test Considerations

- May cause transient increase in AST (SGOT), ALT (SGPT), LDH, and alkaline phosphatase. • May cause false-positive results for Coombs' test and urine glucose when tested with copper sulfate method (Clinitest). Use glucose enzymatic tests (Clinistix or Tes-Tape) to test urine glucose.

Patient/Family Teaching

- Advise patient to report the signs of superinfection (furry overgrowth on the tongue, vaginal itching or discharge, loose or foul-smelling stools) and allergy. • Inform patient that diarrhea is a side effect, but if diarrhea becomes bloody, contains pus or mucus, or is accompanied by fever, contact physician as pseudomembranous colitis has been associated with cephalosporin use. Advise patient not to treat diarrhea without consulting physician or pharmacist.

> • **Home Care Issues:** Instruct family or care-giver on dilution, rate, and administration of drug and proper care of IV equipment.

≋ PHARMACOLOGIC PROFILE

Indications

• Cefonicid is used in the treatment of the following infections due to susceptible organisms: respiratory tract infections, skin and skin structure infections, bone and joint infections, urinary tract and gynecologic infections, and septicemia. It has also been used as a perioperative prophylactic anti-infective.

Action

• Cefonicid binds to the bacterial cell wall membrane, causing cell death. • It is active against many Gram-positive cocci, including *Streptococcus pneumoniae,* group A beta-hemolytic streptococci, and penicillinase-producing staphylococci, while possessing increased activity against several other important Gram-negative pathogens, including *Haemophilus influenzae, Acinetobacter, Enterobacter, Escherichia coli, Klebsiella pneumoniae, Neisseria gonorrhoeae* (including penicillinase-producing strains), *Providencia, Proteus,* and *Serratia.* • It is also active against *Bacteroides fragilis,* but has no activity against methicillin-resistant staphylococci or enterococci.

Time/Action Profile (blood levels)

Onset	Peak
rapid	end of infusion

Pharmacokinetics

• **Distribution:** Cefonicid is widely distributed, crosses the placenta, and enters breast milk in low concentrations. Penetration into CSF is minimal. • **Metabolism and Excretion:** Cefonicid is excreted primarily unchanged by the kidneys. • **Half-life:** 4.5 hours (increased in renal impairment).

Contraindications

• Cefonicid is contraindicated in patients with hypersensitivity to cephalosporins or serious hypersensitivity to penicillins.

Adverse Reactions and Side Effects*

• **CNS:** SEIZURES (high doses) • **Derm:** <u>rashes</u>, urticaria • **GI:** <u>nausea</u>, <u>vomiting</u>, cramps, <u>diarrhea</u>, PSEUDOMEMBRANOUS COLITIS • **Hemat:** blood dyscrasias, hemolytic anemia • **Local:** <u>phlebitis</u> at IV site • **Misc:** superinfection, allergic reactions including ANAPHYLAXIS and serum sickness.

Cefoperazone Sodium	*Anti-infective (third generation cephalosporin)*
Cefobid	**pH 4.5–6.5 contains 1.5 mEq Na/g**

≋ ADMINISTRATION CONSIDERATIONS

Usual Dose

ADULTS: 2–4 g/day in divided doses q 12 hr. For serious infections 2–4 g q 8 hr or 3–6 g q 12 hr (up to 16 g/day).
CHILDREN: 25–50 mg/kg q 6–12 hr (unlabeled).

Dilution

• **Intermittent Infusion:** Reconstitute each gram of cefoperazone with at least 2.8 ml of sterile or bacteriostatic water for injection, D5W, or 0.9% NaCl for a concentration not to exceed 50 mg/ml. Do not use preparations containing benzyl alcohol when used for neonates. Shake vigorously and allow to stand following reconstitution for visualization of clarity. • Each gram should be **further diluted** in 20–40 ml of 0.9% NaCl, D5W, D10W, D5/0.25% NaCl, D5/0.9% NaCl, D5/LR, or lactated Ringer's solution. • Solution is stable for 24 hours at room temperature or 5 days if refrigerated. • **Continuous Infusion:** A concentration of 2–25 mg/ml can be used.

Compatibility

• **Syringe:** heparin.
• **Y-site:** allopurinol sodium ✦ acyclovir ✦ cyclophosphamide ✦ enalaprilat ✦ esmolol ✦ famotidine ✦ fludarabine

---

*<u>Underlines</u> indicate most frequent; CAPITALS indicate life-threatening.

• foscarnet • hydromorphone • magnesium sulfate • melphalan • morphine.
  • **Additive:** cimetidine • clindamycin • furosemide.

Incompatibility
• **Syringe:** doxapram.
• **Y-site:** filgrastim • hetastarch • labetalol • meperidine
  • ondansetron • perphenazine • promethazine • sargramostim • vinorelbine. • If given concurrently, aminoglycosides should be administered at a separate site, at least
1 hour apart.

Rate of Administration
  • **Intermittent Infusion:** Administer over 15–60 minutes.

≋ CLINICAL PRECAUTIONS

• Obtain specimens for culture and sensitivity prior to initiating therapy. First dose may be given before results are
  available.
• Determine history of allergic reactions to penicillins or
  cephalosporins. Persons with a negative history of penicillin sensitivity may still have an allergic response. Observe patient for signs and symptoms of anaphylaxis
  (rash, pruritus, laryngeal edema, wheezing). Discontinue
  the drug immediately if these occur. Keep epinephrine,
  an antihistamine, and resuscitation equipment close by
  in the event of an anaphylactic reaction.
• Assess patient for infection (vital signs; appearance of
  wound, sputum, urine, and stool; WBC).
• Monitor for phlebitis. Change IV site every 48–72 hours
  to prevent phlebitis.
• Assess hepatic function. Cefoperazone is excreted in bile.
  Patients with severe hepatic impairment or biliary obstruction should not receive more than 4 g/day. Patients
  with both hepatic and renal impairment should not receive more than 1–2 g/day.
• Cefoperazone crosses the placenta and enters breast milk
  in low concentrations. Safe use in pregnancy, lactation,
  and children younger than age 12 has not been established (Pregnancy Category B).

Lab Test Considerations

• Cefoperazone may cause hypoprothrombinemia. Monitor prothrombin time and assess for bleeding (guaiac test stools; check for hematuria, bleeding gums, ecchymosis). Risk factors for this adverse reaction are hepatic or renal dysfunction, thrombocytopenia, concurrent anticoagulant or antiplatelet therapy, malnutrition, old age, or the presence of chronic debilitating illness. If bleeding occurs, it can be reversed with vitamin K, or prophylactic vitamin K 10 mg/wk may be given. • May cause increase in BUN, AST (SGOT), ALT (SGPT), LDH, and alkaline phosphatase. Peak and trough levels should be drawn periodically on patients with hepatic, biliary, or renal dysfunction. • May cause false-positive results for Coombs' test and urine glucose when tested with copper sulfate method (Clinitest). Use glucose enzymatic tests (Clinistix or Tes-Tape) to test urine glucose.

Patient/Family Teaching

• Advise patient to report the signs of superinfection (furry overgrowth on the tongue, vaginal itching or discharge, loose or foul-smelling stools) and allergy. • Caution patient that if alcohol is ingested within 48–72 hours of cefoperazone, a disulfiram-like reaction (abdominal cramps, nausea, vomiting, hypotension, palpitations, dyspnea, tachycardia, sweating, flushing) may occur. Alcohol and medications containing alcohol should be avoided during and for several days after therapy. • Inform patient that diarrhea is a side effect, but if diarrhea becomes bloody, contains pus or mucus, or is accompanied by fever, contact physician as pseudomembranous colitis has been associated with cephalosporin use. Advise patient not to treat diarrhea without consulting physician or pharmacist.

 PHARMACOLOGIC PROFILE

Indications

• Cefoperazone is used in the treatment of skin and skin structure infections, bone and joint infections, urinary tract and gynecologic infections, respiratory tract infections, intra-abdominal infections, and septicemia.

Action

- Cefoperazone binds to the bacterial cell wall membrane, causing cell death. • Cefoperazone is noted for activity against *Citrobacter, Enterobacter, Escherichia coli, Klebsiella pneumoniae, Pseudomonas aeruginosa, Haemophilus influenzae, Neisseria, Proteus, Providencia,* and *Serratia.* • In addition, cefoperazone has some activity against anaerobes including *Bacteroides fragilis.* • Its activity against staphylococci is diminished in comparison to second-generation cephalosporins, while action against Gram-negative pathogens is enhanced, even for organisms resistant to first- and second-generation agents.

Time/Action Profile (blood levels)

Onset	Peak
rapid	end of infusion

Pharmacokinetics

- **Distribution:** Cefoperazone is widely distributed, crosses the placenta, and enters breast milk in low concentrations. • **Metabolism and Excretion:** Cefoperazone is excreted in bile. • **Half-life:** 1.6–2 hours.

Contraindications

- Cefoperazone is contraindicated in patients with hypersensitivity to cephalosporins or serious hypersensitivity to penicillins.

Adverse Reactions and Side Effects*

- **Derm:** <u>rashes</u>, urticaria • **GI:** <u>nausea</u>, <u>vomiting</u>, <u>diarrhea</u>, cramps, PSEUDOMEMBRANOUS COLITIS • **Hemat:** blood dyscrasias, hemolytic anemia, bleeding • **Local:** <u>phlebitis</u> at IV site • **Misc:** superinfection, allergic reactions including ANAPHYLAXIS and serum sickness.

---

*<u>Underlines</u> indicate most frequent; CAPITALS indicate life-threatening.

Cefotaxime Sodium

*Anti-infective
(third generation
cephalosporin)*

Claforan

pH 4.5–7.5
contains 2.2 mEq Na/g

 ADMINISTRATION CONSIDERATIONS

Usual Dose

ADULTS AND CHILDREN >50 kg: 500 mg–2 g q 4–12 hr (up to 12 g/day).

CHILDREN >1 mo OR <50 kg: 8.3–30 mg/kg q 4 hr or 12.5–45 mg/kg q 6 hr up to 200 mg/kg/day.

INFANTS 1–4 wk: 50 mg/kg q 8 hr.

INFANTS 0–1 wk: 50 mg/kg q 12 hr.

Dilution

• **Direct IV: Dilute** in 10 ml of sterile or bacteriostatic water for injection for a concentration of 100–200 mg/ml. Do not use preparations with benzyl alcohol for neonates. • **Intermittent Infusion:** Reconstituted solution may be **further diluted** in 50–100 ml of D5W, D10W, lactated Ringer's solution, D5/0.25% NaCl, D5/0.45% NaCl, or D/0.9% NaCl for a concentration of 20–60 mg/ml. • Solution is stable for 24 hours at room temperature and for 5 days if refrigerated.

Compatibility

• **Syringe:** heparin.

• **Y-site:** acyclovir ◆ cyclophosphamide ◆ diltiazem ◆ famotidine ◆ fludarabine ◆ hydromorphone ◆ magnesium sulfate ◆ melphalan ◆ meperidine ◆ morphine ◆ ondansetron ◆ perphenazine ◆ sargramostim ◆ tolazoline ◆ vinorelbine.

• **Additive:** clindamycin ◆ metronidazole.

Incompatibility

• **Syringe:** doxapram.

• **Y-site:** allopurinol sodium ◆ filgrastim ◆ fluconazole ◆ hetastarch. • Aminoglycosides should be administered at a separate site, at least 1 hour apart, if given concurrently.

• **Additive:** aminophylline ◆ sodium bicarbonate.

Rate of Administration

• **Direct IV:** Administer slowly over 3–5 minutes. • **Intermittent Infusion:** Administer over 30 minutes.

≋ CLINICAL PRECAUTIONS

• Obtain specimens for culture and sensitivity prior to initiating therapy. First dose may be given before results are available.
• Determine history of allergic reactions to penicillins or cephalosporins. Persons with a negative history of penicillin sensitivity may still have an allergic response. Observe patient for signs and symptoms of anaphylaxis (rash, pruritus, laryngeal edema, wheezing). Discontinue the drug immediately if these occur. Keep epinephrine, an antihistamine, and resuscitation equipment close by in the event of an anaphylactic reaction.
• Assess patient for infection (vital signs; appearance of wound, sputum, urine, and stool; WBC).
• Monitor for phlebitis. Change IV site every 48–72 hours to prevent phlebitis.
• Assess renal function; monitor intake and output, and daily weight. Cefotaxime is excreted primarily by the kidneys. Dosage adjustment may be necessary in patients with severe renal impairment or geriatric patients. If creatinine clearance is less than 20 ml/min, decrease dose by 50%.
• Probenecid decreases excretion and increases blood levels of cefotaxime.
• Cefotaxime crosses the placenta and enters breast milk in low concentrations. Safe use in pregnancy has not been established (Pregnancy Category B).

Lab Test Considerations

• May cause transient increase in BUN, AST (SGOT), ALT (SGPT), LDH, and alkaline phosphatase. • May cause false-positive results for Coombs' test.

Patient/Family Teaching

• Advise patient to report the signs of superinfection (furry overgrowth on the tongue, vaginal itching or discharge, loose or foul-smelling stools) and allergy. • Inform patient that diarrhea is a side effect, but if diarrhea becomes bloody, contains pus or mucus, or is accompanied by fever, contact physician as pseudomembranous colitis has been associated with cephalosporin use. Advise patient not to treat diarrhea without consulting physician or pharmacist.

 PHARMACOLOGIC PROFILE

Indications

• Cefotaxime is used in the treatment of skin and skin structure infections, bone and joint infections, urinary tract and gynecologic infections, respiratory tract infections, intraabdominal infections, and septicemia and meningitis due to susceptible organisms. • It has also been used as a perioperative prophylactic anti-infective.

Action

• Cefotaxime binds to the bacterial cell wall membrane, causing cell death. The activity of cefotaxime against staphylococci is diminished in comparison to that of second-generation cephalosporins, whereas action against Gram-negative pathogens is enhanced, even for organisms resistant to first- and second-generation agents. Notable is increased action against *Citrobacter, Enterobacter, Escherichia coli, Klebsiella pneumoniae, Pseudomonas aeruginosa, Haemophilus influenzae, Neisseria, Proteus, Providencia,* and *Serratia.* • Cefotaxime has some activity against anaerobes including *Bacteroides fragilis.*

Time/Action Profile (blood levels)

Onset	Peak
rapid	end of infusion

Pharmacokinetics

• **Distribution:** Cefotaxime is widely distributed, crosses the placenta, and enters breast milk in low concentrations. Penetration into CSF is sufficient to treat meningitis. • **Metabolism and Excretion:** Partly metabolized and partly excreted in urine. • **Half-life:** 0.9–1.7 hours.

Contraindications

• Cefotaxime is contraindicated in patients with hypersensitivity to cephalosporins or serious hypersensitivity to penicillins.

Adverse Reactions and Side Effects*

• **Derm:** <u>rashes</u>, urticaria • **GI:** <u>nausea</u>, <u>vomiting</u>, <u>diarrhea</u>, cramps, PSEUDOMEMBRANOUS COLITIS • **Hemat:** blood dyscrasias, hemolytic anemia, bleeding • **Local:** <u>phlebitis</u> at IV site • **Misc:** superinfection, allergic reactions including ANAPHYLAXIS and serum sickness.

Cefotetan Disodium	Anti-infective /(second generation cephalosporin)
Cefotan	pH 4.5–6.5 contains 3.5 mEq Na/g

≋ ADMINISTRATION CONSIDERATIONS

Usual Dose

ADULTS: 0.5–3 g q 12 hr (1–2 g q 24 hr for urinary tract infections). *Perioperative prophylaxis:* 1 g 30–60 min preoperatively.

Dilution

• **Direct IV: Reconstitute** each gram of cefotetan with at least 10 ml of sterile water for injection, D5W, or 0.9% NaCl. Shake well and allow to stand until solution becomes clear. • Solution may range from colorless to yellow in color. • **Intermittent Infusion:** May be **further diluted** with 50–100 ml of D5W or 0.9% NaCl. • Solution is stable for 24 hours at room temperature or 96 hours if refrigerated.

Compatibility

• **Y-site:** allopurinol sodium ✦ amikacin ✦ aminophylline ✦ ampicillin ✦ atropine ✦ cimetidine ✦ digoxin ✦ diltiazem

---

*<u>Underlines</u> indicate most frequent; CAPITALS indicate life-threatening.

✦ dopamine ✦ epinephrine ✦ erythromycin ✦ famotidine ✦ filgrastim ✦ fluconazole ✦ fludarabine ✦ furosemide ✦ insulin ✦ melphalan ✦ meperidine ✦ mezlocillin ✦ morphine ✦ multivitamins ✦ oxytocin ✦ paclitaxel ✦ penicillin G potassium ✦ piperacillin ✦ sargramostim ✦ tacrolimus ✦ ticarcillin ✦ vitamin B complex with C.

Incompatibility
- **Syringe:** doxapram.
- **Y-site:** vinorelbine. Aminoglycosides should be administered at a separate site, at least 1 hour apart, if given concurrently.
- **Additive:** aminoglycosides ✦ heparin.

Rate of Administration
- **Direct IV:** Administer slowly over 3–5 minutes. • **Intermittent Infusion:** Administer over 20–30 minutes.

≋ CLINICAL PRECAUTIONS

- Obtain specimens for culture and sensitivity prior to initiating therapy. First dose may be given before results are available.
- Determine history of allergic reactions to penicillins or cephalosporins. Persons with a negative history of penicillin sensitivity may still have an allergic response. Observe patient for signs and symptoms of anaphylaxis (rash, pruritus, laryngeal edema, wheezing). Discontinue the drug immediately if these occur. Keep epinephrine, an antihistamine, and resuscitation equipment close by in the event of an anaphylactic reaction.
- Assess patient for infection (vital signs; appearance of wound, sputum, urine, and stool; WBC).
- Monitor for phlebitis. Change IV site every 48–72 hours to prevent phlebitis.
- Assess renal function. Cefotetan is excreted primarily by the kidneys. Dosage adjustment may be necessary in renal impairment and in the elderly. If creatinine clearance is 30 ml/min or less, decreased dose and/or increased dosing interval is recommended.
- Probenecid decreases excretion and increases blood levels of cefotetan.
- Cefotetan crosses the placenta and enters breast milk in

low concentrations. Although safety in pregnancy has not been established, cefotetan has been used during obstetrical surgery without adverse effects (Pregnancy Category B).

Lab Test Considerations

• Cefotetan may cause hypoprothrombinemia. Monitor prothrombin time and assess for bleeding (guaiac test stools; check for hematuria, bleeding gums, ecchymosis). Risk factors for this adverse reaction are hepatic or renal dysfunction, thrombocytopenia, concurrent anticoagulant or antiplatelet therapy, malnutrition, old age, or the presence of chronic debilitating illness. If bleeding occurs, it can be reversed with vitamin K, or prophylactic vitamin K 10 mg/wk may be given. • May cause transient increase in AST (SGOT), ALT (SGPT), LDH, and alkaline phosphatase. • May cause false-positive results for Coombs' test and urine glucose when tested with copper sulfate method (Clinitest). Use glucose enzymatic tests (Clinistix or Tes-Tape) to test urine glucose.

Patient/Family Teaching

• Advise patient to report the signs of superinfection (furry overgrowth on the tongue, vaginal itching or discharge, loose or foul-smelling stools) and allergy. • Caution patient that if alcohol is ingested within 48–72 hours of cefotetan, a disulfiram-like reaction (abdominal cramps, nausea, vomiting, hypotension, palpitations, dyspnea, tachycardia, sweating, flushing) may occur. Alcohol and medications containing alcohol should be avoided during and for several days after therapy. • Instruct patient that diarrhea is a side effect, but if diarrhea becomes bloody, contains pus or mucus, or is accompanied by fever, contact physician as pseudomembranous colitis has been associated with cephalosporin use. Advise patient not to treat diarrhea without consulting physician or pharmacist.

☰ PHARMACOLOGIC PROFILE

Indications

• Cefotetan is used in the treatment of the following infections due to susceptible organisms: respiratory tract infections, skin and skin structure infections, bone and joint infections, urinary tract and gynecologic infections, septicemia, and intra-abdominal and biliary tract infections. • It has also been used as a perioperative prophylactic anti-infective.

Action
• Cefotetan binds to the bacterial cell wall membrane, causing cell death. It is active against many Gram-positive cocci including *Streptococcus pneumoniae,* group A beta-hemolytic streptococci, and penicillinase-producing staphylococci, with additional increased activity against several Gram-negative pathogens, including *Haemophilus influenzae, Enterobacter, Escherichia coli, Klebsiella pneumoniae, Neisseria gonorrhoeae* (including penicillinase-producing strains), *Providencia, Proteus,* and *Serratia.* • It is also active against *Bacteroides fragilis,* but has no activity against methicillin-resistant staphylococci or enterococci.

Time/Action Profile

Onset	Peak
rapid	end of infusion

Pharmacokinetics
• **Distribution:** Cefotetan is widely distributed, although penetration into CSF is poor. It crosses the placenta and enters breast milk in low concentrations. • **Metabolism and Excretion:** Elimination of cefotetan occurs primarily through the kidneys as unchanged drug. • **Half-life:** 3–4.6 hours (increased in renal impairment).

Contraindications
• Cefotetan is contraindicated in patients with a history of hypersensitivity to cephalosporins or serious hypersensitivity to penicillins.

Adverse Reactions and Side Effects*
• **Derm:** rashes, urticaria • **GI:** nausea, vomiting, cramps, diarrhea, PSEUDOMEMBRANOUS COLITIS • **Hemat:** blood dyscrasias, hemolytic anemia • **Local:** phlebitis at IV site • **Misc:** superinfection, allergic reactions including ANAPHYLAXIS and serum sickness.

---

*Underlines indicate most frequent; CAPITALS indicate life-threatening.

Cefoxitin Sodium	*Anti-infective (second generation cephalosporin)*
Mefoxin	**pH 4.2–8** **contains 2.3 mEq Na/g**

≋ ADMINISTRATION CONSIDERATIONS

Usual Dose

ADULTS: 1–2 g q 6–8 hr (up to 12 g/day in divided doses q 4–6 hr). *Perioperative prophylaxis:* 2 g 30–60 min preoperatively, then 2 g q 6 hr for up to 24 hr.

CHILDREN ≥3 mo: 80–160 mg/kg/day in divided doses q 4–6 hr.

Dilution

• **Direct IV: Dilute** with 10 ml of sterile water for injection to each 1-g vial and 20 ml to each 2-g vial for a concentration not to exceed 180 mg/ml. Shake well and allow to stand until solution becomes clear. • Darkened powder does not alter potency. Solution may range from colorless to light amber. • **Intermittent Infusion:** May be **further diluted** with 50–100 ml of D5W, D10W, D5/0.25% NaCl, D5/0.45% NaCl, D5/0.9% NaCl, 0.9% NaCl, D5/LR, 5% sodium bicarbonate, or Ringer's or lactated Ringer's solution for a concentration of 10–40 mg/ml. • **Continuous Infusion:** May be diluted in 500–1000 ml.

Compatibility

• **Syringe:** heparin.
• **Y-site:** acyclovir • cyclophosphamide • diltiazem • famotidine • fluconazole • foscarnet • hydromorphone • magnesium sulfate • meperidine • morphine • ondansetron • perphenazine.
• **Additive:** cimetidine • clindamycin • multivitamins • vitamin B complex with C.

Incompatibility

• **Y-site:** filgrastim • hetastarch. Aminoglycosides should be administered at a separate site, at least 1 hour apart, if given concurrently.
• **Additive:** ranitidine.

Rate of Administration

• **Direct IV:** Administer slowly over 3–5 minutes. • **Intermittent Infusion:** Administer over 15–30 minutes.

≋ CLINICAL PRECAUTIONS

- Obtain specimens for culture and sensitivity prior to initiating therapy. First dose may be given before results are available.
- Determine history of allergic reactions to penicillins or cephalosporins. Persons with a negative history of penicillin sensitivity may still have an allergic response. Observe patient for signs and symptoms of anaphylaxis (rash, pruritus, laryngeal edema, wheezing). Discontinue the drug immediately if these occur. Keep epinephrine, an antihistamine, and resuscitation equipment close by in the event of an anaphylactic reaction.
- Assess patient for infection (vital signs; appearance of wound, sputum, urine, and stool; WBC).
- Monitor for phlebitis. Change IV site every 48–72 hours to prevent phlebitis.
- Assess renal function; monitor intake and output, and daily weight. Cefoxitin is excreted primarily by the kidneys. Dosage adjustment may be necessary in renal impairment or geriatric patients. If creatinine clearance is 50 ml/min or less, decreased dose and/or increased dosing interval is recommended.
- Probenecid decreases excretion and increases blood levels of cefoxitin.
- Although safety in pregnancy has not been established, cefoxitin has been used during obstetrical surgery without adverse effects (Pregnancy Category B).

Lab Test Considerations

• May cause transient increase in BUN, AST (SGOT), ALT (SGPT), LDH, and alkaline phosphatase. • May cause false-positive results for Coombs' test and urine glucose when tested with copper sulfate method (Clinitest). Use glucose enzymatic tests (Clinistix or Tes-Tape) to test urine glucose. • May cause falsely elevated serum and urine creatinine concentrations. Do not draw serum samples within 2 hours of administration.

Patient/Family Teaching

• Advise patient to report the signs of superinfection (furry overgrowth on the tongue, vaginal itching or discharge, loose or foul-smelling stools) and allergy. • Inform patient that diarrhea is a side effect, but if diarrhea becomes bloody, contains pus or mucus, or is accompanied by fever, contact physician as pseudomembranous colitis has been associated with cephalosporin use. Advise patient not to treat diarrhea without consulting physician or pharmacist.

PHARMACOLOGIC PROFILE

Indications

• Cefoxitin is used in the treatment of the following infections due to susceptible organisms: respiratory tract infections, skin and skin structure infections, bone and joint infections, urinary tract and gynecologic infections, septicemia, and intra-abdominal infections. • Cefoxitin has also been used as a perioperative prophylactic anti-infective.

Action

• Cefoxitin binds to the bacterial cell wall membrane, causing cell death. It is active against many Gram-positive cocci including *Streptococcus pneumoniae,* group A beta-hemolytic streptococci, and penicillinase-producing staphylococci, and also has increased activity against several Gram-negative pathogens, including *Haemophilus influenzae, Escherichia coli, Klebsiella pneumoniae, Neisseria gonorrhoeae* (including penicillinase-producing strains), *Providencia,* and *Proteus.* • It is also active against *Bacteroides fragilis*, but has no activity against methicillin-resistant staphylococci or enterococci.

Time/Action Profile

Onset	Peak
rapid	end of infusion

Pharmacokinetics

• **Distribution:** Cefoxitin is widely distributed, although penetration into CSF is poor. It crosses the placenta and enters breast milk in low concentrations. • **Metabolism and**

Excretion: Elimination of cefoxitin occurs primarily through the kidneys as unchanged drug. • **Half-life:** 0.7–1.1 hours (increased in renal impairment).

Contraindications

• Cefoxitin is contraindicated in patients with a history of hypersensitivity to cephalosporins or serious hypersensitivity to penicillins.

Adverse Reactions and Side Effects*

• **GI:** <u>nausea</u>, <u>vomiting</u>, cramps, <u>diarrhea</u>, PSEUDOMEMBRA-NOUS COLITIS • **Derm:** <u>rashes</u>, urticaria • **Hemat:** blood dyscrasias, hemolytic anemia, bleeding • **Local:** <u>phlebitis</u> at IV site • **Misc:** superinfection, allergic reactions including ANAPHY-LAXIS and serum sickness.

Ceftazidime	Anti-infective (third generation cephalosporin)
Ceptaz, Fortaz, Tazicef, Tazidime	pH 5–8 2.3 mEq Na/g

≋ ADMINISTRATION CONSIDERATIONS

Usual Dose

ADULTS: 0.5–2 g q 8–12 hr (250–500 mg q 12 hr for urinary tract infections).
GERIATRIC PATIENTS: 0.5–2 g q 12 hr.
CHILDREN 1 mo–12 yr: 30–50 mg/kg q 8 hr.
NEONATES ≤4 wk: 30 mg/kg q 12 hr.

Dilution

• **Direct IV:** Add 5 ml of sterile water for injection to each 500 ml or 10 ml to each 1-g or 2-g vial. Do not use preparations with benzyl alcohol for neonates. Dilution causes car-

---

*<u>Underlines</u> indicate most frequent; CAPITALS indicate life-threatening.

bon dioxide to form inside the vial, resulting in positive pressure; vial may require venting after dissolution to preserve sterility of vial. Venting is not required for Ceptaz preparation. • **Intermittent Infusion:** Reconstituted solution may be **further diluted** in at least 1 g/10 ml of 0.9% NaCl, D5W, D10W, D5/0.25% NaCl, D5/0.45% NaCl, D5/0.9% NaCl, or lactated Ringer's solution for a concentration of 1–40 mg/ml. • Solution is stable for 18 hours at room temperature or 7 days if refrigerated.

Compatibility

• **Y-site:** acyclovir • allopurinol sodium • ciprofloxacin • diltiazem • enalaprilat • esmolol • famotidine • filgrastim • fludarabine • foscarnet • gallium nitrate • hydromorphone • labetalol • melphalan • meperidine • morphine • ondansetron • paclitaxel • ranitidine • tacrolimus • vinorelbine • zidovudine.

• **Additive:** ciprofloxacin • clindamycin • fluconazole • metronidazole • ofloxacin.

Incompatibility

• **Y-site:** fluconazole • idarubicin. • Aminoglycosides should be administered at a separate site, at least 1 hour apart, if given concurrently.
• **Additive:** ranitidine.

Rate of Administration

• **Direct IV:** Administer slowly over 3–5 minutes. • **Intermittent Infusion:** Administer over 30–60 minutes.

≋ CLINICAL PRECAUTIONS

- Obtain specimens for culture and sensitivity prior to initiating therapy. First dose may be given before results are available.
- Determine history of allergic reactions to penicillins or cephalosporins. Persons with a negative history of penicillin sensitivity may still have an allergic response. Observe patient for signs and symptoms of anaphylaxis (rash, pruritus, laryngeal edema, wheezing). Discontinue the drug immediately if these occur. Keep epinephrine,

an antihistamine, and resuscitation equipment close by in the event of an anaphylactic reaction.
- Assess patient for infection (vital signs; appearance of wound, sputum, urine, and stool; WBC).
- Monitor for phlebitis. Change IV site every 48–72 hours to prevent phlebitis.
- Assess renal function; monitor intake and output, and daily weight. Ceftazidime is excreted primarily by the kidneys. Reduced dose and/or increased dosing interval is recommended if creatinine clearance is 50 ml/min or less.
- Safe use of ceftazidime in pregnancy or lactation has not been established (Pregnancy Category B).

Lab Test Consideraions

- May cause transient increase in BUN, AST (SGOT), ALT (SGPT), LDH, and alkaline phosphatase. • May cause false-positive results for Coombs' test and urine glucose when tested with copper sulfate method (Clinitest). Use glucose enzymatic tests (Clinistix or Tes-Tape) to test urine glucose.

Patient/Family Teaching

- Advise patient to report the signs of superinfection (furry overgrowth on the tongue, vaginal itching or discharge, loose or foul-smelling stools) and allergy. • Inform patient that diarrhea is a side effect, but if diarrhea becomes bloody, contains pus or mucus, or is accompanied by fever, contact physician as pseudomembranous colitis has been associated with cephalosporin use. Advise patient not to treat diarrhea without consulting physician or pharmacist.

PHARMACOLOGIC PROFILE

Indications

- Ceftazidime is used in the treatment of the following infections due to susceptible organisms: skin and skin structure infections, bone and joint infections, urinary tract and gynecologic infections, respiratory tract infections, intra-abdominal infections, septicemia, and meningitis.

Action

• Ceftazidime binds to the bacterial cell wall membrane, causing cell death. Its activity against staphylococci is diminished in comparison to that of second-generation cephalosporins, while action against Gram-negative pathogens is enhanced, even for organisms resistant to first- and second-generation agents. Ceftazidime is notable for increased action against *Citrobacter, Acinetobacter, Escherichia coli, Klebsiella pneumoniae, Branhamella catarrhalis, Pseudomonas aeruginosa, Haemophilus influenzae, Neisseria, Proteus, Providencia,* and *Serratia.* • It has some activity against anaerobes, including *Bacteroides fragilis.*

Time/Action Profile

Onset	Peak
rapid	end of infusion

Pharmacokinetics

• **Distribution:** Ceftazidime is widely distributed. It crosses the placenta and enters breast milk in low concentrations. Penetration into CSF is sufficient to treat meningitis.
• **Metabolism and Excretion:** Elimination of ceftazidime occurs primarily (>90%) through the kidneys as unchanged drug. • **Half-life:** 1.4–2 hours (increased in renal impairment).

Contraindications

• Ceftazidime is contraindicated in patients with hypersensitivity to cephalosporins or serious hypersensitivity to penicillins.

Adverse Reactions and Side Effects*

• **Derm:** <u>rashes</u>, urticaria • **GI:** <u>nausea</u>, <u>vomiting</u>, <u>diarrhea</u>, cramps, PSEUDOMEMBRANOUS COLITIS • **Hemat:** blood dyscrasias, hemolytic anemia • **Local:** <u>phlebitis</u> at IV site • **Misc:** superinfection, allergic reactions including ANAPHYLAXIS and serum sickness.

---

*<u>Underlines</u> indicate most frequent; CAPITALS indicate life-threatening.

Ceftizoxime Sodium

*Anti-infective
(third generation
cephalosporin)*

Cefizox

pH 5.5−8
contains 2.6 mEq Na/g

☰ ADMINISTRATION CONSIDERATIONS

Usual Dose

ADULTS: 1−4 g q 8−12 hr (500 mg q 12 hr for urinary tract infections).

CHILDREN >6 mo: 50 mg/kg q 6−8 hr (not to exceed 200 mg/kg/day).

Dilution

• **Direct IV: Reconstitute** each 1 g with 10 ml or each 2-g vial with 20 ml of sterile water for injection. • Solution may vary in color from yellow to amber. • **Intermittent Infusion:** May be **further diluted** in 50−100 ml of D5W, D10W, 0.9% NaCl, D5/0.25% NaCl, D5/0.45% NaCl, D5/0.9% NaCl, or lactated Ringer's solution. • Solution is stable for 8 hours at room temperature or 48 hours if refrigerated.

Compatibility

• **Y-site:** acyclovir ◆ allopurinol sodium ◆ enalaprilat ◆ esmolol ◆ famotidine ◆ fludarabine ◆ foscarnet ◆ hydromorphone ◆ labetalol ◆ melphalan ◆ meperidine ◆ morphine ◆ ondansetron ◆ sargramostim ◆ vinorelbine.

• **Additive:** clindamycin.

Incompatibility

• **Y-site:** filgrastim. Aminoglycosides should be administered at a separate site, at least 1 hour apart, if given concurrently.

Rate of Administration

• **Direct IV:** Administer slowly over 3−5 minutes. • **Intermittent Infusion:** Administer over 15−30 minutes.

☰ CLINICAL PRECAUTIONS

• Obtain specimens for culture and sensitivity prior to initiating therapy. First dose may be given before results are available.

- Determine history of allergic reactions to penicillins or cephalosporins. Persons with a negative history of penicillin sensitivity may still have an allergic response. Observe patient for signs and symptoms of anaphylaxis (rash, pruritus, laryngeal edema, wheezing). Discontinue the drug immediately if these occur. Keep epinephrine, an antihistamine, and resuscitation equipment close by in the event of an anaphylactic reaction.
- Assess patient for infection (vital signs; appearance of wound, sputum, urine, and stool; WBC).
- Monitor for phlebitis. Change IV site every 48–72 hours to prevent phlebitis.
- Assess renal function; monitor intake and output, and daily weight. Ceftizoxime is excreted primarily by the kidneys. Reduced dose and/or increased dosing interval is recommended if creatinine clearance is less than 80 ml/min.
- Probenecid decreases excretion and increases blood levels of ceftizoxime.
- Safe use of ceftizoxime in pregnancy or lactation has not been established (Pregnancy Category B).

Lab Test Considerations

- May cause increase in BUN creatinine, AST (SGOT), ALT (SGPT), and alkaline phosphatase. • May cause false-positive results for Coombs' test.

Patient/Family Teaching

- Advise patient to report the signs of superinfection (furry overgrowth on the tongue, vaginal itching or discharge, loose or foul-smelling stools) and allergy. • Inform patient that diarrhea is a side effect, but if diarrhea becomes bloody, contains pus or mucus, or is accompanied by fever, contact physician as pseudomembranous colitis has been associated with cephalosporin use. Advise patient not to treat diarrhea without consulting physician or pharmacist.

☰ PHARMACOLOGIC PROFILE
Indications

- Ceftizoxime is used in the treatment of the following infections due to susceptible organisms: skin and skin structure infections, bone and joint infections, urinary tract and gynecologic infections, respiratory tract infections, intra-abdominal infections, septicemia, and meningitis.

Action

• Ceftizoxime binds to the bacterial cell wall membrane, causing cell death. Its activity against staphylococci is diminished in comparison to second-generation cephalosporins, whereas action against Gram-negative pathogens is enhanced, even for organisms resistant to first- and second-generation agents. Ceftizoxime is notable for increased action against *Citrobacter, Acinetobacter, Escherichia coli, Klebsiella pneumoniae, Branhamella catarrhalis, Pseudomonas aeruginosa, Haemophilus influenzae, Neisseria, Proteus, Providencia,* and *Serratia.* • It has some activity against anaerobes, including *Bacteroides fragilis.*

Time/Action Profile

Onset	Peak
rapid	end of infusion

Pharmacokinetics

• **Distribution:** Ceftizoxime is widely distributed. It crosses the placenta and enters breast milk in low concentrations. CSF penetration is sufficient to treat meningitis. • **Metabolism and Excretion:** Elimination of ceftizoxime occurs primarily (>90%) through the kidneys as unchanged drug. • **Half-life:** 1.4–1.9 hours (increased in renal impairment).

Contraindications

• Ceftizoxime is contraindicated in patients with hypersensitivity to cephalosporins or serious hypersensitivity to penicillins.

Adverse Reactions and Side Effects*

• **GI:** <u>nausea</u>, <u>vomiting</u>, <u>diarrhea</u>, cramps, PSEUDOMEMBRANOUS COLITIS • **Derm:** <u>rashes</u>, urticaria • **Hemat:** blood dyscrasias, hemolytic anemia, bleeding • **Local:** <u>phlebitis</u> at IV site • **Misc:** superinfection, allergic reactions including ANAPHYLAXIS and serum sickness.

---

*<u>Underlines</u> indicate most frequent; CAPITALS indicate life-threatening.

Ceftriaxone Sodium

*Anti-infective
(third generation
cephalosporin)*

Rocephin

pH 6.6–6.7
contains 3.6 mEq Na/g

≋ ADMINISTRATION CONSIDERATIONS

Usual Dose

ADULTS: 1–2 g q 24 hr or 500 mg–1 g q 12 hr. *Perioperative prophylaxis:* 1 g 30 min–2 hr prior to surgery.

CHILDREN: 25–37.5 mg/kg q 12 hr (100 mg/kg/day for meningitis).

Dilution

• **Intermittent Infusion:** Reconstitute each 250-mg vial with 2.4 ml, each 500-mg vial with 4.8 ml, each 1-g vial with 9.6 ml, and each 2-g vial with 19.2 ml of sterile or bacteriostatic water for injection, D5W, or 0.9% NaCl. Do not use preparations containing benzyl alcohol for neonates. May be **further diluted** in 50–100 ml of 0.9% NaCl, D5W, D10W, D5/0.45% NaCl, or lactated Ringer's solution for a concentration of 10–40 mg/ml. • Solution is stable for 3 days at room temperature.

Compatibility

• **Y-site:** acyclovir • allopurinol sodium • diltiazem • fludarabine • foscarnet • gallium nitrate • melphalan • meperidine • morphine • paclitaxel • sargramostim • tacrolimus • vinorelbine • zidovudine.

Incompatibility

• **Y-site:** filgrastim • fluconazole • vancomycin. • Aminoglycosides should be administered at a separate site, at least 1 hour apart, if given concurrently.

• **Additive:** Manufacturer recommends that ceftriaxone not be physically combined with other drugs.

Rate of Administration

• **Intermittent Infusion:** Administer over 30–60 minutes.

≋ CLINICAL PRECAUTIONS

- Obtain specimens for culture and sensitivity prior to initiating therapy. First dose may be given before results are available.
- Determine history of allergic reactions to penicillins or cephalosporins. Persons with a negative history of penicillin sensitivity may still have an allergic response. Observe patient for signs and symptoms of anaphylaxis (rash, pruritus, laryngeal edema, wheezing). Discontinue the drug immediately if these occur. Keep epinephrine, an antihistamine, and resuscitation equipment close by in the event of an anaphylactic reaction.
- Assess patient for infection (vital signs; appearance of wound, sputum, urine, and stool; WBC).
- Monitor for phlebitis. Change IV site every 48–72 hours to prevent phlebitis.
- Assess renal function; monitor intake and output, and daily weight.
- Ceftriaxone crosses the placenta and enters breast milk in low concentrations. Safe use in pregnancy has not been established (Pregnancy Category B).

Lab Test Considerations

• May cause increase in BUN, creatinine, AST (SGOT), ALT (SGPT), bilirubin, and alkaline phosphatase. • May cause false-positive results for Coombs' test and urine glucose when tested with copper sulfate method (Clinitest). Use glucose enzymatic tests (Clinistix or Tes-Tape) to test urine glucose.

Patient/Family Teaching

• Instruct patient to notify the physician or nurse if signs of pseudolithiasis (epigastric pain, anorexia, nausea, vomiting) occur. This is more common when ceftriaxone is administered as a bolus over 3–5 minutes. • Advise patient to report the signs of superinfection (furry overgrowth on the tongue, vaginal itching or discharge, loose or foul-smelling stools) and allergy. • Inform patient that diarrhea is a side effect, but if diarrhea becomes bloody, contains pus or mucus, or is accompanied by fever, contact physician as pseudomembranous colitis has been associated

with cephalosporin use. Advise patient not to treat diarrhea without consulting physician or pharmacist.
• **Home Care Issues:** Instruct family or care-giver on dilution, rate, and administration of drug and proper care of IV equipment.

≋ PHARMACOLOGIC PROFILE

Indications
• Ceftriaxone is used in the treatment of the following infections due to susceptible organisms: skin and skin structure infections, bone and joint infections, urinary tract and gynecologic infections, respiratory tract infections, intraabdominal infections, and meningitis. • It has also been used as a perioperative prophylactic anti-infective.

Action
• Ceftriaxone binds to the bacterial cell wall membrane, causing cell death. Its activity against staphylococci is diminished in comparison to second-generation cephalosporins, whereas action against Gram-negative pathogens is enhanced, even for organisms resistant to first- and second-generation agents. Ceftriaxone is notable for increased action against *Citrobacter, Acinetobacter, Escherichia coli, Klebsiella pneumoniae, Branhamella catarrhalis, Pseudomonas aeruginosa, Haemophilus influenzae, Neisseria, Proteus, Providencia,* and *Serratia.* • It has some activity against anaerobes including *Bacteroides fragilis.*

Time/Action Profile

Onset	Peak
rapid	end of infusion

Pharmacokinetics
• **Distribution:** Ceftriaxone is widely distributed. It crosses the placenta and enters breast milk in low concentrations. Penetration into CSF is sufficient to treat meningitis.
• **Metabolism and Excretion:** Ceftriaxone is partially metabolized and partially excreted in the urine. • **Half-life:** 5.4–10.9 hours.

Contraindications

• Ceftriaxone is contraindicated in patients with hypersensitivity to cephalosporins or serious hypersensitivity to penicillins.

Adverse Reactions and Side Effects*

• **CNS:** SEIZURES (high doses) • **GI:** <u>nausea</u>, <u>vomiting</u>, <u>diarrhea</u>, cramps, PSEUDOMEMBRANOUS COLITIS, pseudolithiasis • **Derm:** <u>rashes</u>, urticaria • **Hemat:** blood dyscrasias, hemolytic anemia • **Local:** <u>phlebitis</u> at IV site • **Misc:** superinfection, allergic reactions including ANAPHYLAXIS and serum sickness.

Cefuroxime Sodium	*Anti-infective* *(second generation* *cephalosporin)*
Kefurox, Zinacef	pH 5–8.5 contains 2.4 mEq Na/g

 ADMINISTRATION CONSIDERATIONS

Usual Dose

ADULTS: 750–1500 mg q 8 hr (up to 3 g q 8 hr). *Perioperative prophylaxis:* 1 g 30–60 min prior to surgery, then q 8–12 hr for 24 hr.

CHILDREN AND INFANTS >3 mo: 50–100 mg/kg/day in divided doses every 6–8 hr. (For meningitis: 200–240 mg/kg/day.)

NEONATES: 30–100 mg/kg/day in divided doses q 8–12 hr.

Dilution

• **Direct IV:** Add 8 ml of sterile water for injection to each 750-mg vial or 16 ml to each 1.5-g vial for a concentration of 90 mg/ml. • Darkened powder does not alter potency. Solution may vary in color from light yellow to amber. Do not use solution that is cloudy or contains a precipitate. • **Intermit-**

---

*<u>Underlines</u> indicate most frequent; CAPITALS indicate life-threatening.

tent Infusion: May be **further diluted** in 100 ml of 0.9% NaCl, D5W, D10W, D5/0.45% NaCl, or D5/0.9% NaCl. • Solution is stable for 24 hours at room temperature and 1 week if refrigerated.

Compatibility

• **Y-site:** acyclovir ♦ allopurinol sodium ♦ atracurium ♦ cyclophosphamide ♦ diltiazem ♦ famotidine ♦ fludarabine ♦ foscarnet ♦ hydromorphone ♦ melphalan ♦ meperidine ♦ morphine ♦ ondansetron ♦ pancuronium ♦ perphenazine ♦ sargramostim ♦ tacrolimus ♦ vecuronium. However, manufacturer recommends that the primary infusion be temporarily discontinued during infusion of cefuroxime.

• **Additive:** clindamycin ♦ furosemide ♦ heparin ♦ metronidazole ♦ potassium chloride.

Incompatibility

• **Syringe:** doxapram.

• **Y-site:** filgrastim ♦ fluconazole ♦ vinorelbine. • Aminoglycosides should be administered at a separate site, at least 1 hour apart, if given concurrently.

• **Additive:** aminoglycosides ♦ sodium bicarbonate.

Rate of Administration

• **Direct IV:** Administer slowly over 3–5 minutes. • **Intermittent Infusion:** Administer over 15–60 minutes.

≋ CLINICAL PRECAUTIONS

• Obtain specimens for culture and sensitivity prior to initiating therapy. First dose may be given before results are available.

• Determine history of allergic reactions to penicillins or cephalosporins. Persons with a negative history of penicillin sensitivity may still have an allergic response. Observe patient for signs and symptoms of anaphylaxis (rash, pruritus, laryngeal edema, wheezing). Discontinue the drug immediately if these occur. Keep epinephrine, an antihistamine, and resuscitation equipment close by in the event of an anaphylactic reaction.

• Assess patient for infection (vital signs; appearance of wound, sputum, urine, and stool; WBC).

- Change IV site every 48–72 hours to prevent phlebitis.
- Assess renal function; monitor intake and output, and daily weight. Cefuroxime is excreted primarily by the kidneys. Dosage adjustment may be necessary in renal impairment or in elderly patients. Dosing interval should be increased if creatinine clearance is 20 ml/min or less.
- Probenecid decreases excretion and increases blood levels of cefuroxime.
- Although safe use in pregnancy has not been established, cefuroxime has been used during obstetrical surgery (Pregnancy Category B).

Lab Test Considerations

• May cause increase in AST (SGOT), ALT (SGPT), bilirubin, and alkaline phosphatase and decrease in hemoglobin and hematocrit levels. • May cause false-positive results for Coombs' test and urine glucose when tested with copper sulfate method (Clinitest). Use glucose enzymatic tests (Clinistix or Tes-Tape) to test urine glucose. • May cause false-negative blood glucose tests with ferricyanide tests. Use glucose enzymatic or hexokinase tests to determine blood glucose concentrations.

Patient/Family Teaching

• Advise patient to report the signs of superinfection (furry overgrowth on the tongue, vaginal itching or discharge, loose or foul-smelling stools) and allergy. • Inform patient that diarrhea is a side effect, but if diarrhea becomes bloody, contains pus or mucus, or is accompanied by fever, contact physician as pseudomembranous colitis has been associated with cephalosporin use. Advise patient not to treat diarrhea without consulting physician or pharmacist.

≋ PHARMACOLOGIC PROFILE

Indications

• Cefuroxime is used in the treatment of the following infections due to susceptible organisms: respiratory tract infections, skin and skin structure infections, bone and joint infections, urinary tract and gynecologic infections, septicemia, and meningitis. • It has also been used as a perioperative prophylactic anti-infective.

Action

• Cefuroxime binds to the bacterial cell wall membrane, causing cell death. It is active against many Gram-positive cocci including *Streptococcus pneumoniae,* group A beta-hemolytic streptococci, and penicillinase-producing staphylococci, with additional increased activity against several Gram-negative pathogens, including *Haemophilus influenzae, Enterobacter, Escherichia coli, Klebsiella pneumoniae, Neisseria gonorrhoeae* (including penicillinase-producing strains), *Providencia, Proteus,* and *Serratia.* • It is also active against *Bacteroides fragilis,* but has no activity against methicillin-resistant staphylococci or enterococci.

Time/Action Profile

Onset	Peak
rapid	end of infusion

Pharmacokinetics

• **Distribution:** Cefuroxime is widely distributed. It crosses the placenta and enters breast milk in low concentrations. Penetration into CSF is sufficient to treat meningitis. • **Metabolism and Excretion:** Elimination of cefuroxime occurs primarily through the kidneys. • **Half-life:** 1.3 hours (increased in renal impairment).

Contraindications

• Cefuroxime is contraindicated in patients with a history of hypersensitivity to cephalosporins or serious hypersensitivity to penicillins.

Adverse Reactions and Side Effects*

• **CNS:** SEIZURES (high doses) • **GI:** <u>nausea</u>, <u>vomiting</u>, cramps, <u>diarrhea</u>, PSEUDOMEMBRANOUS COLITIS • **Derm:** <u>rashes</u>, urticaria • **Hemat:** blood dyscrasias, hemolytic anemia • **Local:** <u>phlebitis</u> at IV site • **Misc:** superinfection, allergic reactions including ANAPHYLAXIS and serum sickness.

---

*<u>Underlines</u> indicate most frequent; CAPITALS indicate life-threatening.

Cephalothin Sodium

*Anti-infective
(first generation
cephalosporin)*

Keflin

pH 6–8.6
contains 2.4–2.8 mEq Na/g

 ADMINISTRATION CONSIDERATIONS

Usual Dose

ADULTS: 500 mg–2 g q 4–6 hr. *Perioperative prophylaxis:* 1–2 g q 30–60 min preoperatively, 1–2 g during procedure, then 1–2 g q 6 hr for up to 24 hr.

CHILDREN: 13.3–26.6 mg/kg q 4 hr or 20–40 mg/kg q 6 hr. *Perioperative prophylaxis:* 20–30 mg/kg 30–60 min preoperatively, repeated during procedure and then q 6 hr for up to 24 hr.

Dilution

• **Direct IV: Dilute** in at least 1 g/10 ml of sterile water for injection, D5W, or 0.9% NaCl. • Darkened color of solution does not affect potency. Do not administer solutions that are cloudy or contain a precipitate. • **Intermittent Infusion:** Reconstituted 1-g or 2-g solution may be **further diluted** in 50 ml of D5W, D10W, D5/0.9% NaCl, D5/LR, lactated Ringer's solution, or 0.9% NaCl. • **Continuous Infusion:** May be **diluted** in 500–1000 ml. • Solution is stable for 24 hours at room temperature and 96 hours if refrigerated.

Compatibility

• **Syringe:** cimetidine.

• **Y-site:** cyclophosphamide ♦ famotidine ♦ hydromorphone ♦ magnesium sulfate ♦ meperidine ♦ morphine ♦ multivitamins ♦ perphenazine ♦ potassium chloride ♦ vitamin B complex with C.

• **Additive:** ascorbic acid ♦ clindamycin ♦ fluorouracil ♦ hydrocortisone sodium succinate ♦ magnesium sulfate ♦ methicillin ♦ methotrexate ♦ potassium chloride ♦ prednisolone sodium phosphate ♦ sodium bicarbonate ♦ vitamin B complex with C.

Incompatibility

- **Syringe:** metoclopramide.
- **Y-site:** Aminoglycosides should be administered at a separate site, at least 1 hour apart, if given concurrently.
- **Additive:** amikacin ◆ aminophylline ◆ bleomycin ◆ calcium chloride ◆ calcium gluceptate ◆ calcium gluconate ◆ colistimethate ◆ diphenhydramine ◆ doxorubicin ◆ erythromycin lactobionate ◆ gentamicin ◆ kanamycin ◆ penicillin G sodium ◆ polymyxin B ◆ ranitidine.

Rate of Administration

- **Direct IV:** Administer slowly over 3–5 minutes. • **Intermittent Infusion:** Administer over 15–30 minutes.

≋ CLINICAL PRECAUTIONS

- Obtain specimens for culture and sensitivity prior to initiating therapy. First dose may be given before results are available.
- Determine history of allergic reactions to penicillins or cephalosporins. Persons with a negative history of penicillin sensitivity may still have an allergic response. Observe patient for signs and symptoms of anaphylaxis (rash, pruritus, laryngeal edema, wheezing). Discontinue the drug immediately if these occur. Keep epinephrine, an antihistamine, and resuscitation equipment close by in the event of an anaphylactic reaction.
- Assess patient for infection (vital signs; appearance of wound, sputum, urine, and stool; WBC).
- Monitor for phlebitis. Change IV site every 48–72 hours to prevent phlebitis.
- Assess renal function; monitor intake and output, and daily weight. Cephalothin is excreted primarily by the kidneys. Reduced dose and/or increased dosing interval is recommended if creatinine clearance is less than 80 ml/min and in elderly patients. Cephalothin may also potentiate nephrotoxicity from other nephrotoxic agents. Risk of nephrotoxicity is greater in patients over 50 years of age.
- Probenecid decreases excretion and increases blood levels of cephalothin.
- Cephalothin crosses the placenta and enters breast milk

in low concentrations. Safe use in pregnancy has not been established (Pregnancy Category B).

Lab Test Considerations

• May cause transient increase in BUN, AST (SGOT), ALT (SGPT), and alkaline phosphatase. • May cause false-positive results for Coombs' test and urine glucose when tested with copper sulfate method (Clinitest). Use glucose enzymatic tests (Clinistix or Tes-Tape) to test urine glucose.

Patient/Family Teaching

• Advise patient to report the signs of superinfection (furry overgrowth on the tongue, vaginal itching or discharge, loose or foul-smelling stools) and allergy. • Inform patient that diarrhea is a side effect, but if diarrhea becomes bloody, contains pus or mucus, or is accompanied by fever, contact physician as pseudomembranous colitis has been associated with cephalosporin use. Advise patient not to treat diarrhea without consulting physician or pharmacist.

PHARMACOLOGIC PROFILE

Indications

• Cephalothin is used in the treatment of respiratory tract infections, serious skin and soft tissue infections, genito-urinary and gastrointestinal tract infections, bone and joint infections, septicemia, and meningitis. • Cephalothin has also been used as a perioperative prophylactic anti-infective.

Action

• Cephalothin binds to the bacterial cell wall membrane, causing cell death. It displays activity against many Gram-positive cocci including *Streptococcus pneumoniae,* group A beta-hemolytic streptococci, and penicillinase-producing staphylococci. • Cephalothin also has activity against some Gram-negative rods, including *Klebsiella pneumoniae, Proteus mirabilis,* and *Escherichia coli,* but is not active against methicillin-resistant staphylococci, *Bacteroides fragilis,* or enterococci.

Time/Action Profile

Onset	Peak
rapid	end of infusion

Pharmacokinetics

• **Distribution:** Cephalothin is widely distributed, although penetration into CSF is poor. It crosses the placenta and enters breast milk in low concentrations. • **Metabolism and Excretion:** Elimination of cephalothin occurs primarily through the kidneys. • **Half-life:** 0.5–1 hour (increased in renal impairment).

Contraindications

• Cephalothin is contraindicated in patients with a history of hypersensitivity to cephalosporins or serious hypersensitivity to penicillins.

Adverse Reactions and Side Effects*

• **CNS:** SEIZURES (high doses) • **GI:** nausea, vomiting, cramps, diarrhea, PSEUDOMEMBRANOUS COLITIS • **Derm:** rashes, urticaria • **Hemat:** blood dyscrasias, hemolytic anemia, bleeding • **Local:** phlebitis at IV site • **Misc:** superinfection, allergic reactions including ANAPHYLAXIS and serum sickness.

Cephapirin Sodium	*Anti-infective (first generation cephalosporin)*
Cefadyl	pH 6.5–8.5 contains 2.36 mEq Na/g

≋ ADMINISTRATION CONSIDERATIONS

Usual Dose

ADULTS: 500–1000 mg q 4–6 hr (up to 12 g/day). *Perioperative prophylaxis:* 1–2 g 30–60 min preoperatively, repeated during procedure and q 6 hr for up to 24 hr.

CHILDREN >3 mo: 10–20 mg/kg q 6 hr.

---

*Underlines indicate most frequent; CAPITALS indicate life-threatening.

Dilution

• **Direct IV: Dilute** in 10 ml or more of bacteriostatic water for injection, D5W, or 0.9% NaCl. • Solution color changes do not alter potency. • **Intermittent Infusion:** Reconstituted solution may be **further diluted** in 50–100 ml of 0.9% NaCl, D5W, D10W, D20W, D5/0.25% NaCl, D5/0.45% NaCl, D5/0.9% NaCl, or D5/LR. • Solution is stable for 24 hours at room temperature and 10 days if refrigerated.

Compatibility

• **Y-site:** acyclovir ◆ cyclophosphamide ◆ famotidine ◆ heparin ◆ hydrocortisone sodium succinate ◆ hydromorphone ◆ magnesium sulfate ◆ meperidine ◆ morphine ◆ multivitamins ◆ perphenazine ◆ potassium chloride ◆ vitamin B complex with C.

• **Additive:** bleomycin ◆ calcium chloride ◆ calcium gluconate ◆ chloramphenicol ◆ diphenhydramine ◆ heparin ◆ hydrocortisone sodium phosphate ◆ hydrocortisone sodium succinate ◆ oxacillin ◆ penicillin G potassium ◆ potassium chloride ◆ sodium bicarbonate ◆ vitamin B complex with C.

Incompatibility

• **Y-site:** Aminoglycosides should be administered at a separate site, at least 1 hour apart, if given concurrently.

• **Additive:** amikacin ◆ ascorbic acid ◆ gentamicin ◆ kanamycin ◆ phenytoin ◆ thiopental.

Rate of Administration

• **Direct IV:** Administer slowly over 3–5 minutes. • **Intermittent Infusion:** Administer over 15–20 minutes.

≋ CLINICAL PRECAUTIONS

• Obtain specimens for culture and sensitivity prior to initiating therapy. First dose may be given before results are available.

• Determine history of allergic reactions to penicillins or cephalosporins. Persons with a negative history of penicillin sensitivity may still have an allergic response. Observe patient for signs and symptoms of anaphylaxis (rash, pruritus, laryngeal edema, wheezing). Discontinue the drug immediately if these occur. Keep epinephrine, an antihistamine, and resuscitation equipment close by in the event of an anaphylactic reaction.

- Assess patient for infection (vital signs; appearance of wound, sputum, urine, and stool; WBC).
- Monitor for phlebitis. Change IV site every 48–72 hours to prevent phlebitis.
- Assess renal function; monitor intake and output, and daily weight. Cephapirin is excreted primarily by the kidneys. Dosing interval should be increased to every 12 hours if serum creatinine is greater than 5 mg/dl.
- Probenecid decreases excretion and increases blood levels of cephapirin.
- Safe use of cephapirin in pregnancy or lactation has not been established (Pregnancy Category B).

Lab Test Considerations

• May cause transient increase in BUN, AST (SGOT), ALT (SGPT), bilirubin, and alkaline phosphatase. • May cause false-positive results for Coombs' test and urine glucose when tested with copper sulfate method (Clinitest). Use glucose enzymatic tests (Clinistix or Tes-Tape) to test urine glucose.

Patient/Family Teaching

• Advise patient to report the signs of superinfection (furry overgrowth on the tongue, vaginal itching or discharge, loose or foul-smelling stools) and allergy. • Inform patient that diarrhea is a side effect, but if diarrhea becomes bloody, contains pus or mucus, or is accompanied by fever, contact physician as pseudomembranous colitis has been associated with cephalosporin use. Advise patient not to treat diarrhea without consulting physician or pharmacist.

 PHARMACOLOGIC PROFILE

Indications

• Cephapirin is used in the treatment of the following infections due to susceptible organisms: respiratory tract infections, serious skin and skin structure infections, urinary tract infections, bone and joint infections, septicemia, and endocarditis. • Cephapirin has also been used as a perioperative prophylactic anti-infective.

Action

• Cephapirin binds to the bacterial cell wall membrane, causing cell death. It displays activity against many Gram-positive cocci including *Streptococcus pneumoniae,* group A beta-hemolytic streptococci, penicillinase-producing staphylococci. • Cephapirin also has activity against some Gram-negative rods including *Klebsiella pneumoniae, Proteus mirabilis, Escherichia coli,* but is not active against methicillin-resistant staphylococci, *Bacteroides fragilis,* or enterococci.

Time/Action Profile

Onset	Peak
rapid	end of infusion

Pharmacokinetics

• **Distribution:** Cephapirin is widely distributed, although penetration into CSF is minimal. It crosses the placenta and enters breast milk in low concentrations. • **Metabolism and Execretion:** Elimination of cephapirin occurs almost entirely through the kidneys as unchanged drug. • **Half-life:** 0.4–0.8 hours (increased in renal impairment).

Contraindications

• Cephapirin is contraindicated in patients with a history of hypersensitivity to cephalosporins or serious hypersensitivity to penicillins.

Adverse Reactions and Side Effects*

• **CNS:** SEIZURES (high doses) • **GI:** <u>nausea</u>, <u>vomiting</u>, cramps, <u>diarrhea</u>, PSEUDOMEMBRANOUS COLITIS • **Derm:** <u>rashes</u>, urticaria • **Hemat:** blood dyscrasias, hemolytic anemia, bleeding • **Local:** <u>phlebitis</u> at IV site • **Misc:** superinfection, allergic reactions including ANAPHYLAXIS and serum sickness.

---

*<u>Underlines</u> indicate most frequent; CAPITALS indicate life-threatening.

Cephradine Sodium	Anti-infective (first generation cephalosporin)
Velosef	pH 8.5–9.5 contains 6 mEq Na/g

 ADMINISTRATION CONSIDERATIONS

Usual Dose

ADULTS: 500–1000 mg q 6 hr. *Perioperative prophylaxis:* 1 g 30–60 min preoperatively, then 1 g q 4–6 hr for up to 24 hr.

CHILDREN >1 yr: 12.5–25 mg/kg q 6 hr (up to 300 mg/kg/day).

Dilution

• **Direct IV: Dilute** the 250-mg or 500-mg vial with 5 ml, the 1-g vial with 10 ml, or the 2-g vial with 20 ml of sterile water for injection, D5W, or 0.9% NaCl. • Solution may vary in color from light straw to yellow. • **Intermittent Infusion:** Reconstituted solution may be **further diluted** in 50–100 ml of 0.9% NaCl, D5W, D10W, D5/0.45% NaCl, or D5/0.9% NaCl. • Solution is stable for 10 hours at room temperature and 48 hours if refrigerated.

Incompatibility

• **Y-site:** Aminoglycosides should be administered at a separate site, at least 1 hour apart, if given concurrently.

• **Additive:** calcium salts • Ringer's solution • lactated Ringer's solution.

Rate of Administration

• **Direct IV:** Administer slowly over 3–5 minutes. • **Intermittent Infusion:** Administer over 15–20 minutes.

≋ CLINICAL PRECAUTIONS

• Obtain specimens for culture and sensitivity prior to initiating therapy. First dose may be given before results are available.

• Determine history of allergic reactions to penicillins or

cephalosporins. Persons with a negative history of penicillin sensitivity may still have an allergic response. Observe patient for signs and symptoms of anaphylaxis (rash, pruritus, laryngeal edema, wheezing). Discontinue the drug immediately if these occur. Keep epinephrine, an antihistamine, and resuscitation equipment close by in the event of an anaphylactic reaction.

- Assess patient for infection (vital signs; appearance of wound, sputum, urine, and stool; WBC).
- Monitor for phlebitis. Change IV site every 48–72 hours to prevent phlebitis.
- Assess renal function; monitor intake and output, and daily weight. Cephradine is excreted primarily by the kidneys. Decreased dose and/or increased dosing interval is recommended if creatinine clearance is 20 ml/min or less.
- Probenecid decreases excretion and increases blood levels of cephradine.
- Although safe use of cephradine in pregnancy has not been established, cephradine has been used during obstetrical surgery (Pregnancy Category B).

Lab Test Considerations

- May cause transient increase in BUN, AST (SGOT), ALT (SGPT), LDH, bilirubin, and alkaline phosphatase.
- May cause false-positive results for Coombs' test and urine glucose when tested with copper sulfate method (Clinitest). Use glucose enzymatic tests (Clinistix or Tes-Tape) to test urine glucose.

Patient/Family Teaching

- Advise patient to report the signs of superinfection (furry overgrowth on the tongue, vaginal itching or discharge, loose or foul-smelling stools) and allergy. • Inform patient that diarrhea is a side effect, but if diarrhea becomes bloody, contains pus or mucus, or is accompanied by fever, contact physician as pseudomembranous colitis has been associated with cephalosporin use. Advise patient not to treat diarrhea without consulting physician or pharmacist.

≋ PHARMACOLOGIC PROFILE

Indications

• Cephradine is used in the treatment of the following infections due to susceptible organisms: respiratory tract infections, serious skin and skin structure infections, urinary tract infections, bone and joint infections, and septicemia. • Cephradine has also been used as a perioperative prophylactic anti-infective.

Action

• Cephradine binds to the bacterial cell wall membrane, causing cell death. It displays activity against many Gram-positive cocci, including *Streptococcus pneumoniae,* group A beta-hemolytic streptococci, and penicillinase-producing staphylococci. • Cephradine also has activity against some Gram-negative rods, including *Klebsiella pneumoniae, Proteus mirabilis,* and *Escherichia coli,* but is not active against methicillin-resistant staphylococci, *Bacteroides fragilis,* or enterococci.

Time/Action Profile

Onset	Peak
rapid	end of infusion

Pharmacokinetics

• **Distribution:** Cephradine is widely distributed, although penetration into CSF is minimal. It crosses the placenta and enters breast milk in low concentrations. • **Metabolism and Excretion:** Elimination of cephradine occurs almost entirely through the kidneys as unchanged drug. • **Half-life:** 0.7–2 hours (increased in renal impairment).

Contraindications

• Cephradine is contraindicated in patients with a history of hypersensitivity to cephalosporins or serious hypersensitivity to penicillins.

Adverse Reactions and Side Effects*

• **CNS:** SEIZURES (high doses) • **GI:** <u>nausea</u>, <u>vomiting</u>, cramps, <u>diarrhea</u>, PSEUDOMEMBRANOUS COLITIS • **Derm:** <u>rashes</u>,

---

*<u>Underlines</u> indicate most frequent; CAPITALS indicate life-threatening.

urticaria • **Hemat:** blood dyscrasias, hemolytic anemia, bleeding • **Local:** <u>phlebitis</u> at IV site • **Misc:** superinfection, allergic reactions including ANAPHYLAXIS and serum sickness.

Chloramphenicol Sodium Succinate	*Anti-infective*
Chloromycetin	pH 6.4–7 contains 2.25 mEq Na/g

 ADMINISTRATION CONSIDERATIONS

Usual Dose

ADULTS: 12.5 mg/kg q 6 hr (not to exceed 4 g/day).

INFANTS >2 wk AND CHILDREN: 12.5 mg/kg q 6 hr or 25 mg/kg q 12 hr (up to 100 mg/kg/day).

INFANTS ≤2 wk: 6.25 mg/kg q 6 hr (up to 100 mg/kg/day).

Dilution

• **Direct IV: Reconstitute** to a 10% solution (100 mg/ml) by adding 10 ml of sterile water for injection or D5W to each 1 g. For neonates, do not use preparations containing benzyl alcohol. • **Intermittent Infusion:** May be **further diluted** in 50–100 ml of D5W, D10W, D5/0.25% NaCl, D5/0.45% NaCl, D5/0.9% NaCl, D5/LR, 0.45% NaCl, 0.9% NaCl, or lactated Ringer's solution. • Solution may form crystals at low temperatures. Shake well to dissolve crystals. Do not administer cloudy preparations. • **Continuous Infusion:** May also be diluted in 500–1000 ml.

Compatibility

• **Syringe:** ampicillin ♦ heparin ♦ methicillin ♦ penicillin G sodium.

• **Y-site:** acyclovir ♦ cyclophosphamide ♦ enalaprilat ♦ esmolol ♦ foscarnet ♦ hydromorphone ♦ labetalol ♦ magnesium sulfate ♦ meperidine ♦ morphine ♦ perphenazine ♦ tacrolimus.

• **Additive:** amikacin ♦ aminophylline ♦ ascorbic acid ♦ calcium chloride ♦ calcium gluconate ♦ cephalothin ♦ cephapirin ♦ colistimethate ♦ cyanocobalamin ♦ heparin ♦ hydrocortisone ✦ kanamycin ✦ lidocaine ✦ magnesium sulfate ✦ methicillin ✦ methyldopa ✦ methylprednisolone sodium succinate ✦ metronidazole ✦ nafcillin ✦ oxacillin ✦ penicillin G potassium ✦ penicillin G sodium ✦ potassium chloride ✦ ranitidine ✦ sodium bicarbonate ✦ vitamin B complex with C.

Incompatibility

- **Syringe:** glycopyrrolate ✦ metoclopramide.
- **Y-site:** fluconazole.
- **Additive:** chlorpromazine ✦ polymyxin B ✦ vancomycin.

Rate of Administration

- **Direct IV:** Administer slowly over at least 1 minute.
- **Intermittent Infusion:** Administer over 30–60 minutes.

≋ CLINICAL PRECAUTIONS

- Obtain specimens for culture and sensitivity prior to administration. First dose may be given before results are available.
- Parenteral chloramphenicol should be used under close medical supervision. Assess patient for infection (vital signs; wound appearance, sputum, urine, stool; WBC) throughout therapy.
- Assess patient daily for signs of bone marrow depression (petechiae, sore throat, fatigue, unusual bleeding). Monitor hematologic status. Chloramphenicol may cause reversible depression of bone marrow or aplastic anemia and other life-threatening dyscrasias. Bone marrow depression from chloramphenicol may be additive with other bone marrow–depressing agents (antineoplastics).
- Patients with impaired liver or renal function, infants, children, and the elderly are at greatest risk for developing adverse reactions.
- Chloramphenicol inhibits drug-metabolizing ability of the liver and may increase effects of the following drugs: oral hypoglycemic agents, warfarin, phenobarbital, and phenytoin.
- Phenobarbital or rifampin may decrease blood levels of chloramphenicol. Observe for re-emergence of infection. Chloramphenicol may decrease the effectiveness of concurrently administered erythromycin or clindamycin.

- Chloramphenicol may delay the therapeutic response to vitamin B_{12} or folic acid therapy.
- Use cautiously in patients with G6-PD deficiency or acute intermittent porphyria.
- Use cautiously, if at all, and in reduced dosage in premature and full-term infants. Assess for gray syndrome (abdominal distention, drowsiness, low body temperature, cyanosis, hypotension, respiratory distress).
- Chloramphenicol is not recommended for use in pregnant patients near term or during labor or lactation due to the risk of adverse reactions in the infant.

Toxicity and Overdose Alert

- Monitor serum levels weekly. Therapeutic peak level is 5–20 mcg/ml.

Lab Test Considerations

- CBC and platelet count should be monitored every 2 days throughout therapy. The drug should be stopped if anemia, reticulocytopenia, leukopenia, or thrombocytopenia develops. Notify physician promptly. • May cause false-positive copper sulfate urine glucose tests (Clinitest). Test urine glucose with glucose enzymatic tests (Clinistix or Tes-Tape).

Patient/Family Teaching

- Instruct patient to contact physician immediately if signs of unusual bleeding; bruising; fever; sore throat; nausea; vomiting; diarrhea; numbness, tingling, burning pain, or weakness in hands or feet occur. Medication should be discontinued with the onset of any of these symptoms. • Instruct patient to report signs of superinfection (stomatitis, perianal itching, vaginal discharge, fever). • Emphasize the importance of follow-up examinations. Bone marrow depression may develop weeks to months after drug therapy has been discontinued.

≋ PHARMACOLOGIC PROFILE

Indications

- Chloramphenicol has been used in the management of the following serious infections due to susceptible organisms when less toxic agents cannot be used: skin and soft tissue infections, intra-abdominal infections, CNS infections, meningitis, and bacteremia.

Action

• Chloramphenicol inhibits protein synthesis in susceptible bacteria at the level of the 50S bacterial ribosome. It is active against a wide variety of Gram-positive aerobic organisms; including *Streptococcus pneumoniae* and other streptococci; Gram-negative pathogens such as *Haemophilus influenzae, Neisseria meningitidis, Salmonella,* and *Shigella;* and anaerobes including *Bacteroides fragilis* and *B. melaninogenicus.* Other organisms inhibited are *Rickettsia, Chlamydia,* and *Mycoplasma.*

Time/Action Profile

Onset	Peak
rapid	end of infusion

Pharmacokinetics

• **Distribution:** Chloramphenicol is widely distributed. CSF levels are 60% of serum values. It readily crosses the placenta and enters breast milk. • **Metabolism and Excretion:** Metabolism occurs primarily in the liver. Less than 10% is excreted unchanged by the kidneys. • **Half-life:** 1.5–3.5 hours (prolonged in adults with impaired hepatic function, children, and neonates).

Contraindications

• Hypersensitivity to chloramphenicol or history of a previous toxic reaction. Avoid use during lactation.

Adverse Reactions and Side Effects*

• **CNS:** depression, confusion, headache • **EENT:** optic neuritis, blurred vision • **GI:** nausea, vomiting, diarrhea, bitter taste • **Derm:** rashes • **Hemat:** <u>bone marrow depression</u>, APLASTIC ANEMIA • **Neuro:** peripheral neuropathy • **Misc:** GRAY SYNDROME in newborns, fever.

---

*<u>Underlines</u> indicate most frequent; CAPITALS indicate life-threatening.

Chlordiazepoxide Hydrochloride	Sedative/hypnotic (benzodiazepine)
Librium	pH 3.0

≋ ADMINISTRATION CONSIDERATIONS

Usual Dose

Alcohol Withdrawal
ADULTS: 50–100 mg initially; may be repeated in 2–4 hr (not to exceed 300 mg/24 hr).

Severe Anxiety
ADULTS: 50–100 mg initially, then 25–50 mg 3–4 times daily as required (not to exceed 300 mg/24 hr).
CHILDREN >12 yr: 25–50 mg/dose.
GERIATRIC PATIENTS: 25–50 mg/dose.

Dilution
• **Direct IV:** Reconstitute 100 mg in 5 ml of 0.9% NaCl or sterile water for injection for a concentration of 20 mg/ml. Do not use IM diluent. • Use solution immediately after reconstitution and discard any unused portion.

Compatibility
• **Y-site:** heparin ◆ hydrocortisone sodium succinate ◆ potassium chloride ◆ vitamin B complex with C.

Incompatibility
• **Syringe:** benzquinamide.

Rate of Administration
• **Direct IV:** Administer slowly over at least 1 minute. Rapid administration may cause apnea, hypotension, bradycardia, or cardiac arrest.

≋ CLINICAL PRECAUTIONS

• Following administration, have patient remain recumbent and observe for 3 hours.
• Assess patient for anxiety and level of sedation. Observe

for signs of excessive sedation (ataxia, dizziness, slurred speech). Monitor blood pressure, heart rate, and respiratory rate frequently. Total daily dose should not exceed 300 mg.

- Assess patients being treated for alcohol withdrawal for tremors, agitation, delirium, and hallucinations. Protect patient from injury.
- Patients with severe pulmonary disease may experience respiratory depression.
- Use cautiously in patients with hepatic dysfunction, severe renal impairment, geriatric or debilitated patients, and older children. Patients in these groups may be more sensitive to the effects of chlordiazepoxide and require dosage reduction.
- Concurrent use of alcohol, antidepressants, antihistamines, and opioid analgesics results in additive CNS depression.
- Cimetidine, oral contraceptives, disulfiram, fluoxetine, isoniazid, ketoconazole, metoprolol, propoxyphene, propranolol, or valproic acid may decrease the metabolism of chlordiazepoxide, enhancing its actions.
- Chlordiazepoxide may decrease efficacy of levodopa.
- Rifampin or barbiturates may increase the metabolism and decrease effectiveness of chlordiazepoxide.
- Sedative effects may be decreased by theophylline.
- Use of chlordiazepoxide should be avoided during pregnancy or lactation and in children less than 12 years (Pregnancy Category D).

Lab Test Considerations

- Patients on prolonged therapy should have CBC and liver function tests evaluated periodically. May cause an increase in serum bilirubin, AST (SGOT), and ALT (SGPT).

Patient/Family Teaching

- Chlordiazepoxide commonly causes drowsiness and dizziness. Advise patient to request assistance with ambulation and to avoid activities requiring alertness until response to medication is known. • Instruct patient to notify physician if pregnancy is suspected.

≋ PHARMACOLOGIC PROFILE

Indications

• Chlordiazepoxide is used as an adjunct in the management of severe anxiety and in the treatment of symptoms of alcohol withdrawal.

Action

• Chlordiazepoxide acts at many levels of the CNS to produce sedative/anxiolytic effect. It depresses the CNS, probably by potentiating gamma-aminobutyric acid (GABA), an inhibitory neurotransmitter.

Time/Action Profile (sedation)

Onset	Peak	Duration†
1–5 min	UK	15–60 min

†With multiple doses, accumulation may occur, leading to prolonged sedation.

Pharmacokinetics

• **Distribution:** Chlordiazepoxide is widely distributed, crosses the blood–brain barrier and placenta, and enters breast milk. • **Metabolism and Excretion:** Chlordiazepoxide is highly metabolized by the liver. Some products of metabolism have CNS depressant properties. • **Half-life:** 5–30 hours.

Contraindications

• Hypersensitivity to chlordiazepoxide. Cross-sensitivity with other benzodiazepines may occur. • Chlordiazepoxide should not be used in comatose patients, patients with preexisting CNS depression, uncontrolled severe pain or narrow-angle glaucoma.

Adverse Reactions and Side Effects*

• **CNS:** <u>dizziness</u>, <u>drowsiness</u>, <u>lethargy</u>, hangover, paradoxical excitation, mental depression, headache • **EENT:** blurred vision • **GI:** nausea, vomiting, diarrhea, constipation • **Derm:** rashes • **Misc:** tolerance, psychological dependence, physical dependence.

---

*<u>Underlines</u> indicate most frequent; CAPITALS indicate life-threatening.

Chlorpromazine Hydrochloride *Antiemetic, Phenothiazine*

{Largactil}, Ormazine, Thorazine pH 3–5

≋ ADMINISTRATION CONSIDERATIONS

Usual Dose

Antiemetic during Surgery
ADULTS: up to 25 mg as a slow infusion at no more than 1 mg/min.
CHILDREN: 275 mcg (0.275 mg)/kg as a slow infusion at no more than 0.5 mg/min.

Intractable Hiccups
ADULTS: 25–50 mg by slow infusion, rate not to exceed 1 mg/min.

Tetanus
ADULTS: 25–50 mg at a rate of 1 mg/min.
CHILDREN: 550 mcg (0.55 mg)/kg at a rate of 0.5 mg/min.

Dilution
• **Direct IV: Dilute** with 0.9% NaCl to a concentration of 1 mg/ml. • Slightly yellowed solution does not indicate loss of potency. Discard markedly discolored solutions. • **Continuous Infusion:** May **dilute** 25–50 mg in 500–1000 ml of D5W, D10W, 0.45% NaCl, 0.9% NaCl, Ringer's or lactated Ringer's solution, or dextrose/saline, dextrose/Ringer's, or dextrose/lactated Ringer's combinations for a concentration not to exceed 1 mg/ml.

Compatibility
• **Syringe:** atropine • butorphanol • diphenhydramine • doxapram • droperidol • fentanyl • glycopyrrolate • hydromorphone • hydroxyzine • meperidine • metoclopramide • midazolam • morphine • pentazocine • scopolamine.
• **Y-site:** fluconazole • heparin • hydrocortisone sodium succinate • ondansetron • potassium chloride • vitamin B complex with C.
• **Additive:** ascorbic acid • netilmicin • vitamin B complex with C.

{} = Available in Canada only.

Incompatibility

- **Syringe:** cimetidine • dimenhydrinate • heparin • pentobarbital • thiopental.
- **Y-site:** allopurinol sodium • fludarabine • melphalan • methotrexate • paclitaxel • piperacillin/tazobactam • sargramostim.
- **Additive:** aminophylline • amphotericin B • ampicillin • chloramphenicol • chlorothiazide • furosemide • methicillin • penicillin G.

Rate of Administration

- **Direct IV:** Inject slowly at a rate of 1 mg/min for adults or 0.5 mg/min for children. • **Continuous Infusion:** Administer at a rate not to exceed 1 mg/min in adults and 0.5 mg/min in children.

≋ CLINICAL PRECAUTIONS

- Monitor blood pressure and pulse. Hypotension may result in dizziness. Patient should remain recumbent for 30 minutes following administration to minimize hypotensive effects. Additive hypotension may occur with nitrates or antihypertensive agents.
- Geriatric or debilitated patients are at increased risk for hypotensive reactions; lower initial infusion rate is recommended. Elderly patients have an increased risk of dystonias and adverse CNS and cardiovascular reactions. Children are also at increased risk for dystonias. Lower initial doses are also recommended in patients with organic brain syndrome or acute confusion.
- To prevent contact dermatitis, avoid getting solution on hands.
- Observe for excessive sedation. Additive CNS depression may occur with other CNS depressants including alcohol, antidepressants, antihistamines, MAO inhibitors, opioid analgesics, sedative/hypnotics, or general anesthetics.
- Monitor for onset of extrapyramidal reactions (akathisia—restlessness; dystonia—muscle spasms and twisting motions; pseudoparkinsonism—mask facies, rigidity, tremors, drooling, shuffling gait, dysphagia). Reduction in dosage or discontinuation of medication

may be necessary. Antiparkinson agents (trihexyphenidyl or benztropine) or diphenhydramine may be used to control these symptoms.

- Assess patient for tardive dyskinesia (rhythmic movement of mouth, face, and extremities), which may be irreversible, and neuroleptic malignant syndrome (fever, respiratory distress, tachycardia, convulsions, diaphoresis, hypertension or hypotension, pallor, tiredness). The risk of neuroleptic malignant syndrome may be increased by concurrent antidepressant therapy.

- Risk of anticholinergic side effects (dry mouth, dry eyes, blurred vision) is increased by other agents having anticholinergic properties including antihistamines, tricyclic antidepressants, disopyramide, and quinidine.

- Use with caution in patients with severe pulmonary disease.

- Patients with prostatic hypertrophy may experience urinary retention.

- Chlorpromazine may lower seizure threshold; use cautiously in patients with seizure disorders.

- Use cautiously in patients with intestinal obstruction (may cause ileus).

- Concurrent use with lithium may produce any of the following: acute encephalopathy, increased excretion of lithium, increased risk of extrapyramidal reactions, or masking of the early signs of lithium toxicity.

- Chlorpromazine may decrease antiparkinsonian activity of levodopa and bromocriptine.

- The vasopressor response to epinephrine and norepinephrine is decreased by chlorpromazine.

- Decreases antihypertensive effect of guanethidine.

- Concurrent use with beta blockers may result in inhibition of metabolism of one or both drugs, producing an increased response.

- Safe use during pregnancy has not been established. Adverse reactions have occurred in neonates.

Lab Test Considerations

- CBC and liver function tests should be evaluated periodically throughout chronic therapy. May cause decreased hematocrit, hemoglobin, leukocytes, granulocytes, and platelets. May cause elevated bilirubin, AST (SGOT), ALT

(SGPT), and alkaline phosphatase. • May cause false-positive or false-negative pregnancy test results and false-positive urine bilirubin test results.

Patient/Family Teaching

• Inform patient of the possibility of extrapyramidal symptoms and tardive dyskinesia. Advise patient to report symptoms immediately. • Caution patient to make position changes slowly to minimize orthostatic hypotension. • May cause drowsiness. Caution patient to avoid activities requiring alertness until response to medication is known. • Advise patient that frequent mouth rinses, good oral hygiene, and sugarless gum or candy may minimize dry mouth. • Inform patient that medication may turn urine a pink-to-reddish-brown color. • Instruct patient to notify physician promptly if sore throat, fever, unusual bleeding or bruising, rash, weakness, tremors, visual disturbances, dark-colored urine, or clay-colored stools occur.

PHARMACOLOGIC PROFILE

Indications

• Chlorpromazine is used in the management of nausea and vomiting occurring during surgery and to control intractable hiccups. It is also used with a barbiturate in the management of tetanus.

Action

• Chlorpromazine alters the effects of dopamine in the CNS. In addition, it possesses significant anticholinergic and alpha-adrenergic blocking activity. Its antiemetic effect is caused by inhibitory action on dopamine receptors in the chemoreceptor trigger zone of the brain.

Time/Action Profile

Onset	Peak	Duration
rapid	UK	UK

Pharmacokinetics

• **Distribution:** Chlorpromazine is widely distributed, reaching high concentrations in the CNS. It also crosses the placenta and enters breast milk. • **Metabolism and Excretion:** Metabolism occurs in the liver and GI mucosa. Some products of metabolism have CNS activity. • **Half-life:** 30 hours.

Contraindications

• Chlorpromazine is contraindicated in patients with previous hypersensitivity to it or to sulfites or benzyl alcohol. • Cross-sensitivity with other phenothiazines may exist. • Chlorpromazine should be avoided in patients with narrow-angle glaucoma, bone marrow depression, severe liver disease, or severe cardiovascular disease.

Adverse Reactions and Side Effects*

• **CNS:** <u>sedation</u>, <u>extrapyramidal reactions</u>, tardive dyskinesia • **EENT:** <u>dry eyes</u>, <u>blurred vision</u>, lens opacities • **CV:** <u>hypotension</u>, tachycardia • **GI:** <u>constipation</u>, <u>dry mouth</u>, ileus, anorexia, hepatitis • **GU:** urinary retention • **Derm:** rashes, <u>photosensitivity</u>, pigment changes • **Endo:** galactorrhea • **Hemat:** AGRANULOCYTOSIS, leukopenia • **Metab:** hyperthermia • **Misc:** allergic reactions, NEUROLEPTIC MALIGNANT SYNDROME.

Cimetidine Hydrochloride	Antiulcer (H₂ antagonist)
Tagamet	pH 3.8–7

 ADMINISTRATION CONSIDERATIONS

Usual Dose

Short-Term Treatment of Active Ulcers

ADULTS: 300 mg q 6–8 hr (not to exceed 2.4 g/day) or as an infusion at 37.5 mg/hr; may be preceded by a 150-mg bolus dose.

CHILDREN: 5–10 mg/kg q 6–8 hr.

---

*<u>Underlines</u> indicate most frequent; CAPITALS indicate life-threatening.

Gastric Hypersecretory Conditions

ADULTS: 300 mg q 6 hr initially (up to 12 g/day has been used).

Prophylaxis of Stress Ulcers

ADULTS: 50 mg/hr as a continuous infusion.

Prophylaxis of Aspiration Pneumonitis

ADULTS: 300 mg IM 1 hr before anesthesia, then 300 mg IV q 4 hr until patient is conscious (unlabeled use).

Dilution

• **Direct IV: Dilute** each 300 mg in 20 ml of 0.9% NaCl for injection. • **Intermittent Infusion: Dilute** each 300 mg in 50 ml of 0.9% NaCl, D5W, D10W, D5/LR, D5/0.9% NaCl, D5/0.45% NaCl, D5/0.25% NaCl, Ringer's or lactated Ringer's solution. • Diluted solution is stable for 48 hours at room temperature. Refrigeration may cause cloudiness but will not affect potency. Do not use solution that is discolored or contains a precipitate. • **Continuous Infusion:** Dilute cimetidine 900 mg in 100–1000 ml of compatible solution (see Intermittent Infusion).

Compatibility

• **Syringe:** atropine • butorphanol • cephalothin • diazepam • diphenhydramine • doxapram • droperidol • fentanyl • glycopyrrolate • heparin • hydromorphone • hydroxyzine • lorazepam • meperidine • midazolam • morphine • nafcillin • nalbuphine • penicillin G sodium • pentazocine • perphenazine • prochlorperazine • promazine • promethazine • scopolamine • sterile water for injection.

• **Y-site:** acyclovir • aminophylline • amrinone • atracurium • cisplatin • cyclophosphamide • cytarabine • diltiazem • doxorubicin • enalaprilat • esmolol • filgrastim • fluconazole • fludarabine • foscarnet • gallium nitrate • haloperidoxol • heparin • hetastarch • idarubicin • labetalol • melphalan • methotrexate • ondansetron • paclitaxel • pancuronium • piperacillin/tazobactam • sargramostim • tacrolimus • tolazoline • vecuronium • vinorelbine • zidovudine.

• **Additive:** acetazolamide • amikacin • aminophylline • atracurium • cefoperazone • cefoxitin • chlorothiazide • clindamycin • colistimethate • dexamethasone • erythromycin lactobionate • furosemide • gentamicin • insulin • lincomycin • methylprednisolone sodium succinate • penicillin G potassium ✦ phytonadione ✦ polymyxin B ✦ potassium chloride ✦ protamine ✦ quinidine gluconate ✦ vancomycin ✦ vitamin B complex ✦ vitamin B complex with C.

Incompatibility

- **Syringe:** cefamandole ✦ cefazolin ✦ chlorpromazine ✦ pentobarbital ✦ secobarbital.
- **Additive:** amphotericin B.

Rate of Administration

- **Direct IV:** Administer over at least 5 minutes. • **Intermittent Infusion:** Administer over 15–20 minutes. • **Continuous Infusion:** Daily dose may be administered over 24 hours. Rate should be individualized. Use infusion pump, especially for volume <250 ml.

≋ CLINICAL PRECAUTIONS

- Monitor signs of gastritis/ulcer disease by assessing pain and/or gastric pH. Guaiac test stools and gastric aspirate if GI bleeding has occurred.
- Geriatric patients and patients with renal impairment are more susceptible to adverse CNS reactions, especially confusion; increased dosing interval recommended if creatinine clearance is 40 ml/min or less. If creatinine clearance is less than 30 ml/min, continuous infusion rate should be decreased by 50%.
- Cimetidine inhibits drug-metabolizing enzymes in the liver and is likely to lead to increased blood levels and toxicity of the following: oral anticoagulants, phenytoin, lidocaine, and theophylline. There may be a similar but less predictable effect with metronidazole, triamterene, metoprolol, propranolol, mexiletine, flecainide, procainamide, quinidine, quinine, caffeine, some benzodiazepines (chlordiazepoxide, diazepam), succinylcholine, opioid analgesics, pentoxifylline, carbamazepine, chloroquine, calcium channel blockers, some sulfonylureas (glyburide and glipizide), and tricyclic antidepressants. Cimetidine may potentiate myelosuppressive properties of carmustine and may decrease the absorption of iron salts, indomethacin, ketoconazole, and tetracyclines. The pharmacologic effects of tocainide may be decreased by cimetidine.
- In the management of pathologic hypersecretory condi-

tions, when more cimetidine is required, it is recommended that the frequency of dosing be increased.
• Safe use in pregnancy has not been established (Pregnancy Category B).

Lab Test Considerations

• Patients receiving long-term therapy should have periodic blood counts. Aplastic anemia and agranulocytosis are rare but life-threatening complications. • Cimetidine may cause transient increase in serum transaminase and serum creatinine. • Serum prolactin concentrations may be increased following IV bolus. • May also cause decreased parathyroid concentrations. • Antagonizes the effects of pentagastrin and histamine during gastric acid secretion testing. Avoid administration for 24 hours preceding the test. • May cause false-negative results in skin tests using allergenic extracts. Cimetidine should be discontinued 24 hours prior to the test.

Patient/Family Teaching

• Inform the patient that smoking interferes with the nocturnal action of cimetidine. Encourage patient to quit smoking or at least not to smoke after the last dose of the day. • May cause drowsiness. Caution patient to avoid driving or other activities requiring alertness until response to the medication is known. • Advise patient to avoid alcohol, products that contain aspirin, ibuprofen, or naproxen, and foods that may cause GI irritation. • Advise patient to report the onset of black tarry stools, fever, sore throat, diarrhea, dizziness, rash, confusion, or hallucinations promptly.

 PHARMACOLOGIC PROFILE

Indications

• Cimetidine is used in the short-term treatment of active duodenal ulcers and benign gastric ulcers and long-term prophylaxis of duodenal ulcers. • Gastric hypersecretory states (Zollinger-Ellison syndrome) have also been managed chronically with cimetidine. • Cimetidine is used to treat and prevent stress-related mucosal damage. • **Unlabeled Uses:** Treatment of upper GI bleeding • prevention of aspiration pneumonitis.

Action
- Cimetidine inhibits the action of histamine at the H_2 receptor site located primarily in gastric parietal cells, resulting in inhibition of gastric acid secretion.

Time/Action Profile (suppression of gastric acid secretion)

Onset	Peak	Duration
10 min	30 min	4–5 hr

Pharmacokinetics
- **Distribution:** Cimetidine is widely distributed. It enters breast milk and CSF and probably crosses the placenta. • **Metabolism and Excretion:** 30% of cimetidine is metabolized by the liver. The remainder is excreted unchanged by the kidneys. • **Half-life:** 2 hours (increased in renal impairment).

Contraindications
- Hypersensitivity to cimetidine.

Adverse Reactions and Side Effects*
- **CNS:** <u>confusion</u>, dizziness, headache, drowsiness • **CV:** bradycardia • **GI:** nausea, diarrhea, hepatitis • **GU:** nephritis, decreased sperm count • **Derm:** rashes, exfoliative dermatitis, urticaria • **Endo:** gynecomastia • **Hemat:** AGRANULOCYTOSIS, APLASTIC ANEMIA, neutropenia, thrombocytopenia, anemia • **MS:** muscle pain.

Ciprofloxacin Lactate	Anti-infective (fluoroquinolone)
Cipro IV	pH 3.3–4.6

ADMINISTRATION CONSIDERATIONS
Usual Dose
ADULTS: 200–400 mg q 12 hr.

---

 *<u>Underlines</u> indicate most frequent; CAPITALS indicate life-threatening.

Dilution

• **Intermittent Infusion: Dilute** ciprofloxacin to a concentration of 1–2 mg/ml with 0.9% NaCl or D5W. • Solution ranges from clear and colorless to slightly yellow. Stable for 14 days refrigerated or at room temperature.

Compatibility

• **Y-site:** amino acids ✦ aztreonam ✦ calcium gluconate ✦ ceftazidime ✦ digoxin ✦ diltiazem ✦ diphenhydramine ✦ dobutamine ✦ dopamine ✦ gallium nitrate ✦ gentamycin ✦ hydroxyzine ✦ lidocaine ✦ metoclopramide ✦ piperacillin ✦ potassium acetate ✦ potassium chloride ✦ potassium phosphates ✦ promethazine ✦ ranitidine ✦ tacrolimus ✦ tobramycin ✦ verapamil. However, manufacturer recommends temporarily discontinuing other solutions when administering ciprofloxacin.

• **Additive:** amikacin ✦ aztreonam ✦ ceftazidime ✦ gentamycin ✦ metronidazole ✦ piperacillin ✦ tobramycin.

• **Solution:** lactated Ringer's for injection.

Incompatibility

• **Y-site:** aminophylline ✦ dexamethasone ✦ furosemide ✦ heparin ✦ hydrocortisone sodium succinate ✦ mezlocillin ✦ phenytoin.

• **Additive:** aminophylline ✦ clindamycin ✦ mezlocillin.

Rate of Administration

• **Intermittent Infusion:** Administer over 60 minutes into a large vein to minimize venous irritation.

≋ CLINICAL PRECAUTIONS

- Obtain specimens for culture and sensitivity. First dose may be given before results are known.
- Inspect IV site frequently. Phlebitis is associated with infusion times of less than 30 minutes.
- Assess renal function. Patients with severe renal impairment (creatinine clearance less than 30 ml/min) should receive the dosage at increased dosing intervals. Encourage liberal fluid intake (2000–3000 ml/day) to decrease the risk of crystalluria. Assess elderly patients for age-related decrease in renal function and make necessary adjustments.

- Assess patient for infection (vital signs; appearance of wound, sputum, urine, and stool; WBC) at beginning and throughout course of therapy.
- Assess mental status. Restlessness is common. Use cautiously in patients with CNS pathology. Seizures may occasionally occur.
- Assess patient for tendon pain or inflammation.
- The risk of tendon rupture is increased by concurrent glucocorticoid therapy, advanced age, or chronic dialysis.
- Ciprofloxacin increases serum theophylline levels and may lead to toxicity. Monitor serum theophylline levels in patients receiving both drugs.
- Drugs that alkalinize the urine increase the risk of crystalluria from ciprofloxacin.
- Ciprofloxacin may increase nephrotoxicity of cyclosporine.
- Nitrofurantoin may decrease effectiveness of ciprofloxacin.
- Probenecid increases blood levels of ciprofloxacin.
- Ciprofloxacin may increase the effect of warfarin.
- Safe use during lactation has not been established. Ciprofloxacin is not recommended during pregnancy or in children younger than the age of 18 (Pregnancy Category C).

Lab Test Considerations

- May cause elevated AST (SGOT), ALT (SGPT), alkaline phosphatase, bilirubin, BUN, creatinine, and LDH concentrations. • May cause elevated or decreased serum platelets and decreased RBCs and WBCs.

Patient/Family Teaching

- Ciprofloxacin may cause dizziness or light-headedness. Caution patient to avoid driving or other activities requiring alertness until response to medication is known. Instruct the patient to report tendon pain or inflammation. If tendonitis occurs, ciprofloxacin should be discontinued. • Caution patient to use sunscreen and protective clothing to prevent photosensitivity reactions. • Advise patient to report signs of superinfection (furry overgrowth on the tongue, vaginal itching or discharge, loose or foul-smelling stools). • Instruct the patient to notify physician if symptoms do not improve.

≋ PHARMACOLOGIC PROFILE

Indications

• Ciprofloxacin is used in the treatment of the following infections due to susceptible organisms: lower respiratory tract infections, skin and skin structure infections, bone and joint infections, and urinary tract infections.

Action

• Ciprofloxacin inhibits bacterial DNA synthesis by inhibiting the enzyme DNA gyrase. It is active against many Gram-positive pathogens. Staphylococci (including *Staphylococcus epidermidis* and methicillin-resistant strains of *Staphylococcus aureus*), *Streptococcus pyogenes,* and *Streptococcus pneumoniae* are usually susceptible. Its Gram-negative spectrum is notable for activity against *Escherichia coli, Klebsiella* species, *Enterobacter, Salmonella, Shigella, Proteus vulgaris, Providencia stuartii, Providencia rettgeri, Morganella morganii, Pseudomonas aeruginosa, Serratia, Haemophilus* species, *Acinetobacter, Neisseria gonorrhoeae, N. meningitidis, Branhamella catarrhalis, Yersinia, Vibrio, Brucella, Campylobacter, Aeromonas* species.

Time/Action Profile

Onset	Peak
rapid	end of infusion

Pharmacokinetics

• **Distribution:** Ciprofloxacin is widely distributed, achieving high tissue concentrations. It crosses the placenta and enters breast milk. CSF levels are low. • **Metabolism and Excretion:** 15% of ciprofloxacin is metabolized by the liver; 40–50% is excreted unchanged by the kidneys. • **Half-life:** 4 hours (increased in renal impairment).

Contraindications

• Ciprofloxacin should not be used in patients with hypersensitivity to ciprofloxacin or other fluoroquinolones. • Pregnant women and children younger than 18 years should not receive ciprofloxacin.

Adverse Reactions and Side Effects*

• **CNS:** tremors, <u>restlessness</u>, headache, confusion, hallucination, SEIZURES, dizziness • **GI:** <u>nausea</u>, <u>diarrhea</u>, <u>vomiting</u>, <u>abdominal pain</u> • **GU:** crystalluria, cylinduria, hematuria • **Derm:** rash, photosensitivity • **Local:** phlebitis at IV site • **MS:** tendonitis, tendon rupture • **Misc:** allergic reactions including ANAPHYLAXIS.

Cisplatin	Antineoplastic (alkylating agent)
Platinol, Platinol-AQ	pH 3.5–5

ADMINISTRATION CONSIDERATIONS

Usual Dose

Metastatic Testicular Tumors
ADULTS AND CHILDREN: 20 mg/m²/day for 5 days (in combination with other agents) every 3 weeks.

Metastatic Ovarian Cancer
ADULTS AND CHILDREN: 50 mg/m² once every 3 weeks (in combination with other agents) or 100 mg/m² every 3–4 weeks (single agent).

Advanced Bladder Cancer
ADULTS AND CHILDREN: 50–70 mg/m² every 3–4 weeks (single agent). Doses should not exceed 120 mg/m²/course.

Dilution

• **Intermittent Infusion:** Reconstitute 10-mg vial with 10 ml of sterile water for injection and 50-mg vial with 50 ml. • Do not use aluminum needles or equipment during preparation or administration. Aluminum reacts with the drug, forms a black or brown precipitate, and renders it ineffective. Unopened vials of powder must be refrigerated. • Solution should be prepared in a biologic cabinet. Wear gloves, gown, and mask while handling medication. Discard equip-

---

*<u>Underlines</u> indicate most frequent; CAPITALS indicate life-threatening.

ment in specially designated containers (see Appendix F).
• Stable for 2 hours if reconstituted with sterile water, for 72 hours with bacteriostatic water. Do not refrigerate solution, as crystals will form. Solution should be clear and colorless; discard if turbid or if it contains precipitates. • **Dilution** in 2 liters of 5% dextrose in 0.3% or 0.45% NaCl containing 37.5 g of mannitol is recommended. • May also be **diluted** with 0.9% NaCl or D5/0.9% NaCl.

Compatibility

• **Syringe:** bleomycin • cyclophosphamide • doxapram • doxorubicin • droperidol • fluorouracil • furosemide • heparin • leucovorin calcium • methotrexate • metoclopramide • mitomycin • vinblastine • vincristine.

• **Y-site:** allopurinol sodium • bleomycin • chlorpromazine • cimetidine • cyclophosphamide • dexamethasone • diphenhydramine • doxorubicin • droperidol • famotidine • filgrastim • fludarabine • fluorouracil • furosemide • gancyclovir • heparin • hydromorphone • leucovorin calcium • lorazepam • melphalan • methotrexate • methylprednisolone • metoclopramide • mitomycin • morphine • ondansetron • paclitaxel • prochlorperazine • promethazine • ranitidine • sargramostim • vinblastine • vincristine • vinorelbine.

• **Additive:** etoposide • floxuridine • hydroxyzine • ifosfamide • leucovorin • magnesium sulfate • mannitol.

Incompatibility

• **Y-site:** gallium nitrate • piperacillin/tazobactam.
• **Additive:** fluorouracil • mesna • sodium bicarbonate • thiotepa.

Rate of Administration

• **Intermittent Infusion:** Infuse over 6–8 hours. Direct IV injection over 1–5 minutes is associated with increased nephrotoxicity and ototoxicity. • **Continuous Infusion:** Has been administered as continuous infusion over 24 hours–5 days in an effort to decrease nausea and vomiting.

≋ CLINICAL PRECAUTIONS

• Monitor for signs of anaphylaxis (facial edema, wheezing, tachycardia, hypotension). Discontinue medication immediately and notify physician if these occur. Epinephrine and resuscitation equipment should be readily available.

- Assess fluid and electrolyte status, intake and output, and specific gravity of urine prior to and following therapy. Adequate hydration is required to prevent renal damage and hearing loss. To reduce the risk of nephrotoxicity, hydrate patient with at least 1–2 liters of IV fluid 8–12 hours before initiating therapy with cisplatin. A urinary output of at least 100 ml/hr should be maintained for 4 hours before initiating and for at least 24 hours after administration. Encourage patient to drink 2000–3000 ml/day to promote excretion of uric acid. Allopurinol and alkalinization of the urine may be ordered to help prevent uric acid nephropathy. Peak uric acid concentrations occur 3–5 days after a dose.

- Do not confuse *cisplatin* with *carboplatin*. Toxicities, indications, and doses are not the same. See *carboplatin* monograph on page 151.

- Cisplatin may cause ototoxicity (especially in children) and neurotoxicity. Assess patient frequently for dizziness, tinnitus, hearing loss, loss of coordination, or numbness and tingling of extremities. These symptoms may be irreversible. Children are at increased risk for ototoxic effects of cisplatin. Risk of nephrotoxicity and ototoxicity is increased by concurrent use of other nephrotoxic and ototoxic agents. Cisplatin is excreted mainly by the kidneys; dosage reduction is required for patients with renal impairment or elderly patients.

- Assess patency of IV site frequently during therapy. This medication may cause severe irritation and necrosis of tissue if extravasation occurs. If a large amount of highly concentrated solution extravasates, a mixture of 4 ml of 10% sodium thiosulfate with 6 ml of sterile water for injection or 1.6 ml of 25% sodium thiosulfate with 8.4 ml of sterile water for injection may be injected through a cannula (1 ml for each ml extravasated) or SC if the needle has been removed, to inactivate cisplatin.

- Severe and protracted nausea and vomiting may occur as early as 1 hour after therapy and may last for 24 hours. Parenteral antiemetic agents should be administered 30–45 minutes prior to therapy and routinely around the clock for the next 24 hours as indicated. Monitor amount of emesis and follow guidelines to prevent dehydration.

- Severe electrolyte depletion may occur. Monitor for hypomagnesemia, hypokalemia, and hypocalcemia. Hypokalemia increases the risk of cardiac glycoside (digoxin) toxicity.
- Bone marrow depression is common. Assess for fever, chills, sore throat, and signs of infection. Monitor platelet count throughout therapy. Assess for bleeding (bleeding gums, bruising, petechiae; guaiac test stools, urine, and emesis). Avoid administering IM injections and taking rectal temperatures. Apply pressure to venipuncture sites for 10 minutes. Anemia may occur. Monitor for increased fatigue, dyspnea, and orthostatic hypotension. Additive bone marrow depression occurs with concurrent or previous use of other antineoplastic agents or radiation therapy. Dosage reduction may be necessary.
- Use cautiously in patients with active infections, bone marrow depression, or chronic debilitating illnesses.
- Use cautiously in patients with childbearing potential. Pregnant or lactating patients should not receive cisplatin (Pregnancy Category D).

Lab Test Considerations

• Monitor CBC prior to and routinely throughout course of therapy. The nadir of leukopenia, thrombocytopenia, and anemia occurs within 18–23 days. Withhold further doses until WBC is >4,000/mm^3 and platelet count is >100,000/mm^3. • Monitor renal and hepatic function prior to and periodically throughout course of therapy. May cause nephrotoxicity (increased BUN and creatinine, and decreased calcium, magnesium, phosphate, and potassium levels). Do not administer additional doses until BUN is <25 mg/100 ml and serum creatinine is <1.5 mg/100 ml. May cause increased uric acid levels. • Hepatotoxity may be manifested by increased AST (SGOT), ALT (SGPT), and bilirubin.

Patient/Family Teaching

• Instruct patient to report pain at injection site immediately. • Instruct patient to notify physician promptly if fever, sore throat, signs of infection, bleeding gums, bruising, petechiae; blood in stools, urine, or emesis; increased fatigue, dyspnea, or orthostatic hypotension occurs. Caution patient to avoid crowds and persons with known infections. Instruct patient to use soft toothbrush and electric razor, and to avoid falls. Caution patient not to drink alcoholic beverages or take medication containing aspirin, ibuprofen, or naproxen, as these may precipitate gastric bleeding. • Instruct patient to report promptly to the physician any numbness or tingling in extremities or face, difficulty with hearing or tinnitus, unusual swelling, or joint pain. • Instruct patient not to receive any vaccinations without advice of physician. • Advise patients with childbearing potential of the need for a nonhormonal method of contraception. • Emphasize the need for periodic lab tests to monitor therapy.

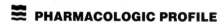

PHARMACOLOGIC PROFILE

Indications

• Cisplatin is used alone or in combination with other antineoplastics, surgery, or radiation in the management of metastatic testicular and ovarian carcinoma, advanced bladder cancer, head and neck cancer, cervical cancer, lung cancer, and other tumors.

Action

• Cisplatin inhibits DNA synthesis by producing cross-linking of parent DNA strands (cell cycle–phase nonspecific). This results in death of rapidly replicating cells, particularly malignant cells.

Time/Action Profile (effect on blood counts)

Onset	Peak	Duration
UK	18–23 days	39 days

Pharmacokinetics

• **Distribution:** Cisplatin is widely distributed. Accumulation continues for months after administration. • **Metabolism and Excretion:** Excretion occurs mainly through the kidneys. • **Half-life:** 30–100 hours.

Contraindications

• Cisplatin is contraindicated in patients with hypersensitivity to cisplatin. • Pregnant or lactating patients should not receive cisplatin.

Adverse Reactions and Side Effects*

• **CNS:** SEIZURES • **EENT:** ototoxicity, tinnitus • **GI:** severe nausea, vomiting, diarrhea, hepatotoxicity • **GU:** nephrotoxicity, infertility • **F and E:** hypomagnesemia, hypokalemia, hypocalcemia • **Hemat:** anemia, leukopenia, thrombocytopenia • **Local:** phlebitis at IV site • **Metab:** hyperuricemia • **Neuro:** peripheral neuropathy • **Misc:** anaphylactoid reactions.

Cladribine	Antineoplastic agent (antimetabolite)
Leustatin	pH 5.5–8

 ADMINISTRATION CONSIDERATIONS

Usual Dose

ADULTS: 0.09 mg/kg/day for 7 days.

Dilution

• **Continuous Infusion:** Add the daily dose to 500 ml of 0.9% NaCl for injection. • Solution for IV administration should be prepared in a biologic cabinet. Wear gloves, gown, and mask while handling IV medication. Discard IV equipment in specially designated containers (see Appendix F). • Solution is stable for 24 hours at room temperature or 8 days if refrigerated. • May also be prepared as a 7-day solution with bacteriostatic 0.9% NaCl for infusion via Pharmacia *Deltec* medication cassettes.

Incompatibility

• **Additive:** D5W. Do not admix with or infuse in the same line as other medications or solutions.

---

*Underlines indicate most frequent; CAPITALS indicate life-threatening.

Rate of Administration

• **Continuous Infusion:** Administer as a continuous infusion over 24 hours.

≋ CLINICAL PRECAUTIONS

• Monitor for bone marrow depression. Assess for fever, chills, sore throat, and signs of infection. Monitor platelet count throughout therapy. Assess for bleeding (bleeding gums, bruising, petechiae, guaiac test stools, urine, and emesis). Avoid administering IM injections and taking rectal temperatures. Apply pressure to venipuncture site for 10 minutes. Anemia may occur. Monitor for increased fatigue, dyspnea, and orthostatic hypotension. Additive bone marrow depression may occur with concurrent use of other antineoplastics or radiation therapy. Cladribine should be used cautiously in patients with active infections, decreased bone marrow reserve, or other chronic debilitating illness.
• Monitor IV site for phlebitis.
• Impaired hepatic or renal function may increase the risk of toxicity of cladribine.
• Safe use of cladribine in children has not been established. Use cladribine cautiously in patients with childbearing potential (Pregnancy Category D).

Toxicity and Overdose Alert

• May cause irreversible neurologic toxicity resulting in motor weakness and progressing to paraparesis or quadriparesis with high doses. If symptoms occur, discontinue cladribine. There is no known antidote.

Lab Test Considerations

• Monitor prior to and periodically throughout therapy, especially during the first 4–8 weeks after treatment. During the first 2 weeks after therapy, platelet counts, absolute neutrophil count (ANC), and hemoglobin levels decrease. Return to normal levels usually occurs by day 12, week 5, and week 8, respectively. • Monitor renal and hepatic function prior to and periodically throughout therapy. May cause nephrotoxicity resulting in elevated serum creatinine levels, anuria, and acidosis.

Patient/Family Teaching

• Instruct patient to notify physician promptly in the event of fever; sore throat; signs of infection; bleeding gums; bruising; petechiae; blood in urine, stool, or emesis; unusual swelling; joint pain; shortness of breath; or confusion. Caution the patient to avoid crowds and persons with known infections. Instruct the patient to use soft toothbrush and electric razor and be especially careful to avoid falls. Patient should also be cautioned not to drink alcoholic beverages or to take products containing aspirin, naproxen, or ibuprofen, because these may precipitate GI hemorrhage. • Advise patient to use nonhormonal contraceptive measures during and for at least 4 months after completion of therapy. • Instruct patient not to receive any vaccinations without advice of physician.

 PHARMACOLOGIC PROFILE

Indications

• Cladribine is used in the management of active hairy-cell leukemia manifested as anemia, leukopenia, thrombocytopenia, or clinical symptoms.

Action

• Cladribine inhibits DNA synthesis and repair, resulting in the death of rapidly replicating cells, particularly malignant ones. Cladribine also has immunosuppressant properties.

Time/Action Profile (noted as effect on peripheral counts)

Parameter	Time to normalization
platelets	2 wk
absolute neutrophil count	5 wk
hemoglobin	8 wk

Pharmacokinetics

• **Distribution:** Distribution of cladribine is not known. • **Metabolism and Excretion:** Metabolism and excretion of cladribine are not known. • **Half-life:** 5.4 hours.

Contraindications

• Cladribine is contraindicated in patients with known hypersensitivity to it. • The diluent provided contains benzyl alcohol and should be avoided in patients with known intolerance. • Pregnant or lactating patients should not receive cladribine.

Adverse Reactions and Side Effects*

• **CNS:** <u>fatigue</u>, <u>headache</u>, dizziness, weakness, malaise, insomnia • **EENT:** epistaxis • **Resp:** <u>abnormal breath sounds</u>, cough, shortness of breath • **CV:** edema, tachycardia • **GI:** <u>nausea</u>, <u>decreased appetite</u>, <u>vomiting</u>, <u>diarrhea</u>, constipation, abdominal pain • **Derm:** rash, sweating, purpura, petechiae, erythema • **Hemat:** <u>neutropenia</u>, <u>anemia</u>, <u>thrombocytopenia</u> • **Local:** injection site reactions, thrombosis, phlebitis • **MS:** myalgia, arthralgia • **Misc:** fever, infection, chills, trunk pain.

Clindamycin Phosphate	Anti-infective
Cleocin Phosphate, {Delacen C Phosphate}	pH 5.5–7

≋ ADMINISTRATION CONSIDERATIONS

Usual Dose

ADULTS: 300–600 mg q 6–8 hr (up to 4.8 g/day or 900 mg q 8 hr.

CHILDREN: 3.75–10 mg/kg (87.5–112.5 mg/m^2) q 6 hr or 5–13.3 mg/kg (116.7–150 mg/m^2) q 8 hr (minimum of 300 mg/day for severe infections).

NEONATES: 3.75–5 mg/kg q 6 hr or 5–6.7 mg/kg q 8 hr.

Dilution

• **Intermittent Infusion:** Do not administer as an undiluted IV bolus. **Dilute** each 300 mg for IV administration with at least 50 ml of D5W, D10W, D5/0.45% NaCl, D5/0.9% NaCl, D5/Ringer's injection, 0.9% NaCl, or lactated

---

*<u>Underlines</u> indicate most frequent; CAPITALS indicate life-threatening.

{} = Available in Canada only.

Ringer's solution for injection. Concentrations must not exceed 12–18 mg/ml. • Stable for 24 hours at room temperature. Crystals may occur if refrigerated but dissolve when warmed to room temperature. Do not administer solution with undissolved crystals.

Compatibility

• **Syringe:** amikacin ◆ aztreonam ◆ gentamicin ◆ heparin.
• **Y-site:** cyclophosphamide ◆ diltiazem ◆ enalaprilat ◆ esmolol ◆ fludarabine ◆ foscarnet ◆ hydromorphone ◆ labetalol ◆ magnesium sulfate ◆ melphalan ◆ meperidine ◆ morphine ◆ multivitamins ◆ ondansetron ◆ perphenazine ◆ piperacillin/tazobactam ◆ sargramostim ◆ tacrolimus ◆ vinorelbine ◆ vitamin B complex with C ◆ zidovudine.
• **Additive:** amikacin ◆ aztreonam ◆ cefamandole ◆ cefazolin ◆ cefonicid ◆ cefoperazone ◆ cefotaxime ◆ cefoxitin ◆ ceftazidime ◆ ceftizoxime ◆ cefuroxime ◆ cephalothin ◆ cimetidine ◆ fluconazole ◆ heparin ◆ hydrocortisone sodium succinate ◆ kanamycin ◆ methylprednisolone ◆ metoclopramide ◆ metronidazole ◆ netilmicin ◆ ofloxacin ◆ penicillin G ◆ piperacillin ◆ potassium chloride ◆ sodium bicarbonate ◆ tobramycin ◆ vitamin B complex with C.

Incompatibility

• **Syringe:** tobramycin.
• **Y-site:** allopurinol sodium ◆ filgrastim ◆ fluconazole ◆ idarubicin.
• **Additive:** aminophylline ◆ barbiturates ◆ calcium gluconate ◆ ceftriaxone ◆ ciprofloxacin ◆ magnesium sulfate ◆ phenytoin ◆ ranitidine.

Rate of Administration

• **Intermittent Infusion:** Administer each 300 mg over a minimum of 10–60 minutes at a rate not exceeding 30 mg/min. Do not give more than 1200 mg in a single 1-hour infusion. • **Continuous Infusion:** May also be initially administered as a single rapid infusion, followed by continuous IV infusion. To maintain serum clindamycin levels of 4 mcg/ml, 5 mcg/ml, or 6 mcg/ml, the rapid infusion rates should be 10 mg/min, 15 mg/min, or 20 mg/min for 30 minutes with maintenance infusion rates of 0.75 mg/min, 1 mg/min, or 1.25 mg/min, respectively.

≋ CLINICAL PRECAUTIONS

- Obtain specimens for culture and sensitivity prior to initiating therapy. First dose may be given before results are available.
- Assess patient for infection (vital signs; appearance of wound, sputum, urine, and stool; WBC) at beginning and throughout therapy.
- Assess bowel status. Diarrhea is a side effect, but diarrhea that is bloody or is accompanied by fever may indicate pseudomembranous colitis that has been associated with clindamycin. This may begin up to several weeks following the cessation of therapy.
- Inspect IV site for redness or irritation. Phlebitis may occur.
- Assess patient for hypersensitivity (skin rash, urticaria).
- Action of neuromuscular blocking agents may be enhanced by clindamycin.
- Safe use in pregnancy or lactation has not been established.

Lab Test Considerations

- Monitor CBC; clindamycin may cause transient decrease in leukocytes, eosinophils, and platelets. • May cause elevated alkaline phosphatase, bilirubin, CPK, AST (SGOT), and ALT (SGPT) concentrations.

Patient/Family Teaching

- Inform patient that bitter taste occurring with IV administration is not significant. • Instruct patient to notify physician immediately if diarrhea, abdominal cramping, fever, or bloody stools occur and not to treat with antidiarrheals without physician's approval. • Advise patient to report signs of superinfection (furry overgrowth on the tongue, vaginal or anal itching or discharge). • Notify physician if there is no improvement within a few days. • Patients with a history of rheumatic heart disease or valve replacement need to be taught the importance of antimicrobial prophylaxis before invasive medical or dental procedures (see Appendix K).

≋ PHARMACOLOGIC PROFILE

Indications

• Clindamycin is used in the treatment of the following serious infections due to susceptible organisms: skin and skin structure infections, respiratory tract infections, septicemia, intra-abdominal infections, gynecologic infections, and osteomyelitis. It is also used for endocarditis prophylaxis. • **Unlabeled Use:** Clindamycin is used in combination with other agents in the treatment of *Pneumocystis carinii* pneumonia (PCP) and CNS toxoplasmosis.

Action

• Clindamycin inhibits protein synthesis in susceptible bacteria at the level of the 50S ribosome, resulting in action that may be bactericidal or bacteriostatic, depending on susceptibility and concentration. It is active against most Gram-positive aerobic cocci including staphylococci, *Streptococcus pneumoniae,* and other streptococci, but not enterococci. Has good activity against many anaerobic bacteria including *Bacteroides fragilis.*

Time/Action Profile

Onset	Peak
rapid	end of infusion

Pharmacokinetics

• **Distribution:** Clindamycin is widely distributed, although it does not significantly cross the blood–brain barrier. It crosses the placenta and enters breast milk. • **Metabolism and Excretion:** Clindamycin is mostly metabolized by the liver. • **Half-life:** 2–3 hours.

Contraindications

• Hypersensitivity to clindamycin or known intolerance to benzyl alcohol. • Patients with a previous history of pseudomembranous colitis or who currently have diarrhea should not receive clindamycin. • Because clindamycin is mostly metabolized by the liver, its use should be avoided in patients with severe liver impairment.

Adverse Reactions and Side Effects*

• **CNS:** dizziness, vertigo, headache • **CV:** hypotension, arrhythmias • **Derm:** rashes • **GI:** <u>diarrhea</u>, nausea, vomiting, PSEUDOMEMBRANOUS COLITIS, bitter taste • **Local:** phlebitis at IV site.

Colchicine	*Antigout agent*
	pH 6–7.2

ADMINISTRATION CONSIDERATIONS

Usual Dose

Acute Gouty Arthritis

ADULTS: 2 mg initially, then 0.5 mg q 6 hr or 1 mg q 6–12 hr until response is obtained (not to exceed 4 mg/day or 4 mg/ treatment course).

GERIATRIC PATIENTS OR PATIENTS WITH CREATININE CLEARANCE OF 10–50 ml/min: 1 mg initially, then 0.25 mg q 6 hr or 0.5 mg q 6–12 hr until response is obtained (not to exceed 2 mg/day or 2 mg/treatment course).

Prevention of Acute Gouty Arthritis

ADULTS: After at least a 1-wk rest period following an acute attack, maintenance therapy of 0.5–1 mg 1–2 times daily may be used.

GERIATRIC PATIENTS OR PATIENTS WITH CREATININE CLEARANCE OF 10–50 ml/min: After at least a 21-day rest period following an acute attack, maintenance therapy of 0.25–0.5 mg 1–2 times daily may be used.

Dilution

• **Direct IV:** May be administered **undiluted.** • If a lower concentration is desired, may **dilute** to a volume of 10–20 ml with sterile water or 0.9% NaCl for injection. • Do not administer solutions that are turbid.

---

*Underlines indicate most frequent; CAPITALS indicate life-threatening.

Incompatibility

- Do not dilute colchicine with or inject into IV tubing containing D5W, solutions containing a bacteriostatic agent, or any other solution that might change the pH of the colchicine solution because precipitation will occur.

Rate of Administration

- **Direct IV:** Administer over 2–5 minutes.

≋ CLINICAL PRECAUTIONS

- Colchicine should be administered at the first sign of an acute attack. Delay in starting treatment reduces the effectiveness of colchicine.
- Assess injection site carefully. Severe local irritation occurs with SC or IM injection. Sloughing of skin and subcutaneous tissues may occur with extravasation.
- Assess involved joints for pain, mobility, and edema every 1–2 hours during initiation of therapy and periodically throughout therapy.
- Monitor intake and output ratios. Fluids should be encouraged to promote a urinary output of at least 2000 ml/day.
- The parenteral route is preferred in patients with active alcoholism. Oral administration increases the risk of GI toxicity in these patients.
- Because toxicity is cumulative, colchicine should be used cautiously in geriatric or debilitated patients or patients with renal or hepatic impairment. Patients who have been on oral colchicine should receive lower initial doses.
- Colchicine may cause reversible malabsorption of vitamin B_{12}. Concurrent use of phenylbutazone, antineoplastic agents, or radiation therapy increases the risk of adverse hematologic reactions.
- Safe use in children or during lactation has not been established. Colchicine may cause fetal harm and should be used during pregnancy only when the potential benefits outweigh the potential risks to the fetus (Pregnancy Category D).

Toxicity and Overdose Alert

• Assess patient for toxicity (weakness, abdominal discomfort, nausea, vomiting, diarrhea). If these symptoms occur, discontinue colchicine. Opioids may be needed to treat diarrhea.

Lab Test Considerations

• May cause a decreased platelet count. • May cause an increase in AST (SGOT) and alkaline phosphatase. • May cause false-positive results for urine hemoglobin. • May interfere with results of urinary 17-hydroxycorticosteroid concentrations.

Patient/Family Teaching

• Advise the patient to follow recommendations regarding weight loss, diet, and alcohol consumption. • Instruct patient to report nausea, vomiting, abdominal pain, diarrhea, unusual bleeding or bruising, sore throat, fatigue, malaise, or rash promptly. Medication should be discontinued if gastric symptoms occur.

≋ PHARMACOLOGIC PROFILE

Indications

• Colchicine is indicated for treatment of acute attacks of gouty arthritis and prevention of recurrent gouty arthritis. Oral therapy should replace IV therapy as soon as possible.

Action

• Colchicine interferes with the function of WBCs in initiating and sustaining the inflammatory response to mono-sodium urate crystals.

Time/Action Profile (anti-inflammatory effect)

Onset	Peak	Duration
6–12 hr	24–48 hr†	UK

†Relief of pain and inflammation; relief of swelling may take up to 72 hr.

Pharmacokinetics

• **Distribution:** Colchicine concentrates in WBCs. • **Metabolism and Excretion:** Colchicine is partially metabolized by the liver, secreted into the GI tract, and is eliminated in feces. Small amounts are excreted in urine. • **Half-life:** 20 minutes in plasma, 60 hours in WBCs.

Contraindications

• Colchicine is contraindicated in patients who exhibit hypersensitivity to it. • Colchicine should be avoided in patients with GI disease or severe renal disease (creatinine clearance less than 10 ml/min).

Adverse Reactions and Side Effects*

• **GI:** <u>nausea</u>, <u>vomiting</u>, <u>diarrhea</u>, abdominal pain • **GU:** anuria, hematuria, renal damage • **Derm:** alopecia • **Hemat:** AGRANULOCYTOSIS, APLASTIC ANEMIA, leukopenia, thrombocytopenia • **Local:** phlebitis at IV site • **Neuro:** peripheral neuritis.

Corticotropin	Hormone (adrenocorticotropic)
ACTH, Acthar	pH 2.5–6

 ADMINISTRATION CONSIDERATIONS

Usual Dose

ADULTS: 10–25 units over 8 hr.
CHILDREN: 1.6 units/kg (50 units/m^2)/day in 3–4 divided doses.

Dilution

• **Reconstitute** 25-unit vial with 1 ml of 0.9% NaCl or sterile water for injection. **Reconstitute** 40-unit vial with 2 ml. • Stable for 24 hours at room temperature and 7 days if refrigerated. • **Direct IV:** May be administered **undiluted**.
• **Intermittent Infusion:** Dilute 10–25 units in 500 ml

---

*<u>Underlines</u> indicate most frequent; CAPITALS indicate life-threatening.

of D5W, D5/0.9% NaCl, 0.9% NaCl, or lactated Ringer's solution.

Compatibility

• **Additive:** calcium gluconate ✦ chloramphenicol ✦ cytarabine (for 8 hours) ✦ erythromycin gluceptate ✦ heparin ✦ hydrocortisone sodium succinate ✦ methicillin ✦ oxytetracycline ✦ penicillin G potassium ✦ potassium chloride ✦ vancomycin ✦ vitamin B complex with C.

Incompatibility

• **Additive:** aminophylline ✦ sodium bicarbonate.

Rate of Administration

• **Direct IV:** Administer over 2 minutes. • **Intermittent Infusion:** Infuse over 8 hours. May also be ordered as 40 units to be infused over 12–48 hours.

≋ CLINICAL PRECAUTIONS

- Because of serious adverse reactions associated with chronic use, this agent is recommended for diagnostic testing of adrenal function only. Because its maximal effect on adrenal function is delayed by several days, it should not be used when a rapid effect is desired.
- In patients with a history of allergic reactions, monitor for hypersensitivity (wheezing, rash or hives, bradycardia, irritability, seizures, nausea, vomiting). These reactions are more likely to occur with SC administration or prolonged therapy. Patients allergic to porcine protein should receive intradermal test dose prior to therapeutic or diagnostic dose.
- Chronic use in children may lead to growth suppression. Chronic treatment will also result in adrenal suppression. If used chronically, do not discontinue abruptly. Additional doses may be needed during stress (infections, surgery). Use lowest possible dose for shortest period of time.
- Monitor mental status. A wide variety of reactions may occur, ranging from depression to acute psychoses.
- Additive hypokalemia may occur with amphotericin B, mezlocillin, piperacillin, ticarcillin, or diuretics. Hypo-

kalemia may increase the risk of cardiac glycoside (digoxin) toxicity.

- Patients with cirrhosis or hypothyroidism may have an exaggerated response to corticotropin.
- Corticotropin may increase requirements for insulin or oral hypoglycemic agents. Monitor diabetic patients carefully.
- Safe use in pregnancy or lactation has not been established. Use in pregnancy only when needed (Pregnancy Category C).

Lab Test Considerations

• When used to diagnose adrenal insufficiency, plasma cortisol concentrations, urine 17-ketosteroids, and 17-hydroxyketosteroids will be measured before and after administration. Therapeutic response is a rise in the plasma and urine steroid concentrations. • Patients on prolonged courses of therapy should routinely have hematologic values, serum electrolytes, and serum and urine glucose evaluated. May decrease WBC counts. May cause hyperglycemia, especially in persons with diabetes. May decrease serum potassium and calcium and increase serum sodium concentrations. • Guaiac test stools. • Corticotropin may increase serum cholesterol and lipid values. • May decrease serum protein-bound iodine and thyroxine concentrations. • Suppresses reactions to allergy skin tests.

Patient/Family Teaching

• This drug causes immunosuppression and may mask symptoms of infection. Instruct patient to avoid people with known contagious illnesses and to report possible infections promptly. • Review side effects with patient. Instruct patient to inform physician promptly if severe abdominal pain or tarry stools occur. Patient should report unusual swelling, weight gain, tiredness, bone pain, bruising, nonhealing sores, visual disturbances, or behavioral changes. • Instruct patient to inform physician if symptoms of underlying disease return or worsen. • Caution patient to avoid vaccinations without first consulting physician. • Explain the purpose of corticotropin and the need for lab tests to patients receiving corticotropin as a diagnostic aid.

≋ PHARMACOLOGIC PROFILE

Indications
• Corticotropin is used in the diagnosis of adrenocortical disorders. • Corticotropin is rarely used as an anti-inflammatory or immunosuppressant unless conventional glucocorticoid therapy has failed.

Action
• Corticotropin, a hormone produced by the pituitary, stimulates the adrenal gland to produce both glucocorticoids (hydrocortisone) and mineralocorticoids (aldosterone). Its action requires intact adrenal responsiveness. • With chronic use, its actions resemble glucocorticoid administration and include suppression of the normal immune response and inflammation. • Chronic use will also result in additional numerous intense metabolic effects including suppression of adrenal function.

Time/Action Profile (effects on plasma cortisol)

Onset	Peak	Duration
UK	1 hr	UK

Pharmacokinetics
• **Distribution:** Corticotropin is removed from plasma to many tissues. It does not cross the placenta. • **Metabolism and Excretion:** The metabolic fate of corticotropin is not known. • **Half-life:** 15 minutes (plasma).

Contraindications
• Corticotropin is contraindicated in patients with hypersensitivity to porcine proteins. It should not be given to patients with serious infections except for some forms of meningitis.

Adverse Reactions and Side Effects*
(seen during high-dose, long-term therapy)
• **CNS:** psychoses, depression, euphoria • **EENT:** cataracts, increased intraocular pressure • **CV:** edema, hypertension, congestive heart failure, thromboembolism • **GI:** nausea, vomiting, increased appetite, weight gain, peptic ul-

---

*Underlines indicate most frequent; CAPITALS indicate life-threatening.

ceration • **Derm:** <u>petechiae</u>, ecchymoses, fragility, <u>decreased wound healing</u>, hirsutism, acne • **Endo:** menstrual irregularities, hyperglycemia, <u>decreased growth in children</u>, ADRENAL SUPPRESSION • **F and E:** <u>hypokalemia</u>, <u>sodium retention</u>, metabolic alkalosis, hypocalcemia • **MS:** weakness, myopathy, aseptic necrosis of joints, osteoporosis • **Misc:** increases susceptibility to infections, pancreatitis, cushingoid appearance (moon face, buffalo hump).

Cosyntropin	Hormone (adrenocorticotropic)
Cortrosyn, synacthen, tetrocosactin	pH 5.5–7.5

 ADMINISTRATION CONSIDERATIONS

Usual Dose

ADULTS AND CHILDREN >**2 yr:** 250 mcg; determine plasma cortisol prior to and 30 min after administration.

CHILDREN <**2 yr:** 125 mcg; determine plasma cortisol prior to and 30 min after administration.

Dilution

• **Direct IV: Reconstitute** 250-mcg vial with 1 ml of 0.9% NaCl for injection. • Solution is stable for 24 hours at room temperature and 21 days if refrigerated. • **Intermittent Infusion:** May be **further diluted** with D5W or 0.9% NaCl. • Solution is stable for 12 hours at room temperature.

Rate of Administration

• **Direct IV:** Administer over 2 minutes. • **Intermittent Infusion:** Infuse at a rate of 40 mcg/hr over 6 hours.

 CLINICAL PRECAUTIONS

- Coordinate laboratory testing of adrenal function to co-incide with drug effect.
- In patients with a history of allergic reactions, monitor for hypersensitivity response (wheezing, rash or hives, bradycardia, irritability, seizures, nausea, vomiting). Co-

syntropin is less likely than ACTH to cause such a response.
- Estrogens may block metabolism and increase the effect of cosyntropin.
- Concurrent glucocorticoid therapy will alter the results of testing.
- Safe use in pregnancy or lactation not established (Pregnancy Category C).

Lab Test Considerations

- Plasma cortisol concentrations will be measured prior to and 30–60 minutes after administration of cosyntropin. Therapeutic response is a rise in the plasma cortisol of at least 7 mcg/100 ml above baseline or a final concentration of at least 18 mcg/100 ml. Administration of glucocorticoids on the day of the test will interfere with test results by causing elevated baseline plasma cortisol concentrations.

Patient/Family Teaching

- Explain the purpose of cosyntropin and the need for lab tests.

≋ PHARMACOLOGIC PROFILE

Indications

- Cosyntropin is used in the diagnosis of adrenocortical disorders.

Action

- A synthetic form of corticotropin, which is normally produced by the pituitary, stimulates the adrenal gland to produce both glucocorticoids (hydrocortisone) and mineralocorticoids (aldosterone). Action requires intact adrenal responsiveness.

Time/Action Profile (effects on plasma cortisol levels)

Onset	Peak	Duration
UK	45–60 min	UK

Pharmacokinetics

- **Distribution:** Cosyntropin is removed from plasma to many tissues. It does not cross the placenta. • **Metabolism**

and Excretion: The metabolic fate of cosyntropin is not known. • **Half-life:** 15 minutes (plasma).

Contraindications

• Cosyntropin is contraindicated in patients with hypersensitivity. • Do not use in patients with serious untreated infections.

Adverse Reactions and Side Effects*

• **Misc:** hypersensitivity reactions including ANAPHYLAXIS.

Cyclophosphamide	Antineoplastic agent (alkylating agent)
Cytoxan, Neosar, {Procytox}	pH 3–7.5

≋ ADMINISTRATION CONSIDERATIONS

Usual Dose

ADULTS: 40–50 mg/kg (1.5–1.8 g/m^2) in divided doses over 2–5 days (up to 100 mg/kg has been used) *or* 10–15 mg/kg (350–550 mg/m^2) every 7–10 days *or* 3–5 mg/kg (110–185 mg/m^2) twice weekly *or* 1.5–3 mg/kg/day.

GERIATRIC PATIENTS: 1–2 mg/kg/day.

CHILDREN: 2–8 mg/kg (60–250 mg/m^2)/day in divided doses for 6 or more days or total dose for 7 days given once weekly. May be followed by maintenance therapy of 10–15 mg/kg q 7–10 days or 30 mg/kg q 3–4 wk.

Dilution

• **Direct IV:** Prepare IV solution by **diluting** each 100 mg with 5 ml of sterile water or bacteriostatic water for injection containing parabens for a concentration of 20 mg/ml. Shake solution gently to dissolve (may be difficult, taking up to 6 minutes) and allow to stand until clear. Use solution prepared without bacteriostatic water within 6 hours. Solution prepared with bacteriostatic water is stable for 24 hours at room

---

*Underlines indicate most frequent; CAPITALS indicate life-threatening.

{} = Available in Canada only.

temperature, 6 days if refrigerated. • Solution for IV administration should be prepared in a biologic cabinet. Wear gloves, gown, and mask while handling IV medication. Discard IV equipment in specially designated containers (see Appendix F). • **Intermittent Infusion:** May be **further diluted** in up to 250 ml of D5W, 0.9% NaCl, D5/0.9% NaCl, 0.45% NaCl, lactated Ringer's solution, or dextrose/Ringer's solution.

Compatibility

• **Syringe:** bleomycin • cisplatin • doxapram • doxorubicin • droperidol • fluorouracil • furosemide • heparin • leucovorin calcium • methotrexate • metoclopramide • mitomycin • vinblastine • vincristine.

• **Y-site:** allopurinol sodium • amikacin • ampicillin • bleomycin • cefamandole • cefazolin • cefoperazone • ceforanide • cefotaxime • cefoxitin • cefuroxime • cephalothin • cephapirin • chloramphenicol • chlorpromazine • cimetidine • cisplatin • clindamycin • dexamethasone • diphenhydramine • doxorubicin • doxycycline • droperidol • erythromycin lactobionate • famotidine • filgrastim • fludarabine • fluorouracil • furosemide • gallium nitrate • gancyclovir • gentamicin • heparin • hydromorphone • idarubicin • kanamycin • leucovorin calcium • lorazepam • melphalan • methotrexate • metoclopramide • metronidazole • mezlocillin • minocycline • mitomycin • morphine • nafcillin • ondansetron • oxacillin • paclitaxel • penicillin G potassium • piperacillin • piperacillin/tazobactam • prochlorperazine • promethazine • ranitidine • sargramostim • ticarcillin • ticarcillin/clavulanate • tobramycin • trimethoprim/sulfamethoxazole • vancomycin • vinblastine • vincristine • vinorelbine.

• **Additive:** fluorouracil • methotrexate • mitoxantrone.

Rate of Administration

• **Direct IV:** Administer reconstituted solution directly at a rate of 100 mg over 1 minute.

≋ CLINICAL PRECAUTIONS

- Monitor blood pressure, pulse, respiratory rate, and temperature frequently during administration.
- Cyclophosphamide is converted by the body to a substance that is irritating to the lining of the bladder and

may produce hemorrhagic cystitis. Monitor urinary output frequently throughout therapy. To reduce the risk of hemorrhagic cystitis, fluid intake should be at least 3000 ml/day for adults and 1000–2000 ml/day for children.

- Fluid intake is also necessary to promote excretion of uric acid. Alkalinization of the urine may be ordered to help prevent uric acid nephropathy.

- Monitor for bone marrow depression. Assess for fever, chills, sore throat, and signs of infection. Monitor platelet count throughout therapy. Assess for bleeding (bleeding gums, bruising, petechiae; guaiac test stools, urine, and emesis). Avoid administering IM injections and taking rectal temperatures. Apply pressure to venipuncture site for 10 minutes. Anemia may occur. Monitor for increased fatigue, dyspnea, and orthostatic hypotension. Additive bone marrow depression may occur with concurrent use of other antineoplastics or radiation therapy.

- Use cyclophosphamide cautiously in patients with active infections, decreased bone marrow reserve, other chronic debilitating illnesses, or elderly patients. Dosage reduction may be required if creatinine clearance is less than 50 ml/min.

- Assess nausea, vomiting, and appetite. Weigh weekly. Antiemetics may be given 30 minutes prior to administration of medication to minimize GI effects. Anorexia and weight loss can be minimized by feeding frequent light meals. Monitor fluid and electrolyte status frequently.

- Assess cardiac and respiratory status for dyspnea, rales/crackles, weight gain, edema. Pulmonary toxicity may occur after prolonged therapy. Cardiotoxicity may occur early in therapy and is characterized by symptoms of congestive heart failure. Cardiotoxicity may be additive with concurrent use of other cardiotoxic agents (doxorubicin).

- Phenobarbital, rifampin, or allopurinol may increase toxicity. Cyclophosphamide may prolong neuromuscular blockade from succinylcholine or delay metabolism of cocaine and may potentiate the effect of oral anticoagulants.

- Use with caution in patients with childbearing potential. Cyclophosphamide should be avoided in pregnant or lactating patients (Pregnancy Category D).

Lab Test Considerations

• Monitor CBC and differential prior to and periodically throughout course of therapy. The nadir of leukopenia occurs in 7–12 days (recovery in 17–21 days). Leukocytes should be maintained between 2500–4000/mm^3. May also cause thrombocytopenia (nadir 10–15 days) and rarely causes anemia. • Monitor BUN, creatinine, and uric acid levels prior to and frequently during course of therapy to detect nephrotoxicity. • Monitor AST (SGOT), ALT (SGPT), LDH, and serum bilirubin prior to and frequently during course of therapy to detect hepatotoxicity. • Urinalysis should be evaluated before initiating therapy and frequently during course of therapy to detect hematuria or change in specific gravity indicative of SIADH. • May suppress positive reactions to skin tests for *Candida,* mumps, *Trichophyton,* and tuberculin PPD. May also produce false-positive results in Pap smear.

Patient/Family Teaching

• Emphasize need for adequate fluid intake prior to and for 72 hours after therapy. Patient should void frequently to decrease bladder irritation from metabolites excreted by the kidneys. Physician should be notified immediately if hematuria is noted. • Instruct patient to notify physician promptly in the event of fever; sore throat; signs of infection; bleeding gums; bruising; petechiae; blood in urine, stool, or emesis; unusual swelling; joint pain; shortness of breath; or confusion. Caution patient to avoid crowds and persons with known infections. Instruct patient to use soft toothbrush and electric razor and be especially careful to avoid falls. Patient should also be cautioned not to drink alcoholic beverages or to take products containing aspirin, ibuprofen, or naproxen, as these may precipitate GI hemorrhage. • Advise patient that this medication may cause sterility and menstrual irregularities or cessation of menses. This drug is also teratogenic, and nonhormonal contraceptive measures should be used during and continue for at least 4 months after completion of therapy. • Discuss with patient the possibility of hair loss. Explore methods of coping. May also cause darkening of skin and fingernails. • Instruct patient not to receive any vaccinations without advice of physician.

PHARMACOLOGIC PROFILE

Indications

• Cyclophosphamide is used alone or with other modalities (other chemotherapeutic agents, radiation therapy, surgery) in the management of ✦ Hodgkin's disease ✦ malignant lymphomas ✦ multiple myeloma ✦ leukemias ✦ mycosis fungoides ✦ neuroblastoma ✦ ovarian carcinoma ✦ breast carcinoma, and a variety of other tumors.

Action

• Cyclophosphamide interferes with protein synthesis, resulting in death of rapidly replicating cells, particularly malignant ones. It also has immunosuppressant action in smaller doses.

Time/Action Profile (effects on blood counts)

Onset	Peak	Duration
7 days	10–14 days	21 days

Pharmacokinetics

• **Distribution:** Cyclophosphamide is widely distributed, crosses the placenta, and enters breast milk. Penetration of the blood–brain barrier is limited. • **Metabolism and Excretion:** Cyclophosphamide is converted to active drug by the liver; 30% is eliminated unchanged by the kidneys. • **Half-life:** 4–6.5 hours.

Contraindications

• Cyclophosphamide should not be given to patients with hypersensitivity to it. • Patients who are pregnant or breast-feeding should avoid cyclophosphamide.

Adverse Reactions and Side Effects*

• **CV:** MYOCARDIAL FIBROSIS, hypotension • **Resp:** pulmonary fibrosis • **GI:** <u>anorexia</u>, <u>nausea</u>, <u>vomiting</u> • **GU:** <u>hemorrhagic cystitis</u>, <u>hematuria</u> • **Derm:** <u>alopecia</u> • **Endo:** SIADH, gonadal suppression • **Hemat:** anemia, <u>thrombocytopenia</u>, <u>leukopenia</u> • **Metab:** hyperuricemia • **Misc:** secondary neoplasms.

---

*<u>Underlines</u> indicate most frequent; CAPITALS indicate life-threatening.

Cyclosporine	*Immunosuppressant*
Sandimmune	**pH UK**

≋ ADMINISTRATION CONSIDERATIONS

Usual Dose

Many other regimens are used.

ADULTS AND CHILDREN: 2–6 mg/kg/day initially; change to oral dosage forms as soon as possible (IV dose is 1/3 of oral dose). Children may require larger or more frequent doses due to more rapid clearance. Initial dose is given 4–12 hr before surgery.

Dilution

• **Intermittent Infusion:** Dilute each 1 ml (50 mg) of IV concentrate immediately before use with 20–100 ml of D5W or 0.9% NaCl for injection. • Solution is stable for 24 hours in D5W. In 0.9% NaCl, it is stable for 6 hours in a polyvinyl-chloride (PVC) container and 12 hours in a glass container at room temperature. Glass containers are recommended because of possible leaching of diethylhexylphthalate into cyclosporine solutions from PVC bags. If PVC bags and tubing are used, administer immediately after preparation to minimize leaching.

Compatibility

• **Y-site:** sargramostim.

Incompatibility

• Information unavailable. Do not mix with other drugs or solutions.
• **Additive:** magnesium sulfate.

Rate of Administration

• **Intermittent Infusion:** Recommended rate of infusion is slowly, over 2–6 hours via infusion pump. • **Continuous Infusion:** May be administered as a continuous infusion over 24 hours.

≋ CLINICAL PRECAUTIONS

• Assess for symptoms of organ rejection throughout therapy.

- Commonly given with other immunosuppressive agents. Protect transplant patients from staff and visitors who may carry infection. Maintain protective isolation as indicated.
- Monitor patient for signs and symptoms of hypersensitivity (wheezing, dyspnea, flushing of face or neck). Oxygen, epinephrine, antihistamines, and equipment for treatment of anaphylaxis should be available with each IV dose.
- Monitor fluid/electrolyte status, renal and hepatic function. Hyperkalemia and hypomagnesemia may occur. Additive hyperkalemia may occur with potassium-sparing diuretics, potassium supplements, or angiotensin-converting enzyme (ACE) inhibitors. In patients with severe hepatic impairment, dosage reduction of cyclosporine may be necessary. Use cautiously in elderly patients and patients with renal impairment. Increased risk of nephrotoxicity occurs with aminoglycosides, amphotericin B, erythromycin, fluoroquinolones, ketoconazole, melphalan, NSAIDs, or sulfonamides. Dosage reduction is required in hepatic impairment.
- Assess nutritional status. Nausea and vomiting commonly complicate therapy. Maintain adequate nutrition and hydration.
- Blood level monitoring is useful in determining dosage and preventing toxicity. Blood levels and risk of toxicity of cyclosporine are increased by anabolic steroids, oral contraceptives, erythromycin, cimetidine, fluconazole, ketoconazole, miconazole, and calcium channel blockers.
- Concurrent use with lovastatin following cardiac transplant may increase the risk of rhabdomyolysis and renal toxicity.
- Use cautiously in patients with active infection. Immunosuppression makes patients more susceptible to infection. Concurrent immunosuppressive therapy increases this risk.
- Monitor mental status and neurological function. Tremors are common. Other psychological changes may occur. The risk of seizures is increased by concurrent use of imipenem-cilastatin.
- Assess skin integrity. Hirsutism, acne, and hypersensitivity skin rashes are common.

- Additive immunosuppression may occur with other immunosuppressants (cyclophosphamide, azathioprine, glucocorticoids) or verapamil.
- Barbiturates, phenytoin, rifampin, carbamazepine, or sulfonamides may decrease the effect of cyclosporine. Cyclosporine increases serum levels and the risk of toxicity from digoxin. Decrease concurrent digoxin dose by 50%. The action of neuromuscular blocking agents may be prolonged by cyclosporine.
- Cyclosporine may decrease antibody response to live virus vaccines and increase the risk of adverse reactions.
- Cyclosporine injection contains 33% alcohol. Use cautiously in patients with known alcohol intolerance.
- Cyclosporine should not be given to pregnant or lactating women unless benefits outweigh risks (Pregnancy Category D).

Lab Test Considerations

- Serum cyclosporine levels should be evaluated periodically during therapy. Dosage may be adjusted daily, in response to levels, during initiation of therapy. Trough levels of 250–800 ng/ml (blood) or 50–300 ng/ml (plasma) 24 hours after a dose is given have been shown to minimize side effects and rejection events. • Nephrotoxicity may occur; monitor BUN and serum creatinine periodically. Notify physician if significant increases occur. May also cause decreased serum magnesium levels. • Cyclosporine may cause hepatotoxicity; monitor for elevated AST (SGOT), ALT (SGPT), alkaline phosphatase, amylase, and bilirubin levels. • May cause increased serum potassium and uric acid levels. • Serum lipid levels may be elevated.

Patient/Family Teaching

- Reinforce the need for lifelong therapy to prevent transplant rejection. Review symptoms of rejection for transplanted organ, and emphasize the need to notify the physician immediately if such symptoms occur. • Advise patient of common side effects (nephrotoxicity, increased blood pressure, hand tremors, increased facial hair, gingival hyperplasia). • Teach patient the correct method for monitoring blood pressure at home. Instruct patient to notify physician of significant changes in blood pressure or if hematuria, urinary frequency, cloudy urine, or decreased urine output occurs. • Instruct patient on proper oral hygiene. Meticulous oral hygiene and regular dental care will help decrease gingival inflammation and hyperplasia. • Instruct patient to consult with physician or pharmacist before taking any over-the-counter medications or receiving any vaccinations while taking this medication. • Advise patient to notify physician if pregnancy is planned or suspected. • Emphasize the importance of follow-up examinations and lab tests.

≋ PHARMACOLOGIC PROFILE

Indications

• Cyclosporine is used with glucocorticoids to prevent rejection in renal, cardiac, and hepatic transplantation. • **Unlabeled Use:** Prevention of rejection in heart-lung, pancreatic, and bone marrow transplantation.

Action

• Cyclosporine inhibits normal immune responses (cellular and humoral) by inhibiting interleukin II, a factor necessary for initiation of cytotoxic T-cell activity.

Time/Action Profile (blood levels)

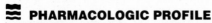

Onset	Peak	Duration
UK	end of infusion	UK

Pharmacokinetics

• **Distribution:** Cyclosporine is widely distributed, mainly into extracellular fluid and blood cells. It crosses the placenta and enters breast milk. • **Metabolism and Excretion:** Extensive metabolism occurs in the liver, with excretion into bile. Small amounts (6%) are eliminated unchanged through the kidneys. • **Half-life:** 19–27 hours.

Contraindications

• Cyclosporine is contraindicated in patients with hypersensitivity to cyclosporine or polyoxethylated castor oil. • Because of its alcohol content, cyclosporine should be avoided in patients on disulfiram therapy.

Adverse Reactions and Side Effects*

• **CNS:** <u>tremor</u>, SEIZURES, headache, flushing, confusion, psychiatric problems • **CV:** <u>hypertension</u> • **Derm:** <u>hirsutism</u>, acne • **GI:** <u>nausea</u>, <u>vomiting</u>, <u>diarrhea</u>, anorexia, abdominal discomfort, <u>gingival hyperplasia</u> • **GU:** <u>nephrotoxicity</u> • **F and E:** hypomagnesemia, hyperkalemia • **Hemat:** leukopenia, anemia, thrombocytopenia • **Metab:** hyperuricemia, hyperlipidemia • **Neuro:** paresthesia, hyperesthesia • **Misc:** <u>hepatoxicity</u>, <u>infections</u>, <u>hypersensitivity reactions</u>, hyperlipidemia.

Cysteine	*Amino acid*
	pH UK

ADMINISTRATION CONSIDERATIONS

Usual Dose

INFANTS: 0.5 g for each 12.5 g of other amino acids in parenteral nutrition solution [up to 1 mMol (121 mg)/kg/day].

Dilution

• **Continuous Infusion: Combine** each 0.5 g of cysteine with 12.5 g of amino acids, as in Aminosyn 5%, then **dilute** with up to 250 ml of 50% dextrose. • Administer prescribed amount within 1 hour of mixing or refrigerate immediately and use within 24 hours.

Incompatibility

• **Continuous Infusion:** Do not admix with other drugs or solutions.

Rate of Administration

• **Continuous Infusion:** Rate should be specified by neonatologist. Administer daily dose as a continuous infusion over 24 hours via central venous catheter. Use an in-line filter and an infusion pump during administration.

---

*<u>Underlines</u> indicate most frequent; CAPITALS indicate life-threatening.

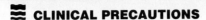 **CLINICAL PRECAUTIONS**

- Solutions must be freshly prepared as cysteine is unstable in combination with crystalline amino acids.

Patient/Family Teaching

- Inform parents of the purpose of this medication.

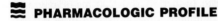 **PHARMACOLOGIC PROFILE**

Indications

- Cysteine is a requirement in the parenteral nutrition of infants.

Action

- Infants lack the enzyme required to convert methionine to cysteine. Cysteine is required for carbohydrate metabolism.

Time/Action Profile

Onset	Peak	Duration
UK	UK	UK

Pharmacokinetics

- **Distribution:** The distribution of cysteine is not known.
- **Metabolism and Excretion:** Cysteine is utilized in carbohydrate metabolism. • **Half-life:** UK.

Contraindications

- There are no known contraindications to the use of cysteine.

Adverse Reactions and Side Effects*

Adverse reactions and side effects noted are those associated with parenteral nutrition.

- **CNS:** headache, confusion • **CV:** congestive heart failure, hypotension, hypertension • **GI:** nausea, vomiting • **F and E:** hypervolemia, hypovolemia, electrolyte disturbances • **Metab:** hyperglycemia, hypoglycemia, azotemia, fatty acid deficiency, hyperammonemia • **Misc:** INFECTION.

---

*Underlines indicate most frequent; CAPITALS indicate life-threatening.

Cytarabine
Antineoplastic
(antimetabolite)

ara-C, cytosine arabinoside, {Cytosar},
Cytosar-U, Tarabine PFS
pH 5

≋ ADMINISTRATION CONSIDERATIONS
Usual Dose
ADULTS AND CHILDREN: Induction 100–200 mg/m²/day or 3 mg/kg/day as a continuous infusion over 24 hr or divided doses by rapid injection for 5–10 days; may be repeated q 2 wk. **High-dose regimen** 2–3 g/m² over 1–3 hr q 12 hr for 2–6 days.

Dilution
• **Reconstitute** 100-mg vials with 5 ml of bacteriostatic water for injection with benzyl alcohol 0.945% for a concentration of 20 mg/ml. **Reconstitute** 500-mg vials with 10 ml for a concentration of 50 mg/ml. • Solution should be prepared in a biologic cabinet. Wear gloves, gown, and mask while handling IV medication. Discard IV equipment in specially designated containers (see Appendix F). • Reconstituted solution is stable for 48 hours. Do not administer a cloudy solution. • **Intermittent Infusion:** May be **further diluted** in 100 ml of 0.9% NaCl or D5W. • May also be diluted in D10W, D5/0.9% NaCl, Ringer's solution, lactated Ringer's solution, or D5/LR.

Compatibility
• **Syringe:** metoclopramide.
• **Y-site:** chlorpromazine ✦ cimetidine ✦ dexamethasone ✦ diphenhydramine ✦ famotidine ✦ filgrastim ✦ fludarabine ✦ furosemide ✦ heparin ✦ hydromorphone ✦ idarubicin ✦ lorazepam ✦ melphalan ✦ methylprednisolone ✦ metoclopramide ✦ morphine ✦ ondansetron ✦ paclitaxel ✦ piperacillin/tazobactam ✦ prochlorperazine ✦ promethazine ✦ ranitidine ✦ sargramostim ✦ vinorelbine.
• **Additive:** methotrexate ✦ mitoxantrone ✦ potassium chloride ✦ prednisolone sodium phosphate ✦ sodium bicarbonate ✦ vincristine.

{} = Available in Canada only.

Incompatibility
- **Y-site:** allopurinol sodium.
- **Additive:** fluorouracil • heparin • regular insulin • nafcillin • oxacillin • penicillin G sodium.

Rate of Administration
- **Direct IV:** Administer each 100 mg direct IV push over 1–3 minutes. • **Intermittent Infusion:** Infuse over 30 minutes. • **Continuous Infusion:** Rate and concentration for IV infusion are ordered individually by physician.

≋ CLINICAL PRECAUTIONS

- Monitor for bone marrow depression. Assess for fever, sore throat, and signs of infection. If these symptoms occur, notify physician immediately. Assess for bleeding (bleeding gums, bruising, petechiae; guaiac test stools, urine, emesis). Avoid administering IM injections and taking rectal temperatures. Hold pressure on all venipuncture sites for at least 10 minutes. Anemia may occur. Monitor for increased fatigue, dyspnea, and orthostatic hypotension. Additive bone marrow depression occurs with other antineoplastics or radiation therapy.
- Monitor intake and output ratios and daily weights. Monitor for symptoms of gout (increased serum acid levels, joint pain, edema). Encourage patient to drink at least 2 liters of fluid each day. Allopurinol may be given to decrease uric acid levels. Alkalinization of urine may be ordered to increase excretion of uric acid.
- Assess nutritional status. Nausea and vomiting may occur within 1 hour of administration of medication, especially if IV dose is administered rapidly. Administering an antiemetic prior to and periodically throughout therapy and adjusting diet as tolerated may help maintain fluid and electrolyte balance and nutritional status.
- Concurrent use with cyclophosphamide increases the risk of cardiotoxicity.
- Use cautiously in patients with active infections, decreased bone marrow reserve, or other chronic debilitating illnesses.
- Cytarabine should be used cautiously in patients with child-bearing potential and should be avoided during pregnancy or lactation (Pregnancy Category D).

Lab Test Considerations

• Monitor CBC and differential prior to and frequently throughout therapy. Leukocyte count begins to drop within 24 hours of administration. The initial nadir occurs in 7–9 days. After a small rise in the count, the second, deeper nadir occurs 15–24 days after administration. Leukocyte and thrombocyte counts usually begin to rise 10 days after the nadirs. Therapy is usually withdrawn if leukocyte count is <1000/mm^3 or platelet count is <50,000/mm^3. Frequent bone marrow examinations are also indicated. • Renal (BUN and creatinine) and hepatic function (AST [SGOT], ALT [SGPT], bilirubin, and LDH) should be monitored prior to and routinely throughout course of therapy. • May cause increased uric acid concentrations.

Patient/Family Teaching

• Caution patient to avoid crowds and persons with known infections. Physician should be informed immediately if symptoms of infection occur. • Instruct patient to report unusual bleeding. Advise patient of thrombocytopenia precautions (use soft toothbrush and electric razor; avoid falls; do not drink alcoholic beverages or take medication containing aspirin, ibuprofen, or naproxen, as these may precipitate gastric bleeding). • Instruct patient to inspect oral mucosa for redness and ulceration. If mouth sores occur, advise patient to use sponge brush and rinse mouth with water after eating and drinking. Consult physician if pain interferes with eating. • Advise patient that this medication may have teratogenic effects. Contraception should be used during therapy and for at least 4 months after therapy is concluded. • Instruct patient not to receive any vaccinations without advice of physician. • Emphasize the need for periodic lab tests to monitor therapy.

≋ PHARMACOLOGIC PROFILE

Indications

• Cytarabine is used mainly in combination chemotherapeutic regimens for the treatment of leukemias and non-Hodgkin's lymphomas.

Action
• Cytarabine inhibits DNA synthesis by inhibiting DNA polymerase (cell cycle–specific for S phase). This results in death of rapidly replicating cells, particularly malignant ones.

Time/Action Profile (effects on WBC counts)

	Onset	Peak	Duration
1st phase	24 hr	7–9 days	12 days
2nd phase	15–24 days	15–24 days	25–34 days

Pharmacokinetics
• **Distribution:** Cytarabine is widely distributed and crosses the placenta. It crosses the blood–brain barrier, but not in sufficient quantities. • **Metabolism and Excretion:** Metabolism occurs mostly in the liver. Small amounts (less than 10%) are excreted unchanged by the kidneys. • **Half-life:** 1–3 hours.

Contraindications
• Cytarabine is contraindicated in patients with hypersensitivity or intolerance to cytarabine or benzyl alcohol. It is also available as a product without benzyl alcohol (Tarabine PFS). • Cytarabine should not be used during pregnancy or lactation (Pregnancy Category D).

Adverse Reactions and Side Effects*
• **CNS:** headache; high dose—CNS dysfunction • **EENT:** high dose—hemorrhagic conjunctivitis, corneal toxicity • **Resp:** high dose—pulmonary edema • **GI:** nausea, vomiting, hepatitis; high dose—severe GI ulceration, hepatotoxicity, stomatitis • **Derm:** rash, alopecia • **Endo:** gonadal suppression • **Hemat:** bone marrow depression • **Metab:** hyperuricemia • **Misc:** fever.

---

*Underlines indicate most frequent; CAPITALS indicate life-threatening.

Cytomegalovirus Immune Globulin	*Vaccine (immune globulin)*
CMV-IGIV, CytoGam (human)	pH NA

≋ ADMINISTRATION CONSIDERATIONS

Usual Dose

ADULTS: 150 mg/kg within 72 hr of transplantation, followed by 100 mg/kg after 2, 4, 6, and 8 wk, then 50 mg/kg at 12 and 16 wk.

Dilution

• **Intermittent Infusion:** Reconstitute with 50 ml of sterile water for injection with a double-ended needle or large syringe. To avoid foaming, do not shake vial. If using a double-ended needle, insert into water first; powder is supplied in an evacuated vial and water will transfer by suction. After water is transferred, release residual vacuum to speed dissolution. Rotate gently to wet undissolved powder. Allow 30 minutes for powder to dissolve. • Solution should be clear, colorless, and free of particulate matter. • Infusion should be started within 6 hours and completed within 12 hours of reconstitution. • Do not use filters.

Compatibility

• **Y-site:** Administer via infusion pump through a separate IV line. If this is not possible, solution may be piggybacked in an IV line containing 0.9% NaCl, D5W, D10W, D20W, or combinations of dextrose and saline, but do not dilute to more than 1/2.

Rate of Administration

• **Intermittent Infusion:** Administer initial dose at 15 mg/kg/hr for first 30 minutes. If no adverse reactions occur, rate may be increased to 30 mg/kg/hr; if no adverse reactions occur in subsequent 30 minutes, rate may be increased to 60 mg/kg/hr. Do not exceed 60-mg/kg/hr rate. During subsequent doses, rate may be increased in same increments every 15 minutes if no adverse reactions occur, until 60-mg/kg/hr maximum is reached.

≋ CLINICAL PRECAUTIONS

- Assess patient during rate changes for pain at injection site.
- Monitor vital signs prior to, during, and following infusion, and before any increases in infusion rate.
- If signs of anaphylaxis or hypotension occur, stop infusion and administer treatment (epinephrine, antihistamines).
- Observe for the development of minor side effects (nausea, muscle cramps, back pain, fever, flushing, chills). If these occur, slow infusion rate or stop temporarily.
- Safe use in pregnancy or lactation has not been established (Pregnancy Category C).

Patient/Family Teaching

- Instruct patient to notify physician if any adverse reactions occur. • May cause drowsiness. Caution patient to avoid driving or other activities requiring alertness after receiving medication until response to medication is known. Advise patient not to receive any live vaccines for 3 months following therapy.

≋ PHARMACOLOGIC PROFILE

Indications

- Cytomegalovirus immune globulin is used to suppress cytomegalovirus (CMV) disease in CMV-negative recipients of transplanted CMV-positive kidneys.

Action

- Cytomegalovirus immune globulin consists of IgG antibodies capable of providing passive immunity against CMV infection. Administering this agent prevents the serious sequelae of CMV disease in renal transplant patients (leukopenia, fever, hepatitis, retinitis, pneumonitis).

Time/Action Profile

Onset	Peak	Duration
rapid	UK	UK

Pharmacokinetics
• **Distribution:** Distribution of cytomegalovirus immune globulin is unknown. • **Metabolism and Excretion:** UK • **Half-life:** UK.

Contraindications
• Cytomegalovirus immune globulin should not be given to patients with previous hypersensitivity to immune globulins or albumin or to those with selective IgA deficiency.

Adverse Reactions and Side Effects*
• **CV:** hypotension • **Resp:** wheezing • **GI:** vomiting, nausea • **Derm:** flushing • **MS:** muscle cramps, back pain • **Misc:** chills, fever, allergic reactions including ANAPHYLAXIS • **Local:** pain at injection site.

Dacarbazine	*Antineoplastic (alkylating agent)*
DTIC-Dome, {DTIC}	pH 3–4

≋ ADMINISTRATION CONSIDERATIONS
Usual Dose
Malignant Melanoma
ADULTS: 2–4.5 mg/kg/day for 10 days repeated q 4 wk, or 250 mg/m²/day for 5 days repeated q 3 wk.

Hodgkin's Disease
ADULTS: 150 mg/m²/day for 5 days as part of combination chemotherapy given q 4 wk, or 375 mg/m² given on the first day with other agents and repeated q 15 days.

Dilution
• **Reconstitute** each 100-mg vial with 9.9 ml of sterile water for injection and each 200-mg vial with 19.7 ml to yield a concentration of 10 mg/ml. • Solution should be prepared

---

*Underlines indicate most frequent; CAPITALS indicate life-threatening.

{} = Available in Canada only.

in a biologic cabinet. Wear gloves, gown, and mask while handling medication. Discard equipment in designated containers (see Appendix F). • Solution is colorless or clear yellow. Do not use solution that has turned pink. Solution is stable for 8 hours at room temperature and for 72 hours if refrigerated. • **Intermittent Infusion:** Further dilute with 250 ml of D5W or 0.9% NaCl. Stable for 24 hours if refrigerated or 8 hours at room temperature.

Compatibility

• **Y-site:** filgrastim • fludarabine • melphalan • ondansetron • paclitaxel • sargramostim • vinorelbine.

• **Additive:** bleomycin • carmustine • cyclophosphamide • cytarabine • dactinomycin • doxorubicin • fluorouracil • mercaptopurine • methotrexate • vinblastine.

Incompatibility

• **Additive:** allopurinol sodium • hydrocortisone sodium succinate • piperacillin/tazobactam.

Rate of Administration

• **Direct IV:** Administer over 1 minute into a free-flowing IV infusion. • **Intermittent Infusion:** Administer over 15–30 minutes.

≋ CLINICAL PRECAUTIONS

- Monitor IV site closely. Dacarbazine is a vesicant. Discontinue IV immediately if infiltration occurs. Protect exposed tissue from light following extravasation. Topical cooling with ice packs or cooling pad may be applied to the site.
- Monitor nutrition and hydration. Nausea and vomiting are common and may be severe and last 1–12 hours. Administration of an antiemetic prior to and periodically during therapy and adjusting diet as tolerated may help maintain fluid and electrolyte balance and nutritional status. Nausea usually decreases on subsequent doses.
- Monitor for bone marrow depression. Assess for fever, chills, sore throat, and signs of infection. Notify physician if these symptoms occur. Assess for bleeding (bleeding gums, bruising, petechiae; guaiac test stools, urine, and emesis). Avoid IM injections and rectal tempera-

tures. Apply pressure to venipuncture sites for 10 minutes. Additive bone marrow depression occurs with concurrent administration of other antineoplastic agents or radiation therapy. Monitor temperature, pulse, and respirations.

- Use cautiously in patients with active infection, decreased bone marrow reserve, renal disease, chronic debilitating illness, or geriatric patients. These patients may be more sensitive to the effects of dacarbazine. Dosage reduction may be required in patients with renal impairment.
- Monitor liver function. Additive hepatotoxicity may occur with other hepatotoxic drugs.
- Phenytoin or phenobarbital may increase metabolism and decrease effectiveness of dacarbazine.
- Use cautiously in patients with childbearing potential. Dacarbazine should be avoided during pregnancy or lactation (Pregnancy Category C).

Lab Test Considerations

- Monitor CBC, differential, and platelet count prior to and periodically throughout therapy. The nadir of thrombocytopenia occurs in 16 days. The nadir of leukopenia occurs in 3–4 weeks. Recovery begins in 5 days. Withhold dose and notify physician if platelet count is <100,000/mm^3 or leukocyte count is <4000/mm^3. • Monitor for increased AST (SGOT), ALT (SGPT), uric acid, and BUN levels.

Patient/Family Teaching

- Instruct patient to notify nurse immediately if discomfort at IV site occurs. • Instruct patient to notify physician in case of fever, chills, sore throat, signs of infection, bleeding gums, bruising, or petechiae; or if blood in urine, stool, or emesis occurs. Caution patient to avoid crowds and persons with known infections. Instruct patient to use soft toothbrush and electric razor. Patients should be cautioned not to drink alcoholic beverages or take products containing aspirin, ibuprofen, or naproxen. • May occasionally cause photosensitivity. Instruct patient to avoid sunlight or wear protective clothing and use sunscreen for 2 days after therapy. • Instruct patient to inform physician if flu-like syndrome occurs. Symptoms include fever, myalgia, and general malaise. May occur after several courses of therapy. Usually occurs 1 week after administration. May persist for 1–3 weeks. Physician may order acetaminophen for relief of symptoms. • Discuss with patient the possibility of hair loss. Explore coping strategies. • Advise patient of the need for a nonhormonal method of contraception. • Instruct patient not to receive any vaccinations without advice of physician.

PHARMACOLOGIC PROFILE

Indications
• Dacarbazine is used alone in the treatment of metastatic malignant melanoma and in combination with other antineoplastic agents in the treatment of advanced Hodgkin's disease.

Action
• Disrupts DNA and RNA synthesis (cell cycle–phase nonspecific) resulting in death of rapidly replicating cells, especially malignant ones.

Time/Action Profile (effects on blood counts)

	Onset	Peak	Duration
WBC	16–20 days	21–25 days	3–5 days
platelets	UK	16 days	3–5 days

Pharmacokinetics
• **Distribution:** Dacarbazine appears to concentrate in the liver. Some penetration into the CSF occurs. • **Metabolism and Excretion:** 50% of dacarbazine is metabolized by the liver; 50% is excreted unchanged by the kidneys. • **Half-life:** 5 hours (increased in renal impairment).

Contraindications
• Dacarbazine is contraindicated in patients with hypersensitivity. • Pregnant or lactating patients should not receive dacarbazine.

Adverse Reactions and Side Effects*
• **GI:** <u>nausea</u>, <u>vomiting</u>, <u>anorexia</u>, diarrhea, hepatic vein thrombosis, HEPATIC NECROSIS • **Derm:** alopecia, photosensitiv-

---

*<u>Underlines</u> indicate most frequent; CAPITALS indicate life-threatening.

ity, facial flushing • **Endo:** gonadal suppression • **Hemat:** bone marrow depression • **Local:** pain at IV site, phlebitis at IV site, tissue necrosis • **MS:** myalgia • **Neuro:** facial paresthesia • **Misc:** facial flushing, flu-like syndrome, malaise, fever, ANAPHYLAXIS.

Dactinomycin	*Antineoplastic agent (antitumor antibiotic)*
actinomycin-D, Cosmegen	pH 5.5–7

ADMINISTRATION CONSIDERATIONS

Usual Dose

ADULTS: 10–15 mcg (0.01–0.015 mg)/kg/day for up to 5 days q 4–6 wk or 500 mcg (0.5 mg)/m^2 once weekly for 3 weeks [not to exceed 2 mg/wk or 15 mcg/kg (600 mcg/m^2)/day for 5 days].

CHILDREN >6 mo: 10–15 mcg/kg or 450 mcg/m^2 daily for up to 5 days or 2.5 mg/m^2 divided into daily doses over 7 days; repeat every 4–6 wk [not to exceed 15 mcg/kg (600 mcg/m^2)/day for 5 days].

Dilution

• **Direct IV:** Reconstitute each 0.5-mg vial with 1.1 ml of sterile water for injection without preservatives for a concentration of 0.5 mg/ml. Use of 0.9% NaCl or preservatives, benzyl alcohol, or parabens for reconstitution causes precipitation. Solution color is gold. Discard any unused solution. Change needle between reconstitution and direct IV administration. • Solution for IV administration should be prepared in a biologic cabinet. Wear gloves, gown, and mask while handling IV medication. Discard IV equipment in specially designated containers (see Appendix F). • **Intermittent Infusion:** May be **further diluted** in 50 ml of 0.9% NaCl or D5W.

Compatibility

• **Y-site:** allopurinol sodium • fludarabine • melphalan • ondansetron • sargramostim • vinorelbine.

Incompatibility

- **Y-site:** filgrastim.

Rate of Administration

- **Direct IV:** May be injected into Y-site or 3-way stopcock of free-flowing infusions of 0.9% NaCl or D5W at a rate of 500 mcg/min. • **Intermittent Infusion:** Infuse over 10–15 minutes.

☰ CLINICAL PRECAUTIONS

- Avoid contact with skin. If spillage occurs, irrigate skin with copious amount of water for 15 minutes. If splashed into eye, irrigate with water and consult ophthalmologist.
- Dactinomycin is a vesicant. Assess IV site frequently for inflammation or infiltration. If extravasation occurs, infusion must be stopped and restarted in another vein to avoid damage to SC tissue. Standard treatments include local injections of glucocorticoids and application of ice compresses.
- Monitor intake and output, appetite, and nutritional intake. Assess for nausea and vomiting, which usually begin a few hours after administration and persist for up to 20 hours. Administration of an antiemetic prior to and periodically during therapy and adjusting diet as tolerated may help maintain fluid and electrolyte balance and nutritional status. Fluids and allopurinol may be given IV to decrease uric acid levels in patients unable to maintain satisfactory oral intake.
- Assess for bone marrow depression. Monitor vital signs prior to and frequently during therapy. Assess for fever, chills, sore throat, and signs of infection. Assess for bleeding (bleeding gums, bruising, petechiae; guaiac test stools, urine, and emesis). Avoid administering IM injections and taking rectal temperatures. Apply pressure to venipuncture sites for 10 minutes. Additive bone marrow depression may occur with concurrent administration of other antineoplastic agents or radiation therapy.
- Use cautiously in patients with active infection, decreased bone marrow reserve, renal disease, chronic debilitating illness, or elderly patients. These patients may be more sensitive to the effects of dactinomycin.

- Use cautiously in patients with childbearing potential. Dactinomycin should be avoided during pregnancy and lactation (Pregnancy Category C).

Lab Test Considerations

- Monitor CBC and differential prior to and throughout therapy. Platelets and leukocyte counts begin to drop 7–10 days after beginning therapy. The nadirs of thrombocytopenia and leukopenia occur in 3 weeks. Recovery occurs 3 weeks later. • Monitor for hepatotoxicity (increased AST [SGOT], ALT [SGPT], LDH, and serum bilirubin). • May cause increased uric acid levels.

Patient/Family Teaching

- Instruct patient to notify nurse if pain or irritation at injection site occurs. • Instruct patient to notify physician if fever, chills, sore throat, signs of infection, bleeding gums, bruising, petechiae, or blood in urine, stool, or emesis occurs. Caution patient to avoid crowds and persons with known infections. Instruct patient to use soft toothbrush and electric razor. Patients should be cautioned not to drink alcoholic beverages or take products containing aspirin, ibuprofen, or naproxen. • Instruct patient to inspect oral mucosa for erythema and ulceration. If ulceration occurs, advise patient to use sponge brush and rinse mouth with water after eating and drinking. • Inform patient that this medication may cause irreversible gonadal suppression. Advise patient that this medication may have teratogenic effects. A nonhormonal method of contraception should be used during therapy and for at least 4 months after therapy is concluded. • Discuss with patient the possibility of hair loss, which usually occurs 7–10 days after administration of dactinomycin. Explore coping strategies. • Instruct patient not to receive any vaccinations without advice of physician. • Emphasize the need for periodic lab tests to monitor for side effects.

≋ PHARMACOLOGIC PROFILE

Indications

- Dactinomycin is used alone and in combination with other treatment modalities (other antineoplastic agents, radiation therapy, surgery) in the management of Wilms' tumor, rhabdomyosarcoma, Ewing's sarcoma, trophoblastic neoplasms, testicular carcinoma, and other malignancies.

Action

- Dactinomycin inhibits RNA synthesis by forming a complex with DNA (cell cycle–phase nonspecific), resulting in death of rapidly replicating cells, particularly malignant ones. It also has immunosuppressive properties.

Time/Action Profile (effects of blood counts)

Onset	Peak	Duration
7 days	14 days	21–28 days

Pharmacokinetics

- **Distribution:** Dactinomycin is widely distributed, but does not cross the blood–brain barrier. It does cross the placenta. • **Metabolism and Excretion:** Dactinomycin is excreted in bile and subsequently in feces as unchanged drug (50%). Small amounts (10%) are excreted unchanged by the kidneys. • **Half-life:** 36 hours.

Contraindications

- Dactinomycin is contraindicated in patients with hypersensitivity. • Pregnant or lactating patients should not receive dacarbazine.

Adverse Reactions and Side Effects*

- **CNS:** lethargy • **GI:** <u>nausea</u>, <u>vomiting</u>, <u>stomatitis</u>, ulceration • **Derm:** <u>alopecia</u>, rashes • **Endo:** gonadal suppression • **Hemat:** <u>anemia</u>, <u>leukopenia</u>, <u>thrombocytopenia</u> • **Local:** <u>phlebitis</u> at IV site • **Misc:** fever.

---

*<u>Underlines</u> indicate most frequent; CAPITALS indicate life-threatening.

Dantrolene Sodium	*Skeletal muscle relaxant (direct-acting)*
Dantrium Intravenous	pH 9.5

≋ ADMINISTRATION CONSIDERATIONS

Usual Dose

Treatment of Malignant Hyperthermia

ADULTS AND CHILDREN: at least 1 mg/kg given repeatedly as symptoms dictate up to cumulative dose of 10 mg/kg, followed by 1–3 days of oral therapy (4–8 mg/kg/day in 4 divided doses).

Prevention of Malignant Hyperthermia

ADULTS AND CHILDREN: 2.5 mg/kg prior to anesthesia.

Dilution

• **Direct IV:** Reconstitute each 20 mg with 60 ml of sterile water for injection without a bacteriostatic agent for a concentration of 333 mcg/ml. Shake until solution is clear. Solution must be used within 6 hours. Protect diluted solution from direct light.

Incompatibility

• **Additive:** acidic solutions, including D5W and 0.9% NaCl.

Rate of Administration

• **Direct IV:** Administer each single dose by rapid continuous IV push through Y-tubing or 3-way stopcock. Follow immediately with subsequent doses as indicated. Medication is very irritating to tissues; observe injection site frequently to avoid extravasation.

≋ CLINICAL PRECAUTIONS

• Assess neuromuscular status and muscle spasticity before initiating therapy and periodically during its course to determine response to therapy.
• Assess previous anesthesia history of all surgical patients. Also assess for family history of reactions to anesthesia (malignant hyperthermia or perioperative death).

- Monitor ECG, vital signs, electrolytes, and urine output continuously when administering for malignant hyperthermia.
- Dantrolene may result in additive CNS depression with other CNS depressants including alcohol, antihistamines, opioid analgesics, sedative/hypnotics, and parenteral magnesium sulfate.
- The risk of hepatotoxicity is increased when used concurrently with other hepatotoxic agents.
- Use cautiously in patients with cardiac, pulmonary, or previous liver disease.
- Concurrent IV adminstration of calcium channel blockers should be avoided. This increases the risk of arrhythmias in hypokalemic patients.
- Safe use in pregnancy has not been established (Pregnancy Category C).

Patient/Family Teaching

- May cause dizziness, drowsiness, light-headedness, visual disturbances, and muscle weakness. Advise patient to avoid activities requiring alertness until response to drug is known. • Patients with malignant hyperthermia should carry identification describing disease process at all times.

PHARMACOLOGIC PROFILE

Indications

- Dantrolene is used intravenously in the emergency treatment and prevention of malignant hyperthermia. • **Unlabeled Use:** Management of neuroleptic malignant syndrome.

Action

- Dantrolene acts directly on skeletal muscle, causing relaxation by decreasing calcium release from sarcoplasmic reticulum in muscle cells. • Dantrolene prevents intense catabolic process associated with malignant hyperthermia.

Time/Action Profile (effects on spasticity)

Onset	Peak	Duration
rapid	rapid	UK

Pharmacokinetics

• **Distribution:** Distribution of dantrolene is not known.
• **Metabolism and Excretion:** Metabolism occurs almost entirely in the liver. • **Half-life:** 4–8 hours.

Contraindications

• There are no known contraindications to the use of IV dantrolene.

Adverse Reactions and Side Effects*

• **CNS:** <u>muscle weakness</u>, <u>drowsiness</u>, dizziness, malaise, headache, confusion, nervousness, insomnia, light-headedness • **EENT:** excessive lacrimation, visual disturbances • **Resp:** pleural effusions • **CV:** tachycardia, changes in blood pressure • **GI:** <u>diarrhea</u>, anorexia, vomiting, cramps, dysphagia, HEPATITIS • **GU:** frequency, incontinence, nocturia, dysuria, crystalluria, impotence • **Derm:** pruritus, urticaria, photosensitivity, sweating • **Hemat:** eosinophilia • **MS:** myalgia • **Misc:** drooling, chills, fever • **Local:** phlebitis.

Daunorubicin Hydrochloride	Antineoplastic agent (antitumor antibiotic)
Cerubidine, daunomycin, rubidomycin	pH 4.5–6.5

 ADMINISTRATION CONSIDERATIONS

Usual Dose

ADULTS: 45 mg/m²/day (range 30–60 mg/m²) for 2–3 days of each course of treatment (total cumulative dose in adults should not exceed 400–550 mg/m²).

GERIATRIC PATIENTS: 30 mg/m² for 2–3 days of each course of treatment.

CHILDREN: 25 mg/m² once weekly (cumulative dose not to exceed 300 mg/m² in children over 2 yr or 10 mg/kg in children less than 2 yr). Dose should be calculated on a mg/kg basis in children under 2 yr or body surface area less than 0.5 m².

---

*<u>Underlines</u> indicate most frequent; CAPITALS indicate life-threatening.

Dilution

• **Direct IV: Reconstitute** each 20 mg with 4 ml of sterile water for injection for a concentration of 5 mg/ml. Shake gently to dissolve. Reconstituted medication is stable for 24 hours at room temperature, 48 hours if refrigerated. Protect from sunlight. • Do not use aluminum needles when reconstituting or injecting daunorubicin, because aluminum darkens the solution. **Further dilute** in 10–15 ml of 0.9% NaCl. • Solution for IV administration should be prepared in a biologic cabinet. Wear gloves, gown, and mask while handling IV medication. Discard IV equipment in specially designated containers (see Appendix F). • **Intermittent Infusion:** May be **further diluted** in 50–100 ml of D5W, 0.9% NaCl, or lactated Ringer's solution.

Compatibility

• **Y-site:** filgrastim ♦ melphalan ♦ ondansetron ♦ vinorelbine.

• **Additive:** hydrocortisone sodium succinate. However, manufacturer does not recommend admixing daunorubicin.

Incompatibility

• **Y-site:** allopurinol sodium ♦ fludarabine ♦ piperacillin/tazobactam.

• **Additive:** dexamethasone ♦ heparin.

Rate of Administration

• **Direct IV:** Administer over at least 3–5 minutes through Y-site or 3-way stopcock into free-flowing infusion of 0.9% NaCl or D5W. Rapid administration rate may cause facial flushing or erythema along the vein. • **Intermittent Infusion:** Infuse 50 ml over 10–15 minutes and 100 ml over 30–45 minutes.

≋ CLINICAL PRECAUTIONS

• Daunorubicin is a vesicant. Assess IV site frequently for inflammation or infiltration. If extravasation occurs, infusion must be stopped and restarted in another vein to avoid damage to tissue. Standard treatments include local injections of steroids and application of ice compresses.

• Do not confuse *daunorubicin* with *doxorubicin*. Doses, indications, and toxicities are not the same. See *doxorubicin* monograph on page 352.

- Monitor intake and output, appetite, and nutritional intake. Assess for nausea and vomiting, which, although mild, may persist for 24–48 hours. Administration of an antiemetic prior to and periodically during therapy and adjusting diet as tolerated may help maintain fluid and electrolyte balance and nutritional status. Encourage fluid intake of 2000–3000 ml/day. Allopurinol and alkalinization of the urine may be used to help prevent urate stone formation.

- Assess for bone marrow depression. Monitor vital signs prior to and frequently during therapy. Assess for fever, chills, sore throat, and signs of infection. Assess for bleeding (bleeding gums, bruising, petechiae; guaiac test stools, urine, and emesis). Avoid administering IM injections and taking rectal temperatures. Apply pressure to venipuncture sites for 10 minutes. Additive bone marrow depression may occur with concurrent use of other antineoplastic agents or radiation therapy.

- Assess patient for evidence of congestive heart failure (peripheral edema, dyspnea, rales/crackles, weight gain, jugular venous distention). Total cumulative doses in excess of 550 mg/m^2 are most likely to result in congestive heart failure that is irreversible. Chest x-ray, echocardiography, ECGs, and radionuclide angiography determination of ejection fraction may be ordered prior to and periodically throughout therapy. A 30% decrease in QRS voltage and decrease in systolic ejection fraction are early signs of cardiomyopathy. Cyclophosphamide and thoracic radiation therapy increase the risk of cardiotoxicity. In these patients the cumulative dose limit is 400 mg/m^2. Cardiomyopathy may not occur until 1–6 months after induction. Non-dose-related reversible arrhythmias may also occur.

- Observe sites of previous radiation therapy. Daunorubicin may produce skin reactions at the sites of previous radiation therapy. Cumulative dose reduction is recommended for patients having chest radiation (not to exceed 450 mg/m^2).

- Use cautiously in patients with active infection, decreased bone marrow reserve, chronic debilitating illness, or elderly patients. Patients with hepatic or renal impairment require dosage reduction if bilirubin is greater than 1.2 mg/dl or serum creatinine is greater than 3 mg/dl.

• Use cautiously in patients with childbearing potential. Daunorubicin should be avoided during pregnancy or lactation (Pregnancy Category D).

Lab Test Considerations

• Monitor CBC and differential prior to and periodically throughout therapy. The leukocyte count nadir occurs 10–14 days after administration. Recovery usually occurs within 21 days after administration of daunorubicin.
• Monitor AST (SGOT), ALT (SGPT), LDH, and serum bilirubin levels. May cause transiently elevated serum phosphatase, bilirubin, and AST (SGOT) concentrations.
• Monitor uric acid levels.

Patient/Family Teaching

• Instruct patient to notify the nurse if pain or irritation at injection site occurs. • Instruct patient to notify physician in case of fever, chills, sore throat, signs of infection, bleeding gums, bruising, or petechiae; or if blood in urine, stool, or emesis occurs. Caution patient to avoid crowds and persons with known infections. Instruct patient to use soft toothbrush and electric razor. Patient should be cautioned not to drink alcoholic beverages or take products containing aspirin, ibuprofen, or naproxen. • Instruct patient to inspect oral mucosa for erythema and ulceration. If ulceration occurs, advise patient to use sponge brush and rinse mouth with water after eating and drinking. Consult physician if mouth pain interferes with eating. Period of highest risk is 3–7 days after administration of dose. • Instruct patient to notify physician immediately if irregular heartbeat, shortness of breath, or swelling of lower extremities occurs. • Discuss with patient possibility of hair loss. Explore methods of coping. Regrowth of hair usually begins within 5 weeks after discontinuing therapy. • Inform patient that medication may turn urine red for 1–2 days following administration. • Inform patient that this medication may cause irreversible gonadal suppression. Advise patient that this medication may have teratogenic effects. A nonhormonal method of contraception should be used during therapy and for at least 4 months after therapy is concluded. • Instruct patient not to receive any vaccinations without advice of physician. • Emphasize the need for periodic lab tests to monitor therapy.

≋ PHARMACOLOGIC PROFILE

Indications
• Daunorubicin is used in combination with other antineoplastic agents in the treatment of leukemias.

Action
• Daunorubicin forms a complex with DNA that subsequently inhibits DNA and RNA synthesis (cell cycle–phase nonspecific). This results in death of rapidly replicating cells, particularly malignant ones. It also has immunosuppressive properties.

Time/Action Profile (effect on blood counts)

Onset	Peak	Duration
7–10 days	10–14 days	21 days

Pharmacokinetics
• **Distribution:** Daunorubicin is widely distributed and crosses the placenta. • **Metabolism and Excretion:** Extensive metabolism occurs in the liver. There is some conversion to a compound, which also has antineoplastic activity. Forty percent of daunorubicin is eliminated by biliary excretion. • **Half-life:** 18.5 hours.

Contraindications
• Daunorubicin is contraindicated in patients with hypersensitivity, underlying congestive heart failure, or cardiac arrhythmias. • Pregnant or lactating women should not receive daunorubicin.

Adverse Reactions and Side Effects*
• **CV:** <u>CONGESTIVE HEART FAILURE</u>, arrhythmias • **GI:** <u>nausea, vomiting</u>, stomatitis, esophagitis • **GU:** red urine • **Derm:** <u>alopecia</u> • **Endo:** gonadal suppression • **Hemat:** <u>bone marrow</u>

---

*<u>Underlines</u> indicate most frequent; CAPITALS indicate life-threatening.

<u>depression</u> • **Local:** <u>phlebitis</u> at IV site • **Metab:** hyperuricemia • **Misc:** fever, chills.

Deferoxamine Mesylate	Antidote (heavy metal antagonist)
Desferal	pH UK

≋ ADMINISTRATION CONSIDERATIONS

Usual Dose
IM route is preferred in acute intoxication unless accompanied by shock.

Test Dose
ADULTS: 0.5–1 g.

Acute Iron Intoxication
ADULTS: 15 mg/kg/hr, up to 90 mg/kg q 8 hr (not to exceed 6 g/day).
CHILDREN: 15 mg/kg/hr.

Chronic Iron Overload
ADULTS: In addition to IM dosage for chronic iron overload, 2-g doses may be given by slow IV infusion at the time each unit of blood is transfused (not in same line). Doses of 2–4 g (40–80 mg/kg) have been given over 12–16 hours.

Dilution
• **Intermittent Infusion: Reconstitute** contents of 500-mg vial with 2 ml and 2-g vial with 8 ml of sterile water for injection. • Solution is stable for 1 week after reconstitution if protected from light. • **Dilute further** in D5W, 0.9% NaCl, or lactated Ringer's solution.

Incompatibility
• Information unavailable. Do not mix with other drugs or solutions.

Rate of Administration
• **Intermittent Infusion:** Maximum infusion rate is 15 mg/kg/hr. Rapid infusion rate may cause hypotension, ery-

thema, urticaria, wheezing, convulsions, tachycardia, or shock.

≋ CLINICAL PRECAUTIONS

- Deferoxamine mesylate is used in conjunction with induction of emesis or gastric aspiration and lavage with sodium bicarbonate, and supportive measures for shock and metabolic acidosis in acute poisoning. IV route is reserved for severe life-threatening poisoning accompanied by shock.
- In acute poisoning, assess time, amount, and type of iron preparation ingested. A trial dose of deferoxamine may be administered between 2 and 4 hours after ingestion of iron and after the GI tract has been cleaned out. Assess for ferrioxamine in the urine (orange-rose color change of urine) until results of serum iron and total iron-binding capacity determinations are available. If unavailable, continue monitoring urine; if color does not appear by 2 hours after injection, usually no further dose is needed.
- Monitor signs of iron toxicity: early acute (abdominal pain, bloody diarrhea, emesis), late acute (decreased level of consciousness, shock, metabolic acidosis).
- May be administered at the same time as blood transfusion in persons with chronically elevated serum iron levels. Use separate site for administration.
- Monitor vital signs closely especially during IV administration for hypotension, erythema, urticaria, or signs of allergic reaction. Keep epinephrine, an antihistamine, and resuscitation equipment close by in the event of an anaphylactic reaction.
- May cause ocular toxicity or ototoxicity. Inform physician if decreased visual acuity or hearing loss occurs. May be reversible with dosage reduction.
- Monitor intake and output and urine color. Chelated iron is excreted primarily by the kidneys; urine may turn red.
- Ascorbic acid may increase the effectiveness of deferoxamine but may also increase cardiac iron toxicity.
- Safe use in pregnancy has not been established (Pregnancy Category C).

Lab Test Considerations

• Monitor serum iron, iron-binding capacity, transferrin levels, and urinary iron excretion prior to and periodically throughout therapy. • Monitor liver function studies to assess damage from iron poisoning.

Patient/Family Teaching

• Reinforce need to keep iron preparations, all medications, and hazardous substances out of the reach of children. • Reassure patient that red coloration of urine is expected and reflects excretion of excess iron. • Advise patient not to take vitamin C preparations without consulting physician, as tissue toxicity may increase. • Encourage patients requiring chronic therapy to keep follow-up appointments for lab tests. Physician may order eye and hearing examinations every 3 months.

PHARMACOLOGIC PROFILE

Indications

• Deferoxamine is used in the management of acute toxic iron ingestion and secondary iron overload syndromes associated with transfusion therapy.

Action

• Deferoxamine chelates unbound iron, forming a water-soluble complex (ferrioxamine) in plasma that is easily excreted by the kidneys. This results in the removal of excess iron. Aluminum is also chelated by deferoxamine.

Time/Action Profile (effects on hematologic parameters)

Onset	Peak	Duration
rapid	UK	UK

Pharmacokinetics

• **Distribution:** Deferoxamine appears to be widely distributed. • **Metabolism and Excretion:** Metabolism occurs via tissues and plasma enzymes. Unchanged drug and chelated form are excreted by the kidneys. Thirty-three percent of iron removed is eliminated in the feces via the biliary excretion. • **Half-life:** 1 hour.

Contraindications

• Deferoxamine use should be avoided during pregnancy or in women who may become pregnant (Pregnancy Category C). • Deferoxamine is contraindicated in patients with severe renal disease or anuria.

Adverse Reactions and Side Effects*

• **CV:** tachycardia • **EENT:** cataracts, blurred vision, ototoxicity • **GI:** abdominal pain, diarrhea • **GU:** <u>red urine</u> • **Local:** pain at injection site, induration at injection site • **MS:** leg cramps • **Misc:** flushing, erythema, urticaria, hypotension, shock following rapid IV administration, allergic reactions, fever.

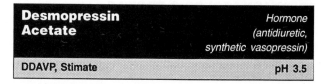

Desmopressin Acetate

Hormone (antidiuretic, synthetic vasopressin)

DDAVP, Stimate   pH 3.5

≋ ADMINISTRATION CONSIDERATIONS

Usual Dose

Diabetes Insipidus

ADULTS: 2–4 mcg/day in 2 divided doses.

Hemophilia A and Type I von Willebrand's Disease

ADULTS AND CHILDREN >3 mo: 0.3 mcg/kg 30 min preoperatively; may be repeated.

Dilution

• **Direct IV:** Administer **undiluted**. • **Intermittent Infusion: Dilute** each dose in 50 ml of 0.9% NaCl for adults and 10 ml in children.

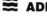

*<u>Underlines</u> indicate most frequent; CAPITALS indicate life-threatening.

Incompatibility

- Information unavailable. Do not mix with other drugs or solutions.

Rate of Administration

- **Direct IV:** Administer each dose over 1 minute for diabetes insipidus. • **Intermittent Infusion:** Infuse slowly over 15–30 minutes for hemophilia.

≋ CLINICAL PRECAUTIONS

- In patients with diabetes insipidus, monitor urine osmolality and urine volume frequently. Assess patient for symptoms of dehydration (excessive thirst, dry skin and mucous membranes, tachycardia, poor skin turgor). Weigh patient daily and assess for edema. IV desmopressin has 10 times the antidiuretic effect of intranasal desmopressin.
- When used in *hemophilia A* and *von Willebrand's disease,* assess patient for signs of bleeding. Monitor ristocetin cofactor and von Willebrand factor when used for von Willebrand's disease. If administered more frequently than every 24–48 hours, tachyphylaxis may develop.
- Monitor blood pressure and pulse during IV infusion.
- Monitor intake and output, and adjust fluid intake (especially in children and elderly) to avoid overhydration in patients receiving desmopressin for hemophilia.
- Use with caution in patients with angina pectoris or hypertension.
- Chlorpropamide, clofibrate, or carbamazepine may enhance the antidiuretic response to desmopressin.
- Demeclocycline, lithium, or norepinephrine may diminish the antidiuretic response to desmopressin.
- Safe use in pregnancy, lactation, or children under 3 months has not been established (Pregnancy Category B).

Toxicity and Overdose Alert

- Signs and symptoms of water intoxication include confusion, drowsiness, headache, weight gain, difficulty urinating, seizures, and coma. • Treatment of overdose includes decreasing dosage and, if symptoms are severe, administration of furosemide.

Lab Test Considerations

• When used for hemophilia A and von Willebrand's disease, monitor plasma Factor VIII concentrations and bleeding time.

Patient/Family Teaching

• Advise patient to notify physician if drowsiness, listlessness, headache, dyspnea, heartburn, nausea, abdominal cramps, vulval pain, or severe nasal congestion or irritation occurs. • Caution patient to avoid concurrent use of alcohol with this medication. • Patients requiring this medication should carry identification describing disease process and medication regimen at all times.

≋ PHARMACOLOGIC PROFILE

Indications

• Desmopressin is used in the treatment of diabetes insipidus caused by a deficiency of vasopressin. • Because of its effect on Factor VIII activity, it is also used to control bleeding in certain types of hemophilia and von Willebrand's disease.

Action

• Desmopressin is an analogue of naturally occurring vasopressin (antidiuretic hormone). Its primary action is enhanced reabsorption of water in the kidneys, which results in maintenance of appropriate body water content in diabetes insipidus. • Large doses increase plasma Factor VIII activity, which helps to control bleeding in certain types of hemophilia and von Willebrand's disease.

Time/Action Profile (effect on Factor VIII activity)

Onset	Peak	Duration
within minutes	15–30 min	3 hr (4–24 hr in mild hemophilia A)

Pharmacokinetics

• **Distribution:** Not fully known; however, desmopressin does enter breast milk. • **Metabolism and Excretion:** Unknown. • **Half-life:** 75 minutes.

Contraindications

• Desmopressin is contraindicated in patients with hypersensitivity to desmopressin or chlorobutanol. • Patients with type IIB or platelet-type (pseudo) von Willebrand's disease should not receive desmopressin.

Adverse Reactions and Side Effects*

• **CNS:** headache, drowsiness, listlessness • **EENT:** rhinitis, nasal congestion • **Resp:** dyspnea • **CV:** hypertension, hypotension, and tachycardia (large dose only) • **GI:** nausea, mild abdominal cramps • **GU:** vulval pain • **Derm:** flushing • **F and E:** water intoxication and hyponatremia • **Local:** phlebitis at IV site.

Dexamethasone Sodium Phosphate	Hormone (glucocorticoid)
Dalalone, Decadron Phosphate, Decaject, Dexacen-4, Dexasone, Dexone, Hexadrol Phosphate, Solurex	pH 7–8.5

☰ ADMINISTRATION CONSIDERATIONS

Usual Dose

0.75 mg dexamethasone is equal to 20 mg hydrocortisone.

Anti-inflammatory and Most Other Uses

ADULTS: 0.5–24 mg/day (up to 1 mg/kg dose has been used).

Cerebral Edema

ADULTS: 10 mg initially; 4–6 mg q 6 hr; may be decreased to 2 mg q 8–12 hr, then change to oral dexamethasone.

Prior to Emetogenic Chemotherapy

ADULTS: 10–20 mg.

Dilution

• **Direct IV:** May be given **undiluted**. Do not administer suspension IV (dexamethasone acetate). • **Intermittent**

---

*Underlines indicate most frequent; CAPITALS indicate life-threatening.

Infusion: May be added to D5W or 0.9% NaCl solution. • Diluted solution should be used within 24 hours.

Compatibility

- **Syringe:** metoclopramide ✦ ranitidine.
- **Y-site:** acyclovir ✦ allopurinol sodium ✦ cisplatin ✦ cyclophosphamide ✦ cytarabine ✦ doxorubicin ✦ famotidine ✦ filgrastim ✦ fluconazole ✦ fludarabine ✦ foscarnet ✦ melphalan ✦ meperidine ✦ methotrexate ✦ morphine ✦ ondansetron ✦ paclitaxel ✦ piperacillin/tazobactam ✦ potassium chloride ✦ sargramostim ✦ tacrolimus ✦ vinorelbine ✦ vitamin B complex with C ✦ zidovudine.
- **Additive:** aminophylline ✦ bleomycin ✦ cimetidine ✦ furosemide ✦ lidocaine ✦ nafcillin ✦ netilmicin ✦ ondansetron ✦ prochlorperazine ✦ ranitidine.

Incompatibility

- **Syringe:** doxapram ✦ glycopyrrolate.
- **Additive:** daunorubicin ✦ doxorubicin ✦ metaraminol ✦ vancomycin.

Rate of Administration

- **Direct IV:** Administer over 1 minute. • **Intermittent Infusion:** Administer infusions at prescribed rate.

≋ CLINICAL PRECAUTIONS

- Assess patients with cerebral edema for changes in level of consciousness and headache.
- Dexamethasone is used in a variety of other conditions. Assess involved systems prior to and periodically during therapy.
- Monitor intake and output ratios, blood pressure, and daily weights. Observe patient for the appearance of peripheral edema, steady weight gain, rales/crackles, or dyspnea.
- Monitor electrolytes. Additive hypokalemia may occur with concurrent administration of diuretics, amphotericin B, mezlocillin, piperacillin, or ticarcillin. Hypokalemia may increase the risk of cardiac glycoside toxicity.
- Chronic treatment will lead to adrenal suppression. Dexamethasone should never be abruptly discontinued.

Supplemental doses may be needed during stress (surgery, infection).

- Use lowest possible dose for shortest period of time.
- May increase requirement for insulin or hypoglycemic agents in patients with diabetes.
- Safe use in pregnancy has not been established. Dexamethasone has been used prenatally to prevent respiratory distress syndrome in premature infants without adverse effects.

Lab Test Considerations

• Monitor serum electrolytes and glucose levels. May cause hyperglycemia, especially in persons with diabetes. May cause hypokalemia. • Promptly report presence of guaiac-positive stools. • Periodic adrenal function tests may be ordered to assess degree of hypothalamic–pituitary–adrenal axis suppression in systemic and chronic topical therapy.

Patient/Family Teaching

• Encourage patient on long-term therapy to eat diet high in protein, calcium, and potassium and low in sodium and carbohydrates (see Appendix H for foods included). • This drug causes immunosuppression and may mask symptoms of infection. Instruct patient to avoid people with known contagious illnesses and to report possible infections immediately. • Review side effects with patient. Instruct patient to inform physician promptly if severe abdominal pain or tarry stools occur. Patient should also report unusual swelling, weight gain, tiredness, bone pain, bruising, nonhealing sores, visual disturbances, or behavior changes. • Instruct patient to inform physician if symptoms of underlying disease return or worsen. • Advise patient to carry identification describing medication regimen in the event of an emergency in which patient cannot relate medical history. • Caution patient to avoid vaccinations without consulting physician. • Explain need for continued medical follow-up to assess effectiveness and possible side effects of medication. Physician may order periodic lab tests and eye examinations. • Emphasize the importance of follow-up examinations to monitor progress and side effects.

≋ PHARMACOLOGIC PROFILE

Indications

• Dexamethasone is used in a wide variety of disorders including ✦ chronic inflammatory conditions ✦ allergies ✦ hematologic diseases ✦ neoplasms ✦ autoimmune diseases. • It is also useful in the management of cerebral edema and as a diagnostic agent in adrenal disorders.

Action

• Dexamethasone suppresses inflammation and the normal immune response and has numerous intense metabolic effects. • Chronic use suppresses adrenal function at doses of 0.75 mg/day. In replacement doses (0.75 mg/day), it is practically devoid of mineralocorticoid (sodium-retaining) activity.

Time/Action Profile (adrenal suppression or anti-inflammatory activity)

Onset	Peak	Duration
rapid	UK	2.75 days

Pharmacokinetics

• **Distribution:** Dexamethasone is widely distributed, crosses the placenta, and probably enters breast milk. • **Metabolism and Excretion:** Dexamethasone is mostly metabolized by the liver; small amounts are excreted unchanged by the kidneys. • **Half-life:** 110–210 minutes; adrenal suppression lasts 2.75 days.

Contraindications

• Dexamethasone is contraindicated in patients with active untreated infections (except for certain forms of meningitis). • Avoid chronic use during lactation. • Some products contain bisulfites, parabens, or alcohol and should be avoided in patients with hypersensitivity to these components.

Adverse Reactions and Side Effects*

Seen with high-dose, chronic therapy.
• **CNS:** headache, restlessness, psychoses, <u>depression</u>, <u>euphoria</u>, personality changes, increased intracranial pressure

---

*<u>Underlines</u> indicate most frequent; CAPITALS indicate life-threatening.

(children only) • **EENT:** cataracts, increased intraocular pressure • **CV:** hypertension, • **GI:** nausea, vomiting, anorexia, peptic ulceration • **Derm:** decreased wound healing, petechiae, ecchymoses, fragility, hirsutism, acne • **Endo:** adrenal suppression, hyperglycemia • **F and E:** hypokalemia, hypokalemic alkalosis, fluid retention (long-term high doses) • **Hemat:** thromboembolism, thrombophlebitis • **Metab:** weight loss, weight gain • **MS:** muscle wasting, muscle pain, aseptic necrosis of joints, osteoporosis • **Misc:** increased susceptibility to infection, cushingoid appearance (moon face, buffalo hump).

Dexpanthenol	*GI stimulant*
D-pantothenyl alcohol, Dexol, Ilopan, pantothenic acid	**pH 5–7**

 ADMINISTRATION CONSIDERATIONS

Usual Dose
ADULTS: 500 mg infused slowly.

Dilution
• **Intermittent Infusion:** Dilute in 500 ml or more of D5W or lactated Ringer's solution. • Do not administer solutions that are discolored or contain a precipitate.

Incompatibility
• Information unavailable.

Rate of Administration
• **Intermittent Infusion:** Infuse slowly over 3–6 hours.

 CLINICAL PRECAUTIONS

• Assess bowel status frequently. Dexpanthenol should not be used for mechanical obstruction of the GI tract.
• Effectiveness has not been clearly demonstrated.

- Dexpanthenol should not be administered within 1 hour of succinylcholine or within 12 hours of neostigmine or other parasympathomimetic agents.
- Safe use in children, pregnancy, or lactation has not been established (Pregnancy Category C).

Patient/Family Teaching

- Instruct patient to report changes in bowel status.

≋ PHARMACOLOGIC PROFILE

Indications

- Dexpanthenol is used to promote GI peristalsis postoperatively or postpartum.

Action

- Dexpanthenol stimulates GI peristalsis by increasing the conversion of choline to acetylcholine.

Time/Action Profile

Onset	Peak	Duration
UK	UK	UK

Pharmacokinetics

- **Distribution:** Following conversion to pantothenic acid, dexpanthenol is widely distributed as coenzyme A, concentrating in the liver, adrenals, heart, and kidneys. • **Metabolism and Excretion:** 70% of dexpanthenol is excreted unchanged by the kidneys; 30% is eliminated in feces. • **Half-life:** UK.

Contraindications

- Dexpanthenol should not be used in patients with previous hypersensitivity or mechanical obstruction of the GI tract.

Adverse Reactions and Side Effects*

- **GI:** abdominal cramping • **Misc:** allergic reactions.

---

*Underlines indicate most frequent; CAPITALS indicate life-threatening.

Dextran 40

Volume expander,
Anticoagulant

low molecular weight dextran,
Gentran 40, Rheomacrodex, 10% LMD   pH 3–7

≋ ADMINISTRATION CONSIDERATIONS

Usual Dose

Shock

Amount and rate depend on severity and response.

ADULTS: Total in first 24 hr should not exceed 2 g/kg (20 ml/kg). Beyond first day, daily dosage should not exceed 1 g/kg (10 ml/kg). Therapy should not exceed 5 days.

Prophylaxis of Thromboembolism

ADULTS: 50–100 g (500–1000 ml) given on day of surgery; 50 g (500 ml) may be given daily for 2–3 days postoperatively, then q 2–3 days during risk period for up to 2 wk.

Dilution

• **Intermittent Infusion:** Solutions are available diluted in 0.9% NaCl or D5W, ready for use. • Crystallization may occur at low temperatures. Submerge container in warm water and dissolve all crystals before administration. Use only clear solutions. Discard remaining solutions.

Compatibility

• **Y-site:** enalaprilat • famotidine.

Incompatibility

• Specific information unavailable. However, manufacturer recommends dextran 40 not be admixed with other solutions.

Rate of Administration

• **Intermittent Infusion:** Initial 500 ml may be administered over 15–30 minutes. Distribute remainder of daily dose over 8–24 hours depending on use.

≋ CLINICAL PRECAUTIONS

• Assess hydration. If dehydration is present, additional fluids will be required. Monitor urine output, specific gravity, and CVP (if available) hourly throughout infusion during treatment of shock. Dosage adjustment may be required if urine output decreases or CVP increases by more than 15 mm H_2O. Dehydration increases the risk of nephrotoxicity.

- Monitor pulse and blood pressure frequently throughout infusion.
- Assess patient for signs of congestive heart failure (dyspnea, coughing, increased pulse and respiratory rate, rales/crackles, jugular venous distention) routinely throughout therapy.
- Assess for signs of hypersensitivity reactions (rash, urticaria, hypotension, nausea, vomiting, headache, tightness in chest, wheezing), especially when infusion is first started. Discontinue therapy and notify physician immediately if these occur. Dextran 1 (Promit) may be administered 1–2 minutes before each dextran infusion to prevent serious anaphylactic reactions.
- Do not confuse dextran 40 with higher molecular weight dextrans (70 and 75). Dextran 40 has different effects on microcirculation and different adverse effects.
- Safe use in pregnancy or lactation has not been established (Pregnancy Category C).

Lab Test Considerations

- Obtain baseline lab data (hemoglobin, hematocrit, serum osmolality) prior to infusion. Monitor these parameters throughout therapy. Hematocrit may be decreased. May cause prolonged bleeding time with high doses. Notify physician if bleeding increases or hematocrit <30%. • May cause unreliable readings for blood typing and crossmatching. Draw blood for type and crossmatch prior to infusion or notify lab of dextran infusion. • May cause false elevations of blood glucose. • May cause an increase in serum AST (SGOT) and ALT (SGPT) concentrations.

Patient/Family Teaching

- Instruct patient to report any discomfort or dyspnea promptly throughout course of therapy.

PHARMACOLOGIC PROFILE

Indications

• Dextran 40 is used in the emergency management of hypovolemic shock when more appropriate products or solutions are unavailable. • Dextran 40 is also used to prevent thromboembolism and subsequent pulmonary emboli after surgical procedures.

Action

• Dextran 40 expands plasma volume by being osmotically active. It consists of polysaccharides whose average molecular weight is 40,000 (range 10,000–90,000). • Its effects on blood include decreased viscosity, decreased RBC aggregation, and decreased rigidity.

Time/Action Profile (hemodynamic effects)

Onset	Peak	Duration
within minutes	UK	UK

Pharmacokinetics

• **Distribution:** UK. • **Metabolism and Excretion:** 70% of dextran 40 is excreted unchanged in the urine. Molecules of higher molecular weight (greater than 70,000) are slowly converted to glucose and then to carbon dioxide and water. Small amounts are excreted in feces. • **Half-life:** UK.

Contraindications

• Patients with previous hypersensitivity to any dextrans should not receive dextran 40. • Use of dextran 40 is contraindicated in patients with bleeding or clotting disorders or thrombocytopenia.

Adverse Reactions and Side Effects*

• **CV:** pulmonary edema (large doses) • **Derm:** urticaria • **GU:** nephrotoxicity • **Misc:** hypersensitivity reactions, including ANAPHYLACTOID REACTIONS.

---

*Underlines indicate most frequent; CAPITALS indicate life-threatening.

Dextrose	*Caloric agent (carbohydrate)*
glucose	pH 3.5–6.5

≋ ADMINISTRATION CONSIDERATIONS

Usual Dose

Hydration (adjust on the basis of clinical situation)

ADULTS AND CHILDREN: 0.5–0.8 g/kg/hr (as 5% dextrose solution).

Hypoglycemia (adjust on the basis of clinical situation)

ADULTS AND CHILDREN: 20–50 ml of 50% (10–25 g) solution infused slowly (3 ml/min). Repeated doses may be given.

INFANTS AND NEONATES: 5–10 ml of 25% solution (250–500 mg/kg) or 2 ml/kg of 10–25% solution infused slowly. Repeated doses may be given.

OLDER INFANTS OR SEVERE HYPOGLYCEMIA: 10–12 ml of 25% solution. Larger or repeated doses may be given.

Dilution

• Hypertonic dextrose solutions may be administered **undiluted** into a central vein or slowly into a large peripheral vein. • Available parenterally in combination with alcohol, dextran, hetastarch, NaCl, potassium, and electrolyte solutions.

Incompatibility

• **Additive:** warfarin • whole blood.

Rate of Administration

• **Direct IV:** Administer at a rate appropriate for the indication.

≋ CLINICAL PRECAUTIONS

• Hypertonic dextrose solutions (>5%) should be administered IV into a central vein. For emergency treatment of hypoglycemia, administer slowly into a large peripheral vein to prevent phlebitis or sclerosis of the vein.

• Assess IV site frequently. Rapid infusions may cause

hyperglycemia or fluid shifts. When hypertonic solution is discontinued, taper solution and administer D5W or D10W to prevent rebound hypoglycemia.

- Patients requiring prolonged infusions of dextrose should have electrolytes added to the dextrose solution to prevent water intoxication and maintain fluid and electrolyte balance.
- Monitor hydration status, intake and output, and electrolytes. Assess for presence of dehydration or edema.
- Assess nutritional status, function of GI tract, and caloric needs of patient. Dextrose solution alone does not contain enough calories to sustain an individual for a prolonged period. Dextrose contains 3.4 cal/g. D5W contains 170 cal/liter and D10W contains 340 cal/liter.
- When glucose solutions are used in diabetic patients, they will alter requirements for insulin or oral hypoglycemic agents. Known diabetic patients should have frequent lab assessment to determine appropriate doses.
- Patients with a history of chronic alcohol abuse or malnutrition should be pretreated with thiamine before receiving infusions of dextrose.
- Has been used safely in children, pregnancy, and lactation (Pregnancy Category C). The infusion rate should not exceed 3.5–7 g/hr in pregnant women, to prevent hyperglycemia in the fetus.

Lab Test Considerations

- May cause elevated serum glucose concentrations.

Patient/Family Teaching

- Explain the purpose of dextrose administration to patient. • Instruct diabetic patient on the correct method for blood glucose monitoring.

≋ PHARMACOLOGIC PROFILE

Indications

- Lower concentration (2.5–11.5%) injections of dextrose solutions are used to provide hydration and calories. Higher concentrations (up to 70%) are used intravenously to treat hyperglycemia and in combination with amino acids to provide calories for parenteral nutrition.

Action

• Dextrose solutions provide calories and hydration and increase blood sugar in hypoglycemic patients.

Time/Action Profile (effects on blood sugar in diabetic patients)

Onset	Peak	Duration
rapid	rapid	brief

Pharmacokinetics

• **Distribution:** Dextrose is widely distributed and rapidly utilized. • **Metabolism and Excretion:** Dextrose is metabolized to carbon dioxide and water. When renal threshold is exceeded, dextrose is excreted unchanged by the kidneys. • **Half-life:** UK.

Contraindications

• Dextrose solutions are contraindicated in patients with allergy to corn and corn products. • Hypertonic solutions (>5%) of dextrose should not be given to patients with central nervous system bleeding, or anuria, or to patients who are at risk of dehydration.

Adverse Reactions and Side Effects*

• **Endo:** inappropriate insulin secretion (long-term use) • **F and E:** hypokalemia, hypophosphatemia, hypomagnesemia, fluid overload • **Local:** local pain and irritation at IV site (hypertonic solutions) • **Metab:** hyperglycemia, glycosuria.

Dezocine	Opioid analgesic (agonist/antagonist)
Dalgan	pH 4

≋ ADMINISTRATION CONSIDERATIONS

Usual Dose

ADULTS: 5 mg initially (range: 2.5–10 mg) q 2–4 hr as needed.

---

*Underlines indicate most frequent; CAPITALS indicate life-threatening.

Dilution
- **Direct IV:** May be given **undiluted**.

Rate of Administration
- **Direct IV:** Administer slowly, each 5 mg over 3–5 minutes.

≋ CLINICAL PRECAUTIONS

- Assess type, location, and intensity of pain prior to and 15 minutes following administration. When titrating opioid doses, increases of 25–50% should be administered until there is either a 50% reduction in the patient's pain rating on a numerical or visual analog scale or the patient reports satisfactory pain relief. Subsequent doses may be safely administered at the time of the peak if the previous dose is ineffective and side effects are minimal. Patients requiring higher doses should be converted to an opioid agonist. Dezocine is not recommended for prolonged use or as first-line therapy for acute or cancer pain.
- Regularly administered doses are more effective than p.r.n. administration. Analgesic is more effective if administered before pain becomes severe. Coadministration with nonopioid analgesics may have additive effects and permit lower opioid doses.
- An equianalgesic chart (Appendix B, page 1045) should be used when changing routes or when changing from one opioid to another.
- Assess level of sedation and mental status. Initial drowsiness will diminish with continued use. Dezocine commonly produces sedation and confusion. Additive CNS depression is likely to occur with concurrent use of alcohol, antihistamines, antidepressants, and sedative/hypnotics.
- Assess blood pressure, pulse, and respiratory rate prior to and periodically during administration. If respiratory rate is less than 10/minute, assess level of sedation. Physical stimulation may be sufficient to prevent significant hypoventilation. Dose may need to be decreased by 25–50%.
- Patient should remain supine during and following administration to minimize adverse effects.

- Avoid using with other opioid analgesics; dezocine will decrease their analgesic properties.
- Obtain analgesic history. Dezocine may precipitate withdrawal symptoms (vomiting, restlessness, abdominal cramps, increased blood pressure and temperature) in patients who are physically dependent on opioid analgesic agonists.
- Although dezocine has a low potential for dependence, prolonged use may lead to physical and psychological dependence and tolerance. Fear of addiction should not prevent patient from receiving adequate analgesia. Most patients who receive dezocine for pain do not develop psychological dependence. If tolerance develops, changing to an opioid agonist may be required to relieve pain.
- Elderly or debilitated patients are more sensitive to the effects of opioid analgesics and may require reduced dosage.
- Exercise caution in administering dezocine to patients with increased intracranial pressure.
- Use cautiously in geriatric patients and patients with severe renal, hepatic, or pulmonary disease, owing to these patients' increased sensitivity to CNS adverse reactions, including respiratory depression. Lower initial doses are recommended. Patients with hypothyroidism, adrenal insufficiency, or alcoholism have an increased risk of adverse reactions to opioid analgesics.
- Dezocine may mask symptoms in patients with undiagnosed abdominal pain.
- Use with caution in patients receiving MAO inhibitors; unpredictable reactions may occur.
- Patients with prostatic hypertrophy may experience urinary retention.
- Safe use during pregnancy, labor, or lactation, or in children under 18 years of age has not been established (Pregnancy Category C).

Toxicity and Overdose Alert

- If an opioid antagonist is required to reverse respiratory depression or coma, naloxone (Narcan) is the antidote. Dilute the 0.4-mg ampule of naloxone in 10 ml of 0.9% NaCl and administer 0.5 ml (0.02 mg) by direct IV push every 2 minutes. For patients weighing less than 40 kg, dilute 0.1 mg of naloxone in 10 ml of NaCl for a concentration of 10 mcg/ml and administer 0.5 mcg every 1–2 minutes. Titrate the dose to avoid withdrawal, seizures, and severe pain.

Lab Test Considerations

• Dezocine may cause elevated serum amylase and lipase levels.

Patient/Family Teaching

• Instruct patient on how and when to ask for pain medication. • Dezocine may cause drowsiness or dizziness. Advise patient to call for assistance when ambulating and to avoid activities requiring alertness until response to medication is known. • Instruct patient to change positions slowly to minimize orthostatic hypotension. • Encourage patient to turn, cough, and deeply breathe every 2 hours to prevent atelectasis. • Advise patient that good oral hygiene, frequent mouth rinses, and sugarless gum or candy may decrease dry mouth. • Advise patient to avoid concurrent use of alcohol or other CNS depressants with dezocine.

PHARMACOLOGIC PROFILE

Indications

• Dezocine is used in the management of moderate to severe pain.

Action

• Dezocine binds to opiate receptors in the CNS, where it alters the perception of and the response to painful stimuli, while causing generalized CNS depression. • In addition, dezocine has partial antagonist properties, which may result in opioid withdrawal in physically dependent patients.

Time/Action Profile (analgesic effect)

Onset	Peak	Duration
within 15 min	UK	2–4 hr

Pharmacokinetics

• **Distribution:** UK. • **Metabolism and Excretion:** Dezocine is mostly metabolized by the liver. Less than 1% is excreted unchanged by the kidneys. • **Half-life:** 2.4 hours (range 1.2–7.4 hours).

Contraindications

• Dezocine is contraindicated in patients with hypersensitivity to dezocine or bisulfites.

Adverse Reactions and Side Effects*

• **CNS:** <u>drowsiness</u>, anxiety, confusion, crying, dizziness, light-headedness, slurred speech • **EENT:** miosis, blurred vision, double vision • **CV:** orthostatic hypotension • **Resp:** respiratory depression • **GI:** nausea, vomiting, abdominal pain, constipation, dry mouth • **GU:** urinary frequency, hesitancy, retention • **Derm:** flushing or redness of skin • **Misc:** tolerance, physical dependence, psychological dependence.

Diazepam	*Sedative/hypnotic (benzodiazepine), Anticonvulsant, Skeletal muscle relaxant*
{Diazemuls}, T-Quil, Valium, Zetran	pH 6.2–6.9

Schedule IV

 ADMINISTRATION CONSIDERATIONS

Usual Dose

Antianxiety, Anticonvulsant, Sedative/Hypnotic
ADULTS: 2–10 mg; may repeat in 3–4 hr if needed.

Precardioversion
ADULTS: 5–15 mg 5–10 min pre-cardioversion.

Pre-endoscopy
ADULTS: up to 20 mg immediately before endoscopy.

---

*<u>Underlines</u> indicate most frequent; CAPITALS indicate life-threatening.

{} = Available in Canada only.

Status Epilepticus

ADULTS: 5–10 mg; additional doses may be given q 10–15 minutes as needed up to 30 mg total; regimen may be repeated in 2–4 hr.

CHILDREN >5 yr: 1 mg; additional doses may be given q 2–5 min to total of 10 mg; repeat q 2–4 hr. One manufacturer recommends that the initial dose should not exceed 250 mcg (0.25 mg)/kg, which may be repeated q 15–30 min to a total of 750 mcg (0.75 mg)/kg.

INFANTS >30 days–CHILDREN 5 yr: 200–500 mcg (0.2–0.5 mg); additional doses may be given q 2–5 min to total of 5 mg. Manufacturer recommends initial dose should not exceed 250 mcg (0.25 mg)/kg, which may be repeated q 15–30 min to a total of 750 mcg (0.75 mg)/kg.

Skeletal Muscle Relaxation

ADULTS: 5–10 mg; may repeat in 3–4 hr.

Tetanic Muscle Spasms

CHILDREN >5 yr: 5–10 mg q 3–4 hr as needed. Manufacturer recommends initial dose should not exceed 250 mcg (0.25 mg)/kg, which may be repeated q 15–30 min to a total of 750 mcg (0.75 mg)/kg.

INFANTS >30 days–CHILDREN 5 yr: 1–2 mg q 3–4 hr as needed. Manufacturer recommends initial dose should not exceed 250 mcg (0.25 mg)/kg, which may be repeated q 15–30 minutes to a total of 750 mcg (0.75 mg)/kg.

Alcohol Withdrawal

ADULTS: 10 mg initially, then 5–10 mg in 3–4 hr as needed.

Dilution

• **Direct IV:** For IV administration, **do not dilute** or mix with any other drug. If administration directly into vein is not feasible, administer IV push into tubing as close to injection site as possible. Continuous infusion is not recommended because of precipitation in IV fluids and absorption of diazepam into infusion bags and tubing. • *Sterile diazepam emulsion* (Diazemuls) may be administered **undiluted** or mixed with its own emulsion base (Intralipid or Nutralipid) only. Use polyethelene-lined or glass infusion sets and polyethylene/polypropylene plastic syringes for administration. Do not use infusion sets containing polyvinyl chloride.

Compatibility
- **Syringe:** cimetidine.
- **Y-site:** dobutamine ✦ nafcillin ✦ quinidine gluconate.

Incompatibility
- **Syringe:** benzquinamide ✦ buprenorphine ✦ doxapram ✦ glycopyrrolate ✦ heparin ✦ nalbuphine. • *Sterile diazepam emulsion* (Diazemuls) is incompatible with glycopyrrolate and morphine.
- **Y-site:** atracurium ✦ diltiazem ✦ fluconazole ✦ foscarnet ✦ heparin ✦ hydromorphone ✦ pancuronium ✦ potassium chloride ✦ vecuronium ✦ vitamin B complex with C.
- **Additive:** bleomycin ✦ dobutamine ✦ doxorubicin ✦ fluorouracil ✦ furosemide.

Rate of Administration
- **Direct IV:** Administer slowly at a rate of 2–5 mg/min. Infants and children should receive total dose over a minimum of 3–5 minutes. Rapid injection may cause apnea, hypotension, bradycardia, or cardiac arrest.

≋ CLINICAL PRECAUTIONS

- Monitor blood pressure, pulse, and respiratory rate prior to and frequently during therapy. Patient should be kept on bed rest and observed for at least 3 hours following parenteral administration. Resuscitation equipment should be available when diazepam is administered IV.
- Assess IV site frequently; diazepam may cause phlebitis and venous thrombosis. Injection may cause burning and venous irritation; avoid small veins.
- Assess level of sedation prior to and periodically during therapy. Concurrent use with alcohol, antidepressants, antihistamines, and opioid analgesics results in additive CNS depression.
- When diazepam is used as an anticonvulsant, observe and record intensity, duration, and location of seizure activity. The initial dose of diazepam offers seizure control for 15–20 minutes after administration. Institute seizure precautions.
- When diazepam is used for muscle spasm, assess spasm, associated pain, and limitation of movement prior to and during therapy.

- When diazepam is used for alcohol withdrawal, assess tremors, agitation, delirium, and hallucinations. Protect patient from injury.
- Use cautiously in patients with hepatic dysfunction or severe renal impairment, and in geriatric or debilitated patients; these patients may require lower initial doses of diazepam. Because of its long duration of action, diazepam should be used with caution in geriatric patients. Initial dose should not exceed 2–5 mg.
- Cimetidine, oral contraceptives, disulfiram, fluoxetine, isoniazid, ketoconazole, metoprolol, propoxyphene, propranolol, or valproic acid may decrease the metabolism of diazepam, thereby enhancing its actions.
- Diazepam may decrease efficacy of levodopa.
- Rifampin or barbiturates may increase the metabolism and thus decrease the effectiveness of diazepam.
- Sedative effects of diazepam may be decreased by theophylline.
- Use cautiously in patients with childbearing potential. Avoid use of diazepam during pregnancy or lactation (Pregnancy Category D). The Canadian product (Diazemuls) is not recommended for use in children.

Lab Test Considerations

- Hepatic and renal function and CBC should be evaluated periodically throughout course of prolonged therapy.

Patient/Family Teaching

- Medication causes drowsiness, clumsiness, and unsteadiness. Advise patient to avoid activities requiring alertness until response to drug is known. • Advise patient to notify physician if pregnancy is suspected. • Patients on anticonvulsant therapy should carry identification describing disease process and medication regimen at all times.

≋ PHARMACOLOGIC PROFILE

Indications

- Diazepam is used in the management of anxiety, as a preoperative sedative, as light anesthesia, and to produce amnesia. • It is also used in the treatment of status epilepticus, as a skeletal muscle relaxant, and in the management of the symptoms of alcohol withdrawal.

Action

• Diazepam depresses the CNS, probably by potentiating gamma-aminobutyric acid (GABA), an inhibitory neurotransmitter. • In addition, it produces skeletal muscle relaxation by inhibiting spinal polysynaptic afferent pathways. • Anticonvulsant properties of diazepam are due to enhanced presynaptic inhibition.

Time/Action Profile (sedation)

Onset	Peak	Duration
1–5 min	15–30 min	15–60 min†

†In status epilepticus, anticonvulsant duration is 15–20 min.

Pharmacokinetics

• **Distribution:** Diazepam is widely distributed. It crosses the blood–brain barrier and the placenta, and enters breast milk. • **Metabolism and Excretion:** Diazepam is highly metabolized by the liver. Some products of metabolism are active as CNS depressants. • **Half-life:** 20–70 hours.

Contraindications

• Diazepam should not be used in patients with hypersensitivity. Cross-sensitivity with other benzodiazepines may occur. • Comatose patients and patients with pre-existing CNS depression or uncontrolled severe pain should not receive diazepam. • Diazepam is contraindicated in patients with narrow-angle glaucoma. • Patients who are pregnant or breast-feeding should not receive diazepam. • Injection contains benzyl alcohol and ethyl alcohol and should be avoided in patients with known intolerance. • Canadian product vehicle contains egg phospholipids and soybean oil and should be avoided in patients with known hypersensitivity.

Adverse Reactions and Side Effects*

• **CNS:** <u>dizziness</u>, <u>drowsiness</u>, <u>lethargy</u>, hangover, paradoxical excitation, mental depression, headache • **CV:** hypotension • **Derm:** rashes • **EENT:** blurred vision • **GI:** nausea, vomiting, diarrhea, constipation • **Local:** venous thrombosis,

---

*<u>Underlines</u> indicate most frequent; CAPITALS indicate life-threatening.

phlebitis • **Resp:** respiratory depression • **Misc:** tolerance, psychological dependence, physical dependence.

Diazoxide	Antihypertensive (vasodilator)
Hyperstat	pH 11.6

≋ ADMINISTRATION CONSIDERATIONS

Usual Dose
ADULTS AND CHILDREN: 1–3 mg/kg (up to 150 mg) q 5–15 min; regimen may be repeated q 4–24 hr as needed.

Dilution
• **Direct IV:** May be administered **undiluted**. Solution must be protected from light. Solution is clear and colorless. Do not administer darkened solution.

Compatibility
• **Syringe:** heparin.

Incompatibility
• **Y-site:** hydralazine • propranolol.

Rate of Administration
• **Direct IV:** Administer rapidly, over 30 seconds or less in adults or children, only into a peripheral vein to prevent cardiac arrhythmias. Slower administration reduces antihypertensive response. May be repeated every 5–15 minutes as indicated.

≋ CLINICAL PRECAUTIONS
• Do not administer SC or IM. Injection may cause warmth and pain along injected vein. Monitor IV site closely; extravasation causes cellulitis and pain. Cold packs may be applied if extravasation occurs.
• Assess patient for previous hypersensitivity to diazoxide or sulfonamides.
• Monitor pulse and blood pressure every 5 minutes until

stable and then hourly. Have patient remain recumbent during and for at least 15–30 minutes following IV administration. Take blood pressure standing prior to ambulation.

- Assess patient for signs and symptoms of congestive heart failure (peripheral edema, dyspnea, rales/crackles, fatigue, weight gain, jugular venous distention). Monitor fluid and electrolyte status. Fluid retention is common and may produce tolerance. Children are especially prone. Pretreatment with a loop diuretic (furosemide or equivalent) is recommended. Use with caution in patients with cardiovascular disease or uremia.
- Use cautiously in diabetic patients, since hyperglycemia routinely occurs.
- Elderly patients and patients with decreased renal function may require dosage adjustment, especially with repeated administration.
- Concurrent diuretic therapy may potentiate hyperglycemic, hyperuricemic, and hypotensive effects of diazoxide. Phenytoin, corticosteroids, and estrogen/progesterone may increase hyperglycemia.
- Diazoxide may increase the metabolism and thus decrease the effectiveness of phenytoin.
- Safe use in pregnancy has not been established. Labor may be inhibited (Pregnancy Category C).

Toxicity and Overdose Alert

- If severe hypotension occurs, treatment includes Trendelenburg position, volume infusion, and sympathomimetics (norepinephrine). • Patients who develop marked hyperglycemia must be monitored for 7 days while blood glucose concentrations stabilize.

Lab Test Considerations

- May cause increased serum glucose, BUN, alkaline phosphatase, AST (SGOT), sodium, and uric acid levels. • Monitor blood glucose levels in diabetic patients requiring frequent parenteral doses. • May cause decreased creatinine clearance, hematocrit, and hemoglobin levels.

Patient/Family Teaching

- Instruct patient to make position changes slowly to minimize orthostatic hypotension. • Caution patient to avoid taking other medications, especially over-the-counter cold medicine, without first consulting physician or pharmacist. • Emphasize the importance of routine follow-up examinations, especially during the first few weeks of antihypertensive therapy.

 PHARMACOLOGIC PROFILE

Indications

• Diazoxide is used in the emergency treatment of malignant hypertension.

Action

• Diazoxide directly relaxes vascular smooth muscle in peripheral arterioles. This results in decreased blood pressure, reflex tachycardia, and increased cardiac output.

Time/Action Profile (effect on blood pressure)

Onset	Peak	Duration
immediate	5 min	3–12 hr

Pharmacokinetics

• **Distribution:** Diazoxide crosses the blood–brain barrier and placenta. • **Metabolism and Excretion:** 50% of diazoxide is metabolized by the liver and 50% is excreted unchanged by the kidneys. • **Half-life:** 21–45 hours.

Contraindications

• Diazoxide should not be used in patients who have known hypersensitivity. Cross-sensitivity with sulfonamides may occur. • Some products contain bisulfites and should be avoided in patients with known intolerance.

Adverse Reactions and Side Effects*

• **CV:** edema, <u>tachycardia</u>, angina, arrhythmias, <u>hypotension</u>, flushing, congestive heart failure, myocardial infarction • **Endo:** <u>hyperglycemia</u> • **F and E:** <u>sodium and water retention</u>, hyperosmolar coma • **Local:** phlebitis at IV site.

---

*<u>Underlines</u> indicate most frequent; capitals indicate life-threatening.

Diethylstilbestrol Diphosphate	*Estrogen*
{Honvol}, Stilphostrol	pH 9–10.5

≋ ADMINISTRATION CONSIDERATIONS

Usual Dose

ADULTS: 500 mg as an infusion on the first day; may be increased to 1 g/day until response is obtained (5 or more days), then 250–500 mg 1–2 times weekly.

Dilution

• **Intermittent Infusion: Dilute** solution in 250–500 ml of D5W or 0.9% NaCl.

Incompatibility

• Information unavailable. Do not mix with other drugs or solutions.

Rate of Administration

• **Intermittent Infusion:** Infuse at a rate of 1–2 ml/min for the first 10–15 minutes. If infusion is tolerated, adjust the rate so that the entire dose has infused within 1 hour.

≋ CLINICAL PRECAUTIONS

• Assess blood pressure prior to and periodically throughout therapy. Monitor intake and output ratios. Assess weekly weight for significant weight changes or steady weight gain. Use cautiously in patients with underlying cardiovascular disease, because of fluid-retaining properties of diethylstilbestrol.

• Assess for the development of thromboembolic phenomenon.

• Use cautiously in patients with severe hepatic or renal disease.

• Diethylstilbestrol may alter requirement for oral anticoagulants, oral hypoglycemic agents, or insulin.

• Barbiturates or rifampin may decrease effectiveness of diethylstilbestrol by increasing its metabolism.

{} = Available in Canada only.

- Monitor tumor response by observing for decreased spread of disease.

Lab Test Considerations

- May cause increased levels of serum glucose, sodium, triglyceride, phospholipid, cortisol, prolactin, prothrombin, and Factors VII, VIII, IX, and X. May decrease serum folate, pyridoxine, antithrombin III, and pregnanediol excretion concentrations. • May alter thyroid hormone assays. • May cause hypercalcemia in patients with metastatic bone lesions.

Patient/Family Teaching

- If nausea becomes a problem, advise patient that eating solid food often provides relief. • Advise patient to report to physician signs and symptoms of fluid retention (swelling of ankles and feet, weight gain), thromboembolic disorders (pain, swelling, tenderness in extremities, headache, chest pain, blurred vision), mental depression, or hepatic dysfunction (yellowed skin or eyes, pruritus, dark urine, light-colored stools). • Diethylstilbestrol may occasionally cause a photosensitivity reaction. Caution patient to use sunscreen and protective clothing. • Emphasize the importance of routine follow-up physical examinations.

 PHARMACOLOGIC PROFILE

Indications

- Diethylstilbestrol diphosphate is used in advanced, inoperable metastatic prostate carcinoma.

Action

- Diethylstilbestrol decreases tumor spread in some androgen-sensitive tumors.

Time/Action Profile (antitumor effect)

Onset	Peak	Duration
4–8 wk	UK	UK

Pharmacokinetics

- **Distribution:** Diethylstilbestrol is widely distributed.
- **Metabolism and Excretion:** Metabolism of diethylstilbestrol occurs in the liver. • **Half-life:** UK.

Contraindications

• Patients with known thromboembolic disease, breast cancer, or other estrogen-dependent tumor should not receive diethylstilbestrol.

Adverse Reactions and Side Effects*

• **CNS:** <u>headache</u>, dizziness, lethargy • **CV:** <u>edema</u>, THROMBOEMBOLISM, <u>hypertension</u>, MYOCARDIAL INFARCTION • **EENT:** worsening of myopia or astigmatism, <u>intolerance to contact lenses</u> • **GI:** <u>nausea</u>, vomiting, anorexia, increased appetite, <u>weight changes</u>, jaundice • **GU:** <u>testicular atrophy</u>, <u>impotence</u> • **Derm:** <u>acne</u>, urticaria, <u>oily skin</u>, pigmentation, photosensitivity • **Endo:** hyperglycemia, <u>gynecomastia</u> • **F and E:** sodium and water retention, hypercalcemia • **MS:** leg cramps • **Misc:** <u>breast tenderness</u>.

Digoxin	Cardiac glycoside, Inotropic agent, Antiarrhythmic
Lanoxin	pH 6.8–7.2

≋ ADMINISTRATION CONSIDERATIONS

Usual Dose

For rapid effect, a larger initial loading or "digitalizing" dose should be administered in several divided doses. Maintenance doses must be determined by renal function. All dosing must be evaluated by individual response.

ADULTS: *Digitalizing dose:* 400–600 mcg (0.4–0.6 mg) initially; additional doses of 100–300 mcg (0.1–0.3 mg) may be given q 4–8 hr until desired clinical effect is achieved. *Maintenance dose:* 125–500 mcg (0.125–0.5 mg)/day given as a single dose or 2 divided doses.

CHILDREN >10 yr: *Digitalizing dose:* 8–12 mcg (0.008–0.012 mg)/kg given as half of this amount initially and the rest divided and given q 4–8 hr. *Maintenance dose:* 25–35% of the digitalizing dose daily, given as a single dose.

---

*<u>Underlines</u> indicate most frequent; CAPITALS indicate life-threatening.

CHILDREN 5–10 yr: *Digitalizing dose:* 15–30 mcg (0.015–0.03 mg)/kg given as half of this amount initially and the rest divided and given q 4–8 hr. *Maintenance dose:* 25–35% of the digitalizing dose daily, given in 2–3 divided doses.

CHILDREN 2–5 yr: *Digitalizing dose:* 25–35 mcg (0.025–0.035 mg)/kg given as half of this amount initially and the rest divided and given q 4–8 hr. *Maintenance dose:* 25–35% of the digitalizing dose daily, given in 2–3 divided doses.

CHILDREN 1–24 mo: *Digitalizing dose:* 30–50 mcg (0.03–0.05 mg)/kg given as half of this amount initially and the rest divided and given q 4–8 hr. *Maintenance dose:* 25–35% of the digitalizing dose daily, given in 2–3 divided doses.

NEONATES: *Digitalizing dose:* 20–30 mcg (0.02–0.03 mg)/kg given as half of this amount initially and the rest divided and given q 4–8 hr. *Maintenance dose:* 25–35% of digitalizing dose daily, given in 2 divided doses.

PREMATURE NEONATES: *Digitalizing dose:* 15–25 mcg (0.015–0.025 mg)/kg given as half of this amount initially and the rest divided and given q 4–8 hr. *Maintenance dose:* 20–30% of digitalizing dose daily, given in 2 divided doses.

Dilution

- **Direct IV:** IV doses may be given **undiluted** or each 1 ml may be **diluted** in 4 ml of sterile water, 0.9% NaCl, D5W, or lactated Ringer's solution for injection. Less diluent will cause precipitation. Use diluted solution immediately. Do not use solution that is discolored or contains precipitate.

Compatibility

- **Syringe:** heparin • milrinone.
- **Y-site:** amrinone • ciprofloxacin • diltiazem • famotidine • meperidine • milrinone • morphine • potassium chloride • tacrolimus • vitamin B complex with C.
- **Additive:** bretylium • cimetidine • furosemide • lidocaine • ranitidine • verapamil. However, mixing with other drugs in the same container or simultaneous administration in the same IV line is not recommended.

Incompatibility

- **Syringe:** doxapram.
- **Y-site:** fluconazole • foscarnet.
- **Additive:** dobutamine.

Rate of Administration

- **Direct IV:** Administer each dose through Y-site injection or 3-way stopcock over at least 5 minutes.

≋ CLINICAL PRECAUTIONS

- Monitor ECG prior to administering and throughout therapy for bradycardia or new arrhythmias. Withhold dose and assess for changes in rhythm or quality of pulse if pulse rate is less than 60 bpm in an adult or 70 bpm in a child or less than 90 bpm in an infant. Additive bradycardia may occur with beta-adrenergic blocking agents and other antiarrhythmic agents (quinidine, disopyramide).
- Before administering loading dose, determine if patient has had any cardiac glycosides in the preceding 2–3 weeks.
- Monitor blood pressure periodically.
- Monitor intake and output ratios and daily weights. Assess for peripheral edema and auscultate lungs for rales/crackles at least every 8 hours.
- Thiazide and loop diuretics, mezlocillin, piperacillin, ticarcillin, amphotericin B, and glucocorticoids may cause hypokalemia and may increase the risk of toxicity.
- Monitor serum digoxin levels during chronic therapy. Quinidine, cyclosporine, amiodarone, verapamil, diltiazem, propafenone, and diclofenac increase serum levels of digoxin and may lead to toxicity. Dosage reduction of digoxin is recommended when used with these agents.
- Use cautiously in geriatric or debilitated patients, who may be particularly sensitive to toxic effects, and in patients with renal impairment. Dosage reduction is required for any decrease in renal function during maintenance therapy. Monitor elderly patients for noncardiac signs of toxicity. Use with caution in patients with functioning artificial pacemakers.
- Dosing should be based on ideal body weight, as digoxin does not penetrate adipose tissue.
- Use cautiously in patients with myocardial infarction.
- Spironolactone increases digoxin half-life (reduced dosage or increased dosing interval may be required).
- Thyroid hormones may decrease therapeutic effects of digoxin.

- Although safety has not been established, digoxin has been used during pregnancy without adverse effects on the fetus (Pregnancy Category C). A dosage increase may be required in the final weeks of pregnancy, and subsequent reduction may be required postpartum. Safe use during lactation has not been established.

Toxicity and Overdose Alert

- Therapeutic serum digoxin levels range from 0.5 to 2 ng/ml. Serum digoxin levels may be drawn 4–10 hours after a dose is administered, although they are usually drawn immediately prior to the next dose. • Observe patient for signs and symptoms of toxicity. In adults and older children, the first signs of toxicity usually include abdominal pain, anorexia, nausea, vomiting, visual disturbances, bradycardia, and other arrhythmias. In infants and small children, the first symptoms of overdose are usually cardiac arrhythmias. Withhold drug if these occur. If signs of toxicity occur and are not severe, discontinuation of digoxin may be all that is required. • If hypokalemia is present and renal function is adequate, potassium salts may be administered. Do not administer if hyperkalemia or heart block exists. • Correction of arrhythmias due to digitalis toxicity may be attempted with lidocaine, procainamide, quinidine, propranolol, or phenytoin. Temporary ventricular pacing may be useful in advanced heart block. • Treatment of life-threatening arrhythmias may include administration of digoxin immune Fab (Digibind), which binds to the digoxin molecule in the blood and is excreted by the kidneys.

Lab Test Considerations

- Serum electrolyte levels, especially potassium, magnesium, and calcium, and renal and hepatic functions should be evaluated periodically during the course of therapy. Hypokalemia, hypomagnesemia, or hypercalcemia may make the patient more susceptible to digitalis toxicity.

Patient/Family Teaching

- Teach patient on chronic therapy to take pulse and to contact physician before taking medication if pulse rate is less than 60 or greater than 100 bpm. • Review signs and symptoms of digitalis toxicity with patient and family. Advise patient to notify physician immediately if these or symptoms of congestive heart failure occur. Inform patient that these symptoms may be mistaken for those of colds or flu. • Caution patient to avoid concurrent use of over-the-counter medications without first consulting physician. • Advise patient to notify physician or dentist of this medication regimen prior to treatment. • Patients taking digoxin should carry identification describing disease process and medication regimen at all times. • Emphasize the importance of routine follow-up examinations to determine effectiveness and to monitor for toxicity.

≋ PHARMACOLOGIC PROFILE

Indications

• Digoxin is used alone or in combination with other agents (diuretics, vasodilators, ACE inhibitors) in the treatment of congestive heart failure. • It is also used to slow the ventricular rate in tachyarrhythmias such as atrial fibrillation and atrial flutter and to terminate paroxysmal atrial tachycardia.

Action

• Digoxin increases the force of myocardial contraction. Electrophysiologic effects of digoxin include prolongation of the refractory period of the AV node and decreased conduction through the SA and AV nodes. These effects result in increased cardiac output and slowing of the heart rate.

Time/Action Profile (for antiarrhythmic or inotropic effects)

Onset†	Peak	Duration‡
5–30 min	1–5 hr	2–4 days

†Provided that a loading dose has been administered.
‡In patients with normal renal function. Duration will be prolonged in patients with any degree of renal impairment.

Pharmacokinetics

• **Distribution:** Digoxin is widely distributed but does not penetrate adipose tissue. It crosses the placenta and enters breast milk. • **Metabolism and Excretion:** Excretion of digoxin occurs almost entirely as unchanged drug via the kidneys. • **Half-life:** 34–44 hours (increased in renal impairment).

Contraindications

• Digoxin is contraindicated in patients with hypersensitivity to digoxin, alcohol, or propylene glycol. • Patients with uncontrolled ventricular arrhythmias, AV block, idiopathic hypertrophic subaortic stenosis, or constrictive pericarditis should not receive digoxin. • Injection contains alcohol and should be avoided in patients with known intolerance.

Adverse Reactions and Side Effects*

• **CNS:** <u>fatigue</u>, weakness, headache • **EENT:** blurred vision, yellow vision • **CV:** ARRHYTHMIAS, <u>bradycardia</u>, ECG changes • **GI:** <u>nausea</u>, <u>vomiting</u>, <u>anorexia</u>, diarrhea • **Endo:** gynecomastia • **Hemat:** thrombocytopenia.

Digoxin Immune Fab	Antidote
	(for digoxin, digitoxin)
Digibind	pH 6–8

≋ ADMINISTRATION CONSIDERATIONS

Usual Dose

When Estimated Digoxin or Digitoxin Dose Is *Not* Known:

ADULTS AND CHILDREN: 800 mg.

When Digoxin or Digitoxin Dose Is Known:

Calculate total dose or body load (TBL) in mg of digoxin or digitoxin. If digoxin was ingested orally as tablets or elixir, multiply the amount ingested by 0.8.

ADULTS AND CHILDREN: Total body load (TBL) × 66.7 = dose of digoxin immune Fab (mg).

---

*<u>Underlines</u> indicate most frequent; CAPITALS indicate life-threatening.

Dosage When Serum Digoxin/Digitoxin Level (SDC) Is Known

Digoxin: Dose (mg) = SDC (ng/ml) × body weight (kg) × 0.4

Digitoxin: Dose (mg) = SDC (ng/ml) × body weight (kg) × 0.04

Dosage for Toxicity during Chronic Therapy

Adults: 240 mg.
Children: 40 mg.

Dilution

• **Intermittent Infusion: Reconstitute** each 40 mg for IV administration in 4 ml of sterile water for injection and mix gently. Solution will contain a concentration of 10 mg/ml. May be **further diluted** with 0.9% NaCl for IV infusion. • Reconstituted solution should be used immediately but is stable for 4 hours if refrigerated. • In infants and small children, monitor for fluid overload. For small doses, a reconstituted 40-mg vial can be diluted with 36 ml of 0.9% NaCl for a concentration of 1 mg/ml. Administer with a tuberculin syringe.

Incompatibility

• Information unavailable. Do not mix with other drugs or solutions.

Rate of Administration

• **Intermittent Infusion:** Administer reconstituted solution by IV infusion through a 0.22-micron membrane filter over 30 minutes. If cardiac arrest is imminent, rapid direct IV injection may be used.

≋ CLINICAL PRECAUTIONS

• Try to obtain history and amount of ingestion of digoxin or digitoxin. Forty mg of digoxin immune Fab is capable of binding approximately 0.6 mg of digoxin or digitoxin.
• Patients with a high risk for allergy to digoxin immune Fab or sheep proteins should have skin testing for allergy prior to administration. Prepare skin test solution by diluting 0.1 ml of the reconstituted solution (10 mg/ml) in 9.9 ml of 0.9% NaCl to produce a 10-ml solution (100 mcg/ml). Testing may be administered by intradermal injection or scratch test. For intradermal use, inject 0.1

ml intradermally. For scratch test, place 1 drop of solution on the skin and make a ¼-inch scratch through the drop with a sterile needle. Following either method, inspect for urticarial wheal surrounded by erythema after 20 minutes. If a positive skin test occurs, use of digoxin immune Fab should be avoided unless absolutely necessary.

- Monitor ECG, pulse, and body temperature prior to and throughout treatment. Patients with atrial fibrillation may develop a rapid ventricular response as a result of decreased digoxin or digitoxin levels, and allergic or febrile reactions may rarely occur.
- Cardiopulmonary resuscitation equipment and medications should be available during administration.
- Assess for increased signs of congestive heart failure (peripheral edema, rales/crackles, weight gain, dyspnea). Smaller amounts of diluent may be used for infants and small children.
- Delay redigitalization for several days until the elimination of digoxin immune Fab from the body is complete.
- Safe use in pregnancy, lactation, or children has not been established (Pregnancy Category C).

Lab Test Considerations

- Monitor serum digoxin or digitoxin levels prior to administration. Initial serum digoxin levels of greater than 5 ng/ml require special assay procedures. • Monitor serum potassium levels frequently during treatment. Prior to treatment, hyperkalemia usually coexists with toxicity. Levels may decrease rapidly; hypokalemia should be treated promptly. • Free serum digoxin or digitoxin levels fall rapidly following administration. Total body concentrations rise suddenly after administration but are bound to the Fab molecule and are inactive. Total body concentrations will decrease to undetectable levels within several days. Serum digoxin or digitoxin levels are not valid for 5–7 days following administration.

Patient/Family Teaching

- Explain the procedure and purpose of the treatment to the patient.

≋ PHARMACOLOGIC PROFILE

Indications
- Digoxin immune Fab is used in the management of potentially life-threatening digoxin or digitoxin toxicity.

Action
- Digoxin immune Fab is an antibody produced in sheep, which binds antigenically to unbound digoxin or digitoxin in serum.

Time/Action Profile (reversal of arrhythmias and hyperkalemia)

Onset	Peak	Duration
30 min (variable)	UK	2–6 hr

Pharmacokinetics
- **Distribution:** Digoxin immune Fab is widely distributed throughout the extracellular space. • **Metabolism and Excretion:** It is excreted by the kidneys as the bound complex (digoxin immune Fab plus digoxin or digitoxin). • **Half-life:** 14–20 hours.

Contraindications
- There are no known contraindications to the use of digoxin immune Fab.

Adverse Reactions and Side Effects*
- **CV:** re-emergence of atrial fibrillation, re-emergence of congestive heart failure • **F and E:** HYPOKALEMIA.

---

*Underlines indicate most frequent; CAPITALS indicate life-threatening.

Dihydroergotamine Mesylate	*Ergot alkaloid* *(headache suppressant)*
D.H.E. 45, {Dihydroergotamine-Sandoz}	pH 3.2–4

ADMINISTRATION CONSIDERATIONS

Usual Dose

Acute Migraine/Cluster Headache (outpatients)

ADULTS: 500 mcg (0.5 mg); may be repeated 1 hr later (not to exceed 2 mg/day or 6 mg/wk). Pretreatment with an antiemetic is recommended.

CHILDREN >6 yr: 250 mcg (0.25 mg); may be repeated in 1 hr. Pretreatment with an antiemetic is recommended (unlabeled).

Chronic Intractable Headache (inpatients)

ADULTS: Following pretreatment with an antiemetic, 500 mcg (0.5 mg). Additional doses of up to 1 mg may be given as needed and tolerated. Regimen may be repeated q 8 hr. To prevent recurrence, it may be repeated q 12 hr for 2–3 additional doses.

Dilution

- **Direct IV:** May be administered **undiluted**.

Incompatibility

- Do not mix with other drugs in syringe or solution.

Rate of Administration

- **Direct IV:** Administer each dose over 1 minute.

☰ CLINICAL PRECAUTIONS

- During acute attack, assess type, location, and intensity of headache prior to and several minutes following administration. Medication is most effective if administered at the first sign of a migraine attack (prodromal stage). Patient should lie down in a quiet, dark room for at least 2 hours following administration.
- Monitor blood pressure prior to and during treatment.

{} = Available in Canada only.

Antihypertensive therapy may be required. Assess peripheral pulses during treatment to detect vasospasm or ischemia.

- Assess for signs of ergotism (cold, numb fingers and toes; nausea; headache; muscle pain; weakness).
- Assess for nausea and vomiting. This agent stimulates the chemoreceptor trigger zone. A phenothiazine antiemetic or metoclopromide is usually given intravenously 3–5 minutes, or orally 1 hour prior to administration of dihydroergotamine.
- Elderly patients may be more susceptible to vasoconstrictive effects. Use with caution in this population. Monitor ECG during first few doses in patients over 60 years of age.
- Concurrent use with beta-adrenergic blockers, oral contraceptives, vasoconstrictors, erythromycin, or heavy cigarette smoking (nicotine) may increase the risk of peripheral vasoconstriction or severe hypertensive reactions.
- Use with vasodilators may result in serious hypertension.
- Although dihydroergotamine has been used in children without adverse effects, safe use in children has not been established. Reserve use for when less toxic agents are ineffective.
- Dihydroergotamine should not be used during pregnancy because it may stimulate uterine musculature and decrease uterine blood flow (Pregnancy Category X).

Patient/Family Teaching

- Advise patient to avoid alcohol (which aggravates headache) and smoking (which constricts blood vessels).
- Instruct patient to avoid exposure to excessive cold, which may aggravate peripheral vasoconstriction.

≋ PHARMACOLOGIC PROFILE

Indications

- Treatment and prevention of vascular headaches, including migraine and cluster headaches.

Action

- Dihydroergotamine produces constriction of dilated vessels in the carotid artery bed, resulting in resolution of vascular headaches.

Time/Action Profile (relief of vascular headache)

Onset	Peak	Duration
less than 5 min	15 min–2 hr	8 hr†

†Following SC administration.

Pharmacokinetics

• **Distribution:** Dihydroergotamine probably enters breast milk. • **Metabolism and Excretion:** Metabolism occurs mostly in the liver, with excretion in feces via biliary elimination. • **Half-life:** 21–32 hours.

Contraindications

• Dihydroergotamine is contraindicated in patients with hypersensitivity to it. Cross-sensitivity with other ergot alkaloids may occur. • Dihydroergotamine injection contains alcohol and should be avoided in patients with known intolerance to alcohol. • Use of dihydroergotamine should be avoided in patients with peripheral vascular disease, cardiovascular disease, uncontrolled hypertension, serious infections, malnutrition, or impaired renal or hepatic function. • Pregnant or lactating patients should not receive dihydroergotamine.

Adverse Reactions and Side Effects*

• **CNS:** headache (due to tolerance), dizziness • **GI:** nausea, vomiting • **Misc:** localized edema of feet or legs, peripheral vasospasm.

Diltiazem Hydrochloride	Calcium channel blocker, Antiarrhythmic
Cardizem	pH 3.7–4.1

☰ ADMINISTRATION CONSIDERATIONS

Usual Dose

ADULTS: 250 mcg (0.25 mg)/kg (20 mg in the average patient). If response is inadequate, dose of 350 mcg (0.35

---

*Underlines indicate most frequent; CAPITALS indicate life-threatening.

mg)/kg (25 mg in the average patient) may be repeated after 15 minutes. Some patients may respond to 150 mcg (0.15 mg)/kg. This may be followed by continuous infusion at 10 mg/hr (range 5–15 mg/hr) for up to 24 hr.

Dilution

• **Direct IV:** May be administered **undiluted**. • **Continuous Infusion: Dilute** 125 mg in 100 ml, 250 mg in 250 ml, or 250 mg in 500 ml of 0.9% NaCl, D5W, or D5/0.45% NaCl for concentrations of 1 mg/ml, 0.83 mg/ml, or 0.45 mg/ml respectively. • Refrigerate after dilution. Administer within 24 hours of dilution.

Compatibility

• **Y-site:** albumin ✦ amikacin ✦ amphotericin B ✦ aztreonam ✦ bretylium ✦ bumetanide ✦cefazolin ✦ cefotaxime ✦ cefotetan ✦ cefoxitin ✦ ceftazidime ✦ ceftriaxone ✦ cefuroxime ✦ cimetidine ✦ ciprofloxacin ✦ clindamycin ✦ digoxin ✦ dobutamine ✦ dopamine ✦ doxycycline ✦ epinephrine ✦ erythromycin lactobionate ✦ esmolol ✦ fluconazole ✦ gentamicin ✦ hetastarch ✦ imipenem/cilastatin ✦ lidocaine ✦ lorazepam ✦ meperidine ✦ metoclopramide ✦ metronidazole ✦ morphine ✦ multivitamins ✦ nitroglycerin ✦ norepinephrine ✦ oxacillin ✦ penicillin G potassium ✦ pentamidine ✦ piperacillin ✦ potassium ✦ ranitidine ✦ sodium nitroprusside ✦ theophylline ✦ ticarcillin ✦ ticarcillin/clavulanate ✦ tobramycin ✦ trimethoprim/sulfamethoxazole ✦ vancomycin.

Incompatibility

• **Syringe:** furosemide.
• **Y-site:** diazepam ✦ furosemide ✦ phenytoin ✦ rifampin.

Rate of Administration

• **Direct IV:** Administer each dose as a bolus over 2 minutes. • **Continuous Infusion:** Initial infusion should be administered at a rate of 10 mg/hr (10 ml/hr of the 1 mg/ml concentration, 12 ml/hr of the 0.83 mg/ml concentration, or 22 ml/hr of the 0.45 mg/ml concentration). May increase in increments of 5 mg/hr, up to 15 mg/hr (15 ml/hr of the 1 mg/ml concentration, 18 ml/hr of the 0.83 mg/ml concentration, or 33 ml/hr of the 0.45 mg/ml concentration) if further reduction in heart rate is required. Some patients may respond to a rate of 5 mg/hr. • Infusion may be continued for up to 24 hours.

≋ CLINICAL PRECAUTIONS

- Monitor ECG continuously during administration for bradycardia or prolonged hypotension. Emergency equipment and medication should be available. Monitor blood pressure and pulse before and frequently during administration. Elderly patients may be more prone to hypotension and constipation.
- Monitor intake and output ratios and daily weights. Assess patient for signs of congestive heart failure (peripheral edema, rales/crackles, dyspnea, weight gain, jugular venous distention).
- Use cautiously in patients with severe hepatic disease; dosage reduction may be required.
- Patients with congestive heart failure should be observed for worsening of condition.
- There is increased risk of bradycardia, conduction defects, or congestive heart failure when diltiazem is used with beta-adrenergic blockers, digoxin, disopyramide, or other cardioactive agents.
- Additive hypotension may occur with other antihypertensives or nitrates.
- Safe use in pregnancy, lactation, or children has not been established (Pregnancy Category C).

Lab Test Considerations

- Total serum calcium concentrations are not affected by calcium channel blockers.

Patient/Family Teaching

- Caution patients to make position changes slowly to minimize orthostatic hypotension. • Medication may cause dizziness. Advise patient to avoid activities requiring alertness until response to medication is known.

≋ PHARMACOLOGIC PROFILE

Indications

- Diltiazem is used to convert atrial arrhythmias including atrial fibrillation, atrial flutter, and paroxysmal supraventricular tachycardia (PSVT).

Action

- Diltiazem increases the refractory period of the AV node. In addition, diltiazem decreases SA node automaticity and AV nodal conduction.

Time/Action Profile (antiarrhythmic effect after rapid IV use)

Onset	Peak	Duration
within 3 min	2–7 min	1–3 hr†

†7 hr after infusion (range 0.5–over 10 hr).

Pharmacokinetics

- **Distribution:** UK. • **Metabolism and Excretion:** Diltiazem is mostly metabolized by the liver. • **Half-life:** 3.4–9 hours.

Contraindications

- Diltiazem is contraindicated in patients with hypersensitivity. • Patients with sick sinus syndrome (without a functioning artificial pacemaker), second- and third-degree heart block, severe hypotension, or atrial arrhythmias associated with accessory bypass tracts (Wolff-Parkinson-White syndrome or short PR interval) should not receive diltiazem.

Adverse Reactions and Side Effects*

- **CNS:** dizziness, <u>headache</u>, tremors, mood changes, <u>fatigue</u>, drowsiness, weakness • **EENT:** decreased visual acuity • **Resp:** dyspnea • **CV:** <u>arrhythmias</u>, <u>edema</u>, <u>hypotension</u>, syncope, palpitations, congestive heart failure, second- and third-degree heart block • **GI:** anorexia, <u>constipation</u>, nausea, abdominal discomfort, hepatitis, gingival hyperplasia • **Derm:** <u>rash</u>, petechiae, photosensitivity, pruritus, sweating, flushing • **Local:** itching and burning at IV site • **Metab:** hyperuricemia • **Neuro:** paresthesia.

---

*<u>Underlines</u> indicate most frequent; CAPITALS indicate life-threatening.

Dimenhydrinate	*Antihistamine, Antiemetic*
Dinate, Dramanate, Dramoject, Dymenate, {Gravol}, Hydrate, Marmine	pH 6.4–7.2

ADMINISTRATION CONSIDERATIONS

Usual Dose

ADULTS: 50–100 mg q 4 hr as needed.
CHILDREN: 1.25 mg/kg (37.5 mg/m^2) q 6 hr as needed (not to exceed 300 mg/day) (unlabeled).

Dilution

• **Direct IV: Dilute** 50 mg in 10 ml of 0.9% NaCl for injection. • May also be diluted within D5W, 0.45% NaCl, 0.9% NaCl, Ringer's solution, lactated Ringer's solution, dextrose/saline combinations, or dextrose/Ringer's combinations.

Compatibility

• **Syringe:** atropine • droperidol • fentanyl • heparin • meperidine • metoclopramide • morphine • pentazocine • perphenazine • ranitidine • scopolamine.
• **Y-site:** acyclovir.
• **Additive:** amikacin • calcium gluconate • chloramphenicol • erythromycin glucceptate • heparin • methicillin • oxytetracycline • penicillin G potassium • potassium chloride • vancomycin • vitamin B complex with C.

Incompatibility

• **Syringe:** butorphanol • chlorpromazine • glycopyrrolate • hydroxyzine • midazolam • pentobarbital • prochlorperazine • promazine • promethazine • thiopental.
• **Y-site:** aminophylline • heparin • hydrocortisone sodium succinate • hydroxyzine • phenobarbital • phenytoin • prednisolone sodium phosphate • prochlorperazine • promazine • promethazine.

Rate of Administration

• **Direct IV:** Inject over 2 minutes.

{} = Available in Canada only.

≋ CLINICAL PRECAUTIONS

- Assess nausea, vomiting, bowel sounds, and abdominal pain before and after the administration of this drug. Dimenhydrinate may mask the signs of an acute abdomen. Monitor intake and output, including emesis. Assess patient for signs of dehydration (excessive thirst, dry skin and mucous membranes, tachycardia, increased urine specific gravity, poor skin turgor).
- Administer before exposure to conditions known to precipitate motion sickness.
- Use cautiously in patients with narrow-angle glaucoma, seizure disorders, or prostatic hypertrophy. Geriatric patients may be more prone to anticholinergic side effects (confusion, constipation).
- Additive CNS depression occurs with concurrent use of other antihistamines, alcohol, opioid analgesics, and sedative/hypnotics.
- May mask signs or symptoms of ototoxicity in patients receiving ototoxic drugs (aminoglycosides, ethacrynic acid).
- Additive anticholinergic properties (dry mouth, dry eyes, blurred vision) may occur with concurrent use of tricyclic antidepressants, quinidine, or disopyramide. MAO inhibitors intensify and prolong the anticholinergic effects of antihistamines.
- Safe use in pregnancy or children has not been established (Pregnancy Category B). Dimenhydrinate is not recommended during lactation (lactation may be inhibited; infant may become excited or irritable).

Lab Test Considerations

- Will cause false-negative allergy skin tests; discontinue 72 hours prior to testing.

Patient/Family Teaching

- Medication may cause drowsiness and sedation. Advise patient to avoid driving or other activities requiring alertness until response to the drug is known. • Inform patient that this medication may cause dry mouth. Frequent oral rinses, good oral hygiene, and sugarless gum or candy may minimize this effect. • Caution patient to avoid alcohol and other CNS depressants concurrently with this medication. • Advise patient to use sunscreen and protective clothing to prevent photosensitivity reactions.

 PHARMACOLOGIC PROFILE

Indications
• Dimenhydrinate is used in the treatment and prevention of nausea, vomiting, dizziness, or vertigo accompanying motion sickness.

Action
• Dimenhydrinate inhibits vestibular stimulation. It also has CNS depressant, anticholinergic, antihistaminic, and antiemetic properties.

Time/Action Profile (antiemetic effect)

Onset	Peak	Duration
rapid	UK	3–6 hr

Pharmacokinetics
• **Distribution:** Dimenhydrinate probably crosses the placenta and enters breast milk. • **Metabolism and Excretion:** Metabolism of dimenhydrinate occurs primarily in the liver. • **Half-life:** UK.

Contraindications
• Contraindicated in patients with hypersensitivity to dimenhydrinate, benzyl alcohol, or propylene glycol.

Adverse Reactions and Side Effects*
• **CNS:** <u>drowsiness</u>, dizziness, headache • **EENT:** blurred vision, tinnitus • **CV:** palpitations, hypotension • **GI:** dry mouth, <u>anorexia</u>, constipation, diarrhea • **GU:** frequency, dysuria • **Derm:** photosensitivity.

---

*<u>Underlines</u> indicate most frequent; CAPITALS indicate life-threatening.

Diphenhydramine Hydrochloride	*Antihistamine, Antiemetic*
Bena-D 10, Bena-D 50, Benadryl, Benahist 10, Benahist 50, Ben-Allergin-50, Benoject-10, Benoject-50, Hyrexin-50, Nordryl, Wehdryl	pH 5–6

 ADMINISTRATION CONSIDERATIONS

Usual Dose

ADULTS: 10–50 mg; up to 100 mg/dose; may be repeated q 2–3 hr (not to exceed 400 mg/day).

CHILDREN: 1.25 mg/kg (37.5 mg/m^2) q 6–8 hr (not to exceed 300 mg/day in 4 divided doses).

Dilution

• **Direct IV:** May give **undiluted**. May be **further diluted** in 0.9% NaCl, 0.45% NaCl, D5W, D10W, D5/0.9% NaCl, D5/0.45% NaCl, D5/0.25% NaCl, Ringer's solution, lactated Ringer's solution, and dextrose/Ringer's combinations.

Compatibility

• **Syringe:** atropine ◆ butorphanol ◆ chlorpromazine ◆ cimetidine ◆ droperidol ◆ fentanyl ◆ glycopyrrolate ◆ hydromorphone ◆ hydroxyzine ◆ meperidine ◆ metoclopramide ◆ midazolam ◆ morphine ◆ nalbuphine ◆ pentazocine ◆ perphenazine ◆ prochlorperazine ◆ promazine ◆ promethazine ◆ ranitidine ◆ scopolamine.

• **Y-site:** acyclovir ◆ ciprofloxacin ◆ cisplatin ◆ cyclophosphamide ◆ cytarabine ◆ doxorubicin ◆ filgrastim ◆ fluconazole ◆ fludarabine ◆ heparin ◆ hydrocortisone ◆ idarubicin ◆ melphalan ◆ meperidine ◆ methotrexate ◆ ondansetron ◆ paclitaxel ◆ piperacillin/tazobactam ◆ potassium chloride ◆ sargramostim ◆ tacrolimus ◆ vinorelbine ◆ vitamin B complex with C.

• **Additive:** amikacin ◆ aminophylline ◆ ascorbic acid ◆ bleomycin ◆ cephapirin ◆ colistimethate ◆ erythromycin lactobionate ◆ lidocaine ◆ methicillin ◆ methyldopate ◆ nafcillin ◆ netilmicin ◆ penicillin G ◆ polymyxin B ◆ vitamin B complex with C.

Incompatibility

- **Syringe:** pentobarbital ◆ thiopental.
- **Y-site:** allopurinol sodium ◆ foscarnet.
- **Additive:** amobarbital ◆ amphotericin B ◆ cephalothin ◆ hydrocortisone sodium succinate ◆ thiopental.

Rate of Administration

- **Direct IV:** Inject each 25 mg over at least 1 minute.

≋ CLINICAL PRECAUTIONS

- Assess for symptoms of allergic reactions including rashes, urticaria, shortness of breath, wheezing, and hypotension when used for this purpose. Emergency equipment and medication should be available.
- Assess for movement disorder prior to and following administration when used for dystonic reactions.
- When used as an antiemetic, assess nausea, vomiting, bowel sounds, abdominal pain, and hydration status. Diphenhydramine may mask the signs of an acute abdomen.
- Geriatric patients are more likely to experience sedation and anticholinergic side effects (constipation, confusion). Increased dosing interval is recommended in this age group and for patients with a creatinine clearance of less than 50 ml/mm.
- Use with caution in patients with severe liver disease, narrow-angle glaucoma, seizure disorders, or prostatic hypertrophy.
- Additive CNS depression will occur with other antihistamines, alcohol, opioid analgesics, and sedative/hypnotics.
- Additive anticholinergic properties (dry mouth, dry eyes, blurred vision) may occur with concurrent use of tricyclic antidepressants, quinidine, or disopyramide. MAO inhibitors intensify and prolong the anticholinergic effects of antihistamines.
- Safe use in pregnancy has not been established (Pregnancy Category B). Diphenhydramine is not recommended during lactation (lactation may be inhibited; infant may become excited or irritable).

Lab Test Considerations

• Diphenhydramine may decrease skin response to allergy tests. Discontinue 4 days prior to skin testing.

Patient/Family Teaching

• Commonly causes drowsiness and sedation. Advise patient to avoid driving or other activities requiring alertness until response to drug is known. • Inform patient that this drug may cause dry mouth. Frequent oral rinses, good oral hygiene, and sugarless gum or candy may minimize this effect. • Advise patient to use sunscreen and protective clothing to prevent photosensitivity reactions. • Caution patient to avoid use of alcohol and other CNS depressants concurrently with this medication.

PHARMACOLOGIC PROFILE

Indications

• Diphenhydramine is used to relieve allergic symptoms caused by histamine release, including anaphylaxis. • Also used in the acute management of Parkinson's disease and dystonic reactions from medications, and as an antiemetic.

Action

• Diphenhydramine blocks the following effects of histamine: vasodilation, increased GI tract secretions, increased heart rate, and hypotension. In addition, it has significant CNS depressant and anticholinergic properties.

Time/Action Profile (antihistaminic effect)

Onset	Peak	Duration
rapid	UK	4–8 hr

Pharmacokinetics

• **Distribution:** Diphenhydramine is widely distributed. It crosses the placenta and enters breast milk. • **Metabolism and Excretion:** Diphenhydramine is metabolized by the liver (95%). • **Half-life:** 2.4–7 hours.

Contraindications

• Diphenhydramine is contraindicated in patients with known hypersensitivity. Some products contain benzethonium chloride or chlorobutanol. Avoid use in patients with known intolerance to these additives. • Diphenhydramine should not be used during acute attacks of asthma or during lactation.

Adverse Reactions and Side Effects*

• **CNS:** <u>drowsiness</u>, paradoxical excitation (children), dizziness, headache • **EENT:** blurred vision, tinnitus • **CV:** palpitations, hypotension • **GI:** <u>dry mouth</u>, <u>anorexia</u>, constipation, diarrhea • **GU:** frequency, dysuria, urinary retention • **Derm:** photosensitivity.

Dipyridamole	*Coronary vasodilator*
IV Persantine, {Persantine}	pH 3.5–4

≋ ADMINISTRATION CONSIDERATIONS

Usual Dose

ADULTS: 570 mcg (0.57 mg)/kg not to exceed 60 mg.

Dilution

• **Direct IV: Dilute** in at least a 1:2 ratio of 0.45% NaCl, 0.9% NaCl, or D5W for a total volume of 20–50 ml. Undiluted dipyridamole may cause venous irritation due to low pH.

Incompatibility

• Information unavailable. Do not mix with other drugs or solutions.

Rate of Administration

• **Direct IV:** Inject dose over 4 minutes into antecubital vein to minimize the effects of acid pH.

≋ CLINICAL PRECAUTIONS

• Monitor vital signs during and 10–15 minutes following infusion. Obtain ECG in at least one lead. If severe chest

---

*<u>Underlines</u> indicate most frequent; CAPITALS indicate life-threatening.

{} = Available in Canada only.

pain or bronchospasm occurs, administer IV aminophylline 50–250 mg at a rate of 50–100 mg over 30–60 seconds. Theophylline negates the effects of dipyridamole during diagnostic thallium imaging. If hypotension is severe, place patient in supine position with head tilting down. If chest pain is unrelieved by aminophylline, administer sublingual nitroglycerin. If chest pain is still unrelieved, treat as if myocardial infarction has occurred.

- Use cautiously in patients who are hypotensive. Elderly patients may be more likely to develop hypotension.
- Dipyridamole has additive effects with aspirin on platelet aggregation. Risk of bleeding may be increased when used with heparin, streptokinase, urokinase or alteplase, some cephalosporins, valproic acid, pentoxifylline, nonsteroidal anti-inflammatory agents, or sulfinpyrazone. Use cautiously in patients who have platelet defects.
- Although safety is not established, dipyridamole has been used without harm during pregnancy (Pregnancy Category B).
- Safe use in lactation or children younger than 12 years has not been established.

Lab Test Considerations

- Bleeding time should be monitored periodically throughout course of therapy.

Patient/Family Teaching

- Instruct patient to notify physician immediately if dyspnea or chest pain occurs. • Caution patient to make position changes slowly to minimize orthostatic hypotension. • Instruct patient to notify physician if unusual bleeding or bruising occurs.

≋ PHARMACOLOGIC PROFILE

Indications

- Dipyridamole is used as a diagnostic agent in lieu of exercise during thallium myocardial perfusion imaging in patients who cannot exercise.

Action

• Dipyridamole produces coronary vasodilation by inhibiting adenosine uptake. During diagnostic thallium imaging, dipyridamole dilates normal coronary arteries, reducing flow to vessels that are narrowed, resulting in abnormal thallium distribution.

Time/Action Profile (coronary vasodilation)

Onset	Peak	Duration
UK	6.5 min†	30 min

†From start of infusion.

Pharmacokinetics

• **Distribution:** Dipyridamole is widely distributed; it crosses the placenta and enters breast milk. • **Metabolism and Excretion:** Dipyridamole is metabolized by the liver and excreted in the bile. • **Half-life:** 10 hours.

Contraindications

• Contraindicated in patients with hypersensitivity to dipyridamole or propylene glycol.

Adverse Reactions and Side Effects*

• **CNS:** <u>headache</u>, <u>dizziness</u>, weakness, syncope, transient cerebral ischemia • **CV:** flushing, <u>hypotension</u>; IV only: MYO-CARDIAL INFARCTION, arrhythmias • **Resp:** bronchospasm • **GI:** GI upset, <u>nausea</u>, vomiting, diarrhea • **Derm:** rash.

Dobutamine	*Inotropic agent*
Dobutrex	**pH 2.5–5.5**

☰ ADMINISTRATION CONSIDERATIONS

Usual Dose

ADULTS: 2.5–10 mcg/kg/min infusion (up to 40 mcg/kg/min).

---

*<u>Underlines</u> indicate most frequent; CAPITALS indicate life-threatening.

Dilution

• **Continuous Infusion:** Reconstitute 250-mg vial with 10 ml of sterile water or D5W for injection. If not completely dissolved, add another 10 ml of diluent. **Dilute** in at least 50 ml of D5W, 0.9% NaCl, sodium lactate, 0.45% NaCl, D5/0.45% NaCl, D5/0.9% NaCl, D5/LR, or lactated Ringer's solution. Standard concentrations range from 250 mcg/ml to 1000 mcg/ml. Concentrations should not exceed 5 mg of dobutamine/ml. • Slight pink color of solution does not alter potency. Solution is stable for 24 hours at room temperature.

Compatibility

• **Syringe:** heparin ♦ ranitidine.
• **Y-site:** amrinone ♦ atracurium ♦ bretylium ♦ calcium chloride ♦ calcium gluconate ♦ ciprofloxacin ♦ diazepam ♦ diltiazem ♦ dopamine ♦ enalaprilat ♦ famotidine ♦ haloperidol ♦ insulin ♦ lidocaine ♦ magnesium sulfate ♦ meperidine ♦ nitroglycerin ♦ pancuronium ♦ potassium chloride ♦ ranitidine ♦ sodium nitroprusside ♦ streptokinase ♦ tacrolimus ♦ tolazoline ♦ vecuronium ♦ verapamil ♦ zidovudine.
• **Additive:** atracurium ♦ atropine ♦ dopamine ♦ enalaprilat ♦ epinephrine ♦ hydralazine ♦ isoproterenol ♦ lidocaine ♦ meperidine ♦ metaraminol ♦ morphine ♦ nitroglycerin ♦ norepinephrine ♦ phentolamine ♦ phenylephrine ♦ procainamide ♦ propranolol ♦ ranitidine. However, it is recommended that dobutamine not be mixed in solution with other medications.

Incompatibility

• **Y-site:** acyclovir ♦ alteplase ♦ aminophylline ♦ foscarnet ♦ indomethacin ♦ phytonadione ♦ piperacillin/tazobactam.
• **Additive:** acyclovir ♦ aminophylline ♦ bumetanide ♦ calcium gluconate ♦ diazepam ♦ digoxin ♦ furosemide ♦ insulin ♦ magnesium sulfate ♦ phenytoin ♦ potassium phosphate ♦ sodium bicarbonate.

Rate of Administration

• **Continuous Infusion:** Administer via infusion pump. Rate of administration is titrated according to patient response (heart rate, presence of ectopic activity, blood pressure, urine output, CVP, PCWP, cardiac output); see Infusion Rate Table.

DOBUTAMINE (Dobutrex) INFUSION RATES AT VARIOUS DILUTIONS

Dilution may be prepared as: 250 mg/1000 ml = 250 mcg/ml
500 mg/1000 ml or 250 mg/500 ml 500 mcg/ml
1000 mg/1000 ml or 250 mg/250 ml = 1000 mcg/ml

	DOBUTAMINE INFUSION RATE (ml/kg/min)		
Dobutamine Infusion Rate (mcg/kg/min)	250 mcg/ml dilution	500 mcg/ml dilution	1000 mcg/ml dilution
2.5 mcg/kg/min	0.01 ml/kg/min	0.005 ml/kg/min	0.0025 ml/kg/min
5 mcg/kg/min	0.02 ml/kg/min	0.01 ml/kg/min	0.005 ml/kg/min
7.5 mcg/kg/min	0.03 ml/kg/min	0.015 ml/kg/min	0.0075 ml/kg/min
10 mcg/kg/min	0.04 ml/kg/min	0.02 ml/kg/min	0.01 ml/kg/min
12.5 mcg/kg/min	0.05 ml/kg/min	0.025 ml/kg/min	0.0125 ml/kg/min
15 mcg/kg/min	0.06 ml/kg/min	0.03 ml/kg/min	0.015 ml/kg/min

≋ CLINICAL PRECAUTIONS

- Hypovolemia should be corrected with volume expanders prior to initiating dobutamine therapy.
- Monitor blood pressure, heart rate, ECG, pulmonary capillary wedge pressure (PCWP), cardiac output, central venous pressure (CVP), and urine output continuously during infusion. An increase in systolic blood pressure of 10–20 mm Hg and an increase in heart rate of 5–15 bpm occur in most patients. Observe patient for extreme increase in blood pressure, heart rate, or ectopy. Dosage reduction may be necessary in these situations. Concurrent use with nitroprusside may have a synergistic effect on increasing cardiac output. Beta-adrenergic blocking agents may negate the effect of dobutamine.
- Use cautiously in patients with myocardial infarction.
- Patients with atrial fibrillation should be pretreated with cardiac glycosides because of the risk of rapid ventricular response. The risk of arrhythmias or hypertension is increased with concurrent use of some general anesthetics (cyclopropane, halothane), MAO inhibitors, oxytocics, or tricyclic antidepressants.
- Safe use in pregnancy, lactation, and children has not been established.

Toxicity and Overdose Alert

• If overdose occurs, reduction or discontinuation of therapy is the only treatment necessary, given the short duration of dobutamine. May cause a decrease in serum potassium.

Lab Test Considerations

• Diabetic patients may require an increase in insulin. Monitor blood glucose levels closely.

Patient/Family Teaching

• Explain to patient the rationale for instituting this medication and the need for frequent monitoring. • Instruct patient to notify nurse immediately of pain or discomfort at the site of administration.

≋ PHARMACOLOGIC PROFILE

Indications

• Dobutamine is used in the short-term management of heart failure due to depressed contractility from organic heart disease or surgical procedures.

Action

• Dobutamine stimulates beta$_1$ (myocardial) adrenergic receptors with relatively minor effect on heart rate or peripheral blood vessels. The result is increased cardiac output without a significantly increased heart rate.

Time/Action Profile (inotropic effects)

Onset	Peak	Duration
1–2 min	10 min	brief (minutes)

Pharmacokinetics

• **Distribution:** UK. • **Metabolism and Excretion:** Dobutamine is metabolized by the liver and other tissues. • **Half-life:** 2 minutes.

Contraindications

• Dobutamine is contraindicated in patients with hypersensitivity to it or bisulfites. • Use of dobutamine should be avoided in patients with idiopathic hypertrophic subaortic stenosis.

Adverse Reactions and Side Effects*

• **CNS:** headache • **Resp:** shortness of breath • **CV:** <u>tachycardia</u>, <u>hypertension</u>, <u>premature ventricular contractions</u>, angina pectoris • **GI:** nausea, vomiting • **Misc:** nonanginal chest pain.

Dopamine	Vasopressor, Inotropic agent
Intropin	pH 2.5 – 4.5

ADMINISTRATION CONSIDERATIONS

Usual Dose

ADULTS: 0.5–5 mcg (0.001–0.005 mg)/kg/min initially; increase at 10–30-min intervals up to 50 mcg/kg/min; titrate by hemodynamic and renal response.

CHILDREN: 0.5–5 mcg/kg/min initially; increase by 1–10 mcg/kg/min at 10–30-min intervals. Titrate to response. Up to 75 mcg/kg/min has been used (unlabeled).

Dilution

• **Continuous Infusion:** Dilute 200–400 mg in 250–500 ml of 0.9% NaCl, D5W, D5/LR, D5/0.45% NaCl, D5/0.9% NaCl, or in lactated Ringer's solution for IV infusion. Concentrations commonly used are 800 mcg/ml or 0.8 mg/ml (200 mg/250 ml) and 1.6 mg/ml (400 mg/250 ml). • Dilute immediately prior to administration. Yellow or brown discoloration indicates decomposition. Discard solution that is cloudy, discolored, or contains a precipitate. Solution is stable for 24 hours.

Compatibility

• **Syringe:** doxapram ✦ heparin ✦ ranitidine.

• **Y-site:** amrinone ✦ atracurium ✦ ciprofloxacin ✦ diltiazem ✦ dobutamine ✦ enalaprilat ✦ esmolol ✦ famotidine ✦ foscarnet ✦ haloperidol ✦ heparin ✦ hydrocortisone sodium succinate ✦ labetalol ✦ lidocaine ✦ meperidine ✦ morphine ✦ nitroglycerin ✦ pancuronium ✦ piperacillin/tazobactam ✦ potassium

---

*<u>Underlines</u> indicate most frequent; CAPITALS indicate life-threatening.

chloride ✦ ranitidine ✦ sargramostim ✦ sodium nitroprusside ✦ streptokinase ✦ tacrolimus ✦ tolazoline ✦ vecuronium ✦ verapamil ✦ vitamin B complex with C ✦ zidovudine.

• Additive: aminophylline ✦ atracurium ✦ bretylium ✦ calcium chloride ✦ chloramphenicol ✦ dobutamine ✦ enalaprilat ✦ heparin ✦ hydrocortisone sodium succinate ✦ kanamycin ✦ lidocaine ✦ methylprednisolone ✦ nitroglycerin ✦ oxacillin ✦ potassium chloride ✦ ranitidine ✦ verapamil.

Incompatibility

• **Y-site:** acyclovir ✦ alteplase ✦ indomethacin.

• **Additive:** acyclovir ✦ amphotericin B ✦ ampicillin ✦ penicillin G potassium. • Dopamine is inactivated (solution turns pink to violet) in alkaline solutions, including sodium bicarbonate.

Rate of Administration

• **Continuous Infusion:** Administer at a rate of 1–5 mcg/min, and increase by 1 mcg/kg/min at 10–30-minute intervals until desired dosage is obtained. Infusion must be administered via infusion pump to ensure precise amount delivered. Rate of administration is titrated according to patient response (blood pressure, heart rate, urine flow, peripheral perfusion, presence of ectopic activity, cardiac output); see Infusion Rate Table below.

DOPAMINE (Intropin) INFUSION RATE TABLE

Dilution may be prepared as: 200 mg/500 ml = 400 mcg/ml
400 mg/500 ml = 800 mcg/ml
800 mg/500 ml = 1600 mcg/ml†

DOPAMINE INFUSION RATE (ml/kg/min)

Dopamine Infusion Rate (mcg/kg/min)	400 mcg/ml dilution	800 mcg/ml dilution	1600 mcg/ml† dilution
0.5 mcg/kg/min	0.0012 ml/kg/min	0.0006 ml/kg/min	0.0003 ml/kg/min
1 mcg/kg/min	0.0025 ml/kg/min	0.0012 ml/kg/min	0.0006 ml/kg/min
2 mcg/kg/min	0.005 ml/kg/min	0.0025 ml/kg/min	0.0012 ml/kg/min
5 mcg/kg/min	0.0125 ml/kg/min	0.0062 ml/kg/min	0.00312 ml/kg/min
10 mcg/kg/min	0.025 ml/kg/min	0.0125 ml/kg/min	0.00625 ml/kg/min
20 mcg/kg/min	0.05 ml/kg/min	0.025 ml/kg/min	0.0125 ml/kg/min
30 mcg/kg/min	0.075 ml/kg/min	0.0375 ml/kg/min	0.02 ml/kg/min
40 mcg/kg/min	0.1 ml/kg/min	0.05 ml/kg/min	0.025 ml/kg/min
50 mcg/kg/min	0.125 ml/kg/min	0.0625 ml/kg/min	0.0312 ml/kg/min

†This concentration is useful in patients with fluid restriction.

≋ CLINICAL PRECAUTIONS

- Hypovolemia should be corrected prior to administration of dopamine.
- Monitor blood pressure, pulse, respiration, ECG, urine output, and hemodynamic parameters every 5–15 minutes during administration. Maintain infusion rate according to preset infusion rate parameters.
- Administer into a large vein, and assess administration site frequently. Extravasation may cause severe irritation, necrosis, and sloughing of tissue. If extravasation occurs, affected area should be infiltrated with 10–15 ml of 0.9% NaCl containing 10–15 mg of phentolamine.
- Palpate peripheral pulses and assess appearance of extremities during infusion. If quality of pulse deteriorates or if extremities become cold or mottled, infusion rate may need to be decreased. Use cautiously in patients with occlusive vascular diseases (initiate therapy with 1 mcg/kg/min). Children are at increased risk of peripheral vascular adverse reactions.
- If hypotension occurs, infusion rate should be increased. If hypotension continues, more potent vasoconstrictors (norepinephrine) may be needed.
- When discontinuing dopamine infusion, reduce dose gradually to prevent severe hypotension.
- Use with MAO inhibitors, doxapram, or ergot alkaloids (ergotamine) results in severe hypertension. Use with IV phenytoin may cause hypotension and bradycardia.
- Concurrent use with general anesthetics or levodopa may increase the risk of arrhythmias. Dosage reduction may be necessary.
- Beta-adrenergic blockers may antagonize cardiac effects of dopamine.
- Safe use in pregnancy, lactation, and children has not been established (Pregnancy Category C).

Toxicity and Overdose Alert

- If excessive hypertension occurs, rate of infusion should be decreased or temporarily discontinued until blood pressure is decreased. Although additional measures are usually not necessary due to short duration of dopamine, phentolamine may be administered if hypertension continues.

Patient/Family Teaching

• Advise patient to inform nurse immediately if chest pain, dyspnea, numbness, tingling, or burning of extremities occurs. • Instruct patient to inform nurse immediately of pain or discomfort at the site of administration.

 PHARMACOLOGIC PROFILE

Indications

• Dopamine is used as an adjunct to standard measures to improve blood pressure, cardiac output, and urine output in the treatment of shock unresponsive to fluid replacement.

Action

• Small doses of dopamine (0.5–2 mcg/kg/min) stimulate dopaminergic receptors, producing renal vasodilation. Larger doses (2–10 mcg/kg/min) stimulate dopaminergic and $beta_1$ adrenergic receptors, producing cardiac stimulation and renal vasodilation. Doses greater than 10 mcg/kg/min stimulate alpha-adrenergic receptors and may cause renal vasoconstriction.

Time/Action Profile (hemodynamic effects)

Onset	Peak	Duration
within 5 min	rapid	<10 min

Pharmacokinetics

• **Distribution:** Dopamine is widely distributed, but does not cross the blood–brain barrier. • **Metabolism and Excretion:** Dopamine is metabolized in the liver, kidneys, and plasma. • **Half-life:** 2 minutes.

Contraindications

• Dopamine is contraindicated in patients with tachyarrhythmias or pheochromocytoma and should also be avoided in patients with bisulfite hypersensitivity.

Adverse Reactions and Side Effects*

• **CNS:** headache • **EENT:** mydriasis (high doses) • **Resp:** dyspnea • **CV:** arrhythmias, hypotension, palpitations, an-

*Underlines indicate most frequent; CAPITALS indicate life-threatening.

gina, ECG changes, vasoconstriction • **GI:** nausea, vomiting
• **GU:** polyuria • **Derm:** piloerection • **Local:** irritation at IV
site.

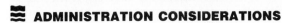

Doxacurium Chloride	*Neuromuscular blocking agent (nondepolarizing)*
Nuromax	**pH 3.9–5**

☰ ADMINISTRATION CONSIDERATIONS

Usual Dose

ADULTS: 50 mcg (0.05 mg)/kg [may need up to 80 mcg (0.08 mg)/kg for prolonged effect] initially, followed 100 minutes later by 5–10 mcg (0.005–0.01 mg)/kg, repeated as required. Decrease dose to 25 mcg (0.025 mg)/kg if succinylcholine is used to facilitate tracheal intubation.

CHILDREN 2–12 yr: 30–50 mcg (0.03–0.05 mg)/kg initially. Maintenance doses may be required more frequently than in adults.

Dilution

• Administer initial IV dose **undiluted** as a bolus. Maintenance dose is usually required 60 minutes following initial dose of 0.025 mg/kg or 100 minutes following initial dose of 0.05 mg/kg. • May be **diluted further** in D5W or 0.9% NaCl. • Use diluted doxacurium within 8 hours. Discard unused diluted doxacurium after 8 hours. • May also be **diluted** with D5/0.9% NaCl or D5/LR.

Compatibility

• **Y-site:** alfentanil ✦ fentanyl ✦ sufentanil.

Incompatibility

• **Syringe/Y-site:** Incompatible with most barbiturates or sodium bicarbonate; do not administer in the same syringe or through the same needle during infusion.

Rate of Administration

• **Direct IV:** Administer bolus doses over 1 minute.

≋ CLINICAL PRECAUTIONS

- Assess respiratory status throughout administration. This agent should only be used by individuals experienced in endotracheal intubation; equipment for this should be readily available.
- Neuromuscular response to doxacurium should be monitored with a peripheral nerve stimulator. Paralysis is initially selective and usually occurs sequentially as follows: levator muscles of the eyelids, muscles of mastication, limb muscles, abdominal muscles, muscles of the glottis, intercostal muscles, and the diaphragm. Recovery of muscle function usually occurs in reverse order. Observe for residual muscle weakness and respiratory distress during recovery period.
- Dose is titrated to patient response.
- Doxacurium has no analgesic or sedative properties. Adequate anesthesia/analgesia should *always* be used when doxacurium is used as an adjunct to surgical procedures.
- Use cautiously in elderly patients due to slower onset of block. Patients with electrolyte or acid–base abnormalities may have unpredictable responses. Correct such abnormalities prior to administration. Burn patients may have resistance to the effects of doxacurium. Patients with neuromuscular diseases may have exaggerated responses.
- Isoflurane, enflurane, halothane, and succinylcholine potentiate effects of doxacurium. Decrease dosage of doxacurium during concurrent use. Carbamazepine and phenytoin decrease duration of block and increase time of onset. Intensity and duration of paralysis may be prolonged by aminoglycoside antibiotics, polymyxin B, colistin, clindamycin, lidocaine, quinidine, procainamide, beta-adrenergic blocking agents, potassium-losing diuretics, and magnesium.
- Safe use in pregnancy, lactation, or children less than 2 years of age has not been established (Pregnancy Category C).

Toxicity and Overdose Alert

- If overdose occurs, use peripheral nerve stimulator to determine the degree of neuromuscular blockade. Maintain airway patency and ventilation until recovery of normal respirations. • Administration of anticholinesterase agents (neostigmine, pyridostigmine) may be used to antagonize the action of doxacurium once the patient has demonstrated some spontaneous recovery from neuromuscular block. Atropine is usually administered prior to or concurrently with anticholinesterase agents to counteract the muscarinic effects. • Administration of fluids and vasopressors may be necessary to treat severe hypotension or shock.

Patient/Family Teaching

• Explain all procedures to patient receiving doxacurium therapy without anesthesia, as consciousness is not affected by doxacurium alone. • Reassure patient that communication abilities will return as the medication wears off.

☰ PHARMACOLOGIC PROFILE

Indications

• Doxacurium is used to produce skeletal muscle paralysis and facilitation of intubation after induction of anesthesia in surgical procedures.

Action

• Doxacurium prevents neuromuscular transmission by blocking the effect of acetylcholine at the myoneural junction, resulting in skeletal muscle paralysis. It has no analgesic or anxiolytic properties.

Time/Action Profile (for a 0.05 mg/kg dose in an adult)

Onset†	Peak‡	Duration‡†
5 min	4–5 min	100 min

†Time to intubating conditions.
‡Maximum suppression of twitch response.
‡†Time to recovery of twitch response to 25% of control.

Pharmacokinetics

• **Distribution:** UK. • **Metabolism and Excretion:** Doxacurium is excreted primarily unchanged in urine and bile. • **Half-life:** 90–120 minutes (increased in kidney transplant patients).

Contraindications

• Doxacurium is contraindicated in patients with hypersensitivity to doxacurium. Preparations containing benzyl alcohol should be avoided in newborn infants; as fatal reactions may occur in this group of patients.

Adverse Reactions and Side Effects*

Note: Almost all adverse reactions to doxacurium are extensions of pharmacologic effects.

• **Resp:** APNEA, respiratory insufficiency • **CV:** hypotension • **Derm:** flushing • **MS:** muscle weakness.

Doxapram Hydrochloride	Respiratory and cerebral stimulant
Dopram	pH 3.5–5

 ADMINISTRATION CONSIDERATIONS

Usual Dose

Respiratory Depression Following Anesthesia

ADULTS: 0.5–1 mg/kg (not to exceed 1.5 mg/kg) initially; may repeat q 5 min to a total of 2 mg/kg or as an infusion at 5 mg/min until response is obtained, then decrease infusion rate to 1–3 mg/min (total dose by infusion method should not exceed 4 mg/kg).

Drug-Induced CNS Depression

ADULTS: Two doses of 2 mg/kg may be repeated at 5-min intervals. Can repeat regimen in 1–2 hr until spontaneous breathing returns or a total of 3 g is given. If response occurs in 1–2 hr, can infuse at rate of 1–3 mg/min for up to 2 hr. The infusion may be repeated after a rest period. Total dose not to exceed 3 g/24 hr.

---

*Underlines indicate most frequent; CAPITALS indicate life-threatening.

Acute Respiratory Insufficiency in COPD

ADULTS: 1–2 mg/min (up to 3 mg/min).

Dilution

• **Direct IV:** Administer **undiluted.** • **Continuous Infusion: Dilute** 250 mg in 250 ml of D5W, D10W, or 0.9% NaCl to yield a concentration of 1 mg/ml. **Dilute** 400 mg (20-mg vial) in 180 ml of IV fluid to yield a 2-mg/ml concentration. Dosages vary with patient's condition.

Compatibility

• **Syringe:** bumetanide ⬩ chlorpromazine ⬩ cimetidine ⬩ hydroxyzine ⬩ imipramine ⬩ isoniazid ⬩ netilmicin ⬩ phytonadione ⬩ pyridoxine ⬩ terbutaline ⬩ thiamine.

Incompatibility

• **Syringe:** aminophylline ⬩ ascorbic acid ⬩ dexamethasone ⬩ folic acid ⬩ furosemide ⬩ hydrocortisone ⬩ methylprednisolone.
• **Additive:** aminophylline ⬩ sodium bicarbonate.

Rate of Administration

• **Direct IV:** Administer over 5 minutes. • **Continuous Infusion:** Administer at an initial rate of 5 mg/min. Once the desired response is obtained, reduce the rate to 1–3 mg/min in patients with respiratory depression. For patients with acute respiratory insufficiency, administer at an initial rate of 1–2 mg/min, increasing to a maximum of 3 mg/min if necessary. Infusion is limited to 2 hours. Administer via infusion pump to ensure accurate dosage.

≋ CLINICAL PRECAUTIONS

• Because of the narrow margin of safety and indications for use, patient must be monitored constantly while receiving doxapram and for 1 hour after medication is discontinued and patient is fully alert. Doxapram should not be used routinely as a respiratory stimulant. Monitor respiratory status (rate, rhythm, depth of respirations) and ABGs. Ensure airway patency and adequate oxygenation. Relapse of respiratory depression may occur if CNS depressant has long duration of action. Position patient on side with head of bed elevated to ensure maximal chest expansion and prevent aspiration. If there is no response to doxapram, other causes for CNS depression should be investigated.

- Monitor level of consciousness and assess deep tendon reflexes for hyperactivity or spasticity.
- Monitor vital signs, ECG, and hemodynamic parameters. Doxapram may cause tachycardia, hypertension, increased cardiac output, and increased pulmonary artery pressure. Assess for changes in parameters, arrhythmias, or chest pain. Use cautiously in patients with COPD or asthma; these patients are at increased risk of arrhythmias secondary to hypoxia. Hypertensive effects may be increased by concurrent use of sympathomimetic amines or MAO inhibitors.
- Monitor IV site frequently for redness or irritation.
- Use cautiously in patients with pre-existing cardiac arrhythmias, increased intracranial pressure, hyperthyroidism, pheochromocytoma, hepatic or renal impairment, or serious uncorrected metabolic disorders.
- Geriatric patients are at increased risk of adverse reactions caused by age-related renal, hepatic, and cardiac disease.
- Doxapram may mask residual effects of skeletal muscle relaxants.
- Safe use in pregnancy, lactation, or children younger than 12 years has not been established (Pregnancy Category B).

Toxicity and Overdose Alert

- Toxicity is manifested by severe hypertension, tachycardia, and hyperactive reflexes or seizures. Infusion should be stopped immediately. Seizures may be controlled with diazepam or a short-acting barbiturate. Resuscitative equipment should be available at all times.

Lab Test Considerations

- Monitor ABGs prior to and every 30 minutes during therapy. Notify physician immediately if ABGs deteriorate. Physician may order cessation of drug, intubation, and mechanical ventilation. • Monitor hemoglobin, hematocrit, erythrocyte, and leukocyte count. Rapid infusion may cause hemolysis. • May cause elevated BUN and proteinuria.

Patient/Family Teaching

• Instruct patient to notify nurse immediately if shortness of breath worsens.

≋ PHARMACOLOGIC PROFILE

Indications

• Doxapram is used in carefully selected short-term situations with other supportive measures to treat postoperative CNS and respiratory depression due to CNS depressants. • It is also used with other supportive maneuvers on a short-term basis in the postoperative period to stimulate deep breathing and to prevent acute hypercapnia during administration of oxygen to patients with acute respiratory insufficiency due to COPD (short-term only—less than 2 hours).

Action

• In low doses, doxapram stimulates breathing by activating carotid receptors. Larger doses directly stimulate the respiratory center in the medulla as well as produce generalized CNS stimulation. The net result is a transient increase in tidal volume and a small increase in respiratory rate. Oxygenation is not increased.

Time/Action Profile (increases in minute volume)

Onset	Peak	Duration
20–40 sec	1–2 min	5–12 min

Pharmacokinetics

• **Distribution:** UK. • **Metabolism and Excretion:** Doxapram is rapidly metabolized, with metabolites mostly excreted by the kidneys. • **Half-life:** 2.4–4.0 hours.

Contraindications

• Doxapram is contraindicated in patients with hypersensitivity to it. It should not be used in patients on ventilators or patients who have had head trauma or seizures. • Use of doxapram should be avoided in patients with flail chest, pulmonary embolism, pneumothorax, pulmonary fibrosis, acute asthma, or extreme dyspnea. • It should also be avoided in patients with cardiovascular or cerebrovascular disease and in newborns. • Some products contain benzyl alcohol and should be avoided in patients with known intolerance to alcohol.

Adverse Reactions and Side Effects*

• **CNS:** SEIZURES†, headache, dizziness, apprehension, disorientation • **EENT:** miosis, sneezing, gagging • **Resp:** dyspnea†, bronchospasm, laryngospasm, coughing, rebound hypoventilation • **CV:** elevated blood pressure†, tachycardia†, arrhythmias†, hypotension, chest pain, changes in heart rate, T-wave inversion • **GI:** nausea, vomiting, diarrhea, urge to defecate • **GU:** perineal or genital burning sensation, urinary retention, spontaneous voiding • **Derm:** flushing, sweating, pruritus • **Hemat:** hemolysis • **Local:** irritation at IV site • **Metab:** hyperpyrexia • **MS:** skeletal muscle hyperactivity†, muscle spasticity†, involuntary movement† • **Neuro:** paresthesia, positive bilateral Babinski's sign, generalized clonus.

Doxorubicin	Antineoplastic (antibiotic)
Adriamycin, Adriamycin PFS, Rubex, RDF	pH 3–6.5

≋ ADMINISTRATION CONSIDERATIONS

Usual Dose

ADULTS: 60–75 mg/m^2, repeat q 21 days or 25–30 mg/m^2 daily for 2–3 days, repeat q 3–4 wk, or 20 mg/m^2 once weekly.

CHILDREN: 30 mg/m^2 daily for 3 days, repeat q 4 wk.

Dilution

• **Direct IV: Dilute** each 10 mg with 5 ml of 0.9% NaCl (nonbacteriostatic) for injection. Shake to dissolve completely. Do not add to IV solution. • Solution should be prepared in a biologic cabinet. Wear gloves, gown, and mask

---

*Underlines indicate most frequent; CAPITALS indicate life-threatening.

†Indicates early signs of toxicity.

while handling medication. Discard IV equipment in specially designated containers (see Appendix F). • Reconstituted medication is stable for 24 hours at room temperature and 48 hours if refrigerated. Protect from sunlight. • Aluminum needles may be used to administer doxorubicin but should not be used during storage, as prolonged contact results in discoloration of solution and formation of a dark precipitate. • The suffix PFS indicates preservative-free solution; RDF indicates rapidly dissolving formulation.

Compatibility

• **Syringe:** bleomycin • cisplatin • cyclophosphamide • droperidol • leucovorin calcium • methotrexate • metoclopramide • mitomycin • vincristine.

• **Y-site:** bleomycin • chlorpromazine • cimetidine • cisplatin • cyclophosphamide • dexamethasone • diphenhydramine • droperidol • famotidine • filgrastim • fludarabine • fluorouracil • hydromorphone • leucovorin calcium • lorazepam • melphalan • methotrexate • methylprednisolone • metoclopramide • mitomycin • morphine • ondansetron • paclitaxel • prochlorperazine • promethazine • ranitidine • sargramostim • vinblastine • vincristine • vinorelbine.

• **Additive:** Manufacturer does not recommend admixture.

Incompatibility

• **Syringe:** furosemide • heparin.

• **Y-site:** allopurinol sodium • gallium nitrate • ganciclovir • piperacillin/tazobactam.

• **Additive:** aminophylline • cephalothin • dexamethasone • diazepam • fluorouracil • hydrocortisone.

Rate of Administration

• **Direct IV:** Administer each dose over 3–5 minutes through Y-site or 3-way stopcock of a free-flowing infusion of 0.9% NaCl or D5W. Facial flushing and erythema along vein involved frequently occur when administration is too rapid.

≋ CLINICAL PRECAUTIONS

• Doxorubicin is a vesicant. Observe IV site frequently for redness or irritation. Medication may infiltrate painlessly even if blood returns on aspiration of infusion needle.

Severe tissue damage may occur if doxorubicin extravasates. If extravasation occurs, stop infusion immediately, restart, and complete dose in another vein. Local infiltration of antidote is not recommended. Apply ice packs and elevate extremity to reduce swelling. Do not apply heat.

- Monitor intake and output ratios, appetite, and nutritional status. Encourage fluid intake of 2000 ml/day. Allopurinol and alkalinization of the urine may be ordered to decrease serum uric acid levels and prevent urate stone formation. Doxorubicin will color urine red. Severe and protracted nausea and vomiting may occur as early as 1 hour after therapy and may last 24 hours. Parenteral antiemetic agents should be administered 30–45 minutes prior to therapy and routinely around the clock for the next 24 hours as indicated. Monitor amount of emesis; if emesis exceeds guidelines, initiate precautions to prevent dehydration.

- Do not confuse doxorubicin with daunorubicin. Indications, dosage, and toxicities are not the same. See *daunorubicin hydrochloride* monograph on page 278.

- Monitor for signs of cardiac toxicity, which can be either acute and transient (ECG abnormalities, sinus tachycardia, extrasystoles) or late in onset (usually occurs 1–6 months after the initiation of therapy) and characterized by the development of intractable congestive heart failure. Total cumulative dose should not exceed 550 mg/m^2 (400 mg/m^2 in patients who have had radiation to the chest or concurrent cardiotoxic medications) without monitoring of cardiac function. ECG should be performed periodically throughout therapy. Cardiac toxicity may be increased by concurrent radiation therapy or cyclophosphamide. Use cautiously in patients with previous history of congestive heart failure or arrhythmias. Cardiac toxicity may be more likely to develop in children younger than 2 and in elderly patients.

- Assess for bone marrow depression. Monitor pulse, blood pressure, and respiratory rate frequently during administration. Assess for signs of infection (fever, tachycardia, cough, dysuria), especially during peak effect on WBCs. Assess for bleeding (bleeding gums, bruising, petechiae; guaiac test stools, urine, and emesis). Avoid IM injections and taking rectal temperatures. Apply pressure to venipuncture sites for 10 minutes. Anemia may occur. Monitor for fatigue, dyspnea, and orthostatic hypotension. Additive bone marrow depression may occur with concurrent administration of other antineoplastics or radiation therapy. Use cautiously in patients with underlying infections, depressed bone marrow reserve, or other chronic debilitating illnesses.

- Patients with liver impairment (serum bilirubin >1.2 mg/dl) require reduced dosage of doxorubicin.
- Observe sites of previous radiation therapy. Doxorubicin may produce skin reactions at sites of previous radiation therapy.
- Doxorubicin may increase risk of hemorrhagic cystitis from cyclophosphamide or hepatitis from mercaptopurine and decrease antibody response to live virus vaccines.
- Use cautiously in patients with childbearing potential. Doxorubicin should be avoided during pregnancy or lactation.

Lab Test Considerations

• Monitor CBC and differential prior to and periodically throughout therapy. The leukocyte count nadir occurs 10–14 days after administration, and recovery usually occurs by the 21st day. Thrombocytopenia and anemia may also occur. • Monitor renal (BUN and creatinine) and hepatic (AST [SGOT], ALT [SGPT], LDH, and serum bilirubin) function prior to and periodically throughout course of therapy. May cause increased uric acid concentrations in serum and urine.

Patient/Family Teaching

• Instruct patient to notify physician promptly if fever; sore throat; signs of infection; bleeding gums; bruising; petechiae; blood in stools, urine, or emesis; increased fatigue; dyspnea; or orthostatic hypotension occurs. Caution patient to avoid crowds and persons with known infections. Instruct patient to use soft toothbrush and electric razor and to avoid falls. Patients should be cautioned not to drink alcoholic beverages or take medication containing aspirin, ibuprofen, or naproxen, as these may precipitate gastric bleeding. • Instruct patient to report pain at injection site immediately. • Instruct patient to inspect oral mucosa for erythema and ulceration. If ulceration occurs, advise patient to use sponge brush, rinse mouth with water after eating and drinking, and confer with physician if mouth pain interferes with eating. The risk of developing stomatitis is greatest 5–10 days after a dose; the usual duration is 3–7 days. • Advise patient that this medication may have teratogenic effects. A nonhormonal method of contraception should be used during therapy and for at least 4 months after therapy is concluded. Inform patient before initiating therapy that this medication may cause irreversible gonadal suppression. • Instruct patient to notify physician immediately if irregular heartbeat, shortness of breath, or swelling of lower extremities occurs. • Discuss the possibility of hair loss with patient. Explore methods of coping. Regrowth usually occurs 2–3 months after discontinuation of therapy. • Instruct patient not to receive any vaccinations without advice of physician. • Inform patient that medication may cause urine to appear red for 1–2 days. • Instruct patient to notify physician if skin irritation occurs at site of previous radiation therapy. • Emphasize the need for periodic lab tests to monitor for side effects.

PHARMACOLOGIC PROFILE

Indications

• Doxorubicin is used alone and in combination with other treatment modalities (surgery, radiation therapy) in the treatment of various solid tumors including breast, ovarian, bladder, and bronchogenic carcinoma. • It is also useful in malignant lymphomas and leukemias.

Action

• Doxorubicin inhibits DNA and RNA synthesis by forming a complex with DNA (cell cycle S–phase specific), which results in death of rapidly replicating cells, particularly malignant ones. It also has immunosuppressive properties.

Time/Action Profile (effect on blood counts)

Onset	Peak	Duration
10 days	14 days	21–24 days

Pharmacokinetics

• **Distribution:** Doxorubicin is widely distributed, but does not cross the blood–brain barrier. • **Metabolism and Excretion:** Doxorubicin is mostly metabolized by the liver, where some of it is converted to a compound that also has antineoplastic activity. It is then excreted predominantly in the bile, 50% as unchanged drug. Less than 5% is eliminated unchanged in the urine. • **Half-life:** 16.7 hours.

Contraindications

• Doxorubicin is contraindicated in patients with hypersensitivity to it. • Doxorubicin should not be given to pregnant or lactating patients.

Adverse Reactions and Side Effects*

• **CV:** CARDIOMYOPATHY, ECG changes • **Derm:** alopecia • **Endo:** gonadal suppression • **GI:** stomatitis, esophagitis, nausea, vomiting, diarrhea • **GU:** red urine • **Hemat:** anemia, leukopenia, thrombocytopenia • **Local:** phlebitis at IV site, tissue necrosis • **Metab:** hyperuricemia • **Misc:** hypersensitivity reactions.

Doxycycline Hyclate	Anti-infective (tetracycline)
Doxy, Doxychel, Vibramycin	pH 1.8–3.3

≋ ADMINISTRATION CONSIDERATIONS

Usual Dose

ADULTS: 200 mg once daily or 100 mg q 12 hr for the first 24 hours, then 100–200 mg q 24 hr or 50–100 mg q 12 hr (150 mg q 12 hr for 10 days for syphilis).

CHILDREN <45 kg AND >8 yr: 4.4–5 mg/kg once daily or 2.2 mg/kg q 12 hr for first 24 hr, then 2.2–4.4 mg/kg q 24 hr or 1.1–2.2 mg/kg q 12 hr.

---

*Underlines indicate most frequent; CAPITALS indicate life-threatening.

Dilution

• **Intermittent Infusion:** Dilute each 100 mg with 10 ml of sterile water or 0.9% NaCl for injection. **Dilute further** in 100–1000 ml of 0.9% NaCl, D5W, D5/LR, Ringer's, or lactated Ringer's solution. • Solution is stable for 12 hours at room temperature and 72 hours if refrigerated. If diluted with D5/LR or lactated Ringer's solution, administer within 6 hours. Protect solution from direct sunlight. Concentrations of less than 1 mcg/ml or greater than 1 mg/ml are not recommended.

Compatibility

• **Y-site:** acyclovir ◆ cyclophosphamide ◆ diltiazem ◆ filgrastim ◆ fludarabine ◆ hydromorphone ◆ magnesium sulfate ◆ melphalan ◆ meperidine ◆ morphine ◆ ondansetron ◆ perphenazine ◆ sargramostim ◆ tacrolimus ◆ vinorelbine.
• **Additive:** ranitidine.

Incompatibility

• **Y-site:** allopurinol sodium ◆ piperacillin/tazobactam.
• **Additive:** barbiturates ◆ erythromycin lactobionate ◆ penicillin G potassium ◆ oxacillin ◆ methicillin ◆ nafcillin.

Rate of Administration

• **Intermittent Infusion:** Administer over a minimum of 1–4 hours. Avoid rapid administration. Avoid extravasation.

≋ CLINICAL PRECAUTIONS

- Obtain specimens for culture and sensitivity prior to initiating therapy. First dose may be given before results are known.
- Assess patient for infection (vital signs; appearance of wound, sputum, urine, stool; WBC) at beginning of and throughout therapy.
- Observe IV site frequently. Doxycycline may cause thrombophlebitis.
- Use cautiously in cachectic or debilitated patients, or patients with hepatic or renal impairment.
- Doxycycline may enhance the effect of oral anticoagulants.
- Barbiturates, phenytoin, or carbamazepine may decrease the activity of doxycycline.

- Doxycycline may decrease the effectiveness of oral contraceptives.
- Pregnant or lactating patients or children under 8 years should not receive doxycycline (Pregnancy Category D).

Lab Test Considerations

- Renal, hepatic, and hematopoietic functions should be monitored periodically during long-term therapy. • May cause increased AST (SGOT), ALT (SGPT), serum alkaline phosphatase, bilirubin, and amylase concentrations. • May interfere with urine glucose testing with copper sulfate method (Clinitest); use glucose enzymatic tests (Tes-Tape, Ketodiastix).

Patient/Family Teaching

- Advise patient to report the signs of superinfection (black, furry overgrowth on the tongue; vaginal itching or discharge; loose or foul-smelling stools). Skin rash, pruritus, and urticaria should also be reported. • Instruct patient to notify physician if symptoms do not improve. • Caution patient to use sunscreen and protective clothing to prevent photosensitivity reactions.

☰ PHARMACOLOGIC PROFILE

Indications

- Doxycycline is used most commonly in the treatment of infections due to unusual organisms including *Mycoplasma*, *Chlamydia*, and *Rickettsia*. • It is also used in the treatment of some sexually transmitted diseases and in the treatment of Lyme disease.

Action

- Doxycycline inhibits bacterial protein synthesis at the level of the 30S ribosome. This results in a bacteriostatic action against susceptible bacteria. It is active against some Gram-positive pathogens (*Bacillus anthracis*, *Clostridium perfringens*, *C. tetani*, *Listeria monocytogenes*, *Nocardia*, *Propionibacterium acnes*, *Actinomyces israelii*) and some Gram-negative pathogens (*Haemophilus influenzae*, *Legionella pneumophila*, *Yersinia enterocolitica*, *Y. pestis*, *Neisseria gonorrhoeae*, *N. meningitidis*). It also possesses activity against several unusual pathogens including *Mycoplasma, Chlamydia, Rickettsia,* and *Borrelia burgdorferi.*

Time/Action Profile

Onset	Peak
rapid	end of infusion

Pharmacokinetics

• **Distribution:** Doxycycline is widely distributed with some penetration into CSF. It also crosses the placenta and enters breast milk. • **Metabolism and Excretion:** 20–40% of doxycycline is excreted unchanged by the kidneys. Some inactivation occurs in the intestine, and some enterohepatic circulation occurs, with excretion in bile and feces. • **Half-life:** 14–17 hours (increased in severe renal impairment).

Contraindications

• Doxycycline should not be used in patients who have hypersensitivity to it. Cross-sensitivity with other tetracyclines may occur. • Because it causes permanent staining of teeth, children younger than 8 years old should not receive doxycycline. • Doxycycline is contraindicated in pregnancy and lactation (Pregnancy Category D).

Adverse Reactions and Side Effects*

• **GI:** <u>nausea</u>, <u>vomiting</u>, <u>diarrhea</u>, pancreatitis, esophagitis, hepatotoxicity • **Hemat:** blood dyscrasias • **Derm:** rashes, photosensitivity • **Local:** phlebitis at IV site • **Misc:** superinfection, hypersensitivity reactions.

Droperidol	*Tranquilizer, Antiemetic*
Inapsine	pH 3–3.8

≋ ADMINISTRATION CONSIDERATIONS

Usual Dose

Premedication

ADULTS: 2.5–10 mg 30–60 min prior to induction of anesthesia.

CHILDREN 2–12 yr: 88–165 mcg (0.088–0.165 mg)/kg.

---

*<u>Underlines</u> indicate most frequent; CAPITALS indicate life-threatening.

Adjunct before Induction of General Anesthesia
ADULTS: 220–275 mcg (0.22–0.275 mg)/kg with anesthetic or analgesic. Additional maintenance doses of 1.25–2.5 mg may be needed.

CHILDREN 2–12 yr: 88–165 mcg (0.088–0.165 mg)/kg.

Adjunct for Maintenance of General Anesthesia
ADULTS: 1.25–2.5 mg.

Adjunct in Regional Anesthesia
ADULTS: 2.5–5 mg.

Use without General Anesthesia (diagnostic procedures)
ADULTS: 1.25–2.5 mg given as additional doses following an initial dose of 2.5–10 mg IM given 30–60 min prior to procedure.

Antiemetic
ADULTS: 0.5–1 mg q 4 hr.

Dilution
• **Direct IV:** May be administered **undiluted.** • **Intermittent Infusion:** May be added to 250 ml of D5W, 0.9% NaCl, or lactated Ringer's solution.

Compatibility
• **Syringe:** atropine • bleomycin • butorphanol • chlorpromazine • cimetidine • cisplatin • cyclophosphamide • dimenhydrinate • diphenhydramine • doxorubicin • fentanyl • glycopyrrolate • hydroxyzine • meperidine • metoclopramide • midazolam • mitomycin • morphine • nalbuphine • pentazocine • perphenazine • prochlorperazine • promazine • promethazine • scopolamine • vinblastine • vincristine.

• **Y-site:** bleomycin • buprenorphine • cisplatin • cyclophosphamide • cytarabine • doxorubicin • filgrastim • fluconazole • fludarabine • hydrocortisone sodium succinate • idarubicin • melphalan • meperidine • metoclopramide • mitomycin • ondansetron • paclitaxel • potassium chloride • sargramostim • vinblastine • vincristine • vinorelbine • vitamin B complex with C.

Incompatibility
• **Syringe:** allopurinol sodium • fluorouracil • furosemide • heparin • leucovorin calcium • methotrexate • pentobarbital.

- **Y-site:** fluorouracil ◆ foscarnet ◆ furosemide ◆ leuco-vorin calcium ◆ methotrexate ◆ nafcillin ◆ piperacillin/tazo-bactam.
  - **Additive:** barbiturates.

Rate of Administration

- **Direct IV:** Administer each dose slowly over at least 1 minute. • **Intermittent Infusion:** Administer by slow infusion. Titrate according to patient response.

≋ CLINICAL PRECAUTIONS

- Monitor blood pressure and heart rate frequently throughout therapy. Risk of hypotension is increased with concurrent use of antihypertensives or nitrates. If hypovolemia occurs, parenteral fluids may be required. Serious hypotension may necessitate use of vasopressors (norepinephrine, phenylephrine). Avoid using epineph-rine, as droperidol reverses its vasopressor effects and may produce paradoxical hypotension.
- Assess patient for level of sedation. Additive CNS de-pression may occur with other CNS depressants includ-ing alcohol, antihistamines, antidepressants, opioid anal-gesics, and other sedatives.
- When used as an antiemetic, assess nausea, vomiting, hydration status, bowel sounds, and abdominal pain prior to and following administration.
- Observe patients for extrapyramidal reactions (dystonia, oculogyric crisis, extended neck, flexed arms, tremor, restlessness, hyperactivity, anxiety) throughout therapy. An anticholinergic or antiparkinsonian agent may be used to treat these symptoms.
- Use cautiously in elderly or debilitated patients, severely ill patients, and diabetics. In elderly or debilitated pa-tients, initial dosage should be reduced. Use with cau-tion in patients with respiratory insufficiency, prostatic hypertrophy, CNS tumors, intestinal obstruction, car-diac disease, seizures (may lower seizure threshold), or severe liver disease.
- Although safety is not established, droperidol has been used during cesarean section without respiratory depres-sion in the newborn (Pregnancy Category C). Safe use in

lactation and in children <2 years has also not been established.

Patient/Family Teaching

• Caution patient to make position changes slowly to minimize orthostatic hypotension. • Medication causes drowsiness. Advise patient to call for assistance during ambulation and transfer.

PHARMACOLOGIC PROFILE

Indications

• Droperidol is used to produce tranquilization and as an adjunct to general and regional anesthesia. • It is also useful in decreasing postoperative or postprocedure nausea and vomiting. • Droperidol may be used in combination with fentanyl (see *droperidol/fentanyl* monograph on page 364).

Action

• Droperidol alters the action of dopamine in the CNS, producing tranquilization and suppression of nausea and vomiting in selected situations.

Time/Action Profile (sedation)

Onset	Peak	Duration†
3–10 min	30 min	2–4 hr

†Listed as duration of tranquilization; alterations in consciousness may last up to 12 hr.

Pharmacokinetics

• **Distribution:** Droperidol appears to cross the blood–brain barrier and placenta. • **Metabolism and Excretion:** Droperidol is mainly metabolized by the liver. Only 10% is excreted unchanged by the kidneys. • **Half-life:** UK.

Contraindications

• Droperidol is contraindicated in patients with hypersensitivity to it or parabens (in Inapsine). • It should be avoided in patients with known intolerance, narrow-angle glaucoma, bone marrow depression, CNS depression, or severe liver or cardiac disease.

Adverse Reactions and Side Effects*

• **CNS:** excessive sedation, <u>extrapyramidal reactions</u>, tardive dyskinesia, restlessness, confusion, hyperactivity, dizziness, nightmares, mental depression, hallucinations, SEIZURES, anxiety, abnormal EEG • **EENT:** dry eyes, blurred vision • **Resp:** bronchospasm, laryngospasm • **CV:** <u>hypotension</u>, <u>tachycardia</u> • **GI:** dry mouth, constipation • **Misc:** chills, shivering, facial sweating.

Droperidol/Fentanyl	Tranquilizer, Opioid analgesic
Innovar	pH 3.5

Schedule II

≋ ADMINISTRATION CONSIDERATIONS

Usual Dose (each ml contains 2.5 mg droperidol and 50 mcg [0.05 mg] fentanyl)

Since droperidol is much longer acting than fentanyl, additional doses of fentanyl alone may be given to prevent accumulation of droperidol.

Adjunct to General Anesthesia

ADULTS: 1 ml/20–25 lb body weight, administered in small increments or as an infusion until somnolence occurs. Additional fentanyl alone is used to maintain analgesia while preventing accumulation of droperidol. In prolonged procedures, additional doses of 0.5–1 ml of droperidol/fentanyl IV may be required if lightening of tranquilization and analgesia occurs.

CHILDREN >2 yr: 0.5 ml/20 lb body weight, administered in small increments or as an infusion until somnolence occurs. Additional fentanyl may be used to maintain analgesia.

---

*<u>Underlines</u> indicate most frequent; CAPITALS indicate lifethreatening.

Adjunct to Regional Anesthesia
ADULTS: 1–2 ml.

Dilution
• **Direct IV:** May be administered **undiluted.** • **Intermittent Infusion:** Droperidol/fentanyl 10 ml may be **added** to 250 ml of D5W.

Compatibility
• **Syringe:** benzquinamide ♦ glycopyrrolate.
• **Y-site:** hydrocortisone sodium succinate ♦ potassium chloride ♦ vitamin B complex with C.
• **Additive:** sodium bicarbonate.

Incompatibility
• **Syringe:** heparin.
• **Y-site:** nafcillin.

Rate of Administration
• **Direct IV:** Direct IV injection should be administered slowly over at least 1 minute. • **Intermittent Infusion:** May be infused until the onset of somnolence as an adjunct to general anesthesia.

≋ CLINICAL PRECAUTIONS

- Monitor blood pressure and heart rate frequently throughout therapy. May cause pronounced respiratory depression. Risk of hypotension is increased with concurrent use of antihypertensives or nitrates. If hypovolemia occurs, parenteral fluids may be required. Serious hypotension may necessitate use of vasopressors (norepinephrine, phenylephrine). Avoid using epinephrine, as droperidol reverses its vasopressor effects and may produce paradoxical hypotension.
- Assess patient for level of sedation. Additive CNS depression may occur with other CNS depressants including alcohol, antihistamines, antidepressants, opioid analgesics, and other sedatives. Decrease dose of opioid analgesics to ¼ to ⅓ of the normal dose if given within 8 hours of droperidol/fentanyl.
- Observe patients for extrapyramidal reactions (dystonia, oculogyric crisis, extended neck, flexed arms, tremor, restlessness, hyperactivity, anxiety) throughout therapy.

Notify physician should any of these occur. An anticholinergic or antiparkinsonian agent may be used to treat these symptoms.

• Use cautiously in elderly or debilitated patients, severely ill patients, and diabetics. Use with caution in patients with respiratory insufficiency, prostatic hypertrophy, CNS tumors, intestinal obstruction, cardiac disease, seizures (may lower seizure threshold), or severe liver disease.

• Although safety is not established, droperidol has been used during cesarean section without respiratory depression in the newborn (Pregnancy Category C). Safe use in lactation and children <2 years of age has also not been established.

Toxicity and Overdose Alert

• Atropine may be used to treat bradycardia. Use of a neuromuscular blocking agent with vagolytic activity, such as pancuronium or gallamine, may prevent bradycardia caused by fentanyl. • If respiratory depression persists following surgery, prolonged mechanical ventilation may be necessary. If an opioid antagonist is required to reverse respiratory depression or coma, naloxone (Narcan) is the antidote. Dilute the 0.4-mg ampule of naloxone in 10 ml of 0.9% NaCl and administer 0.5 ml (0.02 mg) by direct IV push every 2 minutes. For children and patients weighing less than 40 kg, dilute 0.1 mg of naloxone in 10 ml of 0.9% NaCl for a concentration of 10 mcg/ml and administer 0.5 mcg every 2 minutes. Titrate the dose to avoid withdrawal, seizures, and severe pain. Administration of naloxone in these circumstances, especially in cardiac patients, has resulted in hypertension and tachycardia, occasionally causing left ventricular failure and pulmonary edema. Monitor respiratory status continuously; the duration of respiratory depression may exceed the duration of a dose of naloxone. Continuous infusion of naloxone may be required (see *naloxone hydrochloride* monograph on page 690). • If hypotension occurs, administer parenteral fluids, position patient to improve venous return to the heart when surgical conditions permit, and administer a vasopressor as necessary. • If muscle rigidity occurs during surgery, a neuromuscular blocking agent and mechanical ventilation should be used. Muscle rigidity occurring on emergence may be treated with naloxone.

Lab Test Considerations

• May cause elevated serum amylase and lipase concentrations.

Patient/Family Teaching

• Caution patient to make position changes slowly to minimize orthostatic hypotension. • Medication causes drowsiness. Advise patient to call for assistance during ambulation and transfer and to avoid driving or other activities requiring alertness for 24 hours after last dose.

 PHARMACOLOGIC PROFILE

Indications

• Droperidol/fentanyl is used to produce tranquilization and analgesia during diagnostic or surgical procedures and as an adjunct in various types of anesthesia.

Action

• *Droperidol* alters the action of dopamine in the CNS. • *Fentanyl* is an opioid analgesic that binds to opiate receptors in the CNS, altering the response to and perception of pain. The effect of the combination is neuroleptanesthesia (quiescence, decreased motor activity, and analgesia without loss of consciousness).

Time/Action Profile (noted as tranquilizing effects of droperidol, analgesic effects of fentanyl)

	Onset	Peak	Duration†
droperidol	3–10 min	30 min	up to 12 hr
fentanyl	1–2 min	3–5 min	0.5–1 hr

†Listed as duration of tranquilization; alterations in consciousness may last up to 12 hr; effects on respiratory depression outlast analgesic effects.

Pharmacokinetics

• **Distribution:** Droperidol appears to cross the blood–brain barrier and placenta. • **Metabolism and Excretion:** Both droperidol and fentanyl are mainly metabolized by the liver with small amounts (10–20%) excreted unchanged by the kidneys. • **Half-life:** UK.

Contraindications

• Droperidol/fentanyl is contraindicated in patients with hypersensitivity to either agent. • Droperidol/fentanyl should be avoided in patients with known intolerance, narrow-angle glaucoma, bone marrow depression, CNS depression, severe liver or cardiac disease, and in patients who have received MAO inhibitors within 14 days.

Adverse Reactions and Side Effects*

• **CNS:** <u>excessive sedation</u>, <u>extrapyramidal reactions</u>, tardive dyskinesia, restlessness, confusion, hyperactivity, dizziness, nightmares, mental depression, hallucinations, euphoria, floating feeling, dysphoria • **EENT:** dry eyes, blurred vision, miosis, diplopia • **Resp:** bronchospasm, laryngospasm, apnea, respiratory depression • **CV:** <u>hypotension</u>, <u>tachycardia</u>, bradycardia • **GI:** dry mouth, constipation, nausea, vomiting • **GU:** urinary retention • **Derm:** sweating, flushing • **MS:** skeletal and thoracic muscle rigidity • **Misc:** chills, shivering, facial sweating.

Edetate Calcium Disodium	*Antidote* *(lead chelator)*
Calcium Disodium Versenate	pH 6.5–8

ADMINISTRATION CONSIDERATIONS

Consult local protocols for more specific instructions. A variety of regimens has been used.

Usual Dose

Diagnosis of Lead Poisoning
(Ca EDTA mobilization test)
ADULTS AND CHILDREN: 500 mg/m^2 (not to exceed 1 g).

---

*<u>Underlines</u> indicate most frequent; CAPITALS indicate life-threatening.

Lead Poisoning without Encephalopathy

ADULTS: 1 g/m^2/day in divided doses or as a single daily infusion for 3–5 days (not to exceed two courses; wait at least 2–4 days and preferably 2–3 wk between courses).

CHILDREN: 1 g/m^2/day given in divided doses or as a single daily infusion for 3–5 days (wait at least 2–4 days and preferably 2–3 wk between courses).

Lead Poisoning with Encephalopathy

ADULTS AND CHILDREN: Start treatment with dimercaprol; then after 4 hr, begin infusion of edetate calcium disodium at 1.5 g/m^2/day for 5 days. If required, a second course without dimercaprol may be given 5–7 days later.

Dilution

• **Intermittent Infusion: Dilute** 5-ml ampule with 250–500 ml of D5W or 0.9% NaCl to yield a final concentration of 2–4 mg/ml.

Compatibility

• **Additive:** netilmicin.

Incompatibility

• **Additive:** D10W • lactated Ringer's solution • amphotericin B • hydralazine.

Rate of Administration

• **Intermittent Infusion:** Administer over 1 hour in asymptomatic adults and over 2 hours in symptomatic patients. Use infusion pump to control rate accurately. • **Continuous Infusion:** May also be administered as a single daily infusion over 8–24 hours.

≋ CLINICAL PRECAUTIONS

• Assess patient and family members for evidence of lead poisoning prior to and during therapy. Acute lead poisoning is accompanied by a metallic taste, abdominal pain, vomiting, diarrhea, oliguria, and coma. Symptoms of chronic toxicity include anorexia, blue-black gum line, vomiting, paresthesia, encephalopathy, seizures, and coma.

• Monitor intake and output, and daily weights. Use cautiously in renal disease. Dosage reduction is required if serum creatinine is greater than 2 mg/dl. If patient is anuric, edetate calcium disodium should not be given until parenteral hydration establishes urine flow. Risk of nephrotoxicity is increased by concurrent use of gluco-corticoids.

- Assess IV site frequently for redness or irritation.
- Monitor neurologic status closely (level of conscious-ness, pupil response, movement). Notify physician im-mediately of changes. If lead encephalopathy is present, concurrent administration of dimercaprol is required. Infuse slowly, as rapid infusion may increase intracranial pressure. Restricting fluids may decrease the risk of in-tracranial hypertension.
- Monitor vital signs and ECG frequently for hypotension or inverted T waves. Use cautiously in patients with ar-rhythmias or underlying heart disease. Edetate calcium disodium increases the risk of cardiac glycoside toxicity.
- Monitor for fever, chills, malaise, or nasal congestion. This histamine-like reaction usually occurs 4–8 hours after IV infusion and resolves in 48 hours.
- Safe use in pregnancy or lactation has not been estab-lished (Pregnancy Category D).

Lab Test Considerations

- Monitor serum and urine lead levels prior to and peri-odically throughout therapy. Wait at least 1 hour after in-fusing edetate calcium disodium before drawing blood for serum lead level testing. • Monitor urinalysis daily and serum creatinine, BUN, alkaline phosphatase, calcium, and phosphorus levels and hepatocellular enzymes. Both lead and edetate calcium disodium are nephrotoxic. Assess for hematuria, proteinuria, or large renal epithelial cells. • May cause an increase in urine glucose. Edetate calcium diso-dium will decrease the duration of action of zinc insulin preparations. • *Lead mobilization test* (for asymptomatic children with blood lead concentrations of 25–69 mcg/dl and erythrocyte protoporphyrin concentrations greater than 35 mcg/dl of whole blood): IM injections of edetate calcium disodium mixed with 1% procaine are adminis-tered in two equal doses 12 hours apart. A 24-hour urine sample is obtained. If urinary excretion of lead is greater than 1 mcg/mg of edetate calcium disodium administered, or if a control 24-hour urine sample is collected before and after the administration of edetate calcium disodium, and the lead concentration of the second sample is three times greater than the first and contains greater than 50 mcg of lead, the test is considered positive for increased body burden of lead and a 5-day course of therapy is administered. Upper limit of normal for blood lead concentrations is 24 mcg/dl of whole blood. Symptomatic patients or those with whole blood lead concentrations greater than 70 mcg/dl should be given chelation therapy immediately without performing the mobilization test.

Patient/Family Teaching

• Discuss need for follow-up appointments to monitor lead levels. Additional treatments may be necessary. • Consult the public health department regarding potential sources of lead poisoning in the home, workplace, and recreational areas.

PHARMACOLOGIC PROFILE

Indications

• Edetate calcium disodium is used in the management of acute and chronic lead poisoning, including encephalopathy and nephropathy.

Action

• Edetate calcium disodium removes toxic amounts of lead or other divalent or trivalent cations, by their displacement from calcium in edetate calcium disodium. This produces a soluble complex, which is excreted by the kidneys.

Time/Action Profile (urinary lead excretion)

Onset	Peak	Duration
1 hr	24–28 hr	UK

Pharmacokinetics

• **Distribution:** Edetate calcium disodium is distributed to extracellular fluids. It does not cross the blood–brain barrier. • **Metabolism and Excretion:** Edetate calcium disodium is rapidly excreted by the kidneys as unchanged drug or lead complex. • **Half-life:** 90 minutes.

Contraindications

• Edetate calcium disodium is contraindicated in anuric patients.

Adverse Reactions and Side Effects*

• **CNS:** headache, malaise, fatigue • **EENT:** sneezing, lacrimation, nasal congestion • **GI:** nausea, vomiting • **GU:** nephrotoxicity, glycosuria • **F and E:** hypercalcemia • **Local:** phlebitis at IV site • **MS:** myalgia, arthralgia, leg cramps • **Neuro:** numbness, tingling • **Misc:** excessive thirst, fever, chills, histamine-like reaction.

Edrophonium Chloride	*Anticholinesterase*
Enlon, Reversol, Tensilon	pH 5.4

ADMINISTRATION CONSIDERATIONS

Usual Dose

Diagnosis of Myasthenia Gravis

ADULTS: 2 mg; if no response, administer 8 mg; may repeat test in 30 min. If cholinergic response occurs, administer atropine 0.4 mg IV.

CHILDREN ≥34 kg: 2 mg; if no response, may administer 1 mg q 30–45 sec to a total of 10 mg. If cholinergic response occurs, administer atropine IV.

CHILDREN <34 kg: 1 mg; if no response, may administer 1 mg q 30–45 sec to a total of 5 mg. If cholinergic response occurs, administer atropine IV.

INFANTS: 500 mcg (0.5 mg).

Assessment of Anticholinesterase Therapy

ADULTS: 1–2 mg 1 hr after oral anticholinesterase dose.

---

*Underlines indicate most frequent; CAPITALS indicate life-threatening.

Differentiation of Cholinergic from Myasthenic Crises
ADULTS: 1 mg; may give additional 1 mg 1 min later.

Reversal of Nondepolarizing Neuromuscular Blocking Agents (Surgery)
ADULTS: 10 mg or 0.5–1 mg/kg; may repeat q 5–10 min (not to exceed 40 mg).

Termination of Paroxysmal Atrial Tachycardia
ADULTS: 5–10 mg.

Dilution
• **Direct IV:** IV doses are administered **undiluted** with a tuberculin syringe.

Compatibility
• **Y-site:** heparin • hydrocortisone • potassium chloride • vitamin B complex with C.

Rate of Administration
• **Direct IV:** Administer doses over 15–45 seconds; see specific indication.

≋ CLINICAL PRECAUTIONS

- Assess neuromuscular status (ptosis, diplopia, vital capacity, ability to swallow, extremity strength) prior to and immediately following administration.
- When differentiating myasthenic from cholinergic crisis, assess patient for increased weakness, diaphoresis, increased salivation and bronchial secretions, dyspnea, nausea, vomiting, diarrhea, and bradycardia. If these symptoms occur, then patient is in cholinergic crisis. If strength improves, patient is in myasthenic crisis. Action of edrophonium may be antagonized by drugs possessing anticholinergic properties, including antihistamines, antidepressants, atropine, haloperidol, phenothiazines, quinidine, and disopyramide.
- When used for arrhythmias, monitor pulse, blood pressure, and ECG prior to and during administration. Edrophonium may lead to excessive bradycardia in patients receiving cardiac glycosides.
- Edrophonium prolongs action of depolarizing muscle-relaxing agents (succinylcholine, decamethonium).

- Use cautiously in patients with a history of asthma, ulcer disease, cardiovascular disease, epilepsy, or hyperthyroidism. When edrophonium is used for myasthenic testing in patients over 50 years old, pretreatment with atropine is recommended to diminish bradycardia and hypotension.
- Available in combination with atropine sulfate (Enlon-Plus).
- Safe use during pregnancy and lactation has not been established. Edrophonium may cause uterine irritability, and newborns may display muscle weakness (Pregnancy Category C).

Toxicity and Overdose Alert

- Atropine may be used for treatment of cholinergic symptoms. Oxygen and resuscitation equipment should be available.

Patient/Family Teaching

- Inform patient that the effects of this medication last up to 30 minutes.

≋ PHARMACOLOGIC PROFILE

Indications

- Edrophonium is used in the diagnosis of myasthenia gravis, in the assessment of adequacy of anticholinesterase therapy in myasthenia gravis, and to differentiate myasthenic from cholinergic crisis. • It is also used to reverse nondepolarizing neuromuscular blockers. • Edrophonium has also been used to terminate paroxysmal atrial tachycardia.

Action

- Edrophonium inhibits the breakdown of acetylcholine so that it accumulates and has a prolonged effect. Effects include miosis, increased intestinal and skeletal muscle tone, bronchial and ureteral constriction, bradycardia, increased salivation, lacrimation, and sweating. It produces improved but short-lived cranial muscular function in patients with myasthenia gravis, reversal of nondepolarizing neuromuscular blockers, and suppression of certain arrhythmias.

Time/Action Profile (cholinergic activity)

Onset	Peak	Duration
30–60 sec	UK	5–10 min

Pharmacokinetics

• **Distribution:** UK. • **Metabolism and Excretion:** UK.
• **Half-life:** UK.

Contraindications

• Edrophonium is contraindicated in patients who have hypersensitivity to it or to phenol or sulfites. • Its use should be avoided in patients with mechanical obstruction of the GI or GU tract. • Pregnant patients should not receive edrophonium; newborns may display muscle weakness. • Edrophonium should not be given during lactation.

Adverse Reactions and Side Effects*

• **CNS:** dizziness, weakness, SEIZURES • **EENT:** miosis, lacrimation • **Resp:** excess secretions, bronchospasm • **CV:** bradycardia, hypotension • **GI:** abdominal cramps, nausea, vomiting, diarrhea, excess salivation • **Derm:** rashes, sweating • **MS:** fasciculation.

Enalaprilat	Angiotensin-converting enzyme (ACE) inhibitor, Antihypertensive
Vasotec IV	pH 6.5–7.5

 ADMINISTRATION CONSIDERATIONS

Usual Dose

ADULTS: 625 mcg (0.625 mg)–1.25 mg q 6 hr.

Dilution

• **Direct IV:** May be administered **undiluted**. • **Intermittent Infusion:** Dilute in 50 ml of D5W, 0.9% NaCl,

---

*Underlines indicate most frequent; CAPITALS indicate life-threatening.

D5/0.9% NaCl, or D5/LR. • Diluted solution is stable for 24 hours.

Compatibility

• **Y-site:** allopurinol sodium • amikacin • aminophylline • ampicillin • ampicillin/sulbactam • aztreonam • butorphanol • calcium gluconate • cefazolin • cefoperazone • ceftazidime • ceftizoxime • chloramphenicol • cimetidine • clindamycin • dextran 40 • dobutamine • dopamine • erythromycin lactobionate • esmolol • famotidine • fentanyl • filgrastim • ganciclovir • gentamicin • heparin • hetastarch • hydrocortisone sodium succinate • labetalol • lidocaine • magnesium sulfate • melphalan • methylprednisolone sodium succinate • metronidazole • morphine • nafcillin • nitroprusside • penicillin G potassium • phenobarbital • piperacillin • piperacillin/tazobactam • potassium chloride • potassium phosphate • ranitidine • sodium acetate • tobramycin • trimethoprim/sulfamethoxazole • vancomycin • vinorelbine.

Incompatibility

• **Y-site:** amphotericin B • phenytoin.

Rate of Administration

• **Direct IV:** Administer over 5 minutes.

≋ CLINICAL PRECAUTIONS

• Monitor blood pressure and pulse frequently during treatment. Precipitous drop in blood pressure may follow initial dose. Volume expansion with saline may be temporarily required. Hypotension may be exaggerated during surgery/anesthesia. Additive hypotension occurs with other antihypertensives, acute ingestion of alcohol, and vasodilators.

• Monitor weight and assess patient routinely for resolution of fluid overload (peripheral edema, rales/crackles, dyspnea, weight gain, jugular venous distention).

• Use cautiously in patients with renal impairment. Dosage reduction is required if serum creatinine is greater than 3 mg/dl or creatinine clearance is less than 30 ml/min. Lower initial doses are necessary in elderly patients,

patients on concurrent diuretic therapy, patients with renal failure, or patients who are sodium and/or water depleted.

- Use with caution in patients with aortic stenosis, cerebrovascular disease, and cardiac insufficiency. Use with extreme caution in patients with a family history of hereditary angioedema.
- Antihypertensive response may be blunted by nonsteroidal anti-inflammatory agents.
- Renal side effects may be exaggerated by concurrent penicillamine therapy.
- Safe use in pregnancy has not been established. Enalaprilat can cause fetal and neonatal morbidity and mortality (Pregnancy Category D). Safe use during lactation and in children has not been established.

Lab Test Considerations

- Monitor BUN, serum creatinine, and electrolyte levels periodically. Serum potassium may be increased and BUN and creatinine transiently increased, while sodium levels may be decreased. Hyperkalemia may result with concurrent potassium therapy or potassium-sparing diuretics.

Patient/Family Teaching

- Caution patient to change positions slowly to minimize orthostatic hypotension, particularly after initial dose. • Enalaprilat may cause dizziness. Caution patient to avoid activities requiring alertness until response to medication is known. • Advise patient that enalaprilat may cause an impairment of taste that generally reverses itself within 8–12 weeks, even with continued therapy. • Instruct patient to notify physician if rash; mouth sores; sore throat; fever; swelling of hands or feet; irregular heartbeat; chest pain; dry cough; swelling of face, eyes, lips, or tongue; or difficulty breathing occurs. • Inform patient that management of hypertension requires compliance with additional interventions (weight reduction, discontinuation of smoking, moderation of alcohol consumption, regular exercise, and stress management), blood pressure monitoring, and follow-up. • Patient should notify physician if pregnancy is planned or suspected.

≋ PHARMACOLOGIC PROFILE

Indications
• Used alone or in combination with other antihypertensives in the management of hypertension. • Used in combination with other drugs in the treatment of congestive heart failure.

Action
• Enalaprilat prevents the production of angiotensin II, a potent vasoconstrictor that stimulates the production of aldosterone by blocking its conversion to the active form. The result is systemic vasodilation, lowering of blood pressure in hypertensive patients, and decreased preload and afterload in patients with congestive heart failure.

Time/Action Profile (effect on blood pressure)

Onset	Peak	Duration
15 min	1–4 hr	6 hr

Pharmacokinetics
• **Distribution:** Minimal crossing of the blood–brain barrier. Rest of distribution not known. Enalaprilat crosses the placenta, and trace amounts enter breast milk. • **Half-life:** 11 hours (increased in renal impairment).

Contraindications
• Hypersensitivity to enalaprilat or known intolerance to benzyl alcohol. • Cross-sensitivity with other ACE inhibitors may exist.

Adverse Reactions and Side Effects*
• **CNS:** headache, dizziness, fatigue • **Resp:** cough • **CV:** hypotension, tachycardia, angina pectoris • **GI:** anorexia, diarrhea, nausea, impaired taste • **GU:** impotence, proteinuria, renal failure • **Derm:** rashes • **F and E:** hyperkalemia • **Misc:** fever, ANGIOEDEMA with laryngospasm.

---

*Underlines indicate most frequent; CAPITALS indicate life-threatening.

Ephedrine Sulfate	*Vasopressor,*
	Bronchodilator
	pH 4.5–7

≋ ADMINISTRATION CONSIDERATIONS

Usual Dose

Vasopressor

ADULTS: 10–25 mg as a slow injection; additional doses may be given in 5–10 min (not to exceed 150 mg/24 hr).

CHILDREN: 0.75 mg/kg (25 mg/m^2) q 6 hr or 0.5 mg/kg (16.7 mg/m^2) q 4 hr.

Bronchodilator

ADULTS: 12.5–25 mg; additional doses may be given.

CHILDREN: 0.75 mg/kg (25 mg/m^2) q 6 hr or 0.5 mg/kg (16.7 mg/m^2) q 4 hr.

Dilution

• **Direct IV:** Inject **undiluted** through Y-site or 3-way stopcock. • Use only clear solution. Discard any unused solution.

Compatibility

• **Solution:** D5W ✦ D10W ✦ 0.45% NaCl ✦ 0.9% NaCl ✦ Ringer's and lactated Ringer's solution ✦ dextrose/saline combinations ✦ dextrose/Ringer's or lactated Ringer's combinations.

• **Additive:** chloramphenicol ✦ lidocaine ✦ metaraminol ✦ nafcillin ✦ penicillin G potassium.

Incompatibility

• **Syringe:** thiopental.

• **Additive:** hydrocortisone sodium succinate ✦ pentobarbital ✦ phenobarbital ✦ secobarbital.

Rate of Administration

• **Direct IV:** Administer slowly, each 10 mg over at least 1 minute.

≋ CLINICAL PRECAUTIONS

- Monitor blood pressure, pulse, ECG, and respiratory rate frequently when used as a vasopressor. The risk of cardiac arrhythmias is increased by concurrent use of cocaine, cyclopropane, halothane, or cardiac glycosides. Hypertensive crises or increased vasoconstriction may result from concurrent use with ergot alkaloids, guanethidine, guanadrel, or MAO inhibitors. Reserpine, methyldopa, antidepressants, beta-adrenergic blockers, or furosemide may decrease the effects of ephedrine. Atropine increases the risk of bradycardia and decreases pressor response. Ephedrine decreases the hypotensive effects of guanadrel and guanethidine.
- When used as a bronchodilator, assess lung sounds, pulse, and blood pressure before and during administration. Adverse effects are increased by concurrent use of theophylline.
- Agents that acidify urine (ammonium chloride) may decrease the effectiveness of ephedrine. Alkalinizing agents (sodium bicarbonate) may increase effects of ephedrine.
- Use cautiously in patients with cardiovascular disease or prostatic hypertrophy. Elderly patients may be more susceptible to adverse CNS reactions.
- Adrenergic (sympathomimetic) effects will be additive with other adrenergic agents, including decongestants.
- Safe use during pregnancy or lactation has not been established (Pregnancy Category C). Ephedrine should be used during pregnancy only when potential benefits outweigh risks.

Patient/Family Teaching

- Instruct patient to notify nurse immediately if shortness of breath is not relieved by medication or is accompanied by diaphoresis, dizziness, palpitations, or chest pain.

≋ PHARMACOLOGIC PROFILE

Indications

- Ephedrine is used in the management of acute hypotension associated with overdosage of antihypertensive agents.

• It is also used as a bronchodilator in the management of reversible airway obstruction due to asthma or COPD.

Action

• Ephedrine is an alpha- and beta-adrenergic agonist. Beta-adrenergic agonist effects result in accumulation of cyclic AMP at beta-adrenergic receptors producing bronchodilation, CNS and cardiac stimulation, diuresis, and gastric acid secretion. Primary alpha-adrenergic effect is peripheral vasoconstriction.

Time/Action Profile (pressor response)

Onset	Peak	Duration
UK	UK	1 hr

Pharmacokinetics

• **Distribution:** Ephedrine probably crosses the placenta and enters breast milk. • **Metabolism and Excretion:** Small amounts of ephedrine are slowly metabolized by the liver. Most of the drug is excreted unchanged by the kidneys. Excretion of ephedrine is dependent on urine pH. Acidifying urine decreases the duration of action. Alkalinizing urine increases the duration of action. • **Half-life:** 3–6 hours (depends on urine pH).

Contraindications

• Ephedrine is contraindicated in patients with known hypersensitivity or intolerance. • Patients with narrow-angle glaucoma, thyrotoxicosis, diabetes mellitus, hypertension, or severe cardiovascular disease should not receive ephedrine. • Ephedrine should be avoided during cyclopropane or halothane anesthesia.

Adverse Reactions and Side Effects*

• **CNS:** CNS stimulation, nervousness, anxiety, paranoid state (long-term use), dizziness, light-headedness, vertigo • **EENT:** rebound congestion (nasal use), local irritation • **Resp:** breathing difficulties • **CV:** angina pectoris, palpitations, tachycardia, ARRHYTHMIAS • **GU:** urinary retention, decreased urine output • **Misc:** rapid development of tolerance (tachyphylaxis), diaphoresis.

---

*Underlines indicate most frequent; CAPITALS indicate life-threatening.

Epinephrine Hydrochloride	*Cardiac stimulant, Vasopressor (adrenergic)*
Adrenalin	pH 2.5–5

≋ ADMINISTRATION CONSIDERATIONS

Usual Dose

Anaphylaxis

ADULTS: 100–250 mcg (0.1–0.25 mg); may repeat every 5–15 min *or* 1–4 mcg/min infusion.

CHILDREN: 10 mcg (0.01 mg)/kg or 300 mcg (0.3 mg)/m^2 *or* 100 mcg (0.1 mg) over 5 min; may repeat q 30 min *or* 0.1–1.5 mcg (0.0001–0.0015 mg)/kg/min infusion.

Vasopressor (anaphylactic shock)

ADULTS: 100–250 mcg (0.1–0.25 mg); may be repeated q 5–15 min or followed by infusion at 1 mcg/min; may be increased to a maximum of 4 mcg/min.

CHILDREN: 10 mcg (0.01 mg)/kg; may be repeated q 5–15 min.

Cardiac Arrest

ADULTS: 0.5–1 mg; repeat q 3–5 min as needed.

CHILDREN: 5–10 mcg (0.005–0.01 mg)/kg or 150–300 mcg/m^2 q 5 min; may be followed by infusion at an initial rate of 0.1 mcg (0.0001 mg)/kg/min, not to exceed 1 mcg (.001 mg)/kg/min.

Dilution

• **Direct IV:** Dilute 0.5 ml of a 1:1000 (1 mg/ml) solution in 10 ml of 0.9% NaCl for injection to prepare a 1:10,000 solution. • Discard any solution not used within 24 hours of preparation. Do not use solution that is pinkish or brownish or one that contains a precipitate. • **Continuous Infusion:** For maintenance, solution may be further diluted in 500 ml of D5W, D10W, 0.9% NaCl, D5/LR, D5/Ringer's solution, dextrose/saline combinations, or Ringer's or lactated Ringer's solution.

Compatibility

• **Syringe:** doxapram • heparin • milrinone.

• **Y-site:** amrinone • atracurium • calcium chloride • calcium gluconate • diltiazem • famotidine • heparin • hydrocortisone sodium succinate • pancuronium • phytonadione ✦ potassium chloride ✦ vecuronium ✦ vitamin B complex with C.

• **Additive:** amikacin ✦ cimetidine ✦ dobutamine ✦ furosemide ✦ metaraminol ✦ ranitidine ✦ verapamil.

Incompatibility

• **Y-site:** ampicillin.

• **Additive:** aminophylline ✦ cephapirin ✦ sodium bicarbonate.

Rate of Administration

• **Direct IV:** Administer each dose slowly over 5–10 minutes; more rapid administration may be used during cardiac resuscitation. • **Continuous Infusion:** Administer through a Y-site or a 3-way stopcock via infusion pump to ensure accurate dosage. See Infusion Rate Table below.

EPINEPHRINE INFUSION RATE TABLE

EPINEPHRINE INFUSION RATES (ml/hr) *CONCENTRATION = 4 mcg/ml*	
Dose (mcg/ml)	*Dose (ml/hr)*
Dilution: 1 mg/250 ml = 4 mcg/ml.	
1 mcg/min	15 ml/hr
2 mcg/min	30 ml/hr
3 mcg/min	45 ml/hr
4 mcg/min	60 ml/hr

≋ CLINICAL PRECAUTIONS

- Monitor blood pressure, pulse, and respiratory rate prior to and every 5 minutes during administration. Monitor ECG continuously.
- For anaphylactic shock, volume replacement should be administered concurrently with epinephrine. Antihistamines and glucocorticoids may be used in conjunction with epinephrine.
- Concurrent use with beta blockers may result in an initial hypertensive reaction, which may be followed by bradycardia.
- Check dose, concentration, and route of administration carefully prior to administration. Fatalities have occurred from medication errors.

- Use cautiously in patients with cardiovascular disease, arrhythmias, hypertension, or hyperthyroidism due to increased risk of cardiovascular reactions. This risk is also increased with use of general anesthesia or cardiac glycosides.
- Use with caution in patients with glaucoma (except for ophthalmic use in open-angle glaucoma).
- Patients with diabetes mellitus may experience an increased need for insulin or oral hypoglycemic agents.
- Additive effects may occur with other sympathomimetic (adrenergic) agents, including decongestants. Concurrent use with beta-adrenergic blockers may cause hypertension followed by bradycardia.
- Use of epinephrine with MAO inhibitors may lead to hypertensive crisis. Concurrent use with guanethidine guanadrel, antidepressants, reserpine, methyldopa, oxytocics, or ergot alkaloids may result in hypertension. Lithium may decrease vasopressor effects.
- Safe use during pregnancy and lactation has not been established; fetal anoxia may occur (Pregnancy Category C).

Lab Test Considerations

- May cause an increase in blood glucose and serum lactic acid concentrations.

Patient/Family Teaching

- Inform patient of the purpose of this medication.

≋ PHARMACOLOGIC PROFILE

Indications

- Epinephrine is used as part of the emergency treatment of anaphylaxis and in the management of cardiac arrest.

Action

- Epinephrine acts as a beta$_1$- and beta$_2$-adrenergic agonist, which produces an accumulation of cyclic adenosine monophosphate (cAMP). Increased levels of cAMP at beta-adrenergic receptors produce bronchodilation, CNS and cardiac stimulation, vasoconstriction, diuresis, and gastric acid secretion.

Time/Action Profile (bronchodilation)

	Onset	Peak	Duration
IV	rapid	20 min	20–30 min

Pharmacokinetics

• **Distribution:** Epinephrine does not cross the blood–brain barrier. It does cross the placenta and enters breast milk. • **Metabolism and Excretion:** The action of epinephrine is rapidly terminated by metabolism and uptake by nerve endings. • **Half-life:** UK.

Contraindications

• Epinephrine is contraindicated in patients with hypersensitivity to sympathomimetic amines. • Some products may contain bisulfites; avoid use in patients with bisulfite hypersensitivity.

Adverse Reactions and Side Effects*

• **CNS:** <u>nervousness</u>, <u>restlessness</u>, <u>insomnia</u>, <u>tremor</u>, <u>headache</u> • **CV:** hypertension, <u>arrhythmias</u>, angina • **Endo:** hyperglycemia • **GI:** nausea, vomiting • **GU:** urinary retention, hesitancy.

Epoetin Alfa	Hormone (erythropoietin)
Epogen, EPO, {Eprex}, erythropoietin, Procrit	pH 6.6 – 7.2

 ADMINISTRATION CONSIDERATIONS

Usual Dose

Anemia of Chronic Renal Failure

ADULTS: 50–100 units/kg 3 times weekly initially, then adjust dosage by changes of 25 units/kg/dose to maintain target

---

*<u>Underlines</u> indicate most frequent; CAPITALS indicate life-threatening.

{} = Available in Canada only.

range of hematocrit of 30–36%. Usual maintenance dose is 25 units/kg 3 times weekly.

Anemia Secondary to Zidovudine (AZT) Therapy

ADULTS: 100 units/kg 3 times weekly for 8 wk. If inadequate response, may increase by 50–100 units/kg q 4–8 wk, up to 300 units/kg 3 times weekly (if hematocrit >40%, stop therapy until it drops to 36%, then decrease dose by 25% and resume therapy).

Anemia from Chemotherapy

ADULTS: 150 units/kg 3 times weekly for 8 weeks; may be increased up to 300 units/kg weekly.

Dilution

• **Direct IV:** May be administered **undiluted** as direct injection or bolus via venous line at end of dialysis session. • Do not shake vial, as inactivation of medication may occur. Discard vial immediately after withdrawing dose from single-use 1-ml vial. Refrigerate multidose 2-ml vial; stable for 21 days after initial entry.

Compatibility

• **Solution:** 0.9% NaCl.

Incompatibility

• Do not admix or administer through IV lines containing other drug solutions.

Rate of Administration

• **Direct IV:** Administer as a bolus.

≋ CLINICAL PRECAUTIONS

• Monitor blood pressure prior to and throughout course of therapy. If severe hypertension is present or if blood pressure begins to increase, additional antihypertensive therapy may be required during initiation of therapy. Hypertension is more likely to occur in patients with chronic renal failure.
• Use with caution in patients with a history of seizures. Institute seizure precautions in patients who experience greater than 4-point increase in hematocrit in a 2-week period or exhibit any change in neurologic status. Risk of seizures is greatest during the first 90 days of therapy.

- Monitor for symptoms of anemia (fatigue, dyspnea, pallor). Transfusions are still required for severe symptomatic anemia, as several weeks are required before therapeutic response occurs.
- Monitor dialysis shunts (thrill and bruit) and status of artificial kidney during hemodialysis. Heparin dose may need to be increased to prevent clotting. Additional iron supplements may be necessary.
- Patients with underlying vascular disease should be monitored for impaired circulation.
- Monitor renal function studies and electrolytes closely, as resulting increased sense of well-being may lead to decreased compliance with other therapies for renal failure.
- Safe use in pregnancy, lactation, or children has not been established (Pregnancy Category C).

Lab Test Considerations

• **Anemia of Chronic Renal Failure:** Hematocrit should be monitored prior to and twice weekly during initial therapy or for 2–6 weeks after a change in dose, and regularly after target range (30–36%) has been reached and maintenance dose is determined. • Other hemopoietic parameters (CBC with differential and platelet count) also should be monitored prior to and regularly throughout therapy. • If hematocrit increases more than 4 points in a 2-week period, the likelihood of a hypertensive reaction and seizures increases. Dose should be immediately decreased and the hematocrit monitored twice weekly for 2–6 weeks. Adjust dose further as needed. • If the hematocrit is increasing and approaching 36%, reduce the dose to maintain suggested target hematocrit range. If increase in hematocrit continues and exceeds 36%, dose should be temporarily withheld until hematocrit begins to decrease, then reinitiate at a lower dose. • If a hematocrit increase of 5–6 points is not achieved after an 8-week period and iron stores are adequate, the dose may be incrementally increased at 4–6-week intervals until the desired response is attained. • **Anemia Secondary to Zidovudine Therapy:** Before initiating therapy, determine endogenous serum erythropoietin level prior to transfusion. Patients receiving zidovudine with endogenous serum erythropoietin levels >500 mU/ml may not respond to therapy. • Monitor hematocrit weekly during dosage adjustment. If response does not reduce transfusion requirements or increase hematocrit effectively after 8 weeks of therapy, increase the dose by 50–100 units/kg 3 times weekly. Evaluate the response and adjust the dose by 50–100 units/kg 3 times weekly incrementally every 4–8 weeks thereafter. If a satisfactory response is not attained to a dose of 300 units/kg 3 times weekly, it is unlikely a higher dose will produce a response. • Once the desired response is attained, the maintenance dose is titrated based on variations of the zidovudine dose and intercurrent infections. • If the hematocrit exceeds 40%, discontinue dose until hematocrit drops to 36%, then decrease the dose by 25%. • **Anemia from Chemotherapy:** Monitor hematocrit weekly until stable. • Patients with lower baseline serum erythropoietin levels may respond more rapidly; not recommended if levels >200 mU/ml. • If response is not adequate after 8 weeks of therapy, dose may be increased up to 300 units/kg 3 times weekly. If no response is attained to this dose, it is unlikely that a higher dose will produce a response. • If hematocrit exceeds 40%, hold dose until it falls to 36%, then decrease dose by 25%. • If initial dose response is >4 percentage points in any 2-week period, reduce dose. • Serum ferritin, transferrin, and iron levels should also be monitored to assess need for concurrent iron therapy. Transferrin saturation should be at least 20%, and ferritin should be at least 100 ng/ml. • Increases in BUN, creatinine, uric acid, phosphorus, and potassium may occur. • May cause increase in WBCs and platelets. • May decrease bleeding times.

Patient/Family Teaching

• Stress the importance of compliance with dietary restrictions, medications, and dialysis. Foods high in iron and low in potassium include liver, pork, veal, beef, mustard and turnip greens, peas, eggs, broccoli, kale, blackberries, strawberries, apple juice, watermelon, oatmeal, and enriched bread. Epoetin alfa will result in increased sense of well-being, but it does not cure underlying disease. • Explain rationale for concurrent iron therapy (increased red blood cell production requires iron). Instruct patient to notify physician if skin rash, hives, facial swelling, or shortness of breath occurs. • Discuss possible return

of menses and fertility in females of childbearing age. Patients should discuss contraceptive options with physician.
• Discuss ways of preventing self-injury in patients at risk for seizures. Driving and activities requiring continuous alertness should be avoided.

• **Home Care Issues:** Home dialysis patients determined to be able to safely and effectively administer epoetin alfa should be taught the proper dosage and administration of medication and the proper disposal of equipment. "Information for Home Dialysis Patients" should be provided to the patient with the medication.

 PHARMACOLOGIC PROFILE

Indications
• Epoetin is used in the treatment of anemia associated with chronic renal failure and in zidovudine (AZT) therapy or chemotherapy.

Action
• Epoetin stimulates erythropoiesis (production of red blood cells), which may decrease the need for transfusions.

Time/Action Profile (effect on RBCs)

Onset	Peak	Duration†
10 days	2–6 wk	2 wk

†Following discontinuation.

Pharmacokinetics
• **Distribution:** UK. • **Metabolism and Excretion:** UK.
• **Half-life:** 4–13 hours.

Contraindications
• Epoetin should not be used in patients with hypersensitivity to human albumin or mammalian cell–derived products. • Patients with uncontrolled hypertension should not receive epoetin. • In patients who have had chemotherapy, epoetin should not be given if serum erythropoietin level exceeds 200 mU/ml.

Adverse Reactions and Side Effects*

Adverse reaction profiles differ depending on condition being treated; some are consequences of restored hemostasis.

• **CNS:** SEIZURES, headache • **CV:** thrombotic events (hemodialysis patients), hypertension • **Derm:** transient rashes • **Endo:** resumption of menses, restored fertility • **Misc:** fever, allergic reactions including ANAPHYLAXIS.

Erythromycin Gluceptate **Erythromycin Lactobionate**	*Anti-infective* *(macrolide)*
Ilotycin Gluceptate	pH 7.7
Erythrocin Lactobionate	pH 6.5–7.5

ADMINISTRATION CONSIDERATIONS

Usual Dose
ADULTS: 250–500 mg q 6 hr (up to 4–6 g/day).
CHILDREN: 3.75–5 mg/kg q 6 hr.

Dilution
• **Intermittent Infusion:** Add 10 ml of sterile water for injection without preservatives to 250- or 500-mg vials and 20 ml to 1-g vial. Reconstitution is the same for erythromycin gluceptate or erythromycin lactobionate. • Solution is stable for 7 days after reconstitution if refrigerated. • **Dilute** further in 100–250 ml of 0.9% NaCl or D5W. • **Continuous Infusion:** May also be administered as an infusion in a dilution of 1 g/liter for a concentration of 1 mg/ml of 0.9% NaCl, D5W, or lactated Ringer's solution.

Compatibility

Erythromycin Gluceptate

• **Additive:** calcium gluconate ♦ corticotropin ♦ dimenhydrinate ♦ heparin ♦ hydrocortisone sodium succinate ♦ methicillin ♦ penicillin G potassium ♦ potassium chloride ♦ sodium bicarbonate.

---

*Underlines indicate most frequent; CAPITALS indicate life-threatening.

Erythromycin Lactobionate

- **Syringe:** methicillin.
- **Y-site:** acyclovir ◆ cyclophosphamide ◆ diltiazem ◆ enalaprilat ◆ esmolol ◆ famotidine ◆ foscarnet ◆ hydromorphone ◆ idarubicin ◆ labetalol ◆ magnesium sulfate ◆ meperidine ◆ morphine ◆ multivitamins ◆ perphenazine ◆ tacrolimus ◆ vitamin B complex with C ◆ zidovudine.
- **Additive:** aminophylline ◆ cimetidine ◆ diphenhydramine ◆ hydrocortisone sodium succinate ◆ lidocaine ◆ methicillin ◆ penicillin G ◆ pentobarbital ◆ polymyxin B ◆ potassium chloride ◆ prednisolone ◆ prochlorperazine ◆ promazine ◆ ranitidine ◆ sodium bicarbonate ◆ verapamil.

Incompatibility

Erythromycin Gluceptate

- **Syringe:** heparin.
- **Y-site:** chloramphenicol ◆ heparin ◆ phenobarbital ◆ phenytoin.
- **Additive:** aminophylline ◆ pentobarbital ◆ secobarbital ◆ streptomycin.

Erythromycin Lactobionate

- **Syringe:** heparin.
- **Y-site:** fluconazole.
- **Additive:** cephalothin ◆ colistimethate ◆ furosemide ◆ heparin ◆ metaraminol ◆ metoclopramide ◆ vitamin B complex with C.

Rate of Administration

- **Intermittent Infusion:** Administer slowly over 20–60 minutes to avoid phlebitis. Assess for pain along vein; slow rate if pain occurs; apply ice and notify physician if unable to relieve pain. • **Continuous Infusion:** May be administered as a slow continuous infusion in a concentration of 1 mg/ml.

≋ CLINICAL PRECAUTIONS

- Assess patient for infection (vital signs; appearance of wound, sputum, urine, and stool; WBC) prior to and throughout therapy.
- Obtain specimens for culture and sensitivity prior to initiating therapy. First dose may be given before receiving results.

- Observe IV site frequently for signs of redness or irritation. Erythromycin commonly causes phlebitis.
- Use cautiously in patients with a history of liver disease.
- Increases activity and may increase the risk of toxicity from alfentanil, bromocriptine, theophylline, carbamazepine, cyclosporine, disopyramide, ergot alkaloids, triazolam, oral anticoagulants, or methylprednisolone. May increase serum digoxin levels in a small percentage of patients.
- Intravenous erythromycin has been used safely during pregnancy to treat chlamydia and syphilis (Pregnancy Category B).

Lab Test Considerations

- Liver function tests should be performed periodically on patients receiving high-dose, long-term therapy. May cause increased serum bilirubin, AST (SGOT), ALT (SGPT), and alkaline phosphatase concentrations.

Patient/Family Teaching

- May cause nausea, vomiting, diarrhea, or stomach cramps; notify physician if these effects persist or if severe abdominal pain, yellow discoloration of the skin or eyes, darkened urine, pale stools, or unusual tiredness develops.
- Advise patient to report signs of superinfection (black, furry overgrowth on the tongue, vaginal itching or discharge, loose or foul-smelling stools). • Instruct patient to notify the physician if symptoms do not improve.

☰ PHARMACOLOGIC PROFILE

Indications

- Erythromycin is used in the treatment of the following infections due to susceptible organisms: upper and lower respiratory tract infections, otitis media (with sulfonamides), skin and skin structure infections, pertussis, diphtheria, erythrasma, intestinal amebiasis, pelvic inflammatory disease, nongonococcal urethritis, syphilis, Legionnaires' disease, and rheumatic fever. It is useful in situations when penicillin is the most appropriate drug but cannot be used because of previous hypersensitivity reactions, including streptococcal infections, treatment of syphilis or gonorrhea, and endocarditis prophylaxis.

Action

• Erythromycin suppresses protein synthesis at the level of the 50S bacterial ribosome, resulting in bacteriostatic action against susceptible bacteria. • It is active against many Gram-positive cocci, including streptococci, staphylococci, and Gram-positive bacilli including *Clostridium, Corynebacterium*. Several Gram-negative pathogens, notably *Neisseria, Haemophilus influenzae, Legionella pneumophila, Mycoplasma,* and *Chlamydia* are also usually susceptible.

Time/Action Profile (blood levels)

Onset	Peak
rapid	end of infusion

Pharmacokinetics

• **Distribution:** Erythromycin is widely distributed but has minimal penetration into CSF. It crosses the placenta and enters breast milk. • **Metabolism and Excretion:** Erythromycin is partially metabolized by the liver and excreted mainly unchanged in the bile. Small amounts are excreted unchanged in the urine. • **Half-life:** 1.4–2 hours.

Contraindications

• Erythromycin should not be used in patients with previous hypersensitivity to it. Some products contain benzyl alcohol and should be avoided in patients with known intolerance (neonates).

Adverse Reactions and Side Effects*

• **GI:** nausea, vomiting, diarrhea, abdominal pain, cramping, hepatitis • **EENT:** ototoxicity • **Derm:** rashes • **Local:** phlebitis at IV site • **Misc:** allergic reactions, superinfection.

---

*Underlines indicate most frequent; CAPITALS indicate life-threatening.

Esmolol Hydrochloride	Antiarrhythmic (beta blocker)
Brevibloc	pH 3.3–5.5

≋ ADMINISTRATION CONSIDERATIONS

Usual Dose

ADULTS: 500-mcg/kg loading dose over 1 min initially, followed by 50 mcg/kg/min infusion for 4 min; if no response within 5 min, give a second loading dose of 500 mcg/kg over 1 min and increase infusion to 100 mcg/kg/min for 4 min. If no response, repeat loading dose of 500 mcg/kg over 1 min and increase infusion rate by 50-mcg/kg/min increments (not to exceed 200 mcg/kg/min). As therapeutic end point is achieved, eliminate loading doses and decrease dosage increments to 25 mcg/kg/min.

CHILDREN: 50 mcg/kg/min; may be increased q 10 min up to 300 mcg/kg/min.

Dilution

• **Direct IV:** The 10 mg/ml concentration may be administered **undiluted**. • **Intermittent Infusion:** The 250 mg/ml concentration of esmolol must be **diluted** and administered via IV infusion. To **dilute** for infusion, remove 20 ml from a 500-ml container of D5W, D5/LR, D5/0.45% NaCl, D5/0.9% NaCl, 0.45% NaCl, 0.9% NaCl, or lactated Ringer's solution. Add 5 g of esmolol to the container, for a concentration of 10 mg/ml. • Esmolol solution is clear, colorless to light yellow. Solution is stable for 24 hours at room temperature.

Compatibility

• **Y-site:** amikacin ✦ aminophylline ✦ ampicillin ✦ atracurium ✦ butorphanol ✦ calcium chloride ✦ cefazolin ✦ cefoperazone ✦ teftazidime ✦ ceftizoxime ✦ chloramphenicol ✦ cimetidine ✦ clindamycin ✦ diltiazem ✦ dopamine ✦ enalaprilat ✦ erythromycin lactobionate ✦ famotidine ✦ fentanyl ✦ gentamicin ✦ heparin ✦ hydrocortisone sodium succinate ✦ magnesium sulfate ✦ methyldopa ✦ metronidazole ✦ morphine ✦ nafcillin ✦ pancuronium ✦ penicillin G potassium ✦ phenytoin ✦ piperacillin ✦ polymyxin B ✦ potassium chloride ✦ potassium phosphate ✦ ranitidine ✦ sodium acetate

• streptomycin • tacrolimus • tobramycin • trimethoprim/
sulfamethoxazole • vancomycin • vecuronium.
  • **Additive:** aminophylline • atracurium • bretylium
• heparin.

Incompatibility

  • **Y-site:** furosemide.
  • **Additive:** diazepam • procainamide • sodium bicarbonate • thiopental.

Rate of Administration

  • **Intermittent Infusion:** The loading dose of esmolol is
administered over 1 minute, followed by a maintenance dose
via IV infusion over 5 minutes. If the response is not adequate, the procedure is repeated every 5 minutes with an increase in the maintenance dose. Titration of dose is based on
heart rate and blood pressure. The maintenance dose should
not be more than 200 mcg/kg/min and can be administered
for up to 48 hours. Esmolol infusions should not be abruptly
discontinued; decrease dosage by 25 mcg/kg/min (see Infusion Rate Table below).

ESMOLOL (Brevibloc) INFUSION RATE TABLE

Dilution: 5 g/500 ml = 10 mg/ml.
Loading regimen = 500 mcg/kg (0.05 ml/kg) loading dose over 1
  min, followed by 50 mcg/kg/min (0.005 ml/kg/min) infusion over
  4 min. If no response, repeat loading dose over 1 min and increase
  infusion rate to 100 mcg/kg/min for 4–10 min. If no response,
  loading dose may be repeated before increasing infusion rates in 50
  mcg/kg/min increments.

PATIENT WEIGHT

Dose	50 kg	60 kg	70 kg	80 kg	90 kg	100 kg
	ESMOLOL INFUSION RATES CONCENTRATION = 10 mg/ml					
loading dose (ml)†	2.5 ml	3 ml	3.5 ml	4 ml	4.5 ml	5 ml
50 mcg/kg/min	15 ml/hr	18 ml/hr	21 ml/hr	24 ml/hr	27 ml/hr	30 ml/hr
75 mcg/kg/min	22.5 ml/hr	27 ml/hr	31.5 ml/hr	36 mlhr	40.5 ml/hr	45 ml/hr
100 mcg/kg/min	30 ml/hr	36 ml/hr	42 ml/hr	48 ml/hr	54 ml/hr	60 ml/hr
125 mcg/kg/min	37.5 ml/hr	45 ml/hr	52.5 ml/hr	60 ml/hr	67.5 ml/hr	75 ml/hr
150 mcg/kg/min	45 ml/hr	54 ml/hr	63 ml/hr	72 ml/hr	81 ml/hr	90 ml/hr
175 mcg/kg/min	52.5 ml/hr	63 ml/hr	73.5 ml/hr	84 ml/hr	94.5 ml/hr	105 ml/hr
200 mcg/kg/min	60 ml/hr	72 ml/hr	84 ml/hr	96 ml/hr	108 ml/hr	120 ml/hr

†Loading dose given over 1 min.

≋ CLINICAL PRECAUTIONS

- Monitor blood pressure, heart rate, and ECG frequently throughout course of therapy. The risk of hypotension is greatest within the first 30 minutes of initiating esmolol infusion.
- Assess infusion site frequently throughout therapy. Concentrations of greater than 10 mg/ml may cause redness, swelling, skin discoloration, and burning at the injection site. If venous irritation occurs, stop the infusion and resume at another site.
- Monitor intake and output ratios and daily weight. Assess patient for signs and symptoms of congestive heart failure (peripheral edema, dyspnea, rales/crackles, weight gain, jugular venous distention).
- To convert to other antiarrhythmic agents following esmolol administration, administer the first dose of the antiarrhythmic agent and decrease the esmolol dose by 50% after 30 minutes. If an adequate response is maintained for 1 hour following the second dose of the antiarrhythmic agent, discontinue the esmolol.
- General anesthesia, IV phenytoin, or verapamil may cause additive myocardial depression.
- Additive bradycardia may occur with cardiac glycosides.
- Additive hypotension may occur with use of other antihypertensive agents, or with acute ingestion of alcohol or nitrates.
- Concurrent use of esmolol with amphetamines, cocaine, ephedrine, epinephrine, norepinephrine, phenylephrine, or pseudoephedrine may result in excess alpha-adrenergic stimulation, hypertension, and bradycardia.
- Esmolol may negate the beneficial beta$_1$ cardiac effects of dopamine or dobutamine.
- Concurrent thyroid administration may decrease effectiveness.
- Use of esmolol with insulin may result in prolonged hypoglycemia.
- Esmolol may prolong the effects of succinylcholine.
- Concurrent use of esmolol with morphine may increase activity of esmolol.

- Use esmolol cautiously in patients with thyrotoxicosis or hypoglycemia (symptoms may be masked).
- Safe use in pregnancy, lactation, or children younger than 18 years has not been established (Pregnancy Category C).

Toxicity and Overdose Alert

- Monitor patient for signs of overdose (bradycardia, severe dizziness or fainting, severe drowsiness, dyspnea, bluish fingernails or palms, seizures). • Treatment of esmolol overdose is symptomatic and supportive. Due to the short action of esmolol, discontinuation of therapy may relieve acute toxicity. • Symptomatic bradycardia may be treated with atropine, isoproterenol, dobutamine, epinephrine, or a transvenous pacemaker. • Premature ventricular contractions may be treated with lidocaine or phenytoin. Avoid the use of quinidine, procainamide, or disopyramide, because they further depress myocardial function. • Congestive heart failure may be treated with oxygen, cardiac glycosides, and/or diuretics. • Hypotension may be treated with Trendelenburg position and IV fluids unless contraindicated. Vasopressors (epinephrine, norepinephrine, dopamine, dobutamine) may also be used. Hypotension does not respond to beta$_2$ agonists. • Glucagon has been used to treat bradycardia and hypotension. • A beta-adrenergic agonist (isoproterenol) and/or theophylline may be used to treat bronchospasm.

Lab Test Considerations

- Monitor blood sugar closely in diabetic patients, because esmolol may mask signs and symptoms of hypoglycemia and may potentiate insulin-induced hypoglycemia.

Patient/Family Teaching

- Caution patient to make position changes slowly to minimize orthostatic hypotension. • May cause drowsiness and dizziness. Caution patient to call for assistance during ambulation or transfer.

≋ PHARMACOLOGIC PROFILE

Indications
• Esmolol is used in the short-term management of supraventricular tachyarrhythmias. It is also used to lower heart rate and blood pressure during surgical procedures.

Action
• Esmolol blocks stimulation of beta$_1$ (myocardial) receptor sites, with less effect on beta$_2$ (pulmonary and vascular) receptor sites. This results in decreased heart rate, decreased contractility, lowering of blood pressure, and decreased AV conduction. Esmolol slows the ventricular response in supraventricular tachyarrhythmias.

Time/Action Profile (cardiovascular effects)

Onset	Peak	Duration
minutes	UK	1–20 min

Pharmacokinetics
• **Distribution:** Esmolol is rapidly and widely distributed.
• **Metabolism and Excretion:** Metabolism of esmolol is accomplished by enzymes in red blood cells and the liver.
• **Half-life:** 9 minutes.

Contraindications
• Esmolol should not be used in patients with uncompensated congestive heart failure, pulmonary edema, cardiogenic shock, bradycardia, or second- or third-degree heart block. The 250 mg/ml concentration contains alcohol and should be avoided in patients with known intolerance.

Adverse Reactions and Side Effects*
• **CNS:** <u>dizziness</u>, <u>headache</u>, confusion, agitation, somnolence, weakness • **EENT:** visual disturbances • **Resp:** bronchospasm, wheezing • **CV:** <u>hypotension</u>, chest pain, pulmonary edema, PVCs, ECG changes, bradycardia • **GI:** <u>nausea</u>, vomiting, constipation, abdominal pain, dyspepsia • **GU:** urinary retention • **Derm:** rash • **Local:** <u>phlebitis</u> at IV site • **Misc:** peripheral ischemia, fever, chills.

---

*<u>Underlines</u> indicate most frequent; CAPITALS indicate life-threatening.

Ethacrynate Sodium	Diuretic (loop)
Edecrin	pH 6.3–7.7

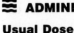 ADMINISTRATION CONSIDERATIONS

Usual Dose
ADULTS: 50 mg or 500 mcg (0.5 mg)–1 mg/kg; may repeat in 2–4 hr, then q 4–6 hr (doses may be repeated hourly in emergent situations).
CHILDREN: 0.5–1 mg/kg q 8–12 hr.

Dilution
• **Direct IV: Reconstitute** with 50 ml of D5W or 0.9% NaCl for a concentration of 1 mg/ml. • Do not use hazy or opalescent solutions. Discard unused solutions after 24 hours.

Compatibility
• **Y-site:** potassium chloride ◆ vitamin B complex with C.
• **Additive:** chlorpromazine ◆ cimetidine ◆ prochlorperazine ◆ promazine.

Incompatibility
• **Additive:** hydralazine ◆ procainamide ◆ ranitidine ◆ tolazoline ◆ triflupromazine.

Rate of Administration
• **Direct IV:** May be injected through Y tubing or a 3-way stopcock at a rate of 10 mg over 2–3 minutes. • Infusion is the preferred route. • **Intermittent Infusion:** Administer total dose over 20–30 minutes.

CLINICAL PRECAUTIONS

• Rotate injection sites with each dose to prevent thrombophlebitis.
• Assess fluid status throughout therapy. Monitor daily weight, intake and output ratios, amount and location of edema, lung sounds, skin turgor, and mucous membranes. If dry mouth, lethargy, weakness, hypotension, or oliguria occurs, dose may need to be reduced or drug discontinued.

- Monitor blood pressure and pulse before and during therapy. Additive hypotension may occur with use of antihypertensives or acute ingestion of alcohol or nitrates.
- Assess for allergy to sulfonamides.
- Assess patients receiving cardiac glycosides for anorexia, vomiting, muscle cramps, paresthesia, or confusion. Hypokalemia increases the risk of cardiac glycoside toxicity. Additive hypokalemia occurs with other diuretics, ticarcillin, mezlocillin, amphotericin B, and glucocorticoids.
- Assess patient for tinnitus and hearing loss. Audiometry is recommended for patients receiving prolonged therapy. Hearing loss is more common following high-dose or rapid IV administration in patients with decreased renal function or those receiving other ototoxic drugs. Assessment of auditory function may be difficult in geriatric or very young patients.
- Use cautiously in patients with severe liver disease, electrolyte depletion, diabetes mellitus, anuria, or increasing azotemia. Elderly patients may be more sensitive to ethacrynate.
- Ethacrynate may increase the effectiveness of oral anticoagulants.
- Ethacrynate increases lithium excretion, may cause toxicity.
- Safe use during pregnancy or lactation has not been established (Pregnancy Category B).

Lab Test Considerations

- Monitor electrolytes, renal and hepatic function, glucose, and uric acid levels prior to and periodically during therapy. • May cause decreased calcium, chloride, magnesium, potassium, and sodium concentrations. • Ethacrynate also may elevate blood glucose, BUN, and uric acid levels.

Patient/Family Teaching

- Caution patient to change positions slowly to minimize orthostatic hypotension. • Advise patient to contact physician immediately if muscle weakness, cramps, nausea, dizziness, numbness, or tingling of extremities occurs.

≋ PHARMACOLOGIC PROFILE

Indications

• Ethacrynate is used to manage edema secondary to congestive heart failure, or to hepatic or renal disease. • Ethacrynate has also been used in the short-term management of pulmonary edema and of ascites due to malignancy, idiopathic edema, and lymphedema.

Action

• Ethacrynate inhibits the resorption of sodium and chloride from the loop of Henle and distal renal tubule, while increasing renal excretion of water, sodium, chloride, magnesium, hydrogen, and calcium. • Its diuretic effect persists despite impaired renal function.

Time/Action Profile (diuresis)

Onset	Peak	Duration
5 min	15–30 min	2 hr

Pharmacokinetics

• **Distribution:** UK. • **Metabolism and Excretion:** Ethacrynate is partially metabolized by the liver; 35–40% is excreted in bile with some renal excretion of unchanged drug. • **Half-life:** 1 hour.

Contraindications

• Ethacrynate should not be used in patients with a history of hypersensitivity to it. Cross-sensitivity with thiazides and sulfonamides may occur.

Adverse Reactions and Side Effects*

• **CNS:** dizziness, headache, encephalopathy • **EENT:** hearing loss, tinnitus • **CV:** hypotension • **GI:** nausea, vomiting, diarrhea, constipation, dry mouth • **GU:** frequency • **F and E:** metabolic alkalosis, hypovolemia, dehydration, hyponatremia, hypokalemia, hypochloremia, hypomagnesemia • **Derm:** rashes • **Metab:** hyperglycemia, hyperuricemia • **MS:** muscle cramps • **Misc:** increased BUN.

---

*Underlines indicate most frequent; CAPITALS indicate life-threatening.

Etidronate Disodium

Hypocalcemic agent (biphosphonate)

Didronel IV   pH 4–5.5

☰ ADMINISTRATION CONSIDERATIONS

Usual Dose

ADULTS: 7.5 mg/kg/day for 3 days. Therapy may be repeated again after 1-wk rest period. If therapy is continued for 7 days, the risk of hypocalcemia is greatly increased.

Dilution

• **Intermittent Infusion: Dilute** in at least 250 ml of 0.9% NaCl. • Solution is stable for 48 hours.

Incompatibility

• Information unavailable. Do not admix with other drugs or solutions.

Rate of Administration

• **Intermittent Infusion:** Infuse over at least 2 hours.

☰ CLINICAL PRECAUTIONS

• Monitor symptoms of hypercalcemia (nausea, vomiting, anorexia, weakness, constipation, thirst, and cardiac arrhythmias).
• Observe patient carefully for evidence of hypocalcemia (paresthesia, muscle twitching, laryngospasm, colic, cardiac arrhythmias, and Chvostek's or Trousseau's sign). Protect symptomatic patients by elevating and padding side rails; keep bed in low position. Risk of hypocalcemia is greatest after 3 days of continuous IV therapy.
• Hypocalcemic effect may be additive with calcitonin.
• Use with caution in patients with long bone fractures, enterocolitis, or congestive heart failure. Patients with moderate renal impairment (serum creatinine 2.5–4.9 mg/dl) may require dosage reduction.
• Safe use in pregnancy, lactation, or children has not been established (Pregnancy Category C).

Lab Test Considerations

• Monitor serum calcium and albumin levels to determine effectiveness of therapy. • Monitor BUN and creatinine levels prior to and periodically throughout course of therapy. • Stable or reversible increases in BUN and creatinine may occur. • Etidronate interferes with bone uptake of technetium Tc 99m in diagnostic scans.

Patient/Family Teaching

• Explain to patient that metallic taste is not uncommon and usually disappears in a few hours. • Advise patient to report signs of hypercalcemic relapse (bone pain, anorexia, nausea, vomiting, thirst, lethargy) to physician promptly. • Emphasize need for keeping follow-up appointments to monitor progress, even after medication is discontinued, in order to detect relapse.

 PHARMACOLOGIC PROFILE

Indications

• Etidronate is used with other agents (saline diuresis) in the management of hypercalcemia associated with malignancies.

Action

• Etidronate blocks the growth of calcium hydroxyapatite crystals by binding to calcium phosphate. This effect results in decreased bone resorption and turnover.

Time/Action Profile (decreased urinary calcium excretion)

Onset	Peak	Duration
24 hr	3 days	11 days

Pharmacokinetics

• **Distribution:** Etidronate is bound to hydroxyapatite crystals in areas of increased osteogenesis. • **Metabolism and Excretion:** 50% of etidronate is excreted unchanged by the kidneys. • **Half-life:** 5–7 hours.

Contraindications

• Etidronate is contraindicated in patients with previous hypersensitivity. • Patients with severe renal impairment (serum creatinine >5 mg/dl) should not receive etidronate. • Etidronate should not be used to manage hypercalcemia due to hyperparathyroidism.

Adverse Reactions and Side Effects*

• **GI:** diarrhea, nausea, loss of taste, metallic taste • **GU:** nephrotoxicity • **Derm:** rash • **MS:** <u>bone pain</u>, <u>bone tenderness</u>, microfractures.

Etomidate	General anesthetic (nonbarbiturate hypnotic)
Amidate	pH 4–7

 ADMINISTRATION CONSIDERATIONS

Usual Dose

Induction

ADULTS AND CHILDREN >**10 yr:** 300 mcg (0.3 mg)/kg (range 200–600 mcg/kg).

Dilution

• **Direct IV:** May be administered **undiluted**.

Rate of Administration

• **Direct IV:** Administer each dose over 30–60 seconds.

 CLINICAL PRECAUTIONS

• Etomidate should be administered only by individuals trained in the administration of general anesthetics and in the management of potential complications of general anesthesia.
• Assess respiratory status throughout use.

---

*<u>Underlines</u> indicate most frequent; CAPITALS indicate life-threatening.

- Administer in large proximal arm vein to minimize pain on injection.
- Monitor pulse and blood pressure continuously during use.
- Opioid analgesics, such as fentanyl, may be administered immediately prior to use of etomidate to minimize pain of injection and involuntary muscle movements. Recovery period is shortened by the use of fentanyl, allowing for lower doses of etomidate. Diazepam may also be used to minimize muscle movements. Dosage of neuromuscular blocking agents does not have to be altered when they are used with etomidate.
- CNS depression may be increased by concurrent use of alcohol, antihistamines, opioid analgesics, or other sedative/hypnotics.
- Concurrent use of antihypertensives may increase the risk of hypotension.
- Safe use in pregnancy, lactation, or children younger than 10 years old has not been established (Pregnancy Category C).

Patient/Family Teaching

- Explain the purpose of the medication to the patient.

PHARMACOLOGIC PROFILE

Indications

- Etomidate is used for the induction of general anesthesia. It has also been used as a supplement to other agents such as nitrous oxide in order to maintain anesthesia during surgical procedures of short duration.

Action

- Etomidate may produce CNS depression by having effects similar to those of gamma-aminobutyric acid (GABA), an inhibitory neurotransmitter. It appears to depress activity/reactivity of the brainstem reticular formation. • Etomidate has no analgesic activity.

Time/Action Profile (hypnotic effect)

Onset	Peak	Duration
within 1 min	UK	3–5 min

Pharmacokinetics
• **Distribution:** UK. • **Metabolism and Excretion:** Etomidate is rapidly metabolized by the liver to inactive metabolites. • **Half-life:** 75 minutes.

Contraindications
• Etomidate is contraindicated in patients with known hypersensitivity to it or propylene glycol.

Adverse Reactions and Side Effects*
• **EENT:** eye movement, snoring • **Resp:** hyperventilation, hypoventilation, brief apnea, laryngospasm • **CV:** hypertension, hypotension, tachycardia, bradycardia, arrhythmias • **GI:** postoperative nausea and vomiting • **Endo:** adrenal suppression • **Local:** <u>transient pain at IV site</u> • **MS:** <u>transient myoclonic muscle movements</u>, tonic movements, averting movements • **Misc:** hiccups.

Etoposide	Antineoplastic (podophyllotoxin derivative)
VP–16, VePesid	pH 3–4

 ADMINISTRATION CONSIDERATIONS

Usual Dose

Testicular Neoplasms
ADULTS: 50–100 mg/m^2 daily for 5 days; repeat q 3–4 wk up to 100 mg/m^2 on days 1, 3, and 5 q 3–4 wk.

Small-Cell Carcinoma of the Lung
ADULTS: from 35 mg/m^2 daily for 4 days up to 50 mg/m^2 daily for 5 days q 3–4 wk.

Dilution
• **Intermittent Infusion:** Dilute 5-ml vial with 250–500 ml of D5W or 0.9% NaCl for a concentration of 0.4–0.2 mg/ml. • Avoid contact with the skin. Use Luer-Lok tubing to

---

*<u>Underlines</u> indicate most frequent; CAPITALS indicate life-threatening.

prevent accidental leakage. If contact with skin occurs, immediately wash skin with soap and water. • Solution should be prepared in a biologic cabinet. Wear gloves, gown, and mask while handling medication. Discard equipment in designated containers. • The 0.2-mg/ml solution is stable for 96 hours. The 0.4-mg/ml solution is stable for 48 hours. Concentrations greater than 0.4 mg/ml are not recommended, as crystallization is likely. Discard solution if crystals are present.

Compatibility

• **Solution:** D5W • 0.9% NaCl • lactated Ringer's injection.

• **Y-site:** allopurinol sodium • fludarabine • melphalan • ondansetron • paclitaxel • piperacillin/tazobactam • sargramostim • vinorelbine.

• **Additive:** cisplatin • floxuridine • fluorouracil • hydroxyzine • ifosfamide.

Incompatibility

• **Y-site:** filgrastim • gallium nitrate • idarubicin.

Rate of Administration

• **Intermittent Infusion:** Infuse slowly over at least 30–60 minutes.

≋ CLINICAL PRECAUTIONS

- Monitor blood pressure prior to and every 15 minutes during infusion. If hypotension occurs, stop the infusion. After stabilizing the blood pressure with IV fluids and supportive measures, infusion may be resumed at slower rate.
- Monitor for hypersensitivity reaction (fever, chills, pruritus, urticaria, bronchospasm, tachycardia, hypotension). If these occur, stop the infusion. Keep epinephrine, an antihistamine, and resuscitative equipment close by in the event of an anaphylactic reaction.
- Monitor IV site carefully; etoposide is an irritant. If solution extravasates, inject 1–4 ml of a mixture of 150 units of hyaluronidase and 1 ml of NaCl through the existing cannula, or if needle has been removed, 1 ml for each ml extravasated. Apply warm compresses to increase systemic absorption of the drug.

- Monitor for bone marrow depression. Assess for fever, chills, sore throat, and signs of infection. Assess for bleeding (bleeding gums, bruising, petechiae; guaiac test stools, urine, and emesis). Avoid giving IM injections and taking rectal temperatures. Apply pressure to venipuncture sites for 10 minutes. Additive bone marrow depression may occur with other antineoplastic agents or radiation therapy.
- Monitor intake and output, appetite, and nutritional intake. Etoposide causes nausea and vomiting in 30% of patients. Prophylactic use of an antiemetic may be helpful. Adjust diet as tolerated to help maintain fluid and electrolyte balance and nutritional status.
- Use cautiously in patients with active infections, decreased bone marrow reserve, or other chronic debilitating illnesses.
- Patients with hepatic or renal impairment may require dosage reduction.
- Use cautiously in patients with child-bearing potential. Etoposide should not be used during pregnancy or lactation (Pregnancy Category D).

Lab Test Considerations

- Monitor CBC and differential prior to and periodically throughout therapy. The nadir of leukopenia occurs in 7–14 days. The nadir of thrombocytopenia occurs in 9–16 days. Recovery of leukopenia and thrombocytopenia occurs in 20 days. • Monitor liver function studies (AST [SGOT], ALT [SGPT], LDH, bilirubin) and renal function studies (BUN, creatinine) prior to and periodically throughout therapy to detect hepatotoxicity and nephrotoxicity.

Patient/Family Teaching

- Advise patient to notify physician in case of fever, chills, sore throat, signs of infection, bleeding gums, bruising, petechiae, or blood in urine, stool, or emesis. • Caution patient to avoid crowds and persons with known infections. Instruct patient to use soft toothbrush and electric razor. • Patient should be cautioned not to drink alcoholic beverages or take products containing aspirin, ibuprofen, or naproxen. • Instruct patient to notify physician if abdominal pain, yellow skin, weakness, paresthesia, or gait disturbances occur. • Instruct patient to inspect oral mucosa for redness and ulceration. If mouth sores occur, advise patient to use sponge brush and rinse mouth with water after eating and drinking. • Discuss with patient the possibility of hair loss; hair usually grows back after treatment ends. Explore coping strategies. • Advise patient to use a nonhormonal method of contraception. • Instruct patient not to receive any vaccinations without advice of physician. • Emphasize the need for periodic lab tests to monitor for side effects.

PHARMACOLOGIC PROFILE

Indications

• Etoposide is used alone and in combination with other treatment modalities (other antineoplastic agents, radiation therapy, surgery) in the management of refractory testicular neoplasms and small-cell carcinoma of the lung.

Action

• Etoposide damages DNA prior to mitosis (cycle-dependent and phase-specific), resulting in death of rapidly replicating cells, particularly malignant ones.

Time/Action Profile (effects on blood counts)

Onset	Peak	Duration
14 days	16 days	20 days

Pharmacokinetics

• **Distribution:** Rapidly distributed; does not appear to enter the CSF significantly but does appear to cross the placenta. Enters breast milk. • **Metabolism and Excretion:** Some metabolism by the liver; 45% excreted unchanged by the kidneys. • **Half-life:** 7 hours (range 3–12 hours).

Contraindications

• Etoposide is contraindicated in patients with hypersensitivity to it or to polysorbates, benzyl alcohol, polyethylene glycol, ethyl alcohol, or citric acid. • It should not be used during pregnancy or lactation.

Adverse Reactions and Side Effects*

• **CNS:** somnolence, fatigue, headache, vertigo • **Resp:** bronchospasm, pulmonary edema • **CV:** <u>hypotension</u>, myocardial infarction, congestive heart failure • **GI:** <u>nausea</u>, <u>vomiting</u> • **Hemat:** <u>leukopenia</u>, <u>thrombocytopenia</u> • **Local:** phlebitis at IV site • **Derm:** <u>alopecia</u> • **Endo:** gonadal suppression • **MS:** muscle cramps • **Neuro:** peripheral neuropathy • **Misc:** allergic reactions, including anaphylaxis, fever.

Factor IX Complex (human) Coagulation Factor IX (human)	*Blood derivative (clotting factor)*
AlphaNine, AlphaNine SD, Bebulin VH, Christmas factor, Konȳne 80, Mononine, Profilnine Heat-Treated, Proplex T	pH 6.4–7.2

 ADMINISTRATION CONSIDERATIONS

Usual Dose

The following formula may be used: Dose (units) = 1 unit/kg body weight (kg) × desired increase (% normal in Factor IX activity).

FACTOR IX COMPLEX (HUMAN)

Bebulin VH, Konȳne 80, Profilnine Heat-Treated, Proplex T

Prevention of Bleeding in Patients with Hemophilia B

ADULTS AND CHILDREN: 20–40 units twice weekly.

Treatment of Severe Bleeding in Patients with Hemophilia B

ADULTS AND CHILDREN: Amount necessary to establish 20–60% of normal Factor IX activity or 60–70 units/kg q 10–12 hr for 2–3 days.

---

*<u>Underlines</u> indicate most frequent; CAPITALS indicate life-threatening.

Treatment of Mild to Moderate Bleeding in Patients with Hemophilia B

ADULTS AND CHILDREN: Amount necessary to establish 20–40% of normal Factor IX activity or 25–55 units/kg once daily for 1–2 days.

Control of Bleeding Following Dental Surgery in Patients with Hemophilia B

ADULTS AND CHILDREN: Amount necessary to establish 40–60% of normal Factor IX activity or 50–60 units/kg given 1 hr prior to procedure; may be repeated.

Control of Bleeding Following Other Surgical Procedures in Patients with Hemophilia B

ADULTS AND CHILDREN: Amount necessary to establish 25–60% of normal Factor IX activity or 50–95 units/kg given 1 hr prior to procedure and q 12–24 hr for at least 7 days.

Treatment of Bleeding in Patients with Hemophilia A and Inhibitors of Factor VIII

ADULTS AND CHILDREN: 75 units/kg; may be repeated in 12 hr.

Reversal of Oral Anticoagulant Activity

ADULTS AND CHILDREN: 1500 units (additional vitamin K may be required).

Control of Bleeding in Patients with Factor VII Deficiency (Proplex T)

ADULTS AND CHILDREN: 0.5 units/kg × body weight (kg) × desired increase in Factor VII (% of normal). For surgical procedures, raise level of Factor VII above 25% (40–60% of normal). Repeat q 4–6 hr for at least 7 days.

COAGULATION FACTOR IX (HUMAN)

AlphaNine SD, Mononine

Prevention of Bleeding in Patients with Hemophilia B

ADULTS AND CHILDREN: Amount necessary to establish 15–25% of normal Factor IX activity or 20–30 units/kg; may be repeated after 24 hr.

Treatment of Severe Bleeding in Patients with Hemophilia B

ADULTS AND CHILDREN: Amount necessary to establish 25–50% of normal Factor IX activity or up to 75 units/kg; may be repeated q 18–30 hr as needed.

Treatment of Mild to Moderate Bleeding in Patients with Hemophilia B

ADULTS AND CHILDREN: Amount necessary to establish 20–30% of normal Factor IX activity.

Control of Bleeding after Dental Surgery in Patients with Hemophilia B

ADULTS AND CHILDREN: Amount necessary to establish 50% of normal Factor IX activity given right before procedure; may be repeated if necessary.

Dilution

• **Direct IV:** Refrigerate concentrate until just prior to reconstitution. Warm diluent (sterile water for injection) to room temperature before reconstituting. Use plastic syringe for preparation and administration. Use the filter needle provided by the manufacturer as an air vent to the vial when reconstituting. After adding diluent, rotate vial gently until completely dissolved. Reconstitution generally requires 5–10 minutes for Factor IX complex and 1–5 minutes for coagulation Factor IX. • Do not refrigerate after reconstitution. Begin administration within 3 hours. • Dry concentrates should be refrigerated, however. *Konȳne 80, Profilnine Heat-Treated,* and *Mononine* can be stored at room temperature for up to 1 month. • Discard partially used vials.

Compatibility

• **Additive:** Heparin may be added to prothrombin complex concentrates at a concentration of 5–10 units/ml of the reconstituted solution. The addition of heparin may reduce the likelihood of the development of thrombotic complications.

Incompatibility

• **Additive:** Reconstitute only with diluent provided. Administer through a separate line. Do not mix with other solutions or medications.

Rate of Administration

• **Direct IV:** Rate of administration should be individualized according to the specific product and the response of the patient. Administer *AlphaNine, AlphaNine SD,* and *Profilnine* at a rate not to exceed 10 ml/min. *Mononine* should be administered at a rate of approximately 2 ml/min. Administer *Konȳne 80* at a rate of 100 units/min. Administer *Proplex T* at a rate of 2–3 ml/min. *Bebulin VH* may be administered at a rate not to exceed 2 ml/min. Temporarily stop infusion and resume at slower rate if facial flushing or tingling occurs.

≋ CLINICAL PRECAUTIONS

- Monitor blood pressure, pulse, and respirations frequently.
- If a hypersensitivity reaction (fever, chills, tingling, headache, urticaria, changes in blood pressure or pulse, nausea and vomiting, lethargy) occurs, slow infusion. Pyrogenic reactions (fever, chills) may also occur and are more common with high doses.
- Obtain history of current trauma; estimate amount of blood loss.
- Monitor for renewed or increased bleeding every 15–30 minutes. Immobilize and apply ice to affected joints.
- Monitor intake and output ratios; note color of the urine. Notify the physician if a significant discrepancy occurs or urine becomes red or orange. Patients with type A, B, or AB blood are particularly at risk for hemolytic reaction.
- Hepatitis B vaccine may be administered prior to therapy to prevent hepatitis.
- Inform all personnel of the patient's bleeding tendency, to prevent further trauma. Apply pressure to all venipuncture sites.
- Use of Factor IX complex with aminocaproic acid may increase the risk of thrombosis.
- Use cautiously following surgical procedures, due to increased risk of thrombosis.
- Safe use in pregnancy or lactation has not been established (Pregnancy Category C).

Lab Test Considerations

- Monitor coagulation studies (activated partial thromboplastin time [APTT], plasma fibrinogen, platelet count, prothrombin time [PT], Factor IX plasma concentrations) before, during, and after therapy to assess effectiveness of therapy. Dosage varies with degree of clotting factor deficit, desired level of clotting factors, and weight. • To control bleeding after major trauma or surgery, Factor IX levels should be maintained at 25–60% of normal for at least 1 week. • Obtain type and crossmatch of blood in case a transfusion is necessary.

Patient/Family Teaching

• Instruct patient to notify nurse immediately if bleeding recurs. • Advise patient to carry identification describing disease process at all times. • Caution patient to avoid products containing aspirin, ibuprofen, or naproxen, as they may further impair clotting. • Review with patient methods of preventing bleeding (use soft toothbrush, avoid IM and SC injections, avoid potentially traumatic activities). • Advise patient that the risk of hepatitis or AIDS transmission may be diminished by the use of heat-treated preparations. Current screening programs and vaccination with hepatitis B vaccine should help decrease the risk.

PHARMACOLOGIC PROFILE

Indications

• Factor IX complex is used in the treatment of active or impending bleeding due to Factor IX deficiency (hemophilia B, Christmas disease), in the treatment of bleeding in patients with Factor VIII inhibitors, and in the prevention and treatment of bleeding in patients with Factor VII deficiency. • It is also used to rapidly reverse the effect of oral anticoagulants in emergency situations.

Action

• Factor IX complex contains blood coagulation Factors II, VII, IX, and X. It provides replacement of deficient Factor IX in hemophilia B, which results in restoration of hemostasis.

Time/Action Profile (hemostasis)

Onset	Peak	Duration
immediate	UK	1–2 days

Pharmacokinetics

• **Distribution:** UK. • **Metabolism and Excretion:** Factor IX is rapidly cleared from plasma by utilization in clotting process. • **Half-life:** *Factor IX* 24–32 hours; *Factor VII* 5–6 hours.

Contraindications

• Factor IX complex should be avoided in patients with Factor VII deficiency (except *Proplex T*), or intravascular coagulation or fibrinolysis associated with liver disease. Mononine is contraindicated in patients with hypersensitivity to mouse protein. Some products contain heparin and should not be used in patients with hypersensitivity.

Adverse Reactions and Side Effects*

• **CNS:** headache, somnolence, lethargy • **CV:** changes in heart rate, changes in blood pressure • **GI:** nausea, vomiting • **Derm:** flushing, urticaria • **Hemat:** thrombosis, disseminated intravascular coagulation • **Neuro:** tingling • **Misc:** fever, chills, risk of transmission of viral hepatitis, risk of transmission of HIV virus, hypersensitivity reactions.

Famotidine	Antiulcer
	(histamine H₂ blocker)
Pepcid	pH 5–5.6

 ADMINISTRATION CONSIDERATIONS

Usual Dose

ADULTS: 20 mg q 12 hr.
CHILDREN: 0.3–0.8 mg/kg q 8 hr (unlabeled).

Dilution

• **Direct IV: Dilute** 2 ml (10 mg/ml solution) in 5 or 10 ml of 0.9% NaCl for injection. • **Intermittent Infusion: Dilute** each 20 mg in 100 ml of 0.9% NaCl, D5W, D10W, lactated Ringer's solution, or sodium bicarbonate. • Diluted solution is stable for 48 hours at room temperature. Do not use solution that is discolored or contains a precipitate.

Compatibility

• **Y-site:** allopurinol sodium ✦ aminophylline ✦ ampicillin ✦ ampicillin/sulbactam ✦ amrinone ✦ atropine ✦ bretylium

---

*Underlines indicate most frequent; CAPITALS indicate life-threatening.

• calcium gluconate • cefazolin • cefoperazone • cefotaxime • cefotetan • cefoxitin • ceftazidime • ceftizoxime • cefurox-ime • cephalothin • cephapirin • cisplatin • cyclophospha-mide • cytarabine • dexamethasone sodium phosphate • dex-tran 40 • digoxin • dobutamine • dopamine • doxorubicin • enalaprilat • epinephrine • erythromycin lactobionate • es-molol • filgrastim • fluconazole • fludarabine • folic acid • furosemide • gentamicin • haloperidol • heparin • hydro-cortisone sodium succinate • imipenem/cilastatin • insulin • isoproterenol • labetalol • lidocaine • magnesium sulfate • melphalan • meperidine • methotrexate • methylpred-nisolone • metoclopramide • mezlocillin • midazolam • mor-phine • nafcillin • nitroglycerin • nitroprusside • norepineph-rine • ondansetron • oxacillin • paclitaxel • perphenazine • phenylephrine • phenytoin • phytonadione • piperacil-lin • potassium chloride • potassium phosphate • procaina-mide • sargramostim • sodium bicarbonate • theophylline • thiamine • ticarcillin • ticarcillin/clavulanate • verapamil • vinorelbine.

Incompatibility
• **Y-site:** piperacillin/tazobactam.

Rate of Administration
• **Direct IV:** Administer over at least 2 minutes. Rapid ad-ministration may cause hypotension. • **Intermittent Infu-sion:** Administer over 15–30 minutes.

≋ CLINICAL PRECAUTIONS

• Assess patient routinely for epigastric or abdominal pain and frank or occult blood in the stool, emesis, or gastric aspirate.
• Elderly patients with active ulcer disease may need a longer course of therapy (more than 6–8 weeks).
• Use cautiously in patients with severe renal impair-ment—dosage reduction or increased dosing interval is recommended if creatinine clearance is less than 10 ml/min.
• Famotidine decreases the absorption of ketoconazole.
• Safe use in pregnancy, lactation, or children is not estab-lished (Pregnancy Category B).

Lab Test Considerations

• CBC with differential should be monitored periodically throughout therapy. • May cause elevated serum transaminase. • Famotidine antagonizes effects of pentagastrin and histamine during gastric acid secretion tests. Avoid administration during the 24 hours preceding the test. • Famotidine may cause false-negative results in skin tests using allergen extracts and should be discontinued prior to the test.

Patient/Family Teaching

• Inform patient that smoking interferes with the action of famotidine. Encourage patient to quit smoking or at least not to smoke after last dose of the day. • Famotidine may cause drowsiness or dizziness. Caution patient to avoid activities requiring alertness until response to the drug is known. • Advise patient to promptly report onset of black, tarry stools; fever; diarrhea; dizziness; or rash.

PHARMACOLOGIC PROFILE

Indications

• Famotidine is used in the short-term and maintenance treatment of active duodenal ulcers. It is also used in the management of gastric hypersecretory states (Zollinger-Ellison syndrome).

Action

• Famotidine inhibits the action of histamine at the H_2 receptor site located primarily in gastric parietal cells, thereby inhibiting gastric acid secretion. Inhibition of gastric acid secretion promotes healing and prevention of ulcers.

Time/Action Profile (inhibition of gastric acid secretion)

Onset	Peak	Duration
within 1 hr	0.5–3 hr	8–15 hr

Pharmacokinetics

• **Distribution:** Famotidine crosses the placenta, but does not enter CSF. • **Metabolism and Excretion:** Up to 70% of famotidine is eliminated unchanged by the kidneys; 30–35%

is metabolized by the liver. • **Half-life:** 2.5–3.5 hours (increased in renal impairment).

Contraindications
• Famotidine is contraindicated in patients with hypersensitivity to it or to benzyl alcohol (multidose vials).

Adverse Reactions and Side Effects*
• **CNS:** <u>dizziness</u>, <u>headache</u>, drowsiness • **EENT:** swelling of eyelids, tinnitus • **Resp:** bronchospasm • **CV:** palpitations, bradycardia, hypotension • **GI:** diarrhea, nausea, <u>constipation</u>, dry mouth • **Derm:** facial edema, loss of hair, rash • **MS:** joint pain, muscle pain • **Misc:** fever.

Fat Emulsion	*Caloric agent*
Intralipid, Liposyn II, Liposyn III	pH 8–8.3

≋ ADMINISTRATION CONSIDERATIONS
Usual Dose

Total Parenteral Nutrition
ADULTS: not to exceed 3 g fat/kg/day.
CHILDREN: not to exceed 4 g fat/kg/day.
PREMATURE INFANTS: 0.5 g fat/kg/day initially; may be increased as tolerated up to 3 g fat/kg/day.

Essential Fatty Acid Deficiency
ADULTS AND CHILDREN: Provide 8–10% of caloric intake as fat.

Dilution
• **Intermittent Infusion:** Emulsions that have separated or appear oily should not be used. • Maximum hang times are 12 hours for *Intralipid,* 24 hours for fat emulsion alone, and 24 hours for admixtures with dextrose and amino acids. Discard all unused portions. • Fat emulsion may be stored at room temperature.

---

*<u>Underlines</u> indicate most frequent; CAPITALS indicate life-threatening.

Compatibility

• **Y-site:** ampicillin • cefamandole • cefazolin • cefoxitin • cephapirin • clindamycin • digoxin • dopamine • erythromycin lactobionate • furosemide • gentamicin • isoproterenol • kanamycin • lidocaine • norepinephrine • oxacillin • penicillin G potassium • ticarcillin • tobramycin.

• **Additive:** Fat emulsion may be admixed ("3-in-1," all-in-one, triple mix total nutrient admixture [TNA]) or administered simultaneously with amino acid and dextrose solution. • Compatible with • Intralipid with FreAmine II 8.5% • FreAmine III 8.5% • Travasol without electrolytes 8.5% and 10% • Veinamine 8% • cimetidine • diphenhydramine • famotidine • hydrocortisone • multivitamins • nizatidine • Dextrose Injection 10% and 70%. • While not generally recommended, heparin may be added in a concentration of 1–2 units/ml prior to administration to increase clearance rate of lipemia, minimize risks associated with hypercoagulability, and prevent catheter thrombosis.

Incompatibility

• **Y-site:** amikacin.

• **Additive:** Although compatibility studies have been done, manufacturer recommends that fat emulsion not be admixed or piggybacked with any other medication.

Rate of Administration

• **Intermittent Infusion:** For adults, the initial infusion rate should be 1 ml/min for the 10% solution and 0.5 ml/min for the 20% solution for the first 15–30 minutes. If no adverse reactions occur, the rate may be increased to infuse 500 ml over 4–6 hours for the 10% solution and 250 ml over 4–6 hours or 500 ml over 8 hours for the 20% solution. Daily dose should not exceed 3 g/kg. • No more than 500 ml of the 10% solution should be infused the first day. Dose may be increased on subsequent days. • No more than 500 ml of the 20% solution of Intralipid should be infused the first day. Dose may be increased the following day. • For children, the initial infusion rate should be 0.1 ml/min of the 10% solution and 0.05 ml/min for the 20% solution for the first 10–15 minutes. If no adverse reactions occur, the rate may be increased to 1 g/kg over 4 hours. Do not exceed a rate of 100 ml/hr for the 10% solution or 50 ml/hr for the 20% solution. Daily dose should not exceed 4 g/kg. • Administer via infusion pump to ensure accurate rate.

≋ CLINICAL PRECAUTIONS

- Monitor weight every other day in adults and daily in infants and children receiving fat emulsion to assist in meeting caloric requirements.
- Assess patient for allergy to eggs prior to initiation of therapy. Acute hypersensitivity reaction with pruritic urticaria may occur in patients allergic to eggs.
- Fat emulsion should comprise no more than 60% of patient's total caloric intake. The remaining 40% should consist of carbohydrates and amino acids.
- Fat emulsion may be administered via peripheral or central venous catheter. Monitor peripheral sites for phlebitis. Manufacturer does not recommend use of filters during administration; but 1.2-micron filters have been used. Use tubing provided by the manufacturer. Change IV tubing after each dose of fat emulsion.
- Due to the lower specific gravity of fat emulsion, it must be hung higher than the amino acid and dextrose to prevent the fat emulsion from backing up into the amino acid and dextrose line. May also be administered in solution with dextrose and amino acids.
- Use cautiously in patients with, or at risk of, thromboembolic disorders including fat embolism, severe liver or pulmonary disease, anemia, or bleeding disorders.
- Use cautiously in preterm infants. Excess infusion rates may lead to pulmonary intravascular fat accumulation and death. Allow for lipemia to clear between daily infusions. Lower infusion rates are recommended.
- Safe use in pregnancy has not been established (Pregnancy Category C).

Toxicity and Overdose Alert

- If signs of overloading syndrome (focal seizures, fever, leukocytosis, splenomegaly, shock) or elevated triglyceride or free fatty acid levels occur, infusion should be stopped and the plasma lipid clearance re-evaluated prior to reinstituting therapy.

Lab Test Considerations

- Monitor triglyceride and fatty acid levels weekly to determine patient's capacity to eliminate infused fat from the circulation. • Monitor hemoglobin, blood coagulation, and platelet count weekly, especially during continuous therapy. • Monitor serum bilirubin, cholesterol, phospholipid, and triglyceride concentrations and hepatic function weekly, especially in premature infants to prevent hyperlipemia.

Patient/Family Teaching

• Explain the purpose of fat emulsion to the patient prior to administration.

PHARMACOLOGIC PROFILE

Indications

• Fat emulsion provides nonprotein calories to patients whose total caloric needs cannot be met by carbohydrate (glucose) alone, usually as part of parenteral nutrition. It is also used in the treatment and prevention of essential fatty acid deficiency in patients receiving long-term parenteral nutrition.

Action

• Fat emulsion acts as a source of nonprotein calories and essential fatty acids.

Time/Action Profile

Onset	Peak	Duration
UK	UK	UK

Pharmacokinetics

• **Distribution:** Fat emulsion distributes into intravascular space. • **Metabolism and Excretion:** Fat emulsion is cleared by conversion to triglycerides, then to free fatty acids and glycerol by lipoprotein lipase. Free fatty acids are transported to tissues, where they may be oxidized as an energy source or restored as triglycerides. • **Half-life:** UK.

Contraindications

• Fat emulsion should not be given to patients with hyperlipidemias, lipoid nephrosis, or acute pancreatitis accompanied by lipemia. • Patients with hypersensitivity to egg products should not receive fat emulsion (emulsifier is egg yolk phospholipid).

Adverse Reactions and Side Effects*

• **CV:** chest pain • **GI:** vomiting, hepatomegaly†, spleno-megaly • **Derm:** jaundice† • **Local:** <u>phlebitis</u> at IV site • **Misc:** <u>fever</u>, chills, shivering, overload syndrome†, <u>infection</u>, hypersensitivity reactions.

Fentanyl Citrate	Opioid analgesic (agonist)
Sublimaze	pH 4–7.5

Schedule II

ADMINISTRATION CONSIDERATIONS

Usual Dose

Adjunct to General Anesthesia (major surgical procedures)

ADULTS: *Low dose*—2 mcg/kg. *Moderate dose*—2–20 mcg/kg; additional doses of 25–100 mcg may be given as necessary. *High dose*—20–50 mcg/kg; additional doses ranging from 25 mcg to 50% of original dose may be repeated as necessary.

Adjunct to General Anesthesia (minor surgical procedures)

ADULTS: 2 mcg (0.002 mg)/kg.

Adjunct to Regional Anesthesia

ADULTS: 50–100 mcg (0.05–0.1 mg).

---

*<u>Underlines</u> indicate most frequent; CAPITALS indicate life-threatening.

†Seen only with long-term use.

To Provide General Anesthesia

ADULTS: 50–100 mcg (0.05–0.1 mg)/kg (up to 150 mcg/kg) with oxygen or oxygen plus nitrous oxide and a neuromuscular blocking agent.

CHILDREN 2–12 yr: 2–3 mcg (0.002–0.003 mg)/kg.

Dilution

• **Direct IV:** May be administered **undiluted**. • **Continuous Infusion:** May also be **diluted** with D5W, 0.9% NaCl, D5/LR, or lactated Ringer's solution for infusion.

Compatibility

• **Syringe:** atracurium • atropine • butorphanol • chlorpromazine • cimetidine • dimenhydrinate • diphenhydramine • droperidol • heparin • hydromorphone • hydroxyzine • meperidine • metoclopramide • midazolam • morphine • pentazocine • perphenazine • prochlorperazine edisylate • promazine • promethazine • ranitidine • scopolamine.

• **Y-site:** atracurium • enalaprilat • esmolol • heparin • hydrocortisone sodium succinate • labetalol • nafcillin • pancuronium • potassium chloride • sargramostim • vecuronium • vitamin B complex with C.

• **Additive:** bupivacaine.

Incompatibility

• **Syringe:** pentobarbital.
• **Additive:** methohexital • pentobarbital • thiopental.

Rate of Administration

• **Direct IV:** Administer slowly over at least 1–2 minutes. Slow IV administration may reduce the incidence or severity of muscle rigidity, bradycardia, or hypotension. • **Continuous Infusion:** Administer until the onset of somnolence, as an adjunct to general anesthesia.

≋ CLINICAL PRECAUTIONS

• Monitor respiratory rate and blood pressure frequently throughout course of therapy. The respiratory depressant effects of fentanyl last longer than the analgesic effects. Subsequent opioid doses should be reduced by ¼ to ½ of the usually recommended dose. Monitor closely.

• Assess type, location, and intensity of pain prior to and

1–2 minutes following IV administration when fentanyl is used to treat pain.

- Benzodiazepines may be administered prior to administration of fentanyl to reduce the induction dose requirements and decrease the time to loss of consciousness. This combination may also increase the risk of hypotension. If benzodiazepines are used, dosage of fentanyl may need to be reduced.

- Opioid antagonist (naloxone), oxygen, and resuscitative equipment should be readily available during the administration of fentanyl.

- Fentanyl may cause additive CNS and respiratory depression with other CNS depressants, including alcohol, antihistamines, antidepresssants, and other sedative/hypnotics.

- Avoid use in patients who have received MAO inhibitors within the previous 14 days (may produce unpredictable, potentially fatal reactions).

- Use cautiously in elderly or debilitated patients, severely ill patients, diabetics; patients with severe pulmonary or hepatic disease, CNS tumors, increased intracranial pressure, head trauma, adrenal insufficiency, undiagnosed abdominal pain, hypothyroidism, alcoholism, or cardiac disease (particularly arrhythmias). Neonates are more likely to experience respiratory depression.

- Safe use in pregnancy, lactation, and children less than 2 years of age is not established (Pregnancy Category C).

Toxicity and Overdose Alert

- Atropine may be used to treat bradycardia. Use of a neuromuscular blocking agent with vagolytic activity, such as pancuronium or gallamine, may prevent bradycardia caused by fentanyl. • If respiratory depression persists following surgery, prolonged mechanical ventilation may be necessary. If an opioid antagonist is required to reverse respiratory depression or coma, naloxone (Narcan) is the antidote. Dilute the 0.4-mg ampule of naloxone in 10 ml of 0.9% NaCl and administer 0.5 ml (0.02 mg) by direct IV push every 2 minutes. For children and patients weighing <40 kg, dilute 0.1 mg of naloxone in 10 ml of 0.9% NaCl for a concentration of 10 mcg/ml and administer 0.5 mcg every 1–2 minutes. Titrate the dose to avoid withdrawal, seizures, and severe pain. Administration of naloxone in these circumstances, especially in cardiac patients, has resulted in hypertension and tachycardia, occasionally causing left ventricular failure and pulmonary edema. Monitor respiratory status continuously; the duration of respiratory depression may exceed the duration of a dose of naloxone. Continuous infusion of naloxone may be required (see *naloxone hydrochloride* monograph on page 690). • If hypotension occurs, administer parenteral fluids, position patient to improve venous return to the heart when surgical conditions permit, and administer a vasopressor as necessary. • If muscle rigidity occurs during surgery, a neuromuscular blocking agent and mechanical ventilation should be used. Muscle rigidity occurring on emergence may be treated with naloxone.

Lab Test Considerations

• Fentanyl may cause elevated serum amylase and lipase concentrations.

Patient/Family Teaching

• Caution patient to make position changes slowly to minimize orthostatic hypotension. • Fentanyl causes dizziness and drowsiness. Advise patient to call for assistance during ambulation and transfer, and to avoid driving or other activities requiring alertness for 24 hours after administration of fentanyl during outpatient surgery. • Instruct patient to avoid alcohol, antihistamines, or other CNS depressants for 24 hours after administration of fentanyl for outpatient surgery, because of additive CNS depression.

☰ PHARMACOLOGIC PROFILE

Indications

• Fentanyl is used in the management of perioperative, intraoperative, and postoperative pain. It is also used in the treatment and prevention of perioperative tachypnea and emergence delirium and as a supplement to general or regional analgesia. • The combination of fentanyl with droperidol produces neuroleptanalgesia (quiescence, decreased motor activity, and analgesia without loss of consciousness). See *droperidol/fentanyl* monograph on page 364.

Action

• Fentanyl binds to opiate receptors in the CNS, altering the response to and perception of pain. It also produces CNS depression.

Time/Action Profile (analgesic effect)

Onset	Peak	Duration
1–2 min	3–5 min	30–60 min

Pharmacokinetics

• **Distribution:** UK. • **Metabolism and Excretion:** Fentanyl is mostly metabolized by the liver; 10–25% is excreted unchanged by the kidneys. • **Half-life:** 3.6 hours (increased after cardiopulmonary bypass and in elderly patients).

Contraindications

• Fentanyl is contraindicated in patients with known hypersensitivity or intolerance.

Adverse Reactions and Side Effects*

• **CNS:** euphoria, floating feeling, dysphoria, hallucinations, depression, excessive sedation • **Resp:** respiratory depression, APNEA, laryngospasm, bronchoconstriction • **CV:** bradycardia • **GI:** constipation, nausea, vomiting • **MS:** skeletal and thoracic muscle rigidity.

Filgrastim   *Colony stimulating factor*

Neupogen, G-CSF, granulocyte-colony
stimulating factor   pH 4

≋ ADMINISTRATION CONSIDERATIONS

Usual Dose

Bone Marrow Depression Following Chemotherapy

ADULTS: 5 mcg (0.005 mg)/kg/day as a single injection daily for up to 2 wk, until absolute neutrophil count reaches

---

*Underlines indicate most frequent; CAPITALS indicate life-threatening.

10,000/mm^3 following expected nadir of chemotherapy-induced neutropenia. Dosage may be increased by 5 mcg/kg during each cycle of chemotherapy, depending on severity of neutropenia.

Bone Marrow Depression Following Bone Marrow Transplant

ADULTS: 10 mcg (0.010 mg)/kg/day. If absolute neutrophil count (ANC) remains >1000/mm^3 for 3 days, decrease to 5 mcg (0.005 mg)/kg/day. If ANC still remains >1000/mm^3 for 3 days, stop filgrastim. If ANC drops to <1000/mm^3 initiate therapy at 5 mcg/kg/day.

Dilution

• **Intermittent Infusion:** Dilute in D5W to produce a concentration of ≥15 mcg of filgrastim/ml. If the final concentration is 2–15 mcg/ml, human albumin, 2 mg/ml (0.2%) or 2 ml of 5% human albumin in 50 ml of D5W, must be added to D5W before filgrastim to prevent absorption of the components of the drug delivery system. Refrigerate; do not freeze. Do not shake. May warm to room temperature for up to 6 hours prior to injection. Discard if left at room temperature for more than 6 hours. Vial is for one-time use only.

Compatibility

• **Y-site:** acyclovir • allopurinol sodium • amikacin • aminophylline • ampicillin • ampicillin/sulbactam • aztreonam • bleomycin • bumetanide • buprenorphine • butorphanol • calcium gluconate • carboplatin • carmustine • cefazolin • cefotetan • ceftazidime • chlorpromazine • cimetidine • cisplatin • cyclophosphamide • cytarabine • dacarbazine • daunorubicin • dexamethasone • diphenhydramine • doxorubicin • doxycycline • droperidol • enalaprilat • famotidine • floxuridine • fluconazole • fludarabine • gallium nitrate • ganciclovir • gentamicin • haloperidol • hydrocortisone • hydromorphone • hydroxyzine • idarubicin • ifosfamide • imipenem/cilastatin • leucovorin calcium • lorazepam • mechlorethamine • melphalan • meperidine • mesna • methotrexate • metoclopramide • miconazole • minocycline • mitoxantrone • morphine • nalbuphine • netilmicin • ondansetron • plicamycin • potassium chloride • promethazine • ranitidine • sodium bicarbonate • streptozocin • ticarcillin • ticarcillin/clavulanate • tobramycin • vancomycin • vinblastine • vincristine • vinorelbine • zidovudine.

Incompatibility

• **Y-site:** amphotericin ♦ cefonicid ♦ cefoperazone ♦ cefotaxime ♦ cefoxitin ♦ ceftizoxime ♦ ceftriaxone ♦ cefuroxime
♦ clindamycin ♦ dactinomycin ♦ etoposide ♦ fluorouracil
♦ furosemide ♦ heparin ♦ mannitol ♦ methylprednisolone
sodium succinate ♦ metronidazole ♦ mezlocillin ♦ mitomycin
♦ piperacillin ♦ prochlorperazine ♦ thiotepa.

Rate of Administration

• **Intermittent Infusion:** *Following chemotherapy,* dose is
administered via infusion over 15–30 minutes. • **Continuous Infusion:** Dose *following chemotherapy* may also be administered as a continuous infusion. *Following bone marrow
transplant,* dose should be administered as an infusion over
4 or 24 hours.

≋ CLINICAL PRECAUTIONS

- Administer no earlier than 24 hours following cytotoxic
  chemotherapy, not during the 24 hours before administration of chemotherapy, and not during 12 hours before
  or after radiotherapy. Simultaneous use with antineoplastic agents may have adverse effects on rapidly prolif-
  erating neutrophils.
- Monitor heart rate, blood pressure, and respiratory status prior to and periodically during therapy.
- Assess pain throughout therapy. Arthralgias or myalgias
  usually occur in the lower extremities when granulocyte
  counts are returning to normal. Medullary bone pain is
  common and dose related, but usually resolves with continued treatment. Bone pain occurs in sites containing
  bone marrow (sternum, spine, pelvis, long bones), is
  probably caused by bone marrow expansion, and occurs
  1–3 days before myeloid recovery. Pain is usually mild to
  moderate and controllable with analgesics.
- Use with caution in patients with malignancies with myeloid characteristics or pre-existing cardiac disease. Cardiac monitoring should be used in patients with pre-
  existing cardiac conditions.
- Safe use in pregnancy, lactation, or children has not
  been established (Pregnancy Category C).

Lab Test Considerations

• *Following chemotherapy,* obtain a CBC with differential, including examination for the presence of blast cells, and platelet count prior to chemotherapy and twice weekly during therapy to avoid leukocytosis. Monitor absolute neutrophil count (ANC). A transient rise is seen 1–2 days after initiation of therapy, but therapy should not be discontinued until ANC is more than $10,000/mm^3$. • *Following bone marrow transplant,* the daily dose is titrated by the neutrophil response. When the ANC is $>1000/mm^3$ for 3 consecutive days, the dose should be reduced to 5 mcg/kg/day. If the ANC remains $>1000/m^3$ for 3 or more consecutive days, filgrastim is discontinued. If the ANC decreases to $<1000/mm^3$, filgrastim should be resumed at 5 mcg/kg/day. • May cause transient increases in uric acid, LDH, and alkaline phosphatase concentrations.

Patient/Family Teaching

• **Home Care Issues:** Instruct patient on correct technique and proper disposal for home administration. Caution patient not to reuse needle, vial, or syringe. Provide patient with a puncture-proof container for needle and syringe disposal.

 PHARMACOLOGIC PROFILE

Indications

• Filgrastim is used in the prevention of febrile neutropenia and associated infection in patients who have received bone marrow–depressing antineoplastic agents for the treatment of nonmyeloid malignancies or who have undergone bone marrow transplantation.

Action

• Filgrastim is a glycoprotein that binds to immature neutrophils and stimulates them to divide and differentiate. It also activates mature neutrophils. This decreases the incidence of infection in patients who received bone marrow–depressing antineoplastic agents.

Time/Action Profile (effect on white blood cell count)

Onset	Peak	Duration
4 hr	within 24 hr	1–7 days†

†Return of neutrophil count to baseline.

Pharmacokinetics
• **Distribution:** UK. • **Metabolism and Excretion:** UK. • **Half-life:** UK.

Contraindications
• Filgrastim is contraindicated in patients with hypersensitivity to *Escherichia coli*–derived proteins or to mannitol.

Adverse Reactions and Side Effects*
• **Resp:** respiratory distress syndrome • **CV:** hypotension, myocardial infarction, arrhythmias • **MS:** medullary bone pain, arthralgias, myalgias.

Fluconazole	*Antifungal*
Diflucan	pH 4–8

≋ ADMINISTRATION CONSIDERATIONS

Usual Dose

Cryptococcal Meningitis
ADULTS: *Treatment*—400 mg once daily (or q 12 hr for first 2 days) until favorable clinical response, then 200–400 mg once daily for at least 10–12 wk following clearing of cerebrospinal fluid; change to oral therapy as soon as possible. *Suppressive therapy*—200 mg once daily.

Oropharyngeal Candidiasis
ADULTS: 200 mg initially, then 100 mg daily for at least 14 days.

---

*Underlines indicate most frequent; CAPITALS indicate life-threatening.

Esophageal Candidiasis
ADULTS: 200 mg initially, then 100 mg once daily for at least 3 wk, or for 2 wk following symptomatic improvement (up to 400 mg/day has been used).

Systemic Candidiasis
ADULTS: *Treatment*—400 mg initially, then 200 mg once daily for 4 wk or for at least 2 wk following symptomatic improvement. *Prevention*—400 mg once daily.

Dilution
• **Intermittent Infusion:** Available in 200 mg/100 ml or 400 mg/200 ml solution. Open overwrap immediately before infusion. Inner bag may have slight opacity that will diminish gradually. Do not administer solution that is cloudy or has a precipitate. Check for leaks by squeezing inner bag. If leak is found, discard container as unsterile. Do not set tubing as part of a series of connections, as this may cause an air embolism.

Compatibility
• **Y-site:** acyclovir • allopurinol sodium • amikacin • aminophylline • ampicillin/sulbactam • aztreonam • benztropine • cefazolin • cefotetan • cefoxitin • chlorpromazine • cimetidine • dexamethasone sodium phosphate • diphenhydramine • droperidol • famotidine • filgrastim • fludarabine • foscarnet • gallium nitrate • ganciclovir • gentamicin • heparin • hydrocortisone sodium phosphate • immune globulin • leucovorin • melphalan • meperidine • metronidazole • midazolam • morphine • nafcillin • ondansetron • oxacillin • paclitaxel • penicillin G potassium • phenytoin • piperacillin/tazobactam • prochlorperazine • promethazine • sargramostim • tacrolimus • ticarcillin/clavulanate • tobramycin • vancomycin • vinorelbine • zidovudine.

• **Additive:** acyclovir • amikacin • amphotericin B • cefazolin • ceftazidime • clindamycin • gentamicin • heparin • metronidazole • morphine • piperacillin • potassium chloride • theophylline. However, manufacturer does not recommend admixing fluconazole with other medications.

Incompatibility
• **Y-site:** amphotericin B • ampicillin • calcium gluconate • cefotaxime • ceftazidime • ceftriaxone • cefuroxime • chloramphenicol • clindamycin • diazepam • digoxin • erythromycin lactobionate • furosemide • haloperidol • hydroxyzine

• imipenem/cilastatin • pentamidine • piperacillin • ticarcillin • trimethoprim/sulfamethoxazole.

• **Additive:** trimethoprim/sulfamethoxazole.

Rate of Administration

• **Intermittent Infusion:** Infuse at a maximum rate of 200 mg/hr.

≋ CLINICAL PRECAUTIONS

• Specimens for culture should be taken prior to instituting therapy. Therapy may be started before results are obtained.
• Assess infected area and monitor CSF cultures prior to and periodically throughout therapy.
• Fluconazole increases the activity of warfarin. Rifampin decreases blood levels of fluconazole. Fluconazole increases the hypoglycemic effects of tolbutamide, glyburide, or glipizide. Fluconazole increases blood levels of cyclosporine and phenytoin.
• Use cautiously in patients with renal impairment. Dosage reduction or increased dosing interval is required if creatinine clearance is 50 ml/min or less. Use cautiously in patients with underlying liver disease and in geriatric patients.
• Safe use in pregnancy, lactation, or children has not been established (Pregnancy Category C).

Lab Test Considerations

• BUN and serum creatinine should be monitored prior to and periodically during therapy; patients with renal dysfunction will require dosage adjustment. • Liver function tests should be monitored prior to and periodically throughout course of therapy. May cause increased AST (SGOT), ALT (SGPT), serum alkaline phosphate, and bilirubin concentrations.

Patient/Family Teaching

• Instruct patient to notify physician if abdominal pain, fever, or diarrhea becomes pronounced or if signs and symptoms of liver dysfunction (unusual fatigue, anorexia, nausea, vomiting, jaundice, dark urine, or pale stools) occur.

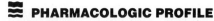 PHARMACOLOGIC PROFILE

Indications

• Fluconazole is used in the treatment of fungal infections due to susceptible organisms, including oropharyngeal or esophageal candidiasis, serious systemic candidal infections, urinary tract infections, peritonitis, and cryptococcal meningitis.

Action

• Fluconazole inhibits synthesis of fungal sterols, a necessary component of the cell wall. It exerts a fungistatic action against susceptible organisms, but may be fungicidal in higher concentrations. Fluconazole is active against *Cryptococcus neoformans* and *Candida* species.

Time/Action Profile (blood levels)

Onset	Peak
rapid	end of infusion

Pharmacokinetics

• **Distribution:** Fluconazole is widely distributed, with good penetration into CSF, eye, and peritoneum. • **Metabolism and Excretion:** More than 80% of fluconazole is excreted unchanged by the kidneys. Less than 10% is metabolized by the liver. • **Half-life:** 30 hours (increased in renal impairment).

Contraindications

• Fluconazole is contraindicated in patients with hypersensitivity to fluconazole or other azole antifungals.

Adverse Reactions and Side Effects*

Note: Incidence of adverse reactions is increased in patients with AIDS.

• **CNS:** headache • **GI:** nausea, vomiting, abdominal discomfort, diarrhea, HEPATOTOXICITY • **Derm:** exfoliative skin disorders including STEVENS-JOHNSON SYNDROME.

---

*Underlines indicate most frequent; CAPITALS indicate life-threatening.

Fludarabine Phosphate	*Antineoplastic agent* *(antimetabolite)*
Fludara	pH 7.2–8.2

≋ ADMINISTRATION CONSIDERATIONS

Usual Dose

ADULTS: 25 mg/m^2 daily for 5 days; repeat course q 28 days.

Dilution

• **Intermittent Infusion: Reconstitute** with 2 ml of sterile water for injection; solid cake should dissolve in less than 15 seconds. • Solution should be prepared in a biologic cabinet. Wear gloves, gown, and mask while handling IV medication. Discard IV equipment in specially designated containers (see Appendix F). • Reconstituted solution is stable for 8 hours. • **Dilute further** in 100–125 ml of 0.9% NaCl or D5W.

Compatibility

• **Y-site:** allopurinol sodium • amikacin • aminophylline • ampicillin • ampicillin/sulbactam • aztreonam • bleomycin • butorphanol • carboplatin • carmustine • cefazolin • cefoperazone • ceforanide • cefotaxime • cefotetan • ceftazidime • ceftizoxime • ceftriaxone • cefuroxime • cimetidine • cisplatin • clindamycin • cyclophosphamide • cytarabine • dacarbazine • dactinomycin • dexamethasone • diphenhydramine • doxorubicin • doxycycline • droperidol • etoposide • famotidine • floxuridine • fluconazole • fluorouracil • furosemide • gentamicin • haloperidol • heparin • hydrocortisone sodium phosphate • hydrocortisone sodium succinate • hydromorphone • ifosfamide • imipenem/cilastatin • lorazepam • magnesium sulfate • mannitol • mechlorethamine • meperidine • mesna • methotrexate • methylprednisolone • metoclopramide • mezlocillin • minocycline • mitoxantrone • morphine • multivitamins • nalbuphine • netilmicin • ondansetron • pentostatin • piperacillin • piperacillin/tazobactam • potassium chloride • promethazine • ranitidine • sodium bicarbonate • ticarcillin • ticarcillin/clavulanate • tobramycin • trimethoprim/sulfamethoxazole • vancomycin • vinblastine • vincristine • vinorelbine • zidovudine.

Incompatibility

• **Y-site:** acyclovir ✦ amphotericin B ✦ chlorpromazine ✦ daunorubicin ✦ ganciclovir ✦ hydroxyzine ✦ miconazole ✦ prochlorperazine.

Rate of Administration

• **Intermittent Infusion:** Infuse over 30 minutes.

≋ CLINICAL PRECAUTIONS

• Monitor respiratory status, intake and output ratios, and daily weights.
• Assess nutritional status. Administering an antiemetic prior to and periodically throughout therapy and adjusting diet as tolerated may help maintain fluid and electrolyte balance and nutritional status.
• May cause tumor lysis syndrome resulting in hyperuricemia, hyperphosphatemia, hypocalcemia, metabolic acidosis, hyperkalemia, hematuria, urate crystalluria, and renal failure. Monitor for flank pain and hematuria.
• Assess patient for visual changes, weakness, confusion, and changes in level of consciousness throughout and for 60 days following therapy; neurologic effects resulting in blindness, coma, and death have been reported.
• Monitor for bone marrow depression. Assess for fever, sore throat, and signs of infection. Assess for bleeding (bleeding gums, bruising, petechiae; guaiac test stools, urine, emesis). Avoid administering IM injections and taking rectal temperatures. Hold pressure on all venipuncture sites for at least 10 minutes. Anemia may occur. Monitor for increased fatigue, dyspnea, and orthostatic hypotension. Additive bone marrow suppression may occur with concurrent use of other antineoplastic agents or radiation therapy.
• Use with caution in patients with pre-existing bone marrow depression or chronic debilitating illness.
• Use cautiously in patients with renal impairment; dosage reduction may be necessary.
• Safe use in children has not been established. Use cautiously in patients with childbearing potential; avoid during pregnancy or lactation (Pregnancy Category D).

Lab Test Considerations

• Monitor CBC, differential, and platelet counts prior to and frequently throughout therapy. The nadir for granulocytes occurs in 13 days (range 3–25 days) and for platelets in 16 days (range 2–32 days) after administration.

Patient/Family Teaching

• Caution patient to avoid crowds and persons with known infections. Physician should be informed immediately if symptoms of infection occur. Instruct patient to report unusual bleeding. Advise patient of thrombocytopenia precautions (use soft toothbrush and electric razor; avoid falls). • Patients should be instructed not to drink alcoholic beverages or take medication containing aspirin, ibuprofen, or naproxen, as these may precipitate gastric bleeding. • Instruct patient to inspect oral mucosa for redness and ulceration. If mouth sores occur, advise patient to use sponge brush and rinse mouth with water after eating and drinking. Consult physician if pain interferes with eating. • Advise patient that this medication may have teratogenic effects. A nonhormonal method of contraception should be used during therapy and for at least 4 months after therapy is concluded. • Instruct patient not to receive any vaccinations without advice of physician. Fludarabine may decrease antibody response to live virus vaccines and increase the risk of adverse reactions. • Emphasize the need for periodic lab tests to monitor for side effects.

≋ PHARMACOLOGIC PROFILE

Indications

• Fludarabine is used in the treatment of B-cell chronic lymphocytic leukemia unresponsive to standard therapy.

Action

• Fludarabine is converted intracellularly to an active phosphorylated metabolite, which then inhibits DNA synthesis. This active compound results in death of rapidly replicating cells, particularly malignant ones.

Time/Action Profile (effect on blood counts)

Onset	Peak	Duration
UK	13–16 days	UK

Pharmacokinetics

• **Distribution:** UK. • **Metabolism and Excretion:** Following administration, fludarabine is rapidly converted to an active metabolite, which when phosphorylated intracellularly exerts antineoplastic activity. Twenty-three percent of initial active metabolite is excreted unchanged by the kidneys. • **Half-life:** 10 hours (for initial active metabolite).

Contraindications

• Fludarabine is contraindicated in patients with hypersensitivity to fludarabine, mannitol, or sodium hydroxide. Fludarabine should not be used during pregnancy or lactation.

Adverse Reactions and Side Effects*

• **CNS:** neurotoxicity, malaise, <u>fatigue</u>, <u>weakness</u>, agitation, confusion, visual disturbances, coma • **EENT:** blindness • **Resp:** pulmonary hypersensitivity, cough dyspnea • **CV:** <u>edema</u> • **GI:** <u>nausea</u>, <u>vomiting</u>, <u>anorexia</u>, <u>diarrhea</u>, GI bleeding, stomatitis • **Derm:** rashes • **Endo:** gonadal suppression • **Hemat:** <u>anemia</u>, <u>leukopenia</u>, <u>thrombocytopenia</u> • **MS:** <u>myalgia</u> • **Neuro:** peripheral neuropathy • **Misc:** tumor lysis syndrome.

Flumazenil	*Benzodiazepine antagonist*
Mazicon	pH 4

ADMINISTRATION CONSIDERATIONS

Usual Dose

Reversal of Benzodiazepine Effects Following Conscious Sedation or General Anesthesia

ADULTS: 0.2 mg; additional doses may be given at 1-min intervals until desired results are obtained, up to a total dose of 1 mg. If resedation occurs, up to 1 mg may be given every 20 min (not to exceed 3 mg/hr).

---

*<u>Underlines</u> indicate most frequent; CAPITALS indicate lifethreatening.

Suspected Benzodiazepine Overdose

ADULTS: 0.2 mg; if desired response is not obtained, a second dose of 0.3 mg may be given 30 sec later. Additional doses of 0.5 mg may be given at 1-min intervals if necessary, to a total dose of 3 mg. Usual dose required is 1–3 mg. If resedation occurs, additional doses may be given at 20-min intervals, giving not more than 1 mg at a time, not to exceed 3 mg in any hr.

Dilution

• **Direct IV:** May be administered **undiluted** or **diluted** in syringe with D5W, 0.9% NaCl, or lactated Ringer's solution.
• Diluted solution should be discarded after 24 hours.

Incompatibility

• Information unavailable. Do not mix with other drugs or solutions. • Flush existing line with 0.9% NaCl prior to administration.

Rate of Administration

• **Direct IV:** Administer each dose over 15 seconds following conscious sedation or general anesthesia. For suspected benzodiazepine overdose, administer over 30 seconds.

≋ CLINICAL PRECAUTIONS

- Ensure that patient has a patent airway and vascular access before administration of flumazenil.
- Observe IV site frequently for redness or irritation. Administer through a free-flowing IV infusion into a large vein to minimize pain at the injection site.
- Optimal emergence should be undertaken slowly to decrease undesirable effects including confusion, agitation, emotional lability, and perceptual distortion.
- Institute seizure precautions. Seizures are more likely to occur in patients who are experiencing sedative/hypnotic withdrawal, patients who have recently received repeated doses of benzodiazepines, or patients who have a prior history of seizure activity. Seizures may be treated with benzodiazepines, barbiturates, or phenytoin. Larger-than-normal doses of benzodiazepines may be required. In these high-risk patients, increasing the interval between flumazenil doses may be necessary.

- In cases of overdose, attempt to assess time of ingestion, and amount and type of benzodiazepine taken. Knowledge of agent ingested allows an estimate of duration of CNS depression, especially in mixed overdoses.
- Observe patient for at least 2 hours for the appearance of resedation. Hypoventilation may occur.
- Safe use in pregnancy, lactation, or children has not been established (Pregnancy Category C). Flumazenil is not recommended for use during labor and delivery.

Patient/Family Teaching

- Flumazenil does not consistently reverse the amnestic effects of benzodiazepines. Provide patient and family with written instructions for postprocedure care. Inform family that patient may appear alert at the time of discharge but the sedative effects of the benzodiazepine may recur. Instruct patient to avoid driving or other activities requiring alertness for at least 18–24 hours after discharge. • Instruct patient not to take any alcohol or nonprescription drugs for at least 18–24 hours after discharge. • Resumption of usual activities should occur only when no residual effects of the benzodiazepine remain.

≋ PHARMACOLOGIC PROFILE

Indications

- Flumazenil is used to completely or partially reverse the effects of benzodiazepines when they are used as general anesthetics, or during diagnostic or therapeutic procedures. Flumazenil is also used in the management of intentional or accidental overdosage of benzodiazepines.

Action

- Flumazenil is a benzodiazepine derivative that antagonizes the CNS depressant effects of benzodiazepine compounds. It has no effect on CNS depression of other causes including opioid analgesics, alcohol, barbiturates, or general anesthetics.

Time/Action Profile

Onset	Peak	Duration
1–2 min	6–10 min	UK

Pharmacokinetics

• **Distribution:** UK. • **Metabolism and Excretion:** Metabolism of flumazenil occurs primarily in the liver. • **Half-life:** 41–79 minutes.

Contraindications

• Flumazenil is contraindicated in patients with hypersensitivity to it, to parabens, or benzodiazepines. • Patients who are receiving chronic benzodiazepine therapy for life-threatening medical problems, including status epilepticus or increased intracranial pressure, should not be given flumazenil. • Cases of serious antidepressant overdosage should not be managed with flumazenil.

Adverse Reactions and Side Effects*

• **CNS:** <u>dizziness</u>, agitation, emotional lability, headache, fatigue, SEIZURES, confusion, somnolence, sleep disorders • **EENT:** abnormal vision, blurred vision, abnormal hearing • **CV:** arrhythmias, chest pain, hypertension • **GI:** <u>nausea</u>, <u>vomiting</u>, hiccups • **Derm:** sweating, flushing • **Local:** pain at injection site, injection site reactions, phlebitis • **Neuro:** paresthesia • **Misc:** rigors, shivering.

Fluorouracil	Antineoplastic agent (antimetabolite)
Adrucil, Efudex, Fluoroplex, 5-Fluorouracil, 5-FU	pH 9.2

ADMINISTRATION CONSIDERATIONS

Usual Dose

Doses may vary greatly, depending on tumor, patient condition, and protocol used.

Advanced Colorectal Cancer

ADULTS: 370 mg/m^2, preceded by leucovorin, or 425 mg/m^2, preceded by leucovorin; daily for 5 days. May be re-

---

*<u>Underlines</u> indicate most frequent; CAPITALS indicate life-threatening.

peated at 4–5 wk intervals. See *leucovorin calcium* monograph on page 554.

Other Tumors

ADULTS: *Initial therapy*—7–12 mg/kg/day for 4 days, followed by a 3-day rest; if no toxicity has occurred, then 7–10 mg/kg q 3–4 days for total of 2 weeks *or* 12 mg/kg/day for 4 days, followed by 1 day of rest; if no toxicity has occurred, then 6 mg/kg every other day for a total of 12 days. *Maintenance therapy*—7–12 mg/kg q 7–16 days *or* 300–500 mg/m²/day for 4–5 days given monthly. *Poor-risk patients*—3–6 mg/kg/day for 3 days; followed by 1 day of rest; if no toxicity has occurred, then 3 mg/kg every other day for 3 doses as initial therapy.

Dilution

• **Direct IV:** May be administered **undiluted.** • **Intermittent Infusion:** May be **diluted** with D5W or 0.9% NaCl. • Solution for IV administration should be prepared in a biologic cabinet. Wear gloves, gown, and mask while handling IV medication. Discard IV equipment in specially designated containers (see Appendix F). • Use plastic IV tubing and IV bags to maintain greater stability of medication. Solution is colorless to light yellow; slight discoloration does not affect potency. Discard highly discolored or cloudy solutions. Solution is stable for 24 hours at room temperature; do not refrigerate. If crystals form, dissolve by warming solution to 140°F, shaking vigorously, and cooling to body temperature.

Compatibility

• **Syringe:** bleomycin ◆ cisplatin ◆ cyclophosphamide ◆ furosemide ◆ heparin ◆ leucovorin ◆ methotrexate ◆ metoclopramide ◆ mitomycin ◆ vinblastine ◆ vincristine. Mix immediately before use.

• **Y-site:** allopurinol sodium ◆ bleomycin ◆ cisplatin ◆ cyclophosphamide ◆ doxorubicin ◆ fludarabine ◆ furosemide ◆ heparin ◆ hydrocortisone sodium succinate ◆ leucovorin ◆ mannitol ◆ melphalan ◆ methotrexate ◆ metoclopramide ◆ mitomycin ◆ paclitaxel ◆ piperacillin/tazobactam ◆ potassium chloride ◆ sargramostim ◆ vinblastine ◆ vincristine ◆ vitamin B complex with C.

• **Additive:** bleomycin ◆ cephalothin ◆ cyclophosphamide ◆ etoposide ◆ floxuridine ◆ ifosfamide ◆ leucovorin ◆ methotrexate ◆ prednisolone ◆ vincristine.

Incompatibility

- **Syringe:** droperidol.
- **Y-site:** droperidol ✦ filgrastim ✦ gallium nitrate ✦ vinorelbine.
- **Additive:** carboplatin ✦ cisplatin ✦ cytarabine ✦ diazepam ✦ doxorubicin.

Rate of Administration

- **Direct IV:** Rapid IV push administration (over 1–2 minutes) is most effective, but there is a more rapid onset of toxicity. • **Intermittent Infusion:** Onset of toxicity is greatly delayed by administering an infusion over 2–8 hours.

≋ CLINICAL PRECAUTIONS

- The number 5 in 5-fluorouracil is part of the drug name and does not refer to the dosage. Dosage of fluorouracil should be based on ideal body weight in obese or edematous patients.
- Monitor vital signs prior to and frequently during therapy.
- Assess mucous membranes, number and consistency of stools, and frequency of vomiting.
- Monitor for bone marrow depression. Assess for fever, chills, sore throat, and signs of infection. Assess for bleeding (bleeding gums, bruising, petechiae; guaiac test stools, urine, and emesis). Avoid IM injections and taking rectal temperatures. Apply pressure to venipuncture sites for 10 minutes. Additional bone marrow depression may occur with other bone marrow depressants (other antineoplastics and radiation therapy).
- Assess IV site frequently for inflammation or infiltration. Patient should notify nurse if pain or irritation at injection site occurs. Fluorouracil may cause thrombophlebitis. If extravasation occurs, infusion must be stopped and restarted in another vein to avoid damage to subcutaneous tissue. Standard treatment includes application of ice compresses.
- Monitor intake and output, appetite, and nutritional intake. GI effects usually occur on fourth day of therapy.

Adjusting diet as tolerated may help maintain fluid and electrolyte balance and nutritional status.

- Monitor patient for cerebellar dysfunction (weakness, ataxia, dizziness). This may persist after discontinuation of therapy.
- Use fluorouracil cautiously in patients with active infections, depressed bone marrow reserve, or other chronic debilitating illnesses.
- Use fluorouracil cautiously in patients with childbearing potential. Avoid during pregnancy or lactation (Pregnancy Category D). Safe use in children has not been established.

Toxicity and Overdose Alert

- If symptoms of toxicity (stomatitis or esophagopharyngitis, uncontrollable vomiting, diarrhea, GI bleeding, leukocyte count less than 3500/mm^3, platelet count less than 100,000/mm^3, or hemorrhage from any site) occur, drug will need to be discontinued. • Pretreatment with leucovorin may prevent some of the toxic effects of fluorouracil.

Lab Test Considerations

- Hepatic, renal, and hematologic functions should be monitored prior to and periodically throughout therapy. CBC should be monitored daily. Criteria for discontinuation of the medication are WBC is less than 3500/mm^3 or platelets are less than 100,000/mm^3. Leukopenia usually occurs in 9–14 days, with the nadir in 21–25 days, and recovery by day 30. Fluorouracil may also cause thrombocytopenia (nadir 7–17 days). • Fluorouracil may cause a decrease in plasma albumin.

Patient/Family Teaching

- Instruct patient to notify physician in case of fever, chills, sore throat, signs of infection, bleeding gums, bruising, petechiae, emesis, or blood in urine or stool. Caution patient to avoid crowds and persons with known infections. Instruct patient to use soft toothbrush and electric razor. Patients should be cautioned not to drink alcoholic beverages or take products containing aspirin, ibuprofen, or naproxen. • Advise patient to rinse mouth with clear water after eating and drinking and to avoid flossing to minimize stomatitis. • Discuss with patient the possibility of hair loss. Explore methods of coping. • Caution patient to use sunscreen and protective clothing to prevent photo-toxicity reactions. • Instruct patient not to receive any vaccinations without advice of physician. Fluorouracil may decrease antibody response to live virus vaccines and increase risk of adverse reactions. • Review with patient the need for nonhormonal method of contraception during therapy. • Emphasize the importance of routine follow-up lab tests to monitor progress and to check for side effects.

 PHARMACOLOGIC PROFILE

Indications

• Fluorouracil is used alone and in combination with other modalities (surgery, radiation therapy, other antineoplastic agents) in the treatment of colon, breast, rectal, gastric, and pancreatic carcinoma. Combination therapy with leucovorin calcium minimizes toxicity.

Action

• Fluorouracil inhibits DNA and RNA synthesis by preventing thymidine production (cell cycle–S phase specific). This results in death of rapidly replicating cells, particularly malignant ones.

Time/Action Profile (effects on blood counts)

Onset	Peak	Duration
1–9 days	9–21 days	30 days

Pharmacokinetics

• **Distribution:** Fluorouracil is widely distributed, concentrating in and persisting in tumors. • **Metabolism and Excretion:** Fluorouracil is converted to floxuridine monophosphate (an active metabolite). This compound undergoes cellular inactivation and metabolism by the liver. Sixty to eighty percent is excreted by the lungs as respiratory CO_2. Small amounts (less than 10–15%) are excreted unchanged by the kidneys. • **Half-life:** 20 hours.

Contraindications

• Fluorouracil is contraindicated in patients with hypersensitivity to it. • Pregnant or lactating patients should not receive fluorouracil (Pregnancy Category D).

Adverse Reactions and Side Effects*

• **CNS:** acute cerebellar dysfunction • **GI:** <u>nausea</u>, <u>vomiting</u>, <u>stomatitis</u>, <u>diarrhea</u> • **Derm:** <u>alopecia</u>, <u>maculopapular rash</u>, nail loss, melanosis of nails, phototoxicity • **Endo:** gonadal suppression • **Hemat:** <u>anemia</u>, <u>leukopenia</u>, <u>thrombocytopenia</u> • **Local:** thrombophlebitis • **Misc:** fever.

Folic Acid	*Vitamin (water soluble), Antianemic*
folate, Folvite, vitamin B₉	pH 8–11

 ADMINISTRATION CONSIDERATIONS

Usual Dose

Initial Therapy
ADULTS AND CHILDREN: up to 1 mg/day.

Maintenance Therapy
ADULTS AND CHILDREN >4 yr: 400 mcg (0.4 mg)/day.
PREGNANT AND LACTATING WOMEN: 800 mcg (0.8 mg)/day.
CHILDREN <4 yr: up to 300 mcg (0.3 mg)/day.
INFANTS: 100 mcg (0.1 mg)/day.

Dilution

• **Intermittent Infusion:** Dilute 5 mg (1 ml) in 49 ml of sterile water for injection. Color of solution ranges from yellow to orange-yellow. • **Continuous Infusion:** May be added to hyperalimentation solution.

Compatibility

• **Y-site:** famotidine.
• **Additive:** D20W.

---

*<u>Underlines</u> indicate most frequent; CAPITALS indicate life-threatening.

Incompatibility
- **Additive:** D50W ◆ calcium gluconate.

Rate of Administration
- **Intermittent Infusion:** Administer at a rate of 5 mg over at least 1 minute.

≋ CLINICAL PRECAUTIONS

- Assess patient for signs of megaloblastic anemia (fatigue, weakness, dyspnea) prior to and periodically throughout therapy.
- Folic acid should be used with caution in patients with undiagnosed anemias.
- Sulfonamides, methotrexate, trimethoprim, and triamterene prevent the activation of folic acid.
- Folic acid requirements are increased by estrogens, phenytoin, or glucocorticoids. Folic acid decreases serum phenytoin levels.
- Do not confuse with folinic acid (leucovorin calcium). See *leucovorin calcium* monograph on page 554.
- Safe use in pregnancy and lactation has been established (Pregnancy Category A). Supplemental amounts are recommended.

Lab Test Considerations

- Monitor plasma folic acid levels, hemoglobin, hematocrit, and reticulocyte count prior to and periodically during course of therapy. ● Folic acid may cause a decrease in serum concentrations of vitamin B_{12} when given in high continuous doses.

Patient/Family Teaching

- Explain that folic acid may make urine more intensely yellow. ● Instruct patient to notify physician if rash occurs, which may indicate hypersensitivity. ● Encourge patient to comply with physician's diet recommendations. Explain that the best source of vitamins is a well-balanced diet with foods from the four basic food groups. Foods high in folic acid include vegetables, fruits, and organ meats; heat destroys folic acid in foods. ● Emphasize the importance of follow-up examinations to evaluate progress.

PHARMACOLOGIC PROFILE

Indications
• Folic acid is used in the treatment of megaloblastic and macrocytic anemias. • Supplements of folic acid are given during pregnancy to promote normal fetal development.

Action
• Folic acid is required for protein synthesis and RBC function. It stimulates the production of RBCs, WBCs, and platelets. Folic acid is necessary for normal fetal development.

Time/Action Profile (increase in reticulocyte count)

Onset	Peak	Duration
3–5 days	5–10 days	UK

Pharmacokinetics
• **Distribution:** Half of all folic acid stores are in the liver. Folic acid enters breast milk and crosses the placenta. • **Metabolism and Excretion:** Folic acid is converted by the liver to its active metabolite, dihydrofolate reductase. Excess amounts are excreted unchanged by the kidneys. • **Half-life:** UK.

Contraindications
• Folic acid should not be used in patients with uncorrected pernicious anemia, as neurologic damage will progress despite correction of hematologic abnormalities. • Preparations containing benzyl alcohol should not be used in newborns.

Adverse Reactions and Side Effects*
• **Derm:** rashes • **Misc:** fever.

---

*Underlines indicate most frequent; CAPITALS indicate life-threatening.

Foscarnet Sodium · *Antiviral*
Foscavir · pH 7.4

≋ ADMINISTRATION CONSIDERATIONS

Usual Dose

ADULTS: 60 mg/kg q 8 hr or 90–120 mg q 12 hr for 2–3 wk initially, then 90–120 mg/kg/day as a single dose.

Dilution

• **Intermittent Infusion:** May be administered via central line in standard 24-mg/ml solution **undiluted**. If administered via peripheral line, must be **diluted** to 12-mg/ml concentration with D5W or 0.9% NaCl to prevent vein irritation. • Do not administer solution that is discolored or contains particulate matter. Use diluted solution within 24 hours. • Dose is based on patient weight; excess solution may be discarded from bottle prior to administration to prevent overdosage.

Compatibility

• **Y-site:** amikacin • aminophylline • ampicillin • aztreonam • benzquinamide • cefazolin • cefoperazone • cefoxitin • ceftazidime • ceftizoxime • ceftriaxone • cefuroxime • chloramphenicol • cimetidine • clindamycin • dexamethasone sodium phosphate • dopamine • erythromycin lactobionate • fluconazole • flucytosine • furosemide • gentamicin • heparin • hydrocortisone sodium succinate • hydromorphone • imipenem/cilastatin • metoclopramide • metronidazole • miconazole • morphine • nafcillin • oxacillin • penicillin G potassium • phenytoin • piperacillin • ranitidine • ticarcillin/clavulanate • tobramycin. • However, manufacturer does not recommend administering other medications or solutions through the same catheter as foscarnet.

Incompatibility

• **Y-site:** acyclovir • amphotericin B • diazepam • digoxin • diphenhydramine • dobutamine • droperidol • ganciclovir • haloperidol • leucovorin • midazolam • pentamidine • prochlorperazine • promethazine • trimetrexate.

• **Solution:** solutions containing calcium • lactated Ringer's • Ringer's solution • parenteral nutrition. • Manufacturer does not recommend admixing foscarnet with other drugs or solutions.

Rate of Administration

• **Intermittent Infusion:** Induction treatment (60 mg/kg) is infused over 1 hour every 8 hours for 2–3 weeks, depending on clinical response. • Maintenance treatment (>60 mg/kg) is infused over 2 hours. • Infuse solution via infusion pump to ensure accurate infusion rate.

≋ CLINICAL PRECAUTIONS

- Diagnosis of cytomegalovirus (CMV) retinitis should be determined by ophthalmoscopy prior to treatment with foscarnet. Culture for CMV (urine, blood, throat) may be taken prior to administration. However, a negative CMV culture does not rule out CMV retinitis. Patients who experience progression of CMV retinitis during maintenance therapy may be re-treated with induction therapy followed by maintenance therapy.
- Patients should be adequately hydrated (500–1000 ml of 0.9% NaCl/dose) prior to and throughout infusion to prevent renal toxicity. Dosage reduction is required for any degree of renal impairment (creatinine clearance less than 1.5 ml/min/kg).
- If signs of electrolyte imbalance (perioral tingling or numbness in the extremities or paresthesia) occur during administration, stop infusion and correct.
- Concurrent use with parenteral pentamidine may result in severe, life-threatening hypocalcemia.
- Use foscarnet with caution in patients with a history of seizure activity.
- Safe use in pregnancy, lactation, or children has not been established (Pregnancy Category C).

Lab Test Considerations

• Monitor serum creatinine prior to and 2 to 3 times weekly during induction therapy and at least every 1–2 weeks during maintenance therapy. Monitor 24-hour creatinine clearance prior to and periodically throughout therapy. If creatinine clearance drops below 0.4 ml/min/kg, foscarnet may need to be discontinued. • Monitor serum calcium, magnesium, potassium, and phosphorus prior to and 2 to 3 times weekly during induction therapy and at least every 1–2 weeks during maintenance therapy. • May cause anemia, granulocytopenia, leukopenia, and thrombocytopenia. • May cause elevated AST (SGOT) and ALT (SGPT) levels and abnormal A-G ratios.

Patient/Family Teaching

• Inform patient that foscarnet is not a cure for CMV retinitis. Progression of retinitis may continue in immunocompromised patients during and following therapy. Advise patients to have regular ophthalmologic examinations. • Advise patient to notify nurse or physician immediately if perioral tingling or numbness in the extremities or paresthesia occurs during or after infusion. Lab samples for serum electrolyte concentrations should be obtained immediately. • Emphasize the importance of frequent follow-up examinations to monitor renal function and electrolytes.

≋ PHARMACOLOGIC PROFILE

Indications

• Foscarnet is used for the treatment of CMV retinitis in patients with the acquired immunodeficiency syndrome. • Foscarnet prevents viral replication by inhibiting viral DNA polymerase and reverse transcriptase.

Time/Action Profile (blood levels)

Onset	Peak
rapid	end of infusion

Pharmacokinetics

• **Distribution:** Foscarnet displays variable penetration into CSF and may concentrate in and be slowly released from bone. The remainder of distribution is not known. • **Metabolism and Excretion:** 80–90% of foscarnet is excreted unchanged in the urine. • **Half-life:** Elimination half-life is 3 hours in patients with normal renal function. A longer terminal half-life of 90 hours may reflect release of the drug from bone.

Contraindications

• Foscarnet is contraindicated in patients with hypersensitivity to it.

Adverse Reactions and Side Effects*

• **CNS:** SEIZURES, headache, fatigue, weakness, malaise, dizziness, depression, confusion, anxiety • **EENT:** vision abnormalities, eye pain, conjunctivitis • **Resp:** coughing, dyspnea • **CV:** edema, chest pain, palpitations, ECG abnormalities • **GI:** nausea, vomiting, diarrhea, anorexia, abdominal pain, constipation, dyspepsia, abnormal taste sensation • **GU:** renal failure, albuminuria, dysuria, polyuria, urinary retention, nocturia • **Derm:** rash, increased sweating, pruritus, skin ulceration • **F and E:** hypocalcemia, hypomagnesemia, hypokalemia, hypophosphatemia, hyperphosphatemia • **Hemat:** anemia, granulocytopenia, leukopenia • **Local:** pain or inflammation at injection site • **MS:** involuntary muscle contraction, back pain, arthralgia, myalgia • **Neuro:** paresthesia, hypoesthesia, neuropathy, tremor, ataxia • **Misc:** fever, chills, flulike syndrome, lymphoma, sarcoma.

Furosemide	Diuretic (loop)
frusemide, Lasix, {Lasix Special}, {Uritol}	pH 8–9.3

ADMINISTRATION CONSIDERATIONS

Usual Dose

ADULTS: 20–80 mg; may be repeated or increased by 20 mg q 12 hr (up to 600 mg/day may be necessary). When the daily maintenance dose is determined, furosemide may be given once daily or in two divided doses. Single doses of 100–200 mg have been used for pulmonary edema.

---

*Underlines indicate most frequent; CAPITALS indicate life-threatening.

{} = Available in Canada only.

CHILDREN: 1–2 mg/kg; may be repeated or increased by 1 mg/kg q 2 hr *or* 1 mg/kg followed by 0.1–0.4 mg/kg/hr (up to 6 mg/kg/day).

Dilution

• **Direct IV:** May be administered **undiluted**. • **Intermittent Infusion: Dilute** large doses in D5W, D10W, D20W, D5/0.9% NaCl, D5/LR, 0.9% NaCl, 3% NaCl, ⅙ M sodium lactate, or lactated Ringer's solution. • Do not use solutions that are yellow. Use diluted solution within 24 hours.

Compatibility

• **Syringe:** bleomycin ◆ cisplatin ◆ cyclophosphamide ◆ fluorouracil ◆ heparin ◆ leucovorin calcium ◆ methotrexate ◆ mitomycin.

• **Y-site:** allopurinol sodium ◆ amikacin ◆ bleomycin ◆ cisplatin ◆ cyclophosphamide ◆ cytarabine ◆ famotidine ◆ fludarabine ◆ fluorouracil ◆ foscarnet ◆ gallium nitrate ◆ heparin ◆ hydrocortisone sodium succinate ◆ indomethacin ◆ kanamycin ◆ leucovorin calcium ◆ methotrexate ◆ mitomycin ◆ paclitaxel ◆ piperacillin/tazobactam ◆ potassium chloride ◆ sargramostim ◆ tacrolimus ◆ tobramycin ◆ tolazoline ◆ vitamin B complex with C.

• **Additive:** amikacin ◆ aminophylline ◆ ampicillin ◆ atropine ◆ bumetanide ◆ calcium gluconate ◆ cefamandole ◆ cefoperazone ◆ cefuroxime ◆ cimetidine ◆ dexamethasone ◆ heparin ◆ kanamycin ◆ morphine ◆ nitroglycerin ◆ penicillin G ◆ potassium chloride ◆ ranitidine ◆ sodium bicarbonate ◆ tobramycin.

Incompatibility

• **Syringe:** doxapram ◆ doxorubicin ◆ droperidol ◆ metoclopramide ◆ milrinone ◆ vinblastine ◆ vincristine.

• **Y-site:** ciprofloxacin ◆ diltiazem ◆ droperidol ◆ esmolol ◆ filgrastim ◆ fluconazole ◆ gentamicin ◆ hydralazine ◆ idarubicin ◆ metoclopramide ◆ morphine ◆ netilmicin ◆ ondansetron ◆ quinidine gluconate ◆ vinblastine ◆ vincristine ◆ vinorelbine.

• **Additive:** buprenorphine ◆ chlorpromazine ◆ dobutamine ◆ erythromycin lactobionate ◆ meperidine ◆ metoclopramide ◆ netilmicin ◆ highly acidic solutions.

Rate of Administration

• **Direct IV:** Administer each 20 mg slowly over 1–2 minutes. • **Intermittent Infusion:** Administer through Y tubing or 3-way stopcock at a rate not to exceed 4 mg/min in adults to prevent ototoxicity. Use an infusion pump to ensure accurate dosage.

≋ CLINICAL PRECAUTIONS

- Assess fluid status throughout therapy. Monitor daily weight, intake and output ratios, amount and location of edema, lung sounds, skin turgor, and mucous membranes. Assess for thirst, dry mouth, lethargy, weakness, hypotension, or oliguria. Monitor blood pressure and pulse before and during administration. Additive hypotension occurs with concurrent administration of antihypertensives or nitrates.
- Assess patients receiving cardiac glycosides for anorexia, nausea, vomiting, muscle cramps, paresthesia, and confusion. Hypokalemia increases the risk of cardiac glycoside toxicity. Additive hypokalemia occurs with other diuretics, mezlocillin, piperacillin, amphotericin B, and glucocorticoids.
- Assess patient for tinnitus and hearing loss. Audiometry is recommended for patients receiving prolonged therapy. Hearing loss is most common following rapid or high-dose IV administration in patients with decreased renal function or those taking other ototoxic drugs (aminoglycosides, cisplatin). Auditory function may be difficult to assess in geriatric or very young patients.
- Assess for allergy to sulfonamides. Cross-sensitivity may occur.
- Furosemide decreases lithium excretion and may cause toxicity. The effects of warfarin or propranolol may be increased by furosemide. Concurrent use with chloral hydrate may result in diaphoresis, hot flashes, hypertension, tachycardia, weakness, and nausea. Diuresis may be enhanced by clofibrate. The risk of electrolyte disturbance or hypotension is increased by concurrent use of thiazide diuretics or other antihypertensives. Salicylates may decrease diuretic response, especially in patients with cirrhosis and ascites.
- Use furosemide cautiously in patients with severe liver disease, electrolyte depletion, diabetes mellitus, anuria, or increasing azotemia. Geriatric patients may be more sensitive to the effects of furosemide.

- Safe use in pregnancy or lactation has not been established (Pregnancy Category C).

Lab Test Considerations

- Monitor electrolytes, renal and hepatic function, serum glucose, and uric acid levels prior to and periodically throughout course of therapy. Glucose tolerance may be decreased in diabetic patients. Furosemide may cause decreased electrolyte levels (especially potassium) and may cause elevated blood glucose, BUN, and uric acid levels.

Patient/Family Teaching

- Caution patient to make position changes slowly to minimize orthostatic hypotension. • Advise patient to contact physician immediately if muscle weakness, cramps, nausea, dizziness, numbness, or tingling of extremities occurs. • Instruct patient to consult physician regarding a diet high in potassium (see Appendix H). • Advise patients on antihypertensive regimen to continue taking medication and monitoring blood pressure routinely, even if feeling better. Furosemide controls but does not cure hypertension. Reinforce the need to continue additional therapies for hypertension (weight loss, restricted sodium intake, stress reduction, regular exercise, moderation of alcohol consumption, cessation of smoking). • Emphasize the importance of routine follow-up examinations.

≋ PHARMACOLOGIC PROFILE

Indications

- Furosemide is used in the management of edema secondary to congestive heart failure or hepatic or renal disease. It is also used in combination with antihypertensives in the treatment of hypertension and in the management of hypercalcemia of malignancy.

Action

- Furosemide inhibits the reabsorption of sodium and chloride from the loop of Henle and distal renal tubule and increases renal excretion of water, sodium, chloride, magnesium, hydrogen, and calcium. It may also have renal and peripheral vasodilatory effects. Effectiveness of furosemide persists in impaired renal function. Furosemide produces diuresis and subsequent mobilization of excess fluid (edema, pleural effusions).

Time/Action Profile (diuretic effect)

Onset	Peak	Duration
5 min	30 min	2 hr

Pharmacokinetics

• **Distribution:** Furosemide crosses the placenta and enters breast milk. The remainder of distribution is not known.
• **Metabolism and Excretion:** Some of furosemide is metabolized by the liver (30–40%). Some undergoes nonhepatic metabolism and renal excretion as unchanged drug. • **Half-life:** 30–60 minutes (increased in renal impairment and neonates, markedly increased in hepatic impairment).

Contraindications

• Furosemide is contraindicated in patients with hypersensitivity to it. Cross-sensitivity with thiazides and sulfonamides may occur. • Products containing benzyl alcohol should not be used in newborns.

Adverse Reactions and Side Effects*

• **CNS:** dizziness, headache, encephalopathy • **EENT:** hearing loss, tinnitus • **CV:** hypotension • **GI:** nausea, vomiting, diarrhea, constipation • **GU:** frequency • **Derm:** rashes, photosensitivity • **Endo:** hyperglycemia • **F and E:** metabolic alkalosis, hypovolemia, dehydration, hyponatremia, hypokalemia, hypochloremia, hypomagnesemia • **Hemat:** blood dyscrasias • **Metab:** hyperuricemia • **MS:** muscle cramps • **Misc:** increased BUN.

---

*Underlines indicate most frequent; CAPITALS indicate life-threatening.

Gallamine Triethiodide	*Neuromuscular blocking agent (nondepolarizing)*
Flaxedil	**pH 6.5–7.5**

 ADMINISTRATION CONSIDERATIONS

Usual Dose

ADULTS AND CHILDREN: 1 mg/kg (not to exceed 100 mg/dose), then 0.5–1 mg may be given 30–40 min later if needed during prolonged procedures.

Dilution

• **Direct IV:** Administer each single dose as an **undiluted** bolus.

Incompatibility

• **Syringe:** barbiturates • meperidine.

Rate of Administration

• **Direct IV:** Each dose should be administered over 30–60 seconds.

 CLINICAL PRECAUTIONS

• Assess respiratory status continuously throughout gallamine therapy. Gallamine should be used only by individuals experienced in endotracheal intubation; equipment for this procedure should be readily available. Respiratory depression is additive with opioid analgesics.

• Neuromuscular response to gallamine should be monitored intraoperatively with a peripheral nerve stimulator. Paralysis is initially selective and usually occurs sequentially in the following muscles: levator muscles of eyelids, muscles of mastication, limb muscles, abdominal muscles, muscles of the glottis, intercostal muscles, and the diaphragm. Recovery of muscle function usually occurs in reverse order. Observe the patient for residual muscle weakness and respiratory distress during the recovery period. Intensity and duration of paralysis may be prolonged by pretreatment with succinylcholine, ether, methoxyflurane (dosage reduction may be necessary), aminoglycoside antibiotics, polymyxin B, colistin, clindamycin, lidocaine, quinidine, procainamide, beta-adrenergic blocking agents, potassium-losing diuretics, and magnesium. Azathioprine may decrease neuromuscular blockade from gallamine.

- Monitor heart rate and ECG throughout therapy. Tachycardia caused by gallamine occurs after doses of 500 mcg/kg. This reaches a maximum within 3 minutes and then declines gradually. Use cautiously in patients with hypertension or shock.
- Dose is titrated to patient response. Gallamine has no effect on consciousness or the pain threshold. Adequate anesthesia and analgesia should *always* be used when gallamine is used as an adjunct to surgical procedures.
- Use with caution in patients with a history of pulmonary disease, or of renal or liver impairment; in elderly or debilitated patients; and in patients with electrolyte disturbances, fractures, or muscular spasm.
- Use with **extreme caution** in patients with myasthenia gravis or myasthenic syndrome.
- Do not confuse gallamine with gallium (see *gallium nitrate* monograph on page 458).
- Use gallamine cautiously in pregnant patients and children weighing less than 5 kg.

Toxicity and Overdose Alert

- If overdose occurs, use peripheral nerve stimulator to determine the degree of neuromuscular blockade. Maintain airway patency and ventilation until recovery of normal respirations occurs. Administration of anticholinesterase agents (edrophonium, neostigmine, pyridostigmine) may be used to antagonize the action of gallamine. Atropine is usually administered prior to or concurrently with anticholinesterase agents to counteract muscarinic effects. Administration of fluids and vasopressors may be necessary to treat severe hypotension or shock.

Patient/Family Teaching

- Explain all procedures to patient receiving gallamine therapy without anesthesia, as consciousness is not affected by gallamine alone. • Reassure patient that communication abilities will return as the medication wears off.

≋ PHARMACOLOGIC PROFILE

Indications
• Gallamine triethiodide is used to produce skeletal muscle paralysis after the induction of anesthesia.

Action
• Gallamine triethiodide prevents neuromuscular transmission by blocking the effect of acetylcholine at the myoneural junction.

Time/Action Profile (muscle relaxation)

Onset	Peak	Duration
1–2 min	3–5 min	15–30 min

Pharmacokinetics
• **Distribution:** Gallium triethiodide distributes into extracellular space and crosses the placenta. • **Metabolism and Excretion:** Excretion occurs almost entirely as unchanged drug by the kidneys. • **Half-life:** 2.5 hours.

Contraindications
• Gallium triethiodide is contraindicated in patients with hypersensitivity to it or to iodides or bisulfites.

Adverse Reactions and Side Effects*
• **CV:** tachycardia, hypertension • **Resp:** wheezing, increased bronchial secretions • **Derm:** skin flushing, erythema, pruritus, urticaria • **Misc:** allergic reactions, including ANAPHYLAXIS.

Gallium Nitrate	*Hypocalcemic agent*
Ganite	pH 6–7

≋ ADMINISTRATION CONSIDERATIONS

Usual Dose
ADULTS: 100–200 mg/m^2 daily for 5 days. A waiting period of 3–4 wk between courses is recommended.

---

*Underlines indicate most frequent; CAPITALS indicate life-threatening.

Dilution

• **Continuous Infusion:** Dilute daily dose in 1000 ml of 0.9% NaCl or D5W. • Solution is stable for 48 hours at room temperature and 7 days if refrigerated.

Compatibility

• **Y-site:** acyclovir ✦ allopurinol sodium ✦ aminophylline ✦ ampicillin/sulbactam ✦ cefazolin ✦ ceftazidime ✦ ceftriaxone ✦ cimetidine ✦ ciprofloxacin ✦ cyclophosphamide ✦ dexamethasone sodium phosphate ✦ diphenhydramine ✦ filgrastim ✦ fluconazole ✦ furosemide ✦ heparin ✦ hydrocortisone sodium succinate ✦ ifosfamide ✦ magnesium sulfate ✦ mannitol ✦ melphalan ✦ meperidine ✦ mesna ✦ methotrexate ✦ metoclopramide ✦ ondansetron ✦ piperacillin ✦ piperacillin/tazobactam ✦ potassium chloride ✦ ranitidine ✦ sodium bicarbonate ✦ ticarcillin/clavulanate ✦ trimethoprim/sulfamethoxazole ✦ vancomycin ✦ vinorelbine.

Incompatibility

• **Y-site:** cisplatin ✦ cytarabine ✦ doxorubicin ✦ etoposide ✦ fluorouracil ✦ haloperidol ✦ hydromorphone ✦ imipenem/cilastatin ✦ lorazepam ✦ morphine ✦ prochlorperazine.

Rate of Administration

• **Continuous Infusion:** Infuse over 24 hours.

≋ CLINICAL PRECAUTIONS

• Gallium nitrate should be instituted after adequate hydration with IV saline has been established. Saline promotes the renal excretion of calcium. Diuretics may also be used following correction of hypovolemia. Adequate hydration and urine output should be maintained at 2000 ml/day throughout therapy. Risk of nephrotoxicity is increased with concurrent use of other nephrotoxic agents, amphotericin B, or aminoglycosides. If patient requires other nephrotoxic drugs, discontinue gallium nitrate and continue hydration for several days following administration of potentially nephrotoxic drug. Monitor serum creatinine and urine output during and after this period.

• Monitor symptoms of hypercalcemia (nausea, vomiting, anorexia, lethargy, fatigue, weakness, constipation, thirst, dehydration, impaired mental status, and cardiac arrhythmias).

- Observe patient carefully for evidence of hypocalcemia (paresthesia, muscle twitching, laryngospasm, abdominal cramps, confusion, cardiac arrhythmias, and Chvostek's or Trousseau's sign). Protect symptomatic patients by elevating and padding side rails; keep bed in low position. If hypocalcemia occurs, stop gallium nitrate therapy. Temporary calcium therapy may be needed.
- Use gallium nitrate cautiously in patients with any degree of renal impairment.
- Do not confuse gallium with gallamine (see *gallamine triethiodide* monograph on page 456).
- Safe use in pregnancy, lactation, or children has not been established (Pregnancy Category C).

Lab Test Considerations

• Monitor BUN and serum creatinine prior to and every 2–3 days throughout therapy. Gallium nitrate therapy should be discontinued if serum creatinine is more than 2.5 mg/dl. • Monitor serum calcium daily and serum phosphate levels twice weekly to determine effectiveness of therapy. Oral phosphate therapy may be needed for hypophosphatemia. If serum calcium drops to normal levels in less than 5 days, gallium should be discontinued. • Monitor serum albumin before and after each course of therapy. • May also cause decreased serum bicarbonate concentrations.

Patient/Family Teaching

• Encourage patient to comply with physician's diet recommendations. Foods high in calcium that should be avoided include dairy products, canned salmon and sardines, broccoli, bok choy, tofu, molasses, and cream soups (see Appendix H). • Emphasize need for keeping follow-up appointments to monitor progress, even after medication is discontinued, in order to detect possible relapse.

≋ PHARMACOLOGIC PROFILE

Indications
• Gallium nitrate is used in the management of cancer-related hypercalcemia.

Action
• Gallium nitrate inhibits calcium resorption from bone, thus lowering serum calcium levels.

Time/Action Profile (effect on serum calcium)

Onset	Peak	Duration
within 24 hr	5 days	6–7.5 days

Pharmacokinetics
• **Distribution:** UK. • **Metabolism and Excretion:** Gallium nitrate is mostly excreted unchanged by the kidneys. • **Half-life:** UK.

Contraindications
• Gallium nitrate is contraindicated in patients with severe renal impairment (serum creatinine more than 2.5 mg/dl).

Adverse Reactions and Side Effects*
• **EENT:** hearing loss, optic neuritis, visual impairment • **F and E:** hypocalcemia, hypophosphatemia • **GU:** renal toxicity.

Ganciclovir Sodium	_Antiviral_
Cytovene	pH 11

≋ ADMINISTRATION CONSIDERATIONS

Usual Dose
ADULTS: 5 mg/kg q 12 hr for 14–21 days initially (up to 15 mg/kg/day), then 5 mg/kg/day or 6 mg/kg for 5 days of each wk. If disease progression occurs, repeat initial twice-daily regimen.

CHILDREN: 2.5–3.3 mg/kg q 8 hr or 3.75–5 mg q 12 hr initially, then 2.5–5 mg/kg once daily (unlabeled).

---

*Underlines indicate most frequent; CAPITALS indicate life-threatening.

Dilution

• **Intermittent Infusion: Reconstitute** 500 mg with 10 ml of sterile water for injection for a concentration of 50 mg/ml. Do not reconstitute with bacteriostatic water with parabens; precipitation will occur. Shake well to dissolve completely. Discard vial if particulate matter or discoloration occurs. • Solution should be prepared in a biologic cabinet. Wear gloves, gown, and mask while handling medication. Discard IV equipment in specially designated containers (see Appendix F). • Reconstituted solution is stable for 12 hours at room temperature; do not refrigerate. • **Dilute** in 100 ml of D5W, 0.9% NaCl, Ringer's or lactated Ringer's solution for a concentration not to exceed 10 mg/ml. • Once diluted for infusion, solution should be used within 24 hours. Refrigerate but do not freeze.

Compatibility

• **Y-site:** allopurinol sodium • cisplatin • cyclophospha-mide • enalaprilat • filgrastim • fluconazole • melphalan • methotrexate • paclitaxel • tacrolimus.

Incompatibility

• **Y-site:** cytarabine • doxorubicin • fludarabine • foscar-net • ondansetron • piperacillin/tazobactam • sargramostim.

Rate of Administration

• **Intermittent Infusion:** Administer slowly, via infusion pump, over 1 hour using an in-line filter. Rapid administration may increase toxicity.

≋ CLINICAL PRECAUTIONS

• Diagnosis of cytomegalovirus (CMV) retinitis should be determined by ophthalmoscopy prior to treatment with ganciclovir. Culture for CMV (urine, blood, throat) may be taken prior to administration. However, a negative CMV culture does not rule out CMV retinitis. If symptoms do not respond after several weeks, resistance to ganciclovir may have occurred. Ophthalmologic examinations should be performed weekly during induction and every 2 weeks during maintenance, or more frequently if the macula or optic nerve is threatened. Progression of CMV retinitis may occur during or following ganciclovir treatment.

- Do not administer by rapid IV injection. Observe infusion site for phlebitis. Infusion site should be rotated to prevent phlebitis.
- Assess for fever, chills, sore throat, and signs of infection. Assess for bleeding (bleeding gums, bruising, petechiae; guaiac test stools, urine, and emesis). Avoid giving IM injections and taking rectal temperatures. Apply pressure to venipuncture sites for 10 minutes. The risk of bone marrow depression is increased with concurrent use of antineoplastic agents, radiation therapy, or zidovudine. Toxicity may be increased by probenecid.
- The risk of seizures is increased with concurrent use of imipenem/cilastatin.
- Use cautiously in patients with renal impairment. Dosage reduction is required if creatinine clearance is less than 80 ml/min. Use with caution in elderly patients. Dosage reduction is also recommended in this population due to age-related decrease in renal function.
- Use cautiously in patients with bone marrow depression or immunosuppression.
- Ganciclovir should not be used during pregnancy or lactation (Pregnancy Category C). Use cautiously in patients with childbearing potential.

Lab Test Considerations

- Monitor neutrophil and platelet count at least every 2 days during twice-daily therapy and weekly thereafter. Granulocytopenia usually occurs during the first 2 weeks of treatment but may occur at any time during therapy. Do not administer if neutrophil count is less than $500/mm^3$ or if platelet count is less than $25,000/mm^3$. Recovery begins within 3–7 days of discontinuation of therapy. • Monitor BUN and serum creatinine level at least once every 2 weeks throughout therapy. • Monitor liver function tests (ALT [SGPT], AST [SGOT], serum bilirubin) periodically during therapy. Ganciclovir may cause elevated levels.

Patient/Family Teaching

- Inform patient that ganciclovir is not a cure for CMV retinitis. Progression of retinitis may continue in immunocompromised patients during and following therapy. Advise patient to have regular ophthalmic examinations.

- Advise patients that ganciclovir may have teratogenic effects. A nonhormonal method of contraception should be used during and for at least 90 days following therapy.
- Emphasize the importance of frequent follow-up examinations to monitor blood counts.

≋ PHARMACOLOGIC PROFILE

Indications

- Ganciclovir sodium is used in the treatment of CMV retinitis in immunocompromised patients, including HIV-infected patients. • It is also used to prevent CMV retinitis in transplant patients.

Action

- CMV virus converts ganciclovir to its active form (ganciclovir phosphate) inside the host cell, where it inhibits viral DNA polymerase. This produces an antiviral effect directed preferentially against CMV-infected cells.

Time/Action Profile

Onset	Peak
rapid	end of infusion

Pharmacokinetics

- **Distribution:** Ganciclovir enters the CSF. The remainder of its distribution is not known. • **Metabolism and Excretion:** 90% of ganciclovir is excreted unchanged by the kidneys. • **Half-life:** 2.9 hours (increased in renal impairment).

Contraindications

- Ganciclovir is contraindicated in patients with hypersensitivity to ganiclovir or acyclovir. • Pregnant or lactating patients should not receive ganciclovir.

Adverse Reactions and Side Effects*

- **CNS:** malaise, abnormal dreams, confusion, dizziness, headache, coma, nervousness, drowsiness • **EENT:** retinal detachment • **Resp:** dyspnea • **CV:** arrhythmias, hyperten-

---

*Underlines indicate most frequent; CAPITALS indicate life-threatening.

sion, hypotension, edema • **GI:** nausea, vomiting, gastric bleeding, abdominal pain, increased liver enzymes • **GU:** hematuria, gonadal suppression • **Derm:** rash, alopecia, pruritus, urticaria • **Endo:** hypoglycemia • **Hemat:** neutropenia, thrombocytopenia, anemia, eosinophilia • **Local:** pain, phlebitis at IV site • **Neuro:** tremor, ataxia • **Misc:** fever.

Gentamicin Sulfate	Anti-infective (aminoglycoside)
{Cidomycin}, Garamycin, Jenamicin	pH 3.5–5.5

≋ ADMINISTRATION CONSIDERATIONS

Usual Dose

All doses after initial loading dose should be determined by renal function and/or gentamicin blood levels.

ADULTS: 1–1.7 mg/kg q 8 hr. Higher doses (up to 15 mg/kg/day) have been used to treat life-threatening infections and intraocular infections. Lower doses have been used to treat uncomplicated urinary tract infections (3 mg/kg/day in 1–2 divided doses).

CHILDREN: 2–2.5 mg/kg q 8 hr.

INFANTS AND OLDER NEONATES: 2.5 mg/kg q 8–16 hr.

PREMATURE OR FULL-TERM NEONATES <7 days: 2.5 mg/kg q 12–24 hr.

Dilution

• **Intermittent Infusion: Dilute** each dose of gentamicin in 50–200 ml of D5W, 0.9% NaCl, or Ringer's solution to provide a concentration not to exceed 1 mg/ml (0.1%). Also available in commercially mixed piggyback injections. Volume of diluent should be reduced for children, but sufficient to infuse over 30 minutes–2 hours. • Do not use solutions that are discolored or contain a precipitate.

{} = Available in Canada only.

Compatibility

- **Syringe:** clindamycin.
- **Y-site:** acyclovir ✦ atracurium ✦ ciprofloxacin ✦ cyclophosphamide ✦ diltiazem ✦ enalaprilat ✦ esmolol ✦ famotidine ✦ filgrastim ✦ fluconazole ✦ fludarabine ✦ foscarnet ✦ hydromorphone ✦ insulin ✦ labetalol ✦ magnesium sulfate ✦ melphalan ✦ meperidine ✦ morphine ✦ multivitamins ✦ ondansetron ✦ paclitaxel ✦ pancuronium ✦ perphenazine ✦ sargramostim ✦ tacrolimus ✦ tolazoline ✦ vecuronium ✦ vinorelbine ✦ vitamin B complex with C ✦ zidovudine. ● If aminoglycosides and penicillins or cephalosporins must be given concurrently, administer in separate sites at least 1 hour apart.
- **Additive:** atracurium ✦ aztreonam ✦ bleomycin ✦ cimetidine ✦ fluconazole ✦ metronidazole ✦ ofloxacin ✦ ranitidine ✦ verapamil.

Incompatibility

- **Syringe:** allopurinol sodium ✦ ampicillin ✦ cefamandole ✦ heparin.
- **Y-site:** furosemide ✦ heparin ✦ hetastarch ✦ idarubicin ✦ indomethacin.
- **Additive:** amphotericin B ✦ ampicillin ✦ cefamandole ✦ cephalothin ✦ cephapirin ✦ heparin ✦ nafcillin ✦ ticarcillin.

Rate of Administration

- **Intermittent Infusion:** Infuse slowly over 30 minutes–2 hours for adults and children. Flush IV line with D5W or 0.9% NaCl following administration.

≋ CLINICAL PRECAUTIONS

- Assess patient for infection (vital signs; appearance of wound, sputum, urine, and stool; WBC) at the beginning and throughout the course of therapy. Obtain specimens for culture and sensitivity prior to initiating therapy. First dose may be given before receiving results. Doses in obese patients should be based on ideal body weight.
- Evaluate eighth cranial nerve function by audiometry prior to and throughout the course of therapy. Hearing loss is usually in the high-frequency range. Eighth cranial nerve dysfunction is associated with persistently elevated peak gentamicin levels. Prompt recognition and intervention is essential in preventing permanent dam-

age. Also monitor for vestibular dysfunction (vertigo, ataxia, nausea, vomiting). The risk of ototoxicity is increased by concurrent use of loop diuretics (bumetanide, furosemide).

- Monitor intake and output ratio, and daily weight to assess hydration status and renal function. Keep patient well hydrated (1500–2000 ml/day) during therapy. The incidence of nephrotoxicity may be increased by concurrent use of other potentially nephrotic drugs. Dosage adjustments are required for any decrease in renal function.
- Elderly patients may be more prone to nephrotoxicity and ototoxicity due to age-related decreases in renal function and difficulty in assessing hearing status.
- Gentamicin may be inactivated by penicillins when co-administered to patients with renal insufficiency.
- Respiratory paralysis may occur after concurrent use of gentamicin with inhalation anesthetics (ether, cyclopropane, halothane, or nitrous oxide) or neuromuscular blockers (atracurium, tubocurarine, gallamine, succinylcholine, decamethonium). The possibility of neuromuscular blockade is increased with concurrent use of other aminoglycoside antibiotics.
- Safe use in pregnancy or lactation has not been established (Pregnancy Category C).

Toxicity and Overdose Alert

- Blood levels should be monitored periodically during therapy. Timing of blood levels is important in interpreting results. Draw blood for peak levels 30 minutes after a 30-minute infusion is completed. Blood samples for trough levels should be drawn just prior to next dose. Acceptable peak level is 4–12 mcg/ml; trough level should not exceed 2 mcg/ml.

Lab Test Considerations

- Monitor renal function by urinalysis, specific gravity, BUN, creatinine, and creatinine clearance prior to and throughout therapy. • Gentamicin may cause increased AST (SGOT), ALT (SGPT), LDH, bilirubin, and serum alkaline phosphatase levels. • Gentamicin may cause decreased serum calcium, magnesium, sodium, and potassium levels.

Patient/Family Teaching

• Instruct patient to report signs of superinfection (fever, upper respiratory infection, vaginal itching or discharge, increasing malaise, diarrhea). • Instruct patient to report signs of hypersensitivity, tinnitus, vertigo, or hearing loss. • Patients with a history of rheumatic heart disease or valve replacement should be taught the importance of using antimicrobial prophylaxis before invasive medical or dental procedures (see Appendix K).

≋ PHARMACOLOGIC PROFILE

Indications

• Gentamicin is used in the treatment of Gram-negative bacillary infections and infections due to staphylococci when penicillins or other less toxic drugs are contraindicated. Especially useful in the following serious Gram-negative bacillary infections due to susceptible organisms: bone infections, CNS infections (additional intrathecal administration required), respiratory tract infections, skin and soft tissue infections, abdominal infections, complicated urinary tract infections, endocarditis, and septicemia. It is also used as part of a regimen for endocarditis prophylaxis in certain patient populations.

Action

• Gentamicin inhibits protein synthesis in bacteria at the level of the 30S ribosome, resulting in bactericidal action against susceptible bacteria. It is active against *Pseudomonas aeruginosa, Klebsiella pneumoniae, Escherichia coli, Serratia, Acinetobacter,* and *Staphylococcus aureus.* In the treatment of enterococcal infections, synergy with a penicillin is required.

Time/Action Profile (blood levels)

Onset	Peak
rapid	end of infusion

Pharmacokinetics

• **Distribution:** Gentamicin is widely distributed in extracellular fluids. It crosses the placenta, but has poor penetration into CSF. • **Metabolism and Excretion:** Excretion of gentamicin is mainly renal (more than 90%). Minimal amounts metabolized by the liver. • **Half-life:** 2–3 hours (increased in renal impairment).

Contraindications

• Gentamicin is contraindicated in patients with hypersensitivity to it. Cross-sensitivity with other aminoglycosides may occur. • Parenteral product contains parabens, bisulfites, and edetate. Avoid using in patients with hypersensitivity or intolerance to these preservatives/additives.

Adverse Reactions and Side Effects*

• **EENT:** <u>ototoxicity</u> (vestibular and cochlear) • **GU:** <u>nephrotoxicity</u> • **Neuro:** enhanced neuromuscular blockade • **Misc:** hypersensitivity reactions, superinfection.

Glucagon Hydrochloride	*Hormone (hyperglycemic)*
	pH 2.5–3

≋ ADMINISTRATION CONSIDERATIONS

Usual Dose
1 USP unit = 1 mg.

Management of Hypoglycemia
ADULTS: 0.5–1 mg (0.5–1 unit); if no response, may repeat in 20 min.

CHILDREN: 25 mcg (0.025 unit)/kg; if no response, may repeat in 20 min (not to exceed 1 mg/dose).

Diagnostic Use—GI X-rays
ADULTS: 250 mcg (0.25 mg)–1 mg.

Dilution
• **Direct IV: Reconstitute** with diluent supplied in kit by manufacturer. With doses greater than 2 units (2 mg), use sterile water for injection instead of diluent supplied by manufacturer to minimize risk of thrombophlebitis, CNS tox-

---

*<u>Underlines</u> indicate most frequent; CAPITALS indicate life-threatening.

icity, or myocardial depression from phenol preservative in diluent supplied by manufacturer. Use immediately after reconstituting. Final concentration should not exceed 1 unit (1 mg)/ml. • Inspect solution prior to use; use only clear, water-like solution.

Incompatibility

• **Additive:** 0.9% NaCl ◆ potassium chloride ◆ calcium chloride.

Rate of Administration

• **Direct IV:** Administer at a rate not exceeding 1 unit (1 mg)/min. May be administered through IV line containing D5W.

≋ CLINICAL PRECAUTIONS

- Assess patient for signs of hypoglycemia (sweating, hunger, weakness, headache, dizziness, tremor, irritability, tachycardia, anxiety) prior to and periodically during course of therapy.
- Assess neurologic status throughout course of therapy. Institute safety precautions to protect patient from injury caused by seizures, falling, or aspiration.
- Assess nutritional status. Patients who lack liver glycogen stores (as in starvation, chronic hypoglycemia, and adrenal insufficiency) will require administration of glucose instead of glucagon.
- Assess for nausea and vomiting after administration of dose. Protect patients with depressed level of consciousness from aspiration by positioning on side; ensure that a suction unit is available. If vomiting occurs, patient will require parenteral glucose to prevent recurrent hypoglycemia.
- Administer supplemental carbohydrates IV or orally to facilitate increase of serum glucose levels. May be given at the same time as a bolus of dextrose.
- Large doses of glucagon may enhance the effect of oral anticoagulants. Glucagon negates the response to insulin or oral hypoglycemic agents. Hyperglycemic effect is intensified and prolonged by epinephrine.
- Use cautiously in patients with a history of insulinoma or pheochromocytoma.

• Safe use in pregnancy or lactation has not been established (Pregnancy Category B).

Lab Test Considerations

• Monitor serum glucose levels to determine effectiveness of therapy. Use of bedside finger-stick blood glucose determination methods is recommended for rapid results.
• Follow-up lab results may be ordered to validate finger-stick glucose values, but do not delay treatment while awaiting lab results, as this could result in neurologic injury or death.

Patient/Family Teaching

• Teach patient and family signs and symptoms of hypoglycemia. Instruct patient to take oral glucose as soon as symptoms of hypoglycemia occur. Glucagon is reserved for episodes when patient is unable to swallow due to decreased level of consciousness.
• **Home Care Issues:** Instruct family on correct technique to prepare, draw up, and administer injection. Physician must be contacted immediately after each dose for orders regarding further therapy or adjustment of insulin dose or diet. • Advise family that patient should receive oral glucose when alertness returns. • Instruct family to position patient on side until fully alert. Explain that glucagon may cause nausea and vomiting. Aspiration may occur if patient vomits while lying on back. • Instruct patient to check expiration date monthly and to replace outdated medication immediately. • Patients with diabetes mellitus should carry a source of sugar (such as a packet of sugar or candy) and identification describing disease process and treatment regimen at all times.

≋ PHARMACOLOGIC PROFILE

Indications

• Glucagon is used in the acute management of severe hypoglycemia when administration of glucose is not feasible. It is also used to terminate insulin shock therapy in psychiatric patients.

Action

• Glucagon stimulates hepatic production of glucose from glycogen stores (glycogenolysis), thus increasing blood glucose in hypoglycemic patients. It also relaxes the musculature of the GI tract and has positive inotropic and chronotropic effects.

Time/Action Profile

	Onset	Peak	Duration
hyperglycemic effect	5–20 min	30 min	90 min
effect on GI musculature	45 sec	UK	9–17 min

Pharmacokinetics

• **Distribution:** UK. • **Metabolism and Excretion:** Glucagon is extensively metabolized by the liver and kidneys. • **Half-life:** 3–10 minutes.

Contraindications

• Glucagon is contraindicated in patients with hypersensitivity to beef or pork protein. • The diluent for glucagon contains glycerin and phenol; avoid use in patients with hypersensitivities to these ingredients.

Adverse Reactions and Side Effects*

• **GI:** <u>nausea</u>, <u>vomiting</u> • **Misc:** hypersensitivity reactions.

Glycopyrrolate	Anticholinergic (antimuscarinic)
Robinul	pH 2–3

ADMINISTRATION CONSIDERATIONS

Usual Dose

Cholinergic Adjunct

ADULTS AND CHILDREN: 200 mcg for each 1 mg of neostigmine or 5 mg of pyridostigmine given at the same time.

---

*<u>Underlines</u> indicate most frequent; CAPITALS indicate life-threatening.

Peptic Ulcer
ADULTS: 100–200 mcg (0.1–0.2 mg); may be repeated q 4 hr up to 4 times daily.

Antiarrhythmic
ADULTS: 100 mcg (0.1 mg); may be repeated q 2–3 min.
CHILDREN: 4.4 mcg (0.0044 mg)/kg; may be repeated q 2–3 min.

Dilution
• **Direct IV:** May be given **undiluted** through Y-site injection or 3-way stopcock. • Do not administer cloudy or discolored solution.

Compatibility
• **Syringe:** atropine • benzquinamide • buprenorphine • chlorpromazine • cimetidine • codeine • diphenhydramine • droperidol • droperidol/fentanyl • hydromorphone • hydroxyzine • levorphanol • lidocaine • meperidine • midazolam • morphine • nalbuphine • neostigmine • oxymorphone • procaine • prochlorperazine • promazine • promethazine • propiomazine • pyridostigmine • ranitidine • scopolamine • triflupromazine • trimethobenzamide.

• **Solution:** D5/0.45% NaCl • D5W • 0.9% NaCl • Ringer's solution. Administer immediately after admixing.

Incompatibility
• **Syringe:** chloramphenicol • dexamethasone sodium phosphate • diazepam • dimenhydrinate • methohexital • pentazocine • pentobarbital • secobarbital • sodium bicarbonate • thiopental.

Rate of Administration
• **Direct IV:** Administer at a rate of 0.2 mg over 1–2 minutes.

≋ CLINICAL PRECAUTIONS
- Assess heart rate, blood pressure, and respiratory rate prior to and periodically during parenteral therapy.
- Monitor intake and output ratios in elderly or surgical patients as glycopyrrolate may cause urinary retention. Instruct patient to void prior to administration.
- Assess patient routinely for abdominal distention and auscultate for bowel sounds.

- Geriatric patients and children may be more sensitive to the effects of glycopyrrolate and more susceptible to adverse reactions.
- Safe use during pregnancy or lactation has not been established (Pregnancy Category B).

Toxicity and Overdose Alert

- If overdosage occurs, neostigmine is the antidote.

Lab Test Considerations

- Glycopyrrolate antagonizes effects of pentagastrin and histamine during the gastric acid secretion test. Avoid administration for 24 hours preceding the test. • May cause decreased uric acid levels in patients with gout or hyperuricemia.

Patient/Family Teaching

- Advise patient receiving glycopyrrolate to make position changes slowly to minimize the effects of drug-induced orthostatic hypotension. • Glycopyrrolate may cause drowsiness and blurred vision. Caution patient to avoid activities requiring alertness until response to the medication is known. • Advise patient to notify physician immediately if eye pain or increased sensitivity to light occurs.

 PHARMACOLOGIC PROFILE

Indications

- Glycopyrrolate is used to treat some of the secretory and vagal actions of cholinesterase inhibitors during reversal of nondepolarizing neuromuscular blockade (cholinergic adjunct). • During anesthesia or surgical procedures, glycopyrrolate has been used as an antiarrhythmic, to counteract excessive vagal reactions. • Also used as an adjunct in the management of peptic ulcer disease.

Action

- Inhibits the action of acetylcholine at postganglionic sites located in smooth muscle, secretory glands, and the CNS (antimuscarinic activity). Low doses decrease sweating, salivation, and respiratory secretions. Intermediate doses result in increased heart rate. GI and GU tract motility are decreased at larger doses. • **Therapeutic Effects:** Decreased GI and respiratory secretions.

Time/Action Profile (anticholinergic effects)

Onset	Peak	Duration
1 min	UK	2–7 hr

Pharmacokinetics

• **Distribution:** Distribution not fully known. Does not significantly cross the blood–brain barrier or enter the eye. Crosses the placenta. • **Metabolism and Excretion:** Eliminated primarily unchanged in the feces, via biliary excretion. • **Half-life:** 1.7 hours.

Contraindications

• Glycopyrrolate is contraindicated in patients with hypersensitivity, narrow-angle glaucoma, acute hemorrhage, tachycardia secondary to cardiac insufficiency, or thyrotoxicosis.

Adverse Reactions and Side Effects*

• **CNS:** drowsiness, confusion • **EENT:** dry eyes, blurred vision, mydriasis, cycloplegia • **CV:** palpitations, tachycardia, orthostatic hypotension • **GI:** dry mouth, constipation • **GU:** urinary hesitancy, retention.

Gonadorelin Acetate	*Gonadotropin-releasing hormone*
Lutrepulse	pH 4.4

≋ **ADMINISTRATION CONSIDERATIONS**

Usual Dose

Adults: 5 mcg q 90 min (range 1–20 mcg q 90 min) for 21 days. If ovulation occurs, continue for 2 wk to maintain corpus luteum.

---

*<u>Underlines</u> indicate most frequent; CAPITALS indicate life-threatening.

Dilution

• **Continuous Infusion: Dilute** each vial with 8 ml of the saline diluent immediately prior to use. Shake for a few seconds to produce a clear, colorless solution. Do not use solution if particulate matter or discoloration is present. • Fill reservoir bag with reconstituted solution. • The 8 ml of solution will supply 90-minute pulsatile doses for approximately 7 consecutive days.

Rate of Administration

• **Continuous Infusion:** *Lutrepulse* pump should be set to deliver 25 or 50 microliters of solution, based on the dose selected, over a pulse period of 1 minute and a pulse frequency of 90 minutes.

≋ CLINICAL PRECAUTIONS

• Cannula and IV site should be changed every 48 hours. Observe site for any redness or irritation.
• Observe patient for the development of ovarian hyperstimulation syndrome (sudden ovarian enlargement, ascites, or pleural effusion). If these signs develop, discontinue treatment. If unchecked, this syndrome may proceed to fluid imbalance, ovarian rupture, or sepsis.
• Ovarian ultrasound should be performed before therapy, on day 7, and again on day 14.
• Regular physical examinations, including pelvic examination, should be performed throughout therapy.
• Safe use in patients younger than 18 years old has not been established.
• Do not confuse with gonadorelin hydrochloride (Factrel). See *gonadorelin hydrochloride* monograph on page 478.
• Gonadorelin acetate has been used safely in pregnancy (Pregnancy Category B).

Lab Test Considerations

• Monitor midluteal phase serum progesterone levels.

Patient/Family Teaching

• Instruct patient regarding proper reconstitution of gonadorelin acetate and use of *Lutrepulse* pump. • Advise pa-

tient to report any redness or inflammation at IV site.
• Counsel patient regarding the need for follow-up if
pregnancy occurs and of the possibility of multiple pregnancies.

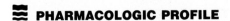

PHARMACOLOGIC PROFILE

Indications

• Gonadorelin acetate is used to produce ovulation in patients with primary hypothalamic amenorrhea. It also helps to
maintain the corpus luteum during pregnancy.

Action

• Gonadorelin acetate causes the release of luteinizing hormone and follicle-stimulating hormone, which promote ovulation.

Time/Action Profile (ovulation)

Onset	Peak	Duration
UK	2–3 wk	UK

Pharmacokinetics

• **Distribution:** UK. • **Metabolism and Excretion:** Gonadorelin acetate is rapidly metabolized to inactive compounds. • **Half-life:** 10–40 minutes.

Contraindications

• Gonadorelin acetate should not be used in patients with
hypersensitivity to it. • Do not use gonadorelin acetate concurrently with ovarian stimulators. • Gonadorelin acetate is
contraindicated in patients with conditions that pregnancy
would exacerbate and in patients with ovarian cysts, hormon-
ally sensitive tumors, or other conditions worsened by repro-
ductive hormones.

Adverse Reactions and Side Effects*

• **Endo:** multiple pregnancies, ovarian hyperstimulation
• **Local:** inflammation, infection, mild phlebitis, hematomas
at IV site.

---

*Underlines indicate most frequent; CAPITALS indicate life-
threatening.

Gonadorelin Hydrochloride	Gonadotropin-releasing hormone
Factrel	pH 4.0–8.0

 ADMINISTRATION CONSIDERATIONS

Usual Dose
ADULTS: 100 mcg (0.1 mg).

Dilution
• **Direct IV: Dilute** the 100-mcg vial with 1 ml or the 500-mcg vial with 2 ml of the diluent provided by the manufacturer. Administer immediately after dilution. Discard unused solution or diluent.

Incompatibility
• Information unavailable. Do not mix with other drugs or solutions.

Rate of Administration
• **Direct IV:** Administer as a bolus.

≋ CLINICAL PRECAUTIONS

• Blood for luteinizing hormone (LH) concentration levels should be drawn 15 minutes prior to, and immediately prior to, administration of gonadorelin to determine the baseline LH concentration. Following administration of gonadorelin, venous blood samples should be drawn at regular intervals.
• Androgens, digoxin, estrogens, oral contraceptives, levodopa, dopamine agonists, progestin, phenothiazines, spironolactone, and glucocorticoids interfere with normal gonadotropin release. The test should not be performed if the patient is taking any of these agents.
• Do not confuse with gonadorelin acetate (Lutrepulse). See *gonadorelin acetate* monograph on page 475.

Lab Test Considerations
• Normal serum LH concentrations are usually 5–25 mIU/ml in postpubertal males and females and in pre-

menopausal females. • Testing of response to gonadorelin hydrochloride should be done during the first 7 days of the menstrual cycle. • Safe use in pregnancy or lactation has not been established (Pregnancy Category B).

Patient/Family Teaching

• Inform patient of the purpose for this medication. • Instruct patient to report the symptoms of anaphylaxis (difficulty breathing, persistent flushing, hives) immediately if they occur.

≋ PHARMACOLOGIC PROFILE

Indications

• Gonadorelin hydrochloride is used to test the gonadotropin-producing capacity of the anterior pituitary.

Action

• Gonadorelin hydrochloride causes the release of gonadotropin (LH) from the anterior pituitary.

Time/Action Profile (increase in LH levels)

Onset	Peak	Duration
within minutes	15 min (males) 30 min (females)	>2 hr

Pharmacokinetics

• **Distribution:** UK. • **Metabolism and Excretion:** The metabolism of gonadorelin hydrochloride is not known. • **Half-life:** UK.

Contraindications

• Gonadorelin hydrochloride should not be given to patients with hypersensitivity to it or to benzyl alcohol.

Adverse Reactions and Side Effects*

• **Misc:** hypersensitivity reactions (multiple-dose use), antibody formation (large multiple doses).

---

*Underlines indicate most frequent; CAPITALS indicate life-threatening.

Granisetron Hydrochloride	Antiemetic
Kytril	pH 4.7–7.3

 ADMINISTRATION CONSIDERATIONS

Usual Dose
ADULTS AND CHILDREN **2–16 yr:** 10 mcg/kg.

Dilution
• **Direct IV: Dilute** in 20–50 ml of 0.9% NaCl or D5W. Solution should be prepared at the time of administration but is stable for 24 hours at room temperature.

Incompatibility
• **Additive:** Granisetron should not be admixed with other medications.

Rate of Administration
• **Direct IV:** Administer over 5 minutes.

 CLINICAL PRECAUTIONS

• Assess patient for nausea, vomiting, abdominal distention, and bowel sounds prior to and following administration.
• Granisetron is administered within 30 minutes before chemotherapy as a single dose and only on the days the patient is to receive chemotherapy.
• Assess for extrapyramidal effects (involuntary movements, facial grimacing, rigidity, shuffling walk, trembling of hands) throughout therapy. This occurs rarely and usually is associated with concurrent use of other drugs known to cause this effect.
• Safe use during pregnancy, lactation, or in children less than 2 years of age has not been established (Pregnancy Category B).

Lab Test Considerations
• May cause elevated AST (SGOT) and ALT (SGPT) levels.

Patient/Family Teaching

• Advise patient to notify physician immediately if involuntary movement of eyes, face, or limbs occurs.

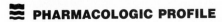
PHARMACOLOGIC PROFILE

Indications

• Granisetron is used to prevent nausea and vomiting associated with emetogenic chemotherapy.

Action

• Granisetron blocks the effects of serotonin at 5-HT$_3$ receptor sites (selective antagonist) located in vagal nerve terminals and the chemoreceptor trigger zone in the CNS.

Time/Action Profile (antiemetic effect)

Onset	Peak	Duration
rapid	30 min	up to 24 hr

Pharmacokinetics

• **Distribution:** Distribution of granisetron is not known.
• **Metabolism and Excretion:** Granisetron is mostly metabolized by the liver; 12% is excreted unchanged by the kidneys. • **Half-life:** 8–9 hours for patients with cancer (range 0.9–31.1 hours), 4.9 hours for healthy volunteers (range 0.9–15.2 hours), 7.7 hours for elderly patients (range 2.6–17.7 hours).

Contraindications

• Granisetron is contraindicated in patients with known hypersensitivity.

Adverse Reactions and Side Effects*

• **CNS:** <u>headache</u>, weakness, somnolence • **CV:** hypertension • **GI:** diarrhea, constipation, taste disorder • **Misc:** fever.

---

*<u>Underlines</u> indicate most frequent; CAPITALS indicate life-threatening.

Haloperidol Lactate
Butyrophenone antipsychotic

Haldol
pH 3–3.8

≋ ADMINISTRATION CONSIDERATIONS

Usual Dose
Haloperidol is not approved for IV use. All doses are unlabeled.

ADULTS: 0.5–50 mg; may be repeated q 30 min.

Dilution
• **Direct IV:** Administer **undiluted.** • **Intermittent/Continuous Infusion:** May be **diluted** in 30–50 ml of D5W or 0.9% NaCl.

Compatibility
• **Y-site:** cimetidine • dobutamine • dopamine • famotidine • filgrastim • fludarabine • lidocaine • melphalan • nitroglycerin • norepinephrine • ondansetron • paclitaxel • phenylephrine • tacrolimus • theophylline • vinorelbine.

Incompatibility
• **Syringe:** heparin.
• **Y-site:** allopurinol sodium • fluconazole • foscarnet • gallium nitrate • heparin • piperacillin/tazobactam • sargramostim.

Rate of Administration
• **Direct IV:** Administer at a rate of 5 mg/min. • **Intermittent Infusion:** Administer over 30 minutes. • **Continuous Infusion:** Has been administered at a rate of 25 mg/hr. Titrate rate to desired response.

≋ CLINICAL PRECAUTIONS

• Assess patient's mental status (orientation, mood, behavior) prior to and periodically throughout therapy.
• Monitor blood pressure (sitting, standing, lying) and pulse prior to and frequently during the period of dosage adjustment. Keep patient recumbent for at least 30 min-

utes following injection to minimize hypotensive effects. Geriatric or debilitated patients may be more sensitive to the effects of haloperidol (dosage reduction may be necessary).

- Use cautiously in patients with cardiac disease, severely ill patients, patients with diabetes, respiratory insufficiency, prostatic hypertrophy, CNS tumors, intestinal obstruction, or history of seizures. Because of its effects on serum prolactin levels, haloperidol should be used with caution in patients with a history of breast cancer.
- Monitor patient for symptoms of dehydration (decreased thirst, lethargy, hemoconcentration).
- Assess fluid intake and bowel function. Increased bulk and fluids in the diet help minimize the constipating effects of this medication.
- Observe patient carefully for extrapyramidal symptoms (pill-rolling motions, drooling, tremors, rigidity, shuffling gait), tardive dyskinesia (uncontrolled movements of face, mouth, tongue, or jaw and involuntary movements of extremities), and neuroleptic malignant syndrome (pale skin, hyperthermia, skeletal muscle rigidity, autonomic dysfunction, altered consciousness, leukocytosis, elevated liver function tests, elevated CPK). Trihexyphenidyl or diphenhydramine may be used to control extrapyramidal symptoms.
- Additive hypotension may occur with concurrent use of antihypertensives, nitrates, or acute ingestion of alcohol. Additive anticholinergic effects may occur with drugs having anticholinergic properties, including antihistamines, antidepressants, atropine, phenothiazines, quinidine, and disopyramide. Additive CNS depression may occur with concurrent use of other CNS depressants, including alcohol, antihistamines, opioid analgesics, and sedative/hypnotics. Concurrent use with epinephrine may result in severe hypotension and tachycardia. Haloperidol may decrease therapeutic effects of levodopa. Concurrent use with lithium may result in acute encephalopathic syndrome. Dementia may occur with concurrent use of methyldopa.
- Safe use in pregnancy, lactation, or children has not been established. Use of haloperidol may result in maternal hypotension and extrapyramidal reactions in the newborn. Use only when benefits outweigh risks.

Lab Test Considerations

• CBC and liver function tests should be evaluated periodically throughout course of therapy.

Patient/Family Teaching

• Inform patient of possibility of extrapyramidal symptoms and tardive dyskinesia. Caution patient to report these symptoms immediately to physician. • Advise patient to make position changes slowly to minimize orthostatic hypotension. • Medication may cause drowsiness. Caution patient to avoid activities requiring alertness until response to medication is known. • Caution patient to avoid taking alcohol or other CNS depressants concurrently with this medication. • Advise patient that extremes of temperature should be avoided, as this drug impairs body temperature regulation. • Instruct patient to use frequent mouth rinses, good oral hygiene, and sugarless gum or candy to minimize dry mouth. • Instruct patient to notify physician promptly if weakness, tremors, visual disturbances, dark-colored urine or clay-colored stools, sore throat, or fever is noted. • Emphasize the importance of routine follow-up examinations.

PHARMACOLOGIC PROFILE

Indications

• IV haloperidol is used for rapid control of acute psychoses or delirium.

Action

• Haloperidol alters the effects of dopamine in the CNS. In addition, it also has anticholinergic and alpha-adrenergic blocking activity.

Time/Action Profile

Onset	Peak	Duration
UK	UK	UK

Pharmacokinetics

• **Distribution:** The distribution of haloperidol is not fully known. High concentrations are achieved in the liver. Haloperidol crosses the placenta and enters breast milk.

• **Metabolism and Excretion:** Haloperidol is mostly metabolized by the liver. • **Half-life:** 21–24 hours.

Contraindications

• Haloperidol should not be used in patients with known hypersensitivity to it. Patients with narrow-angle glaucoma, bone marrow depression, CNS depression, or severe liver or cardiovascular disease should not receive haloperidol. Some injectables contain parabens or benzyl alcohol and should be avoided in patients with known intolerance or hypersensitivity.

Adverse Reactions and Side Effects*

• **CNS:** sedation, extrapyramidal reactions, tardive dyskinesia, restlessness, confusion, seizures • **EENT:** dry eyes, blurred vision • **Resp:** respiratory depression • **CV:** hypotension, tachycardia • **GI:** constipation, ileus, anorexia, dry mouth, hepatitis • **GU:** urinary retention • **Derm:** rashes, photosensitivity, diaphoresis • **Endo:** galactorrhea • **Hemat:** anemia, leukopenia • **Metab:** hyperpyrexia • **Misc:** hypersensitivity reactions, NEUROLEPTIC MALIGNANT SYNDROME.

Heparin Sodium **Heparin Calcium**	*Anticoagulant*
Calciparine, {Hepalean}, {Heparin Leo}, Liquaemin Sodium	pH 5–7.5

ADMINISTRATION CONSIDERATIONS

Usual Dose

THERAPEUTIC ANTICOAGULATION

Dosage depends on results of partial thromboplastin time (PTT).

Intermittent IV Bolus

ADULTS: 10,000 units, followed by 5000–10,000 units q 4–6 hr or 100 units/kg q 4 hr.

---

*Underlines indicate most frequent; CAPITALS indicate life-threatening.

{} = Available in Canada only.

CHILDREN: 50–100 units/kg, followed by 50–100 units/kg q 4 hr.

IV Infusion

ADULTS: 5000 units (35–70 units/kg), followed by 20,000–40,000 units infused over 24 hr (approx. 1000 units/hr).

CHILDREN: 50 units/kg followed by 100 units/kg q 4 hr or 20,000 units/m^2/24 hr.

HEPARIN FLUSH

ADULTS AND CHILDREN: 10–100 units.

DISSEMINATED INTRAVASCULAR COAGULATION (DIC)

ADULTS: 50–100 units/kg q 4 hr as a continuous infusion or intermittent injection. Discontinue within 4–8 hr if no clinical improvement occurs.

CHILDREN: 25–50 units/kg q 4 hr as a continuous infusion or intermittent injection. Discontinue within 4–8 hr if no clinical improvement occurs.

VASCULAR SURGERY

ADULTS: At least 150 units/kg (300 units/kg if procedure lasts less than 60 min, 400 units/kg if procedure lasts more than 60 min) initially; subsequent doses determined by coagulation tests.

CHILDREN: At least 150 units/kg (300 units/kg if procedure lasts less than 60 min); subsequent doses determined by coagulation tests.

Dilution

• **Direct IV:** May be administered **undiluted**. • **Intermittent Infusion: Dilute** in 50–100 ml of 0.9% NaCl, D5/saline combinations, D5/Ringer's or lactated Ringer's combinations, or Ringer's solution for injection. • **Continuous Infusion: Dilute** in 1000 ml of 0.9% NaCl, D5/saline combinations, D5/Ringer's or lactated Ringer's combinations, or Ringer's solution for injection. • Ensure adequate mixing of heparin in solution. • **Heparin Lock:** To prevent clot formation in intermittent infusion (heparin lock) sets, inject dilute heparin solution of 10–100 units/0.5–1 ml after each medication injection or every 8–12 hours. To prevent incompatibility of heparin with medication, flush heparin lock set with sterile water or 0.9% NaCl for injection before and after medication is administered.

Compatibility

*   **Syringe:** aminophylline • amphotericin B • ampicillin • atropine • bleomycin • cefamandole • cefazolin • cefoperazone • cefotaxime • cefoxitin • chloramphenicol • cimetidine • cisplatin • clindamycin • cyclophosphamide • diazoxide • digoxin • dimenhydrinate • dobutamine • dopamine • epinephrine • fentanyl • fluorouracil • furosemide • leucovorin • lidocaine • lincomycin • methotrexate • metoclopramide • mezlocillin • mitomycin • nafcillin • naloxone • neostigmine • nitroglycerin • nitroprusside • norepinephrine • pancuronium • penicillin G • phenobarbital • piperacillin • succinylcholine • trimethoprim/sulfamethoxazole • verapamil • vincristine.

*   **Y-site:** acyclovir • allopurinol sodium • aminophylline • ampicillin • atracurium • atropine • betamethasone • bleomycin • calcium gluconate • cephalothin • cephapirin • chlordiazepoxide • chlorpromazine • cimetidine • cisplatin • cyanocobalamin • cyclophosphamide • cytarabine • dexamethasone • digoxin • diphenhydramine • dopamine • edrophonium • enalaprilat • epinephrine • esmolol • conjugated estrogens • ethacrynate • famotidine • fentanyl • fluconazole • fludarabine • fluorouracil • foscarnet • furosemide • hydralazine • insulin • isoproterenol • kanamycin • labetalol • leucovorin • lidocaine • magnesium sulfate • melphalan • menadiol sodium • meperidine • methicillin • methotrexate • methoxamine • methylergonovine • metoclopramide • minocycline • mitomycin • morphine • neostigmine • norepinephrine • ondansetron • oxacillin • oxytocin • paclitaxel • pancuronium • penicillin G potassium • pentazocine • phytonadione • piperacillin/tazobactam • prednisolone • procainamide • prochlorperazine • propranolol • pyridostigmine • ranitidine • sargramostim • scopolamine • sodium bicarbonate • streptokinase • succinylcholine • tacrolimus • trimethobenzamide • trimethaphan camsylate • vecuronium • vinblastine • vincristine • vinorelbine • zidovudine.

*   **Additive:** aminophylline • amphotericin B • ascorbic acid • bleomycin • calcium gluconate • cephapirin • chloramphenicol • clindamycin • colistimethate • dimenhydrinate • dopamine • erythromycin gluceptate • esmolol • fluconazole • furosemide • isoproterenol • lidocaine • methyldopate • methylprednisolone • nafcillin • norepinephrine • octreotide • potassium chloride • prednisolone • promazine • ranitidine • sodium bicarbonate • verapamil • vitamin B complex

• vitamin B complex with C. • Also compatible with TPN solutions or fat emulsion.

Incompatibility

• **Syringe:** amikacin • chlorpromazine • diazepam • doxorubicin • droperidol • droperidol/fentanyl • erythromycin • gentamicin • haloperidol • kanamycin • meperidine • methicillin • methotrimeprazine • netilmicin • pentazocine • promethazine • streptomycin • tobramycin • triflupromazine • vancomycin.

• **Y-site:** alteplase • ciprofloxacin • diazepam • dimenhydrinate • ergotamine tartrate • erythromycin glucceptate • gentamicin • haloperidol • hydroxyzine • idarubicin • kanamycin • methotrimeprazine • phenytoin • promazine • triflupromazine • tobramycin • vancomycin.

• **Additive:** amikacin • atracurium • codeine • cytarabine • daunorubicin • erythromycin lactobionate • gentamicin • hyaluronidase • kanamycin • levorphanol • meperidine • methadone • morphine • polymyxin B • promethazine • streptomycin.

Rate of Administration

• **Direct IV:** May be given undiluted over at least 1 minute. • **Intermittent Infusion:** Infusion may be administered over 4–24 hours. Use an infusion pump to ensure accuracy.

≋ CLINICAL PRECAUTIONS

• Inform all personnel caring for the patient of anticoagulant therapy. Venipunctures and injection sites require application of pressure to prevent bleeding or hematoma formation. IM injections of other medications should be avoided, as hematomas may develop.

• Assess patient for signs of bleeding and hemorrhage (bleeding gums, nosebleed, unusual bruising, black tarry stools, hematuria, fall in hematocrit or blood pressure, guaiac-positive stools). Assess patient for evidence of additional or increased thrombosis. Symptoms will depend on area of involvement. Monitor patient for hypersensitivity reactions (chills, fever, urticaria).

• Patients requiring long-term anticoagulation should have oral anticoagulant therapy instituted 4–5 days prior to discontinuing heparin therapy.

- Heparin should be used cautiously in patients with untreated hypertension, ulcer disease, spinal cord or brain injury, or malignancy.
- The risk of bleeding from heparin may be increased by concurrent use of drugs that affect platelet function, including aspirin, nonsteroidal anti-inflammatory agents, dipyridamole, large doses of penicillin, and dextran. This risk may also be increased by concurrent use of drugs that cause hypoprothrombinemia, including quinidine, cefamandole, cefmetazole, cefoperazone, cefotetan, and plicamycin. Concurrent use of thrombolytic agents may increase the risk of bleeding, although concurrent or sequential use is often employed.
- Probenecid increases the intensity and duration of the action of heparin.
- Elderly patients may be more sensitive to heparin, especially after 24–48 hours of therapy. Dosage reduction may be necessary. Elderly female patients are more susceptible to bleeding complications.
- When heparin is used in the management of disseminated intravascular coagulation, the underlying cause should be treated concurrently.
- Heparin may be used during pregnancy, but use with caution during the last trimester and in the immediate postpartum period. Dosage adjustments may be necessary (Pregnancy Category C).

Toxicity and Overdose Alert

- Protamine sulfate is the antidote. See *protamine sulfate* monograph, page 869. However, because of heparin's short half-life, overdosage can often be treated by simply discontinuing the drug.

Lab Test Considerations

- Activated PTT (aPTT) and hematocrit should be monitored prior to and periodically throughout course of therapy. When intermittent IV therapy is used, draw aPTT levels 30 minutes before next dose. During continuous administration, blood for aPTT levels can be drawn 1.5–2 hours after initiation of heparin therapy. • Monitor platelet count every 2–3 days throughout course of therapy. May cause mild thrombocytopenia, which appears on fourth day and resolves despite continued heparin therapy. Thrombocytopenia, which necessitates discontinuing medication, may develop on eighth day of therapy. Patients who have received a previous course of heparin may be at higher risk for severe thrombocytopenia for several months after the initial course. Heparin may cause prolonged PT levels (used in monitoring warfarin response); false elevations of serum thyroxine, T_3 resin uptake, and sulfobromophthalein (BSP); and false-negative ^{125}I fibrinogen uptake tests. • Heparin may cause decreased serum triglyceride and cholesterol levels and increased plasma free fatty acid concentrations. • Heparin may also cause elevated AST (SGOT) and ALT (SGPT) levels.

Patient/Family Teaching

• Caution patient to avoid IM injections and activities leading to injury and to use a soft toothbrush and electric razor during heparin therapy. • Advise patient to report any symptoms of unusual bleeding or bruising to physician immediately. • Instruct patient not to take medications containing aspirin, ibuprofen, or naproxen while on heparin therapy. • Patients on anticoagulant therapy should carry an identification card with this information at all times.

≋ PHARMACOLOGIC PROFILE

Indications

• Heparin is used in the prophylaxis and treatment of various thromboembolic disorders including venous thromboembolism, pulmonary emboli, atrial fibrillation with embolization, acute and chronic consumptive coagulopathies, and peripheral arterial thromboembolism. It is used in very low doses (10–100 units) to maintain patency of IV catheters ("heparin flush"). It is also used in the management of disseminated intravascular coagulation (DIC).

Action

• Heparin potentiates the effects of antithrombin III. • In low doses, heparin prevents the conversion of prothrombin to thrombin. Higher doses neutralize thrombin, preventing the conversion of fibrinogen to fibrin. • These actions prevent thrombus formation and prevent extension of existing thrombi. Heparin does not lyse existing thrombi.

Time/Action Profile (effects on aPTT)

Onset	Peak	Duration
immediate	5–10 min	2–6 hr

Pharmacokinetics

• **Distribution:** Heparin does not cross the placenta or enter breast milk. • **Metabolism and Excretion:** Heparin appears to be removed by the reticuloendothelial system (lymph nodes, spleen). • **Half-life:** 1–2 hours (increases with increasing dosage).

Contraindications

• Heparin is contraindicated in patients with hypersensitivity to heparin or to pig or beef proteins (some products are derived from hog intestinal mucosa, others from beef lung). • Heparin should not be used in patients with uncontrolled bleeding, open wounds, or severe liver or kidney disease. • Products containing benzyl alcohol should not be used in premature infants.

Adverse Reactions and Side Effects*

• **GI:** hepatitis • **Hemat:** BLEEDING, thrombocytopenia • **Derm:** rashes, urticaria • **Misc:** hypersensitivity, fever.

Hetastarch	Volume expander
HES, Hespan, Hydroxyethyl starch	pH 5.5, contains 154 mEq Na/L

 ADMINISTRATION CONSIDERATIONS

Usual Dose

ADULTS: 30–60 g (500–1000 ml of 6% solution). May be repeated, but should not exceed 90 g (1500 ml) day. In acute hemorrhagic shock, up to 20 ml/kg/hr may be used.

---

*Underlines indicate most frequent; CAPITALS indicate life-threatening.

Dilution

• **Continuous Infusion:** Administer hetastarch **undiluted** by IV infusion. • Available in a 6% solution diluted with 0.9% NaCl. Solution should be clear pale yellow to amber; do not administer solution that is cloudy, discolored, or that contains a precipitate. Store at room temperature. Discard unused solution.

Compatibility

• **Y-site:** cimetidine ✦ doxycycline ✦ enalaprilat.

Incompatibility

• **Y-site:** amikacin ✦ cefamandole ✦ cefoperazone ✦ cefotaxime ✦ cefoxitin ✦ gentamicin ✦ theophylline ✦ tobramycin.

Rate of Administration

• **Continuous Infusion:** Rate of administration is determined by blood volume, indication, and patient response. • In acute hemorrhagic shock, hetastarch may be administered up to 1.2 g/kg (20 ml/kg)/hr. • Slower rates are generally used in patients with burns or septic shock.

≋ CLINICAL PRECAUTIONS

- Monitor vital signs, central venous pressure (CVP), cardiac output, pulmonary capillary wedge pressure, and urinary output prior to and frequently throughout therapy. Assess patient for signs of vascular overload (elevated CVP, rales/crackles, dyspnea, hypertension, jugular venous distention) during and following administration.
- If fever, wheezing, flu-like symptoms, urticaria, periorbital edema, or submaxillary and parotid gland enlargement occur, stop infusion immediately. Antihistamines, epinephrine, glucocorticoids, and airway management may be required to suppress this response.
- Assess surgical patients for increased bleeding following administration caused by interference with platelet function and clotting factors. Use hetastarch cautiously in elderly patients or patients with thrombocytopenia.
- There is no danger of serum hepatitis or HIV infection from hetastarch. Crossmatching is not required.

- Safe use in pregnancy, lactation, or children has not been established.

Lab Test Considerations

- Monitor CBC with differential, hemoglobin, hematocrit, platelet count, prothrombin time, partial thromboplastin time, and clotting time throughout course of therapy. Large volumes of hetastarch may cause hemodilution; do not allow hematocrit to drop below 30% by volume. May cause increased erythrocyte sedimentation rate; prolonged bleeding time; and prolonged prothrombin, partial thromboplastin, and clotting times. • Hetastarch may cause elevated indirect serum bilirubin and amylase concentrations.

Patient/Family Teaching

- Explain to patient the rationale for use of hetastarch. Instruct patient to notify physician or nurse if dyspnea, itching, or flu-like symptoms occur.

 PHARMACOLOGIC PROFILE

Indications

- Hetastarch is used as an adjunct in the early management of shock or impending shock due to burns, hemorrhage, surgery, sepsis, or trauma when fluid replacement and plasma volume expansion are needed.

Action

- Hetastarch is a synthetic molecule that acts as a colloidal osmotic agent similar to albumin.

Time/Action Profile (volume expansion)

Onset	Peak	Duration
rapid	end of infusion	24 hr or longer

Pharmacokinetics

- **Distribution:** UK. • **Metabolism and Excretion:** Molecules of hetastarch with a molecular weight of 50,000 or less are excreted unchanged by the kidneys. Larger molecules are slowly degraded before excretion. • **Half-life:** 90% of hetastarch has a half-life of 17 days; the remaining 10% has a half-life of 48 days.

Contraindications

• Hetastarch is contraindicated in patients with hypersensitivity to it. • Patients with severe bleeding disorders, congestive heart failure, pulmonary edema, oliguric or anuric renal failure, or early pregnancy should not receive hetastarch.

Adverse Reactions and Side Effects*

• **CNS:** headache • **CV:** pulmonary edema, congestive heart failure • **GI:** vomiting • **Hemat:** decreased platelet function, decreased hematocrit • **Derm:** pruritus, urticaria • **F and E:** fluid overload, peripheral edema of the lower extremities • **MS:** myalgia • **Misc:** hypersensitivity reactions, including ANAPHYLACTOID REACTIONS; chills, fever, parotid and submaxillary gland enlargement.

Hydralazine Hydrochloride	Antihypertensive (vasodilator)
Apresoline	pH 3.4–4

≋ ADMINISTRATION CONSIDERATIONS

Usual Dose

ADULTS: 5–20 mg repeated as needed.
CHILDREN: 425–875 mcg (0.425–0.875 mg)/kg (12.5–25 mg/m²) q 6 hr or 283–617 mcg (0.283–0.617 mg)/kg (8.3–16.7 mg/m²) q 4 hr.

Dilution

• **Direct IV:** Inject **undiluted** through Y-tubing or 3-way stopcock. • Use solution as quickly as possible after drawing through needle into syringe. Hydralazine changes color after contact with a metal filter.

---

*Underlines indicate most frequent; CAPITALS indicate life-threatening.

Compatibility

- **Y-site:** heparin ◆ hydrocortisone sodium succinate ◆ potassium chloride ◆ verapamil ◆ vitamin B complex with C.
- **Additive:** dobutamine.
- **Solution:** dextrose/saline combinations ◆ dextrose/Ringer's or lactated Ringer's solution combinations ◆ D5/LR ◆ D5W ◆ D10W ◆ D10/LR ◆ 0.45% NaCl ◆ 0.9% NaCl ◆ Ringer's or lactated Ringer's solution. However, manufacturer does not recommend admixture in infusion solutions.

Incompatibility

- **Y-site:** aminophylline ◆ ampicillin ◆ diazoxide ◆ furosemide.
- **Additive:** aminophylline ◆ ampicillin ◆ chlorothiazide ◆ edetate calcium disodium ◆ ethacrynate sodium ◆ hydrocortisone sodium succinate ◆ methohexital ◆ nitroglycerin ◆ phenobarbital ◆ verapamil.

Rate of Administration

- **Direct IV:** Administer at a rate of 10 mg over at least 1 minute for adults. Administer at a rate of 0.2 mg/kg/minute in children.

≋ CLINICAL PRECAUTIONS

- Monitor blood pressure and pulse frequently during initial dosage adjustment and periodically throughout course of therapy. Notify physician of significant changes. Geriatric patients are less likely to develop reflex tachycardia, making them more prone to orthostatic hypotension.
- Parenteral route should be used only when drug cannot be given orally. Oral and intravenous doses are not interchangeable. IV doses are smaller.
- Additive hypotension occurs with other antihypertensive agents, or nitrates. MAO inhibitors may exaggerate hypotension. Hydralazine may reduce the pressor response to epinephrine. Nonsteroidal anti-inflammatory agents may decrease antihypertensive response. Beta-adrenergic blockers decrease tachycardia from hydralazine (therapy may be combined for this reason).

- Use hydralazine cautiously in patients with cardiovascular or cerebrovascular disease or severe renal or hepatic disease.
- Safe use in pregnancy, lactation, or children has not been established (Pregnancy Category C).

Lab Test Considerations

- CBC, electrolytes, LE cell prep, and antinuclear antibody (ANA) titer should be monitored prior to and periodically during prolonged therapy. • Hydralazine may cause a positive direct Coombs' test.

Patient/Family Teaching

- Caution patient to avoid sudden changes in position to minimize orthostatic hypotension. • Hydralazine may occasionally cause drowsiness. Advise patient to avoid activities requiring alertness until response to medication is known. • Encourage patient to comply with additional interventions for hypertension (weight reduction, low-sodium diet, discontinuation of smoking, moderation of alcohol intake, regular exercise, and stress management). Instruct patient and family on proper technique for blood pressure monitoring. Advise them to check blood pressure at least weekly and report significant changes to physician. Patients should weigh themselves twice weekly and assess feet and ankles for fluid retention. • Advise patient to notify physician immediately if general tiredness, fever, muscle or joint aching, chest pain, skin rash, sore throat or numbness, tingling, pain, or weakness of hands and feet occur. Vitamin B_6 (pyridoxine) may be used to treat peripheral neuritis. • Emphasize the importance of follow-up examinations to evaluate effectiveness of medication.

≋ PHARMACOLOGIC PROFILE

Indications

- Hydralazine is used in combination with a diuretic to lower blood pressure in moderate to severely hypertensive patients. It is also used to decrease afterload in the treatment of congestive heart failure unresponsive to conventional therapy with cardiac glycosides and diuretics.

Action

• Hydralazine is a direct-acting peripheral arteriolar vaso-dilator.

Time/Action Profile (antihypertensive effect)

Onset	Peak	Duration
5–20 min	10–80 min	4–6 hr

Pharmacokinetics

• **Distribution:** Hydralazine is widely distributed. It crosses the placenta and enters breast milk in minimal concentrations. • **Metabolism and Excretion:** Hydralazine is mostly metabolized by the GI mucosa and liver. • **Half-life:** 2–8 hours.

Contraindications

• Hydralazine is contraindicated in patients with hypersensitivity to it. • Injectable product contains parabens and propylene glycol; avoid use in patients with hypersensitivity to these additives.

Adverse Reactions and Side Effects*

• **CNS:** headache, peripheral neuropathy, dizziness, drowsiness • **CV:** <u>tachycardia</u>, angina, arrhythmias, orthostatic hypotension, edema • **GI:** nausea, vomiting, diarrhea • **Derm:** rashes • **F and E:** <u>sodium retention</u> • **MS:** arthritis, arthralgias • **Neuro:** peripheral neuropathy • **Misc:** <u>drug-induced lupus syndrome</u>.

Hydrocortisone Sodium Phosphate	*Glucocorticoid (short-acting)*
Hydrocortone phosphate	pH 7.5–8.5

≋ ADMINISTRATION CONSIDERATIONS

Usual Dose

ADULTS: 15–500 mg; may be repeated q 2–6 hr.

CHILDREN: *Adrenocortical insufficiency:* 62–93 mcg (0.062–0.093 mg)/kg or 3.3–4 mg/m^2 3 times daily. *Other indica-*

---

*<u>Underlines</u> indicate most frequent; CAPITALS indicate life-threatening.

tions: 666 mcg (0.666 mg)–4 mg/kg or 20–120 mg/m^2 q 12–24 hr.

Dilution

• **Direct IV:** Reconstitute with provided solution or 2 ml of bacteriostatic water or saline for injection. • **Intermittent Infusion:** May be added to 50–1000 ml of D5W, 0.9% NaCl, or D5/0.9% NaCl. • Diluted solution should be used within 24 hours.

Compatibility

• **Syringe:** metoclopramide.

• **Y-site:** allopurinol sodium ♦ filgrastim ♦ fluconazole ♦ fludarabine ♦ melphalan ♦ ondansetron ♦ paclitaxel ♦ piperacillin/tazobactam ♦ vinorelbine.

• **Additive:** amikacin ♦ amphotericin B ♦ bleomycin ♦ cephapirin ♦ dacarbazine ♦ heparin ♦ metaraminol ♦ sodium bicarbonate ♦ verapamil.

Incompatibility

• **Y-site:** sargramostim.

Rate of Administration

• **Direct IV:** Administer each 100 mg over at least 30 seconds. Doses 500 mg and larger should be infused over at least 10 minutes. • **Intermittent Infusion:** Administer infusions at prescribed rate.

≋ CLINICAL PRECAUTIONS

- Hydrocortisone is indicated for many conditions. Assess involved systems prior to and periodically throughout course of therapy.
- Assess patient for signs of adrenal insufficiency (hypotension, weight loss, weakness, nausea, vomiting, anorexia, lethargy, confusion, restlessness) prior to and periodically throughout chronic therapy.
- Monitor intake and output ratios and daily weights. Observe patient for the appearance of peripheral edema, steady weight gain, rales/crackles, or dyspnea. Hydrocortisone may mask signs of infection.
- Phenytoin, phenobarbital, and rifampin stimulate metabolism of hydrocortisone and may decrease effectiveness.

- Oral contraceptives may block metabolism of hydrocortisone.
- Live vaccines should not be administered to patients receiving more than 20 mg/day due to increased risk of adverse reactions and decreased antibody response.
- Use cautiously in children (chronic use may lead to growth suppression). Children receiving prolonged therapy should have periodic evaluations of growth.
- Chronic treatment with doses greater than 20 mg/day results in adrenal suppression. Do not discontinue abruptly. During periods of stress (infections, surgery) additional doses may be required. Use lowest possible dose for shortest period of time.
- The risk of developing hypertension or hyperglycemia is increased in geriatric patients.
- Safe use in pregnancy or lactation has not been established. Chronic use during pregnancy may result in hypoadrenalism in the infant.

Lab Test Considerations

- Patients on prolonged courses of hydrocortisone should routinely have hematologic values, serum electrolytes, and serum and urine glucose evaluated. Hydrocortisone may decrease serum potassium and calcium and increase serum sodium concentrations. Additive hypokalemia may occur with amphotericin B, mezlocillin, piperacillin, ticarcillin, or diuretics. Hypokalemia may increase the risk of cardiac glycoside toxicity. Glucocorticoids may cause hyperglycemia, especially in persons with diabetes, and may increase requirements for insulin or oral hypoglycemic agents. • Guaiac-test stools. • Hydrocortisone may increase serum cholesterol and lipid values and decrease serum protein-bound iodine and thyroxine concentrations. • Hydrocortisone suppresses reactions to allergy skin tests and may cause decreased WBC counts. • Periodic adrenal function tests may be ordered during long-term therapy to assess degree of hypothalamic–pituitary–adrenal (HPA) axis suppression.

Patient/Family Teaching

- Inform patients that stopping hydrocortisone suddenly if it has been taken on a chronic basis may result in adrenal insufficiency (anorexia, nausea, fatigue, weakness, hypotension, dyspnea, and hypoglycemia). If these signs appear, notify physician immediately. This condition can be life-threatening. • Encourage patients on long-term therapy to eat a diet high in protein, calcium, and potassium and low in sodium and carbohydrates (see Appendix H for foods included). • Hydrocortisone causes immunosuppression and may mask symptoms of infection. Instruct patient to avoid people with known contagious illnesses and to report possible infections. Caution patient to avoid vaccinations without consulting physician. • Review side effects with patient. Instruct patient to inform physician promptly if severe abdominal pain or tarry stools occur. Patient should also report unusual swelling, weight gain, tiredness, bone pain, bruising, nonhealing sores, visual disturbances, or behavior changes. • Instruct patient to inform physician if symptoms of underlying disease return or worsen. • Advise patient to carry identification in the event of an emergency in which patient cannot relate medical history. • Emphasize the importance of follow-up examinations to monitor progress and side effects.

 PHARMACOLOGIC PROFILE

Indications

• Hydrocortisone is used in the short-term management of a variety of inflammatory and allergic conditions, including asthma and ulcerative colitis. It is also used in the management of adrenocortical insufficiency. Hydrocortisone is not suitable for alternate-day therapy.

Action

• Hydrocortisone replaces cortisol in deficiency states. It suppresses the normal immune response and inflammation and has additional profound and varied metabolic effects. Hydrocortisone is a potent mineralocorticoid (sodium retention). It will also suppress adrenal function with chronic use at doses of more than 20 mg/day.

Time/Action Profile (anti-inflammatory effects)

Onset	Peak	Duration
rapid	UK	1.25–1.5 days

Pharmacokinetics

• **Distribution:** Hydrocortisone is widely distributed. It crosses the placenta and probably enters breast milk. • **Metabolism and Excretion:** Hydrocortisone is metabolized by the liver. • **Half-life:** 80–120 minutes.

Contraindications

• Hydrocortisone is contraindicated in patients with serious infections, except for some forms of meningitis. • Injectable product contains bisulfites and should be avoided in patients with known hypersensitivity.

Adverse Reactions and Side Effects*

These are seen mostly with chronic therapy.

• **CNS:** psychoses, depression, euphoria • **EENT:** cataracts, increased intraocular pressure • **CV:** edema, hypertension, congestive heart failure, thromboembolism • **GI:** nausea, vomiting, increased appetite, weight gain, GI bleeding, peptic ulceration • **Derm:** petechiae, ecchymoses, fragility, decreased wound healing; hirsutism, acne • **Endo:** menstrual irregularities, hyperglycemia, decreased growth in children, adrenal suppression • **F and E:** hypokalemia, sodium retention, metabolic alkalosis, hypocalcemia • **MS:** weakness, myopathy, aseptic necrosis of joints, osteoporosis • **Misc:** increased susceptibility to infections; pancreatitis, cushingoid appearance (moon face, buffalo hump).

Hydrocortisone Sodium Succinate	Glucocorticoid (short-acting)
A-Hydrocort, Solu-Cortef	pH 7–8

≋ ADMINISTRATION CONSIDERATIONS

Usual Dose

Adults: 100–500 mg; may be repeated q 2–6 hr.

Children: *Adrenocortical insufficiency:* 62–93 mcg (0.062–0.093 mg)/kg or 3.3–4 mg/m² 3 times daily. *Other indica-*

---

*Underlines indicate most frequent; CAPITALS indicate life-threatening.

tions: 666 mcg (0.666 mg)−4 mg/kg or 20−120 mg/m^2 q 12−24 hr.

Dilution

• **Direct IV:** Reconstitute with provided solution or 2 ml of bacteriostatic water or saline for injection. • **Intermittent Infusion:** May be added to 50−1000 ml of D5W, 0.9% NaCl, dextrose/saline combinations, dextrose/Ringer's or lactated Ringer's combinations, D10W, D20W, Ringer's or lactated Ringer's injection, 3% NaCl, sodium lactate ⅙ M, or D5/0.9% NaCl for a concentration of 0.1−1 mg/ml. • Diluted solution should be used within 24 hours.

Compatibility

• **Syringe:** metoclopramide ♦ thiopental.

• **Y-site:** acyclovir ♦ allopurinol sodium ♦ aminophylline ♦ ampicillin ♦ amrinone ♦ atracurium ♦ atropine ♦ betamethasone ♦ calcium gluconate ♦ cephalothin ♦ cephapirin ♦ chlordiazepoxide ♦ chlorpromazine ♦ cyanocobalamin ♦ dexamethasone ♦ digoxin ♦ diphenhydramine ♦ dopamine ♦ droperidol ♦ edrophonium ♦ enalaprilat ♦ epinephrine ♦ esmolol ♦ conjugated estrogens ♦ ethacrynate ♦ famotidine ♦ fentanyl ♦ fentanyl/droperidol ♦ filgrastim ♦ fludarabine ♦ fluorouracil ♦ foscarnet ♦ furosemide ♦ gallium nitrate ♦ hydralazine ♦ insulin ♦ isoproterenol ♦ kanamycin ♦ lidocaine ♦ magnesium sulfate ♦ melphalan ♦ menadiol ♦ methicillin ♦ methoxamine ♦ methylergonovine ♦ minocycline ♦ morphine ♦ neostigmine ♦ norepinephrine ♦ ondansetron ♦ oxacillin ♦ oxytocin ♦ paclitaxel ♦ pancuronium ♦ penicillin G potassium ♦ pentazocine ♦ phytonadione ♦ piperacillin/tazobactam ♦ prednisolone ♦ procainamide ♦ prochlorperazine ♦ propranolol ♦ pyridostigmine ♦ scopolamine ♦ sodium bicarbonate ♦ succinylcholine ♦ tacrolimus ♦ trimethobenzamide ♦ trimethaphan camsylate ♦ vecuronium ♦ vinorelbine.

• **Additive:** amikacin ♦ aminophylline ♦ amphotericin ♦ calcium chloride ♦ calcium gluconate ♦ cephalothin ♦ cephapirin ♦ chloramphenicol ♦ clindamycin ♦ daunorubicin ♦ dopamine ♦ erythromycin ♦ lidocaine ♦ magnesium sulfate ♦ mitoxantrone ♦ netilmicin ♦ norepinephrine ♦ penicillin G ♦ piperacillin ♦ polymyxin B ♦ potassium chloride ♦ procaine ♦ sodium bicarbonate ♦ thiopental ♦ vancomycin ♦ verapamil ♦ vitamin B complex with C.

Incompatibility

- **Y-site:** ciprofloxacin ✦ diazepam ✦ ergotamine tartrate ✦ idarubicin ✦ phenytoin ✦ sargramostim.
- **Additive:** bleomycin ✦ colistimethate ✦ diphenhydramine ✦ doxorubicin ✦ ephedrine ✦ hydralazine ✦ nafcillin ✦ pentobarbital ✦ phenobarbital ✦ prochlorperazine ✦ promethazine ✦ secobarbital.

Rate of Administration

- **Direct IV:** Administer each 100 mg over at least 30 seconds. Doses 500 mg and larger should be infused over at least 10 minutes. • **Intermittent Infusion:** Administer infusions at prescribed rate.

≋ CLINICAL PRECAUTIONS

- Hydrocortisone is indicated for many conditions. Assess involved systems prior to and periodically throughout course of therapy.
- Assess patient for signs of adrenal insufficiency (hypotension, weight loss, weakness, nausea, vomiting, anorexia, lethargy, confusion, restlessness) prior to and periodically throughout chronic therapy.
- Monitor intake and output ratios and daily weights. Observe patient for the appearance of peripheral edema, steady weight gain, rales/crackles, or dyspnea. Hydrocortisone may mask signs of infection.
- Phenytoin, phenobarbital, and rifampin stimulate metabolism of hydrocortisone and may decrease effectiveness.
- Oral contraceptives may block metabolism of hydrocortisone.
- Live vaccines should not be administered to patients receiving more than 20 mg/day due to increased risk of adverse reactions and decreased antibody response.
- Use cautiously in children (chronic use may lead to growth suppression). Children receiving prolonged therapy should also have periodic evaluations of growth.
- Chronic treatment with doses greater than 20 mg/day results in adrenal suppression. Do not discontinue abruptly. During periods of stress (infections, surgery)

additional doses may be required. Use lowest possible dose for shortest period of time.
- The risk of developing hypertension is increased in geriatric patients.
- Safe use in pregnancy or lactation has not been established. Chronic use during pregnancy may result in hypoadrenalism in the infant.

Lab Test Considerations

• Patients on prolonged courses of hydrocortisone should routinely have hematologic values, serum electrolytes, and serum and urine glucose levels evaluated. Hydrocortisone may decrease serum potassium and calcium and increase serum sodium concentrations. Additive hypokalemia may occur with amphotericin B, mezlocillin, piperacillin, ticarcillin, or diuretics. Hypokalemia may increase the risk of cardiac glycoside toxicity. Glucocorticoids may cause hyperglycemia, especially in persons with diabetes, and may increase requirements for insulin or oral hypoglycemic agents. • Guaiac-test stools. • Hydrocortisone may increase serum cholesterol and lipid values and decrease serum protein-bound iodine and thyroxine concentrations. • Hydrocortisone suppresses reactions to allergy skin tests and may cause decreased WBC counts. • Periodic adrenal function tests may be ordered during long-term therapy to assess degree of hypothalamic–pituitary–adrenal (HPA) axis suppression.

Patient/Family Teaching

• Inform patients that stopping hydrocortisone suddenly if it has been taken on a chronic basis may result in adrenal insufficiency (anorexia, nausea, fatigue, weakness, hypotension, dyspnea, and hypoglycemia). If these signs appear, notify physician immediately. This condition can be life-threatening. • Encourage patients on long-term therapy to eat a diet high in protein, calcium, and potassium and low in sodium and carbohydrates (see Appendix H for foods included). • Hydrocortisone causes immunosuppression and may mask symptoms of infection. Instruct patient to avoid people with known contagious illnesses and to report possible infections. Caution patient to avoid vaccinations without first consulting physician. • Review side effects with patient. Instruct patient to inform physician promptly if severe abdominal pain or tarry stools occur. Patient should also report any unusual swelling, weight gain, tiredness, bone pain, bruising, nonhealing sores, visual disturbances, or behavior changes. • Instruct patient to inform physician if symptoms of underlying disease return or worsen. • Advise patient to carry identification in the event of an emergency in which patient cannot relate medical history. • Emphasize the importance of follow-up examinations to monitor progress and side effects.

≋ PHARMACOLOGIC PROFILE

Indications
• Hydrocortisone is used in the short-term management of a variety of inflammatory and allergic conditions, including asthma and ulcerative colitis. It is also used in the management of adrenocortical insufficiency. Hydrocortisone is not suitable for alternate-day therapy.

Action
• Hydrocortisone replaces cortisol in deficiency states. It suppresses the normal immune response and inflammation and has additional profound and varied metabolic effects. Hydrocortisone is a potent mineralocorticoid (sodium retention). It will also suppress adrenal function with chronic use at doses of more than 20 mg/day.

Time/Action Profile (anti-inflammatory effects)

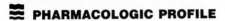

Onset	Peak	Duration
rapid	UK	1.25–1.5 days

Pharmacokinetics
• **Distribution:** Hydrocortisone is widely distributed. It crosses the placenta and probably enters breast milk. • **Metabolism and Excretion:** Hydrocortisone is metabolized by the liver. • **Half-life:** 80–120 minutes.

Contraindications
• Hydrocortisone is contraindicated in patients with serious infections, except for some forms of meningitis.

Adverse Reactions and Side Effects*

These are seen mostly with chronic therapy.

• **CNS:** psychoses, <u>depression</u>, euphoria • **EENT:** cataracts, increased intraocular pressure • **CV:** edema, hypertension, congestive heart failure, thromboembolism • **GI:** <u>nausea</u>, vomiting, increased appetite, weight gain, GI bleeding, peptic ulceration • **Derm:** <u>petechiae</u>, ecchymoses, fragility, <u>decreased wound healing</u>; hirsutism, acne • **Endo:** menstrual irregularities, hyperglycemia, <u>decreased growth in children</u>, <u>adrenal suppression</u> • **F and E:** <u>hypokalemia</u>, <u>sodium retention</u>, metabolic alkalosis, hypocalcemia • **MS:** weakness, myopathy, aseptic necrosis of joints, osteoporosis • **Misc:** increased susceptibility to infections; pancreatitis, cushingoid appearance (moon face, buffalo hump).

Hydromorphone Hydrochloride	Opioid analgesic (agonist)
Dilaudid HCl, Dilaudid HP	pH 4–5.5

Schedule II

ADMINISTRATION CONSIDERATIONS

Usual Dose

Intermittent Injection

ADULTS: 1–4 mg q 4–6 hr as needed initially. Larger doses may be required.

Continuous Infusion (unlabeled use)

ADULTS: Range 0.2–30 mg/hr depending on previous opioid use. An initial bolus of twice the hourly rate in mg may be

---

*<u>Underlines</u> indicate most frequent; CAPITALS indicate life-threatening.

given, with subsequent boluses of 50–100% of the hourly rate in mg.

Dilution

• **Direct IV: Dilute** with at least 5 ml of sterile water or 0.9% NaCl for injection. • Inspect solution for particulate matter. Slight yellow color does not alter potency. Store at room temperature.

Compatibility

• **Syringe:** atropine • chlorpromazine • cimetidine • diphenhydramine • fentanyl • glycopyrrolate • hydroxyzine • midazolam • pentazocine • pentobarbital • promethazine • ranitidine • scopolamine • tetracaine • thiethylperazine • trimethobenzamide.

• **Y-site:** acyclovir • allopurinol sodium • amikacin • ampicillin • cefamandole • cefoperazone • cefotaxime • cefoxitin • ceftizoxime • cefuroxime • cephalothin • cephapirin • chloramphenicol • cisplatin • clindamycin • cyclophosphamide • cytarabine • doxorubicin • doxycycline • erythromycin lactobionate • filgrastim • fludarabine • foscarnet • gentamicin • kanamycin • magnesium sulfate • melphalan • methotrexate • metronidazole • mezlocillin • nafcillin • ondansetron • oxacillin • paclitaxel • penicillin G potassium • piperacillin • piperacillin/tazobactam • ticarcillin • tobramycin • trimethoprim/sulfamethoxazole • vancomycin • vinorelbine.

• **Additive:** ondansetron • verapamil.

• **Solution:** D5W • D5/0.45% NaCl • D5/0.9% NaCl • D5/LR • D5/Ringer's injection • 0.45% NaCl • 0.9% NaCl • Ringer's and lactated Ringer's injection.

Incompatibility

• **Y-site:** diazepam • gallium nitrate • minocycline • phenobarbital • phenytoin • sargramostim.

• **Additive:** sodium bicarbonate • thiopental.

Rate of Administration

• **Direct IV:** Administer slowly, at a rate not to exceed 2 mg over 3–5 minutes. Rapid administration may lead to increased respiratory depression, hypotension, and circulatory collapse.

≋ CLINICAL PRECAUTIONS

- Assess type, location, and intensity of pain prior to and 15–30 minutes (peak) following administration. When titrating opioid doses, increases of 25–50% should be administered until there is a 50% reduction in the patient's pain rating on a numerical or visual analog scale or the patient reports satisfactory pain relief. Subsequent doses may be safely administered at the time of the peak if the previous dose is ineffective and side effects are minimal.

- Patients on continuous infusion should have additional bolus doses provided every 15–30 minutes as needed for breakthrough pain. The bolus dose is usually set to the amount of drug administered each hour by continuous infusion.

- An equianalgesic chart (Appendix B, page 1045) should be used when changing routes or when changing from one opioid to another.

- Regularly administered doses may be more effective than p.r.n. administration. Analgesic is more effective if given before pain becomes severe. Coadministration with nonopioid analgesics may have additive analgesic effects and permit lower opioid doses.

- Assess blood pressure, pulse, and respiratory rate before and periodically during administration. If respiratory rate is less than 10/minute, assess level of sedation. Physical stimulation may be sufficient to prevent significant hypoventilation. Dose may need to be decreased by 25–50%.

- Assess bowel function routinely. Prevention of constipation should be instituted with increased intake of fluids and bulk, stool softeners, and laxatives to minimize constipating effects. Stimulant laxatives should be administered routinely if opioid use exceeds 2–3 days, unless contraindicated.

- Prolonged use may lead to physical and psychological dependence and tolerance. This should not prevent patient from receiving adequate analgesia. Most patients who receive hydromorphone for medical reasons do not develop psychological dependence. Progressively higher doses may be required to relieve pain with long-term therapy. Medication should be discontinued gradually after long-term use to prevent withdrawal symptoms. High potency concentration (HP) should only be used in patients who are tolerant to lower doses of opioids.

- Assess level of sedation. Initial drowsiness will diminish with continued use. Additive CNS depression my occur with alcohol, antidepressants, antihistamines, and sedative/hypnotics.

- Use with extreme caution in patients receiving MAO inhibitors (may produce severe, unpredictable reactions; reduce initial dose of hydromorphone to 25% of usual dose).

- Use cautiously in patients with head trauma; increased intracranial pressure; severe renal, hepatic, or pulmonary disease; hypothyroidism; adrenal insufficiency; alcoholism; elderly or debilitated patients (dosage reduction recommended); undiagnosed abdominal pain; or prostatic hypertrophy. Elderly patients are more likely to have CNS depression and constipation during hydromorphone therapy.

- Administration of partial-antagonist opioid analgesics may precipitate opioid withdrawal in physically dependent patients.

- Nalbuphine or pentazocine may decrease analgesia.

- Safe use in pregnancy, lactation, or children has not been established. Chronic use should be avoided (Pregnancy Category C).

Toxicity and Overdose Alert

- If an opioid antagonist is required to reverse respiratory depression or coma, naloxone (Narcan) is the antidote. Dilute the 0.4-mg ampule of naloxone in 10 ml of 0.9% NaCl and administer 0.5 ml (0.02 mg) by direct IV push every 2 minutes. For children and patients weighing <40 kg, dilute 0.1 mg of naloxone in 10 ml of 0.9% NaCl for a concentration of 10 mcg/ml and administer 0.5 mcg every 1–2 minutes. Titrate the dose to avoid withdrawal, seizures, and severe pain.

Lab Test Considerations

- May increase plasma amylase and lipase concentrations.

Patient/Family Teaching

• Instruct patient on how and when to ask for p.r.n. pain medication. • Medication may cause drowsiness or dizziness. Advise patient to call for assistance when ambulating or smoking. Caution patient to avoid activities requiring alertness until response to medication is known. • Advise patient to make position changes slowly to minimize orthostatic hypotension. • Instruct patient to avoid concurrent use of alcohol or other CNS depressants. • Encourage patient to turn, cough, and breathe deeply every 2 hours to prevent atelectasis.

• **Home Care Issues:** Explain to patient and family how and when to administer hydromorphone and how to take care of the equipment. • Emphasize the importance of aggressive prevention of constipation with the use of this drug.

≋ PHARMACOLOGIC PROFILE

Indications

• Hydromorphone is used alone and in combination with nonopioid analgesics in the management of moderate to severe pain.

Action

• Hydromorphone binds to opiate receptors in the CNS, where it alters the perception of and response to painful stimuli while producing generalized CNS depression.

Time/Action Profile (analgesic effect)

Onset	Peak	Duration
10–15 min	15–30 min	2–3 hr

Pharmacokinetics

• **Distribution:** Hydromorphone is widely distributed. It crosses the placenta and enters breast milk. • **Metabolism and Excretion:** Hydromorphone is mostly metabolized by the liver. • **Half-life:** 2–4 hours.

Contraindications

• Hydromorphone is contraindicated in patients with hypersensitivity to it. • Chronic use of hydromorphone should be avoided during pregnancy or lactation (Pregnancy Category C). • Hydromorphone may contain benzyl alcohol; avoid use in patients with hypersensitivity or known intolerance to alcohol. Products containing benzyl alcohol should not be used in infants.

Adverse Reactions and Side Effects*

• **CNS:** sedation, confusion, headache, euphoria, floating feeling, unusual dreams, hallucinations, dysphoria, dizziness • **EENT:** miosis, diplopia, blurred vision • **Resp:** respiratory depression • **CV:** hypotension, bradycardia • **GI:** nausea, vomiting, constipation • **GU:** urinary retention • **Derm:** sweating, flushing • **Misc:** tolerance, physical dependence, psychological dependence.

Idarubicin Hydrochloride	*Antineoplastic (antitumor antibiotic)*
Idamycin	pH 5–7

≋ ADMINISTRATION CONSIDERATIONS

Usual Dose

ADULTS: 12 mg/m^2 daily for 3 days in combination with cytarabine (see *cytarabine* monograph on page 262).

Dilution

• **Direct IV:** Reconstitute 5-mg and 10-mg vials with 5 ml and 10 ml, respectively, of 0.9% NaCl (nonbacteriostatic) for injection for a concentration of 1 mg/ml. Vial contents are under pressure; use care when inserting needle. • Solution should be prepared in a biologic cabinet. Wear gloves, gown, and mask while handling medication. Discard IV equipment in specially designated containers (see Appendix F). • When diluted in 0.9% NaCl in concentrations of 0.05–0.5 mg/ml, idarubicin solution may develop a haze, which is normal. • Reconstituted medication is stable for 72 hours at room temperature and 7 days if refrigerated.

---

*Underlines indicate most frequent; CAPITALS indicate life-threatening.

Compatibility

- **Y-site:** amikacin • cimetidine • cyclophosphamide • cytarabine • diphenhydramine • droperidol • erythromycin lactobionate • filgrastim • imipenem/cilastatin • magnesium sulfate • mannitol • melphalan • metoclopramide • potassium chloride • ranitidine • sargramostim • vinorelbine.

Incompatibility

- **Syringe:** heparin.
- **Y-site:** acyclovir • allopurinol sodium • ampicillin/sulbactam • cefazolin • ceftazidine • clindamycin • dexamethasone • etoposide • furosemide • gentamicin • heparin • hydrocortisone sodium succinate • lorazepam • meperidine • methotrexate • mezlocillin • piperacillin/tazobactam • sodium bicarbonate • vancomycin • vincristine.
- **Additive:** Do not add to IV solution. Manufacturer does not recommend mixture.

Rate of Administration

- **Direct IV:** Administer each dose slowly over 10–15 minutes through Y-site or 3-way stopcock of a free-flowing infusion of 0.9% NaCl or D5W. Tubing may be attached to a butterfly needle and injected into a large vein.

≋ CLINICAL PRECAUTIONS

- Assess injection site frequently for redness, irritation, or inflammation. Medication may infiltrate painlessly or cause burning or stinging. If extravasation occurs, infusion must be stopped and restarted elsewhere to avoid damage to SC tissue. Treatment of extravasation includes elevation and rest of extremity for 24–48 hours, then resumption of normal activity, and intermittent ice packs (apply for 30 minutes immediately and 30 minutes q.i.d. for 3 days). If pain, erythema, or vesication occurs, early plastic surgery may be warranted.
- Monitor blood pressure, pulse, respiratory rate, and temperature frequently during administration.
- Severe and protracted nausea and vomiting may occur as early as 1 hour after therapy and may last 24 hours. Parenteral antiemetic agents should be administered 30–45 minutes prior to therapy and routinely around the clock for the next 24 hours as indicated. Monitor amount of emesis, and follow guidelines to prevent dehydration.

- Assess oral mucosa for redness or irritation. Further courses of idarubicin should be withheld until recovery from mucositis, and subsequent doses should be decreased by 25%.
- Monitor for development of signs of myocardial toxicity manifested by life-threatening arrhythmias, cardiomyopathy, and congestive heart failure (peripheral edema, dyspnea, rales/crackles, weight gain). Elderly patients are at increased risk. Chest x-ray, ECG, echocardiography, and radionuclide angiography determinations of ejection fraction should be monitored prior to and periodically throughout therapy.
- Monitor for development of bone marrow depression. Assess for fever, chills, sore throat, and signs of infection. Monitor platelet count throughout therapy. Assess for bleeding (bleeding gums, bruising, petechiae; guaiac test stools, urine, and emesis). Avoid giving IM injections and taking rectal temperatures. Apply pressure to venipuncture sites for 10 minutes. Anemia may occur. Monitor for increased fatigue, dyspnea, and orthostatic hypotension. Additive myelosuppression may occur with concurrent use of other antineoplastic agents or radiation therapy.
- Monitor intake and output ratios. Encourage fluid intake of 2000–3000 ml/day. Allopurinol and alkalinization of the urine may be used to decrease serum uric acid levels and to help prevent urate stone formation.
- Use cautiously in patients with active infection, decreased bone marrow reserve, other chronic debilitating illness, hepatic impairment (dosage reduction may be required; avoid if bilirubin is more than 5 mg/dl), renal impairment (dosage reduction recommended if serum creatinine is more than 2.5 mg/100 ml), pre-existing cardiac disease, or previous daunorubicin or doxorubicin therapy.
- Use with caution in patients with childbearing potential. Safe use in children has not been established.

Lab Test Considerations

- Monitor CBC, differential, and platelet count prior to and periodically during therapy. Nadirs of leukopenia and thrombocytopenia are 10–14 days, with recovery occurring 21 days after a dose. • Monitor renal and hepatic function prior to and frequently throughout therapy. Idarubicin may cause hyperuricemia. May also cause transient increases in AST (SGOT), ALT (SGPT), serum alkaline phosphatase, and bilirubin.

Patient/Family Teaching

• Instruct patient to notify physician promptly in case of fever, sore throat, signs of infection, bleeding gums, bruising, petechiae; blood in stools, urine, or emesis; increased fatigue, dyspnea, or orthostatic hypotension. Caution patient to avoid crowds and persons with known infections. Instruct patient to use a soft toothbrush and electric razor and to be especially careful to avoid falls. Patients should be cautioned not to drink alcoholic beverages or take medication containing aspirin, ibuprofen, or naproxen as these may precipitate gastric bleeding. • Instruct patient to report pain at injection site immediately. • Instruct patient to inspect oral mucosa for erythema and ulceration. If ulceration occurs, advise patient to use sponge brush, rinse mouth with water after eating and drinking, and confer with physician if mouth pain interferes with eating. • Advise patient that this medication may have teratogenic effects. Nonhormonal contraception should be used during therapy and for at least 4 months after therapy is concluded. • Instruct patient to notify physician immediately if irregular heart beat, shortness of breath, or swelling of lower extremities occurs. • Discuss the possibility of hair loss with patient. Explore methods of coping. • Instruct patient not to receive any vaccinations without advice of physician. Idarubicin may decrease antibody response to, and increase risk of adverse reactions from, live virus vaccines. • Emphasize the need for periodic lab tests to monitor for side effects.

≋ PHARMACOLOGIC PROFILE

Indications

• Idarubicin is used as part of combination chemotherapy in the treatment of acute myelogenous leukemia in adults.

Action

• Idarubicin inhibits nucleic acid synthesis. This results in death of rapidly replicating cells, particularly malignant ones.

Time/Action Profile (effect on WBC, platelet counts)

Onset	Peak	Duration
within days	10–14 days	21 days†

†After dose.

Pharmacokinetics

• **Distribution:** Idarubicin is rapidly distributed, with extensive tissue binding and a high degree of cellular uptake. • **Metabolism and Excretion:** Idarubicin undergoes extensive hepatic and extrahepatic metabolism. One metabolite is active (idarubicinol). It is primarily eliminated via biliary excretion. • **Half-life:** 22 hours (range 4–46 hours).

Contraindications

• Idarubicin is contraindicated in pregnancy or lactation (Pregnancy Category D).

Adverse Reactions and Side Effects*

• **CNS:** headache, mental status changes • **Resp:** pulmonary toxicity, pulmonary allergic reactions • **CV:** cardiotoxicity, congestive heart failure, arrhythmia • **GI:** nausea, vomiting, abdominal cramps, diarrhea, mucositis • **Derm:** alopecia, rashes • **Endo:** gonadal suppression • **Hemat:** anemia, leukopenia, thrombocytopenia, bleeding • **Local:** phlebitis • **Metab:** hyperuricemia • **Neuro:** peripheral neuropathy • **Misc:** fever.

Ifosfamide	Antineoplastic (alkylating agent)
Ifex	pH 6

 ADMINISTRATION CONSIDERATIONS

Usual Dose

ADULTS: 1.2 g/m²/day for 5 days; coadminister with mesna. May repeat cycle q 3 wk. (See *mesna* monograph on page 595.)

---

*Underlines indicate most frequent; CAPITALS indicate life-threatening.

Dilution

• **Intermittent Infusion:** Prepare solution by **diluting** each 1-g vial with 20 ml of sterile water or bacteriostatic water for injection containing parabens. • Solution should be prepared in a biologic cabinet. Wear gloves, gown, and mask while handling IV medication. Discard IV equipment in specially designated containers (see Appendix F). • Use solution prepared without bacteriostatic water within 6 hours. Solution prepared with bacteriostatic water is stable for 1 week at 30°C or 6 weeks at 5°C. • May be **further diluted** to a concentration of 0.6 to 20 mg/ml in D5W, 0.9% NaCl, 0.45% NaCl, lactated Ringer's solution, D5/Ringer's injection, D5/0.9% NaCl, or sterile water for injection.

Compatibility

• **Syringe:** mesna.
• **Y-site:** allopurinol sodium ◆ filgrastim ◆ fludarabine ◆ gallium nitrate ◆ melphalan ◆ ondansetron ◆ paclitaxel ◆ piperacillin/tazobactam ◆ sargramostim ◆ vinorelbine.
• **Additive:** carboplatin ◆ cisplatin ◆ etoposide ◆ fluorouracil ◆ mesna.

Rate of Administration

• **Intermittent Infusion:** Administer over a minimum of 30 minutes.

≋ CLINICAL PRECAUTIONS

• Monitor blood pressure, pulse, respiratory rate, and temperature frequently during administration.
• Monitor urinary output frequently throughout therapy. To reduce the risk of hemorrhagic cystitis, fluid intake should be at least 3000 ml/day for adults prior to and for at least 72 hours following treatment. Mesna is given concurrently to prevent hemorrhagic cystitis.
• Monitor neurologic status. Ifosfamide should be discontinued if severe CNS symptoms (agitation, confusion, hallucinations, unusual tiredness) occur. Symptoms usually return to normal within 3 days of discontinuation of ifosfamide, but may persist for longer; fatalities have been reported.
• Assess patient for nausea, vomiting, and appetite, and

weigh weekly. Premedication with an antiemetic may be used to minimize GI effects. Adjust diet as tolerated.

- Monitor for development of bone marrow depression. Assess for fever, chills, sore throat, and signs of infection. Additive myelosuppression may occur with other antineoplastic agents or radiation therapy. Monitor platelet count throughout therapy. Assess for bleeding (bleeding gums, bruising, petechiae; guaiac test stools, urine, and emesis). Avoid giving IM injections and taking rectal temperatures. Apply pressure to venipuncture sites for 10 minutes.
- Use cautiously in patients with active infections, decreased bone marrow reserve, other chronic debilitating illness, or impaired renal function.
- Ifosfamide should be used cautiously in patients with childbearing potential. Avoid during pregnancy or lactation (Pregnancy Category D). Safe use in children has not been established.

Lab Test Considerations

- Monitor CBC, differential, and platelet count prior to and periodically throughout course of therapy. Withhold dose if WBC is less than 2000/mm^3 or platelet count is less than 50,000/mm^3. Nadir of leukopenia and thrombocytopenia occurs within 7–14 days and usually recovers within 21 days of a course of therapy. • Urinalysis should be evaluated before each dose. Withhold dose if urinalysis shows more than 10 RBCs per high-power field. • Monitor AST (SGOT), ALT (SGPT), serum alkaline phosphatase, bilirubin, and LDH prior to and periodically during therapy. Ifosfamide may cause elevation in liver enzymes and serum bilirubin. • Monitor BUN, serum creatinine, phosphate, and potassium periodically during therapy.

Patient/Family Teaching

- Emphasize need for adequate fluid intake throughout course of therapy. Patient should void frequently to decrease bladder irritation from metabolites excreted by the kidneys. Physician should be notified immediately if hematuria is noted. • Instruct patient to notify physician promptly in case of fever, sore throat, signs of infection, bleeding gums, bruising, petechiae; blood in urine, stool, or emesis; or confusion. Caution patient to avoid crowds and persons with known infections. Instruct patient to use a soft toothbrush and electric razor and to avoid falls. Patients should also be cautioned not to drink alcoholic beverages or to take products containing aspirin, ibuprofen, or naproxen, as these may precipitate GI hemorrhage. • Review with patient the need for nonhormonal contraception during therapy. • Discuss with patient the possibility of hair loss. Explore methods of coping. • Instruct patient not to receive any vaccinations without advice of physician, as ifosfamide may decrease antibody response to and increase risk of adverse reactions from live virus vaccines.

 PHARMACOLOGIC PROFILE

Indications

• Ifosfamide is used along with mesna, which prevents ifosfamide-induced hemorrhagic cystitis, in combination with other antineoplastic agents in the treatment of germ cell testicular carcinoma.

Action

• Following conversion to active compounds, ifosfamide interferes with DNA replication and RNA transcription, ultimately disrupting protein synthesis (cell cycle–phase nonspecific). This results in death of rapidly replicating cells, particularly malignant ones.

Time/Action Profile (effect on WBC counts)

Onset	Peak	Duration
within days	7–14 days	21 days†

†After dose.

Pharmacokinetics

• **Distribution:** Ifosfamide is excreted in breast milk. • **Metabolism and Excretion:** Ifosfamide is metabolized by the liver to active antineoplastic compounds. • **Half-life:** 15 hours.

Contraindications

• Patients with previous hypersensitivity to ifosfamide should not be given ifosfamide. It should not be used in pregnancy, lactation, or children (Pregnancy Category D).

Adverse Reactions and Side Effects*

• **CNS:** CNS toxicity (somnolence, confusion, hallucinations, coma), dizziness, disorientation, cranial nerve dysfunction • **CV:** cardiotoxicity • **GI:** nausea, vomiting, anorexia, diarrhea, constipation, liver dysfunction • **GU:** hemorrhagic cystitis, renal toxicity, dysuria, gonadal suppression • **Derm:** alopecia • **Hemat:** leukopenia, thrombocytopenia, anemia • **Local:** phlebitis • **Misc:** allergic reactions.

Imipenem/Cilastatin Sodium	Anti-infective (carbapenem)
Primaxin IV	pH 6.5–7.5

≋ ADMINISTRATION CONSIDERATIONS

Usual Dose (based on imipenem)

ADULTS: *Mild infections*—250–500 mg q 6 hr. *Moderate infections*—500 mg q 6–8 hr (up to 1 g q 6–8 hr). *Severe infections*—500 mg q 6 hr–1 g q 6–8 hr.

Dilution

• **Intermittent Infusion: Reconstitute** each 250- or 500-mg vial with 10 ml of compatible diluent and shake well. Transfer the resulting suspension to not less than 100 ml of compatible diluent. Add an additional 10 ml to each previously reconstituted vial and shake well to ensure all medication is used. Transfer the remaining contents of the vial to the infusion container. *Do not* administer suspension by direct injection. **Reconstitute** 120-ml infusion bottles with 100 ml of a compatible diluent. Shake well until clear. • Compatible diluents include 0.9% NaCl, D5W, D10W, D5/0.2% sodium bicarbonate, D5/0.9% NaCl, D5/0.45% NaCl, D5/0.225% NaCl, or mannitol 2.5%, 5%, or 10%. • Solution may range from clear to yellow in color. Do not administer cloudy solution. Solution is stable for 4 hours at room temperature and 24 hours if refrigerated.

---

*Underlines indicate most frequent; CAPITALS indicate life-threatening.

Compatibility

Y-site: acyclovir ♦ diltiazem ♦ famotidine ♦ filgrastim ♦ fludarabine ♦ foscarnet ♦ idarubicin ♦ insulin ♦ melphalan ♦ ondansetron ♦ tacrolimus ♦ vinorelbine ♦ zidovudine.

Incompatibility

• **Y-site:** allopurinol sodium ♦ fluconazole ♦ gallium nitrate ♦ meperidine ♦ sargramostim.

• **Additive:** Do not admix with other antibiotics.

Rate of Administration

• **Intermittent Infusion:** Administer each 250- or 500-mg dose over 20–30 minutes and each 1-g dose over 40–60 minutes. Do not administer direct IV.

≋ CLINICAL PRECAUTIONS

• Obtain a history before initiating therapy to determine previous use of and reactions to penicillins or cephalosporins. Persons with a negative history of penicillin sensitivity may still have an allergic response.

• Obtain specimens for culture and sensitivity prior to initiating therapy. First dose may be given before receiving results.

• Assess patient for infection (vital signs; appearance of wound, sputum, urine, and stool; WBC) at beginning and throughout course of therapy.

• Observe patient for signs and symptoms of anaphylaxis (rash, pruritus, laryngeal edema, wheezing). Discontinue the drug immediately if these occur. Have epinephrine, an antihistamine, and resuscitative equipment close by in the event of an anaphylactic reaction.

• Intramuscular imipenem/cilastatin is a different dosage form (Primaxin IM).

• Probenecid decreases renal excretion and increases blood levels of imipenem/cilastatin. The risk of seizures from imipenem/cilastatin is increased by concurrent ganciclovir and should be avoided. Imipenem/cilastatin may antagonize the action of penicillins and cephalosporins.

• Use cautiously in patients with a previous history of multiple hypersensitivity reactions, seizure disorders, or renal impairment (dosage reduction required if creatinine clearance is 70 ml/min/1.73 m^2 or less).

- Safe use in pregnancy, lactation, or children has not been established (Pregnancy Category C).

Lab Test Considerations

- BUN, AST (SGOT), ALT (SGPT), LDH, serum alkaline phosphatase, bilirubin, and creatinine may be transiently increased by imipenem/cilastatin. • Hemoglobin and hematocrit concentrations may be decreased. • Imipenem/cilastatin may cause a positive direct Coombs' test.

Patient/Family Teaching

- Advise patient to report the signs of superinfection (black, furry overgrowth on the tongue; vaginal itching or discharge; loose or foul-smelling stools) and allergy.

≋ PHARMACOLOGIC PROFILE

Indications

- Imipenem/cilastatin is used in the treatment of the following serious infections due to susceptible organisms: lower respiratory tract infections, urinary tract infections, abdominal infections, gynecologic infections, skin and skin structure infections, bone and joint infections, bacteremia, endocarditis, and polymicrobic infections.

Action

- Imipenem binds to bacterial cell wall, resulting in cell death. Combination with cilastatin prevents renal inactivation of imipenem, resulting in high urinary concentrations. Imipenem/cilastatin resists the actions of many enzymes that degrade other penicillins and penicillinlike anti-infectives. Its action is bactericidal against susceptible bacteria. Imipenem/cilastatin has a broad spectrum and is active against most Gram-positive aerobic cocci including *Streptococcus pneumoniae,* group A beta-hemolytic streptococci, *Enterococcus,* and *Staphylococcus aureus.* It is also active against many Gram-negative bacillary organisms: *Escherichia coli, Klebsiella, Acinetobacter, Proteus, Serratia,* and *Pseudomonas aeruginosa.* It also displays activity against *Salmonella, Shigella, Neisseria gonorrhoeae,* and numerous anaerobes.

Time/Action Profile (blood levels)

Onset	Peak
rapid	end of infusion

Pharmacokinetics

• **Distribution:** Imipenem/cilastatin is widely distributed. It crosses the placenta and enters breast milk. • **Metabolism and Excretion:** 70% of imipenem/cilastatin is excreted unchanged by the kidneys. • **Half-life:** 1 hour (prolonged in renal impairment).

Contraindications

• Imipenem/cilastatin is contraindicated in patients with hypersensitivity to it. Cross-sensitivity may occur with penicillins and cephalosporins.

Adverse Reactions and Side Effects*

• **CNS:** SEIZURES, dizziness, somnolence • **CV:** hypotension • **GI:** <u>nausea</u>, <u>diarrhea</u>, <u>vomiting</u> • **Derm:** <u>rash</u>, pruritus, urticaria, sweating • **Hemat:** eosinophilia • **Local:** <u>phlebitis</u> at IV site • **Misc:** allergic reactions including ANAPHYLAXIS, fever, superinfection.

Immune Globulin Intravenous	Serum (immune globulin)
Gamimune N, Gammar-IV, IGIV, Iveegam, IVIG, Sandoglobulin, Venoglobulin-I	pH Gamimune N 4–4.5; Sandoglobulin 6.4–6.8

≋ ADMINISTRATION CONSIDERATIONS

Usual Dose

Immunodeficiency Syndrome

ADULTS AND CHILDREN: 200–800 mg/kg/mo.

---

*<u>Underlines</u> indicate most frequent; CAPITALS indicate life-threatening.

Idiopathic Thrombocytopenic Purpura
ADULTS AND CHILDREN: 400 mg/kg/day for 2–5 days or 1 g/kg/ day for 1–2 days. Regimen may be repeated q 10–21 days.

Prevention of Bacterial Infections in HIV-infected Children
CHILDREN: 400 mg/kg q 28 days.

Kawasaki Disease
CHILDREN: 400 mg/kg/day for 4 days or 2 g/day single dose.

Prevention of Bacterial Infections in Patients with B-cell Chronic Lymphocytic Leukemia
ADULTS: 400 mg/kg q 21–28 days.

Dilution
• **Intermittent Infusion:** Reconstituted solutions should be swirled to mix. Do not shake to prevent foaming. • *Gamimune N* should be **diluted** with D5W. Solutions of *Gamimune N* should be refrigerated but not frozen. Discard solution that has been frozen. • *Gammar-IV* should be **reconstituted** with 50 ml of sterile water for injection. Refrigerate, do not freeze. Discard unused solution. • *Iveegam* should be **reconstituted** with 10 ml or 20 ml of sterile water for injection for the 500-mg and 1-g vials, respectively, and 50 ml and 100 ml for the 2.5-g and 5-g infusion bottles, respectively. • Refrigerate; do not freeze or use solution that has been frozen. Discard unused solution. • *Sandoglobulin* should be **reconstituted** with the 0.9% NaCl provided by the manufacturer for a solution containing 30 or 60 mg of protein per ml. For patients with agammaglobulinemia or hypogammaglobulinemia, use a solution containing 30 mg/ml for the initial dose. Solutions of *Sandoglobulin* should be stored at room temperature. • Do not use turbid solutions. • *Venoglobulin-I* should be **reconstituted** with 50 ml and 100 ml of sterile water for injection for the 2.5-g and 5-g vials, respectively. Prior to reconstitution, powder and diluent should be warmed to room temperature.

Incompatibility
• **Additive:** Manufacturer recommends not mixing with other drugs or solutions. Immune globulin IV (IGIV) should be administered by IV infusion using separate tubing.

Rate of Administration
• **Intermittent Infusion:** *Gamimune N* should be infused at a rate of 0.01–0.02 ml/kg/min for 30 minutes. If no adverse

reactions occur, the infusion rate may be gradually increased to a maximum of 0.08 ml/kg/hr. • *Gammar-IV* should be infused at a rate of 0.01 ml/kg/min, gradually increasing to 0.3–0.6 ml/kg/min after 15–30 minutes. • *Iveegam* should be infused at 1 ml/min, up to a maximum of 2 ml/min. • *Sandoglobulin* should be infused at an initial rate of 0.5–1 ml/min. After 15–30 minutes, the rate may be increased to 1.5–2.5 ml/min, and subsequent infusions may be given at a rate of 2–2.5 ml/min. • *Venoglobulin-I* should be infused at 0.01–0.02 ml/kg/min for the first 30 minutes. If the rate does not cause the patient distress, it may be increased to 0.04 ml/kg/min. • If adverse reactions occur during infusion, decrease the rate of infusion or stop the infusion until the adverse reactions subside. The infusion may then be resumed at a rate of tolerance for the individual.

≋ CLINICAL PRECAUTIONS

- Monitor vital signs continuously during infusion of immune globulin IV and assess patient for signs of anaphylaxis (hypotension, flushing, chest tightness, wheezing, fever, dizziness, nausea, vomiting, diaphoresis) for 1 hour following initiation of infusion. Epinephrine and antihistamines should be available for treatment of anaphylactic reactions.
- For passive immunity, determine the date of exposure to infection. Immune globulin should be administered within 2 weeks of exposure to hepatitis A, within 6 days after exposure to measles, and within 7 days after exposure to hepatitis B.
- Immune globulin may interfere with the normal immune response to some live vaccines, including measles, mumps, and rubella virus vaccine (do not administer within 3 months of immune globulin).
- Use immune globulin cautiously in patients with acid-base disorders (*Gamimune N* product only), agammaglobulinemia, or hypogammaglobulinemia (increased risk of hypotension and anaphylaxis following rapid IV administration).
- Immune globulin has been used during pregnancy, though safety is not established (Pregnancy Category C).

Lab Test Considerations

• Monitor platelet count in patients being treated for idiopathic thrombocytopenic purpura.

Patient/Family Teaching

• Explain the use and purpose of immune globulin therapy to the patient. • Advise patient to report symptoms of anaphylaxis immediately.

 PHARMACOLOGIC PROFILE

Indications

• Immune globulin provides passive immunity to a variety of infections including hepatitis A, hepatitis B, and measles (rubeola) when immune sera are unavailable or when there is insufficient time for active immunization to take place. It is useful in patients with immunodeficiency syndromes (HIV, Kawasaki disease, B-cell chronic lymphocytic leukemia) who are unable to produce IgG-type antibodies. Immune globulin is also used to treat idiopathic thrombocytopenic purpura (ITP).

Action

• Immune globulin is a human serum fraction containing gamma globulin antibodies (IgG). It provides passive immunity against many infections.

Time/Action Profile (antibody levels)

Onset	Peak	Duration†
immediate	UK	several days–several weeks

†Effect on platelet count in ITP.

Pharmacokinetics

• **Distribution:** Rapidly and evenly distributed. Crosses the placenta. • **Metabolism and Excretion:** Removed by redistribution, tissue binding, and catabolism. • **Half-life:** 21–24 days.

Contraindications

• Immune globulin IV is contraindicated in patients with hypersensitivity to immune globulins or additives (maltose, thimerosal, glycine, polyethylene glycol, albumin) or in patients with selective IgA deficiency.

Adverse Reactions and Side Effects*

• **CNS:** faintness, light-headedness, headache, malaise • **Resp:** dyspnea, wheezing • **CV:** chest pain • **GI:** nausea • **GU:** diuresis (if preparation contains maltose), nephrotic syndrome • **Derm:** urticaria, cyanosis • **Local:** local inflammation, urticaria at site, phlebitis • **MS:** hip pain, back pain, arthralgia • **Misc:** allergic reactions including ANAPHYLAXIS, angioedema, fever, chills, sweating.

Indomethacin Sodium Trihydrate	Nonsteroidal anti-inflammatory agent
Indocin IV, {Indocin PDA}	pH 6–7.5

ADMINISTRATION CONSIDERATIONS

Usual Dose

NEONATES: 200 mcg (0.2 mg)/kg initially. **If age is younger than 48 hours** at time of initial dose, then 1–2 additional doses of 100 mcg (0.1 mg)/kg may be given q 12–24 hr; **if age is 2–7 days** at time of initial dose, then 1–2 additional doses of 200 mcg (0.2 mg)/kg may be given q 12–24 hr; **if age is greater than 7 days** at time of initial dose, then 1–2 additional doses of 250 mcg (0.25 mg)/kg may be given q 12–24 hr (up to 300 mcg/kg/dose has been used).

Dilution

• **Direct IV: Reconstitute** with 1 or 2 ml of preservative-free 0.9% NaCl or preservative-free sterile water for injection for a concentration of 0.1 mg/ml or 0.05 mg/ml, respectively. • Reconstitute immediately prior to use and discard any unused solution. Do not dilute further or admix.

---

*Underlines indicate most frequent; CAPITALS indicate life-threatening.

{} = Available in Canada only.

Rate of Administration

• **Direct IV:** Although the manufacturer recommends administering over 5–10 seconds, administration over 20–35 minutes may decrease the incidence of necrotizing enterocolitis or cerebral ischemia. Avoid extravasation, as solution is irritating to tissues.

≋ CLINICAL PRECAUTIONS

• Monitor respiratory status and heart sounds routinely throughout therapy.
• Monitor intake and output, fluid, and electrolyte status throughout therapy. Fluid restriction is usually instituted concurrently.
• Indomethacin may increase serum levels and risk of toxicity from zidovudine, digoxin, or aminoglycosides (dosage adjustments may be necessary).
• Indomethacin may increase the risk of bleeding with cefamandole, cefotetan, cefoperazone, plicamycin, thrombolytic agents, or anticoagulants. Use cautiously in patients with decreased platelet counts or coagulation deficits.

Lab Test Considerations

• Monitor serum electrolyte concentrations and renal function tests during and following administration. If renal function impairment occurs (serum creatinine $>1.2–1.4$ mg/dl), therapy should be withheld until adequate renal function is restored. • Serum potassium, BUN, serum creatinine, AST (SGOT), and ALT (SGPT) tests may show increased levels. • Blood glucose concentrations may be altered. Urine glucose and urine protein concentrations may be increased. • Indomethacin may cause decreased creatinine clearance; serum sodium concentrations; urine chloride, potassium, and sodium concentrations; urine osmolality; and urine volume. • Leukocyte and platelet count may be decreased. • Bleeding time may be prolonged for 1 day after discontinuation.

Patient/Family Teaching

• Explain to parents the purpose of medication and the need for frequent monitoring.

≋ PHARMACOLOGIC PROFILE

Indications

- Indomethacin is an alternative to surgery in the management of patent ductus arteriosus in premature neonates.

Action

- Indomethacin inhibits prostaglandin synthesis. E-type prostaglandins maintain a patent ductus arteriosus in certain congenital cardiac defects. Inhibition of prostaglandin synthesis results in closure of patent ductus arteriosus.

Time/Action Profile (closure of patent ductus arteriosus)

Onset	Peak	Duration
within 48 hr	UK	UK

Pharmacokinetics

- **Distribution:** Indomethacin crosses the blood–brain barrier and the placenta and enters breast milk. • **Metabolism and Excretion:** Indomethacin is mostly metabolized by the liver. • **Half-life:** 2.6–11 hours (may be up to 60 hours in neonates) (range 12–21 hours).

Contraindications

- Indomethacin in contraindicated in patients with hypersensitivity. Cross-sensitivity may exist with other nonsteroidal anti-inflammatory agents, including aspirin. Indomethacin should be avoided in patients with active GI bleeding, ulcer disease, proctitis, or a recent history of rectal bleeding.

Adverse Reactions and Side Effects*

- **Resp:** apnea, exacerbation of pulmonary infection • **CV:** bradycardia, pulmonary hypertension • **GI:** necrotizing enterocolitis, GI bleeding • **GU:** impaired renal function • **F and E:** dilutional hyponatremia • **Hemat:** disseminated intravascular coagulation, bleeding problems • **Metab:** acidosis, alkalosis, hypoglycemia.

---

*Underlines indicate most frequent; CAPITALS indicate life-threatening.

Insulin, Regular

Hormone
(hypoglycemic)

Humulin R, {Insulin Toronto},
Regular Iletin I, Regular Iletin II (Pork),
{Novolin ge Toronto}, Novolin R,
Velosulin Human   pH 7–7.8

≋ ADMINISTRATION CONSIDERATIONS

Usual Dose

Note: Dose depends on blood sugar, response, and many
other factors.

Ketoacidosis

ADULTS AND CHILDREN: 0.1 units/kg/hr. May be preceded by
bolus of 0.1 units/kg.

Dilution

• **Direct IV:** May be administered IV **undiluted** directly
into vein or through Y-site injection or 3-way stopcock. • Use
only insulin syringes to draw up the dose. The unit markings
on the insulin syringe must match the insulin's units/ml. Special syringes for doses less than 50 units are available. Prior to
withdrawing dose, rotate vial between palms to ensure a uni-
form solution; do not shake. • Do not use if insulin is cloudy,
discolored, or unusually viscous. Insulin should be stored in
a cool place but does not need to be refrigerated. • **Continuous Infusion:** May be diluted in 0.45% NaCl or 0.9%
NaCl as an infusion; however, insulin potency may be reduced by at least 20–80% by the plastic or glass container or
tubing before reaching the venous system.

Compatibility

• **Syringe:** metoclopramide.
• **Y-site:** ampicillin • ampicillin sulbactam • aztreonam
• cefazolin • cefotetan • dobutamine • famotidine • gentamicin • heparin • imipenem/cilastatin • indomethacin • magnesium sulfate • meperidine • morphine • oxytocin • pentobarbital • potassium chloride • ritodrine • sodium bicarbonate
• tacrolimus • terbutaline • ticarcillin • ticarcillin/clavulanate
• tobramycin • vancomycin • vitamin B complex with C.

{} = Available in Canada only.

- **Additive:** bretylium ⬥ cimetidine ⬥ lidocaine ⬥ ranitidine ⬥ verapamil. ⬥ May be added to TPN solutions.

Incompatibility

- **Additive:** aminophylline ⬥ amobarbital ⬥ chlorothiazide ⬥ cytarabine ⬥ dobutamine ⬥ pentobarbital ⬥ phenobarbital ⬥ phenytoin ⬥ secobarbital ⬥ sodium bicarbonate ⬥ thiopental.

Rate of Administration

- **Direct IV:** Administer each 50 units over 1 minute.
- **Continuous Infusion:** When administered as an infusion, rate should be ordered by physician, and infusion should be placed on an IV pump for accurate administration. ⬥ Rate of administration should be decreased when serum glucose level reaches 250 mg/100 ml.

≋ CLINICAL PRECAUTIONS

- Regular insulin is the *only* insulin that can be administered IV. Regular insulin U500 is not intended for IV route.
- Check type, species source, dose, and expiration date of insulin with another licensed nurse. Do not interchange insulins.
- Assess patient periodically throughout therapy for signs and symptoms of hypoglycemia (anxiety, chills, cold sweats, confusion, cool pale skin, difficulty in concentration, drowsiness, excessive hunger, headache, irritability, nausea, nervousness, rapid pulse, shakiness, unusual tiredness or weakness) and hyperglycemia (drowsiness, flushed dry skin, fruitlike breath odor, frequent urination, loss of appetite, tiredness, unusual thirst).
- Monitor body weight periodically. Changes in weight may necessitate changes in insulin dosage.
- Beta blockers may block some signs of hypoglycemia (shaking, tachycardia).
- Insulin requirements may be increased by thiazide diuretics, acute alcohol ingestion, glucocorticoids, thyroid preparations, smoking, estrogens, or rifampin.
- Insulin requirements may be decreased by anabolic steroids (testosterone), clofibrate, guanethidine, some antidepressants, MAO inhibitors, salicylates, phenylbutazone, and oral anticoagulants.

- When writing insulin doses, do not abbreviate units in order to prevent medication errors.
- Insulin requirements are altered during stress, pregnancy, and infection. Closer monitoring is necessary during these times.

Toxicity and Overdose Alert

- Overdose of insulin is manifested by symptoms of hypoglycemia. Mild hypoglycemia may be treated by ingestion of oral glucose. Severe hypoglycemia is a life-threatening emergency; treatment consists of IV glucose, glucagon, or epinephrine.

Lab Test Considerations

- Monitor blood glucose or urine glucose and ketones frequently in ketoacidosis and times of stress, and every 6 hours throughout course of therapy. • Insulin may cause decreased serum inorganic phosphate, magnesium, and potassium levels. • Glycosylated hemoglobin may also be monitored to determine effectiveness of therapy.

Patient/Family Teaching

- Explain to patient that this medication controls hyperglycemia but does not cure diabetes. Therapy is long-term. Instruct patient in proper testing of serum glucose or urine glucose and ketones. Stress the importance of double-voided specimens for accuracy. • Emphasize the importance of compliance with diabetic diet and exchange system for meals, and of regular exercise. • Advise patient to notify physician if nausea, vomiting, or fever develops, if he or she is unable to eat regular diet, or if blood sugar levels are not controlled. • Instruct patient on signs and symptoms of hypoglycemia and hyperglycemia and what to do if they occur. • Patients with diabetes mellitus should carry at all times a source of sugar (candy, sugar packets) and identification describing their disease and treatment regimen.

☰ PHARMACOLOGIC PROFILE

Indications

- Insulin is used in the treatment of insulin-dependent diabetes mellitus (IDDM, type I) and in the management of non-insulin-dependent diabetes mellitus (NIDDM, type II) unresponsive to treatment with diet and/or oral hypoglycemic agents.

Action

• Insulin lowers blood glucose by increasing transport of glucose into cells, promoting the conversion of glucose to glycogen, promoting the conversion of amino acids to proteins in muscle, and stimulating triglyceride formation. Insulin also inhibits the release of free fatty acids. Sources include beef and pork, semisynthetic, and human insulin prepared by recombinant DNA technology (biosynthetic).

Time/Action Profile (effect on blood glucose)

Onset	Peak	Duration
10–30 min	15–30 min	30–60 min

Pharmacokinetics

• **Distribution:** Insulin is widely distributed. • **Metabolism and Excretion:** Insulin is metabolized by liver, kidney, and muscle. • **Half-life:** 9 minutes (prolonged in diabetics).

Contraindications

• Some types of insulin may be contraindicated in patients with allergy or hypersensitivity to a particular type of insulin, preservatives, or other additives.

Adverse Reactions and Side Effects*

• **Derm:** urticaria • **Endo:** hypoglycemia, rebound hyperglycemia (Somogyi effect) • **Misc:** allergic reactions, including ANAPHYLAXIS.

---

*Underlines indicate most frequent; CAPITALS indicate life-threatening.

Iron Dextran   *Iron supplement*
{Imferon}, InFeD   pH 5.2–6.5

☰ ADMINISTRATION CONSIDERATIONS

Usual Dose

Each ml contains 50 mg elemental iron. A test dose of 25 mg (0.5 ml) over 5 min is recommended prior to therapy.

Iron Deficiency Anemia (chronic)

ADULTS AND CHILDREN >15 kg: Total dose (ml) = $0.0476 \times$ weight (kg) $\times$ (14.8 −Hgb) + 1 ml/5 kg weight (up to 14 ml). This total dose is divided up and given in small daily doses until total is reached; not to exceed 100 mg/day.
• *Unlabeled Use:* Total dose is diluted in 500 ml normal saline and infused over 1–8 hr, preceded by a test dose of 10 drops/min for 10 min.

CHILDREN 5–15 kg: Total dose (ml) = $0.0476 \times$ weight (kg) $\times$ (12 −Hgb) + iron stores. This total dose is divided up and given in small daily doses until total is reached; not to exceed 100 mg/day.

Anemia Secondary to Blood Loss (acute)

ADULTS AND CHILDREN: Total dose (ml) = $0.02 \times$ blood loss (ml) $\times$ Hct (%); not to exceed 100 mg/day.

Dilution

• **Direct IV:** Administer **undiluted.** • **Intermittent Infusion:** Dilute dose in 200–1000 ml of 0.9% NaCl. Do not dilute in D5W, as increased pain and phlebitis may occur.
• Multidose vials are not intended for IV use.

Incompatibility

• **Y-site:** Discontinue other IV solutions during infusion.
• **Additive:** The manufacturer does not recommend mixing with other medications or adding to parenteral nutrition solutions.

Rate of Administration

• **Direct IV:** Administer at a rate of 1 ml (50 mg)/min.
• **Intermittent Infusion:** Infuse over 1–8 hours. Flush line with 10 ml of 0.9% NaCl at completion of infusion.

{} = Available in Canada only.

≋ CLINICAL PRECAUTIONS

- Prior to initial dose, a test dose of 25 mg (0.5 ml) should be given by the same route as the dose is to be given, to determine the potential for reactions. The IV test dose should be administered over 5 minutes. The remaining portion may be administered after 1 hour, if no adverse reactions have occurred.
- Monitor blood pressure and heart rate frequently following administration until stable. Rapid infusion rate may cause hypotension and flushing. Following administration, patient should remain recumbent for at least 30 minutes to prevent orthostatic hypotension.
- Assess patient for signs and symptoms of anaphylaxis (rash, pruritus, laryngeal edema, wheezing). Keep epinephrine and resuscitation equipment close by in the event of an anaphylactic reaction.
- Assess patient's nutritional status and dietary history to determine possible cause of anemia and need for patient teaching.
- Oral iron preparations should be discontinued prior to parenteral administration.
- Chloramphenicol and vitamin E may impair the normal hematologic response to parenteral iron.
- Use iron dextran cautiously in patients with autoimmune disorders or rheumatoid arthritis, as they may be more susceptible to allergic reactions.
- Use in pregnancy or women of childbearing potential only if benefits outweigh risks (Pregnancy Category C).

Lab Test Considertions

- Monitor hemoglobin, hematocrit, reticulocyte values, transferrin, ferritin, total iron-binding capacity, and plasma iron concentrations periodically throughout therapy. Serum ferritin levels peak in 7–9 days and return to normal in 3 weeks. Serum iron determinations may be inaccurate for 1–2 weeks after therapy with large doses; therefore, hemoglobin and hematocrit are used to gauge initial response. Normal hemoglobin concentrations of 14.8 g/100 ml should be used for patients weighing >15 kg, while 12 g/100 ml should be used for patients weighing 15 kg or less. • Iron dextran may impart a brownish hue to serum

when blood is drawn within 4 hours of administration.
• Iron dextran may cause false increase in serum bilirubin and false decrease in serum calcium values. • Prolonged PTT may be calculated when blood sample is anticoagulated with citrate dextrose solution; use sodium citrate instead. • The diagnosis of iron-deficiency anemia should be reconfirmed if hemoglobin has not increased by 1 g/100 ml in 2 weeks.

Patient/Family Teaching

• Delayed reaction may occur 1–2 days after administration and last 3–4 days. Instruct patient to contact physician if fever, chills, malaise, muscle and joint aches, nausea, vomiting, dizziness, or backache occurs. • Instruct patient to follow a diet high in iron (organ meat, leafy green vegetables, dried beans and peas, dried fruit, cereals).

PHARMACOLOGIC PROFILE

Indications

• Iron dextran is used in the treatment and prevention of iron-deficiency anemia in patients who are unable to tolerate oral iron preparations.

Action

• Iron dextran enters the bloodstream and organs of the reticuloendothelial system (liver, spleen, bone marrow), where iron is separated from the dextran complex and becomes part of the body's iron stores.

Time/Action Profile (effect on reticulocyte counts)

Onset	Peak	Duration
4 days	1–2 wk	weeks–months

Pharmacokinetics

• **Distribution:** Iron dextran remains in the body for many months. It crosses the placenta and enters breast milk. • **Metabolism and Excretion:** Iron dextran is lost slowly from the body through desquamation or blood loss. • **Half-life:** 6 hours.

Contraindications

• Iron dextran should not be used in patients with a previous history of hypersensitivity to it, and it is contraindicated in patients with all other types of anemias.

Adverse Reactions and Side Effects*

• **CNS:** headache, dizziness, SEIZURES, syncope • **EENT:** bad taste • **CV:** <u>hypotension</u>, tachycardia • **GI:** nausea, vomiting • **Derm:** urticaria, flushing • **Local:** phlebitis at IV site • **MS:** arthralgia • **Misc:** allergic reactions including ANAPHYLAXIS, fever, lymphadenopathy.

Isoproterenol Hydrochloride	*Antiarrhythmic, Inotropic agent, Bronchodilator (beta-adrenergic amine)*
Isoprenaline, Isuprel HCl	pH 3.5–4.5

 ADMINISTRATION CONSIDERATIONS

Usual Dose

Bronchodilation (during anesthesia)
ADULTS: 10–20 mcg (0.01–0.02 mg); repeated as needed.

Cardiac Stimulant
ADULTS: 20–60 mcg (0.02–0.06 mg) initially; then 10–200 mcg (0.010–0.2 mg) as needed *or* 5 mcg (0.005 mg)/min infusion (range 2–20 mcg/min).

Shock Secondary to Hypoperfusion
ADULTS: 0.5–5 mcg (0.0005–0.005 mg)/min, up to 30 mcg (0.03 mg)/min.

CHILDREN: 0.1 mcg (0.0001 mg)/kg/min initially, up to 1 mcg (0.001 mg)/kg/min infusion.

Dilution

• **Direct IV:** May be administered by diluting 0.2 mg (1 ml) of a 1:5000 solution with 10 ml of 0.9% NaCl for injection or D5W, to make a 1:50,000 solution of 20 mcg/ml.

---

*<u>Underlines</u> indicate most frequent; CAPITALS indicate life-threatening.

• Do not use if solution is pinkish to brownish or contains a precipitate. • **Continuous Infusion:** Prepare by adding 1–10 ml of a 1:5000 solution to 500 ml of D5W, D10W, 0.9% NaCl, 0.45% NaCl, dextrose/saline combinations, dextrose/Ringer's or lactated Ringer's combinations, Ringer's or lactated Ringer's solution. • Usual dilution is 2 mg (10 ml) of a 1:5000 solution in 500 ml, which provides a 1:250,000 solution (4 mcg/ml).

Compatibility

• **Syringe:** ranitidine.

• **Y-site:** amrinone • atracurium • bretylium • famotidine • heparin • hydrocortisone sodium succinate • pancuronium • potassium chloride • tacrolimus • vecuronium • vitamin B complex with C.

• **Additive:** atracurium • calcium chloride • calcium gluceptate • cephalothin • cimetidine • dobutamine • heparin • magnesium sulfate • multivitamins • netilmicin • potassium chloride • ranitidine • succinylcholine • verapamil • vitamin B complex with C.

Incompatibility

• **Additive:** aminophylline • barbiturates • furosemide • lidocaine • sodium bicarbonate.

Rate of Administration

• **Direct IV:** Administer each 1 ml of 1:50,000 solution (0.02 mg) over 1 minute. • **Continuous Infusion:** Administer at a rate of 5 mcg/min in adults and 2.5 mcg/min or 0.1 mcg/kg/min in children, adjusting according to patient response and desired parameters for blood pressure, hemodynamic values, and urine output. Administer via infusion pump to ensure delivery of precise amounts of medication. (See Infusion Rate Table below.)

ISOPROTERENOL (Isuprel) INFUSION RATE TABLE

Dilution: 2 mg/500 ml

ISOPROTERENOL INFUSION RATES (ml/hr) *CONCENTRATION = 4 mcg/ml*	
Dose (mcg/min)	*Dose (ml/hr)*
2 mcg/min	30 ml/hr
5 mcg/min	75 ml/hr
10 mcg/min	150 ml/hr
15 mcg min	225 ml/hr
20 mcg/min	300 ml/hr

≋ CLINICAL PRECAUTIONS

- ECG, hemodynamic parameters, and urine output should be monitored continuously.
- Assess blood pressure, pulse, respiratory pattern, lung sounds, arterial blood gases, and character of secretions frequently during course of therapy when isoproterenol is used as a bronchodilator. Monitor for chest pain, arrhythmias, heart rate greater than 110 bpm, and hypertension. Follow parameters of pulse, blood pressure, and ECG changes for adjusting dosage or discontinuing medication.
- Assess volume status. Hypovolemia should be corrected prior to administering isoproterenol IV.
- Additive adrenergic effects may be seen with other adrenergic (sympathomimetic agents). Hypertensive crisis may occur when isoproterenol is used with MAO. Therapeutic effects of isoproterenol may be blocked by beta-blocking agents. The risk of arrhythmias is increased by concurrent use of cyclopropane or halothane anesthesia.
- Use cautiously with elderly patients, who are more susceptible to adverse reactions. Dosage reduction may be warranted.
- Use with caution in patients with cardiac disease, hypertension, hyperthyroidism, diabetes, glaucoma, or pregnancy near term.
- Safe use during pregnancy or lactation has not been established (Pregnancy Category C).

Lab Test Considerations

- Isoproterenol may decrease serum potassium concentration.

Patient/Family Teaching

- Patient should inform physician if chest pain, headache, severe dizziness, palpitations, nervousness, or weakness occurs.

≋ PHARMACOLOGIC PROFILE

Indications

- Isoproterenol is used in the management of ventricular arrhythmias due to AV nodal block and in the treatment of shock associated with decreased cardiac output and vasoconstriction. It is also used as a bronchodilator in reversible airway obstruction during general anesthesia.

Action

- Isoproterenol is a beta-adrenergic agonist that results in the accumulation of cyclic adenosine monophosphate (cAMP). Results of increased levels of cAMP at beta-adrenergic receptors include bronchodilation, CNS and cardiac stimulation, diuresis, and gastric acid secretion. Isoproterenol stimulates both $beta_1$ (myocardial) and $beta_2$ (pulmonary) adrenergic receptors.

Time/Action Profile (cardiovascular effects)

Onset	Peak	Duration
rapid	UK	min

Pharmacokinetics

- **Distribution:** UK. • **Metabolism and Excretion:** Isoproterenol is metabolized by the lung, liver, and other tissues. Fifty percent is excreted unchanged by the kidneys. • **Half-life:** UK.

Contraindications

- Isoproterenol should not be used in patients with hypersensitivity to adrenergic amines or bisulfites.

Adverse Reactions and Side Effects*

- **CNS:** <u>nervousness</u>, <u>restlessness</u>, insomnia, <u>tremor</u>, headache • **Resp:** paradoxical bronchospasm (with excessive use) • **CV:** hypertension, arrhythmias, angina • **GI:** nausea, vomiting • **Endo:** hyperglycemia.

---

*<u>Underlines</u> indicate most frequent; CAPITALS indicate life-threatening.

Kanamycin Sulfate	Anti-infective (aminoglycoside)
Kantrex	pH 4.5

ADMINISTRATION CONSIDERATIONS

Usual Dose

ADULTS, CHILDREN, AND INFANTS: 5 mg/kg q 8 hr or 7.5 mg/kg q 12 hr, not to exceed 1.5 g/day in adults or 30 mg/kg/day in children, although up to 2 g/day has been used in adults with intraocular infections.

Dilution

• **Intermittent Infusion:** Dilute each 500 mg of kanamycin in 100–200 ml or each 1 g in 200–400 ml of D5W, D10W, D5/0.9% NaCl, 0.9% NaCl, or lactated Ringer's solution. • Volume of diluent should be decreased proportionately for children, but sufficient to infuse over 30–60 minutes. Darkening of solution does not alter potency.

Compatibility

• **Y-site:** cyclophosphamide • furosemide • hydromorphone • magnesium sulfate • meperidine • morphine • perphenazine • potassium chloride • vitamin B complex with C.

• **Additive:** ascorbic acid • chloramphenicol • clindamycin • dopamine • furosemide • polymyxin B • sodium bicarbonate • vitamin B complex with C.

Incompatibility

• **Syringe:** heparin.

• **Additive:** amphotericin B • cephalothin • cephapirin • chlorpheniramine • colistimethate • heparin • methohexital. • If penicillins or cephalosporins must be given concurrently with aminoglycosides, administer in separate sites.

Rate of Administration

• **Intermittent Infusion:** Infuse slowly over 30–60 minutes for adults or children. Flush IV line with D5W or 0.9% NaCl following administration.

≋ CLINICAL PRECAUTIONS

- Assess patient for infection (vital signs; appearance of wound, sputum, urine, and stool; WBC) at beginning and throughout course of therapy.
- Obtain specimens for culture and sensitivity prior to initiating therapy. First dose may be given before receiving results.
- Evaluate eighth cranial nerve function by audiometry prior to and throughout course of therapy. Hearing loss is usually of the high-frequency type. Prompt recognition and intervention is essential in preventing permanent damage. Incidence of ototoxicity is increased with loop diuretics (bumetanide, furosemide, torsemide). Also monitor for vestibular dysfunction (vertigo, ataxia, nausea, vomiting). Eighth cranial nerve dysfunction is associated with persistently elevated peak kanamycin levels. Geriatric patients are at increased risk for ototoxicity and nephrotoxicity. Auditory assessment may be difficult in geriatric or very young patients.
- Monitor intake and output and daily weight to assess hydration status and renal function. Maintain adequate hydration (1500–2000 ml/day). The risk of nephrotoxicity is increased by concurrent therapy with other nephrotoxic agents.
- Assess patient for signs of superinfection (fever, upper respiratory infection, vaginal itching or discharge, increasing malaise, diarrhea).
- Use kanamycin cautiously in renal impairment of any kind (dosage adjustments necessary). Kanamycin is inactivated by penicillins when coadministered to patients with renal insufficiency.
- Kanamycin has neuromuscular blocking properties. Possible respiratory paralysis may occur after administration of inhalation anesthetics (ether, cyclopropane, halothane, nitrous oxide) or neuromuscular blockers (tubocurarine, succinylcholine, decamethonium).
- Safe use in pregnancy and lactation has not been established (Pregnancy Category D).

Lab Test Considerations

- Monitor renal function by urinalysis, specific gravity, BUN, creatinine, and creatinine clearance prior to and throughout therapy. • Kanamycin may cause increased AST (SGOT), ALT (SGPT), LDH, bilirubin, and serum alkaline phosphatase levels and may cause decreased serum calcium, magnesium, sodium, and potassium levels. • Blood levels should be monitored periodically during therapy. Timing of blood levels is important in interpreting results. Draw blood for peak levels 30 minutes after a 30-minute IV infusion is completed. Trough levels should be drawn just prior to next dose. Acceptable peak level is 15–30 mcg/ml; trough level should not exceed 5–10 mcg/ml.

Patient/Family Teaching

• Instruct patient to report signs of hypersensitivity, tinnitus, vertigo, or hearing loss.

≋ PHARMACOLOGIC PROFILE

Indications

• Kanamycin is used in the treatment of Gram-negative bacillary infections and infections due to staphylococci when penicillins or other less toxic drugs are contraindicated. It is used to treat the following infections due to susceptible organisms: bone infections, respiratory tract infections, skin and soft tissue infections, abdominal infections, complicated urinary tract infections, endocarditis, and septicemia. Treatment of enterococcal infections requires synergy with a penicillin.

Action

• Kanamycin inhibits protein synthesis in bacteria at the level of the 30S ribosome, resulting in bactericidal action against susceptible bacteria. It is active against staphylococci, *Pseudomonas aeruginosa, Klebsiella pneumoniae, Escherichia coli, Proteus, Serratia,* and *Acinetobacter.*

Time/Action Profile (blood levels)

Onset	Peak
rapid	end of infusion

Pharmacokinetics

• **Distribution:** Kanamycin is widely distributed into extracellular fluids. It crosses the placenta, but has poor penetration into CSF. • **Metabolism and Excretion:** Excretion of kanamycin is mainly (>90%) renal. Minimal amounts are metabolized by the liver. • **Half-life:** 2–4 hours (increased in renal impairment).

Contraindications

• Kanamycin is contraindicated in patients with hypersensitivity to it or bisulfites. Cross-sensitivity with other aminoglycosides may occur.

Adverse Reactions and Side Effects*

• **EENT:** <u>ototoxicity</u> (vestibular and cochlear) • **GU:** <u>nephrotoxicity</u> • **Neuro:** enhanced neuromuscular blockade • **Misc:** hypersensitivity reactions.

Ketamine Hydrochloride	General anesthetic
Ketalar	pH 3.5–5.5

≈ ADMINISTRATION CONSIDERATIONS

Usual Dose

General Anesthesia

ADULTS AND CHILDREN: *Induction*—1–4.5 mg/kg (average dose of 2 mg produces 5–10 min of surgical anesthesia) *or* 1–2 mg as a single dose given as a 500 mcg (0.5 mg)/kg/min infusion along with diazepam 2–5 mg, up to 15 mg total of diazepam (see *diazepam* monograph on page 304). *Maintenance*—10–50 mcg (0.01–0.05 mg)/kg given as an infusion of 1–2 mg/min *or* 0.1–0.5 mg (100–500 mcg)/min along with 2–5 mg diazepam as needed (usual total dose of diazepam for induction and maintenance is 15–20 mg).

Local Anesthesia Adjunct (unlabeled)

ADULTS: 5–30 mg prior to local anesthesia; may be repeated.

---

*<u>Underlines</u> indicate most frequent; CAPITALS indicate life-threatening.

Sedation and Analgesia (unlabeled)

ADULTS: 200–750 mcg (0.2–0.75 mg)/kg initially, then 5–20 mcg (0.005–0.02 mg)/kg/min as an infusion.

Dilution

• **Direct IV:** Dilute 100-mg/ml concentration with equal parts of sterile water for injection, 0.9% NaCl, or D5W.
• **Continuous Infusion:** Dilute 10 ml of 50-mg/ml concentration or 5 ml of 100-mg/ml concentration with 500 ml of 0.9% NaCl or D5W and mix well, for a concentration of 1 mg/ml. Dilution with 250 ml may be used if fluid restriction is needed.

Compatibility

• **Syringe:** benzquinamide.

Incompatibility

• **Syringe:** barbiturates ◆ diazepam ◆ doxapram.

Rate of Administration

• **Direct IV:** Administer slowly over at least 60 seconds. More rapid administration may cause respiratory depression, apnea, and hypertension. • **Continuous Infusion:** Administer at a rate of 0.5 mg/kg/min for induction. Maintenance infusion may be administered at a rate of 1–2 mg/min, or 0.1–0.5 mg/min given concurrently with diazepam. Dosage must be titrated according to individual patient requirements. Tonic-clonic movements during anesthesia do not indicate the need for more ketamine.

≋ CLINICAL PRECAUTIONS

- Assess level of consciousness frequently throughout therapy. Ketamine produces a dissociative state. The patient does not appear to be asleep and experiences a feeling of dissociation from the environment.
- Monitor blood pressure, ECG, and respiratory status frequently throughout therapy. Ketamine may cause hypertension and tachycardia and may cause increased CSF pressure and increased intraocular pressure.
- Ketamine should be administered on an empty stomach to prevent vomiting and aspiration.
- Ketamine may be administered concurrently with a dry-

ing agent (atropine, scopolamine), as ketamine increases salivary and tracheobronchial mucous gland secretions. However, atropine may also increase the incidence of unpleasant dreams.

- Patients may experience a state of confusion (emergence delirium) during recovery from ketamine. Administration of a benzodiazepine and minimizing verbal, tactile, and visual stimulation may prevent emergence delirium. Severe emergence delirium may be treated with short- or ultra-short-acting barbiturates.

- Use ketamine cautiously in patients with cardiovascular disease; during procedures involving larynx, pharynx, or bronchial tree (muscle relaxants are required); and in patients with a history of alcohol abuse, cerebral trauma, intracerebral mass or hemorrhage, hyperthyroidism, history of psychiatric problems, increased CSF or intraocular pressure, or severe eye trauma.

- Use of ketamine with barbiturates or opioid analgesics may result in prolonged recovery time. Use with halothane may result in decreased blood pressure, cardiac output, and heart rate. Use with tubocurarine or nondepolarizing neuromuscular blocking agents may result in prolonged respiratory depression. Concurrent use with thyroid hormone increases the risk of tachycardia and hypertension. Concurrent administration with diazepam may decrease the incidence of emergence reactions.

- Ketamine has been used in low doses in obstetrical surgery without adverse effects on the newborn, but is not recommended in pregnant or lactating patients.

Toxicity and Overdose Alert

- Respiratory depression or apnea may be treated with mechanical ventilation or analeptics.

Patient/Family Teaching

- Psychomotor impairment may last for 24 hours following anesthesia. Caution patient to avoid driving or other activities requiring alertness until response to medication is known. • Advise patient to avoid alcohol or other CNS depressants for 24 hours following anesthesia.

≋ PHARMACOLOGIC PROFILE

Indications

• Ketamine provides anesthesia for short procedures. It is also used as induction prior to the use of other anesthetics and as a supplement to other anesthetics.

Action

• Ketamine blocks afferent impulses of pain perception, suppresses spinal cord activity, and affects CNS transmitter systems, producing anesthesia with profound analgesia, minimal respiratory depression, and minimal skeletal muscle relaxation.

Time/Action Profile (anesthesia)

Onset	Peak	Duration
15–30 sec	UK	5–10 min

Pharmacokinetics

• **Distribution:** Ketamine is rapidly distributed, enters the CNS, and crosses the placenta. • **Metabolism and Excretion:** Ketamine is mostly metabolized by the liver, with some conversion to another active compound. • **Half-life:** 2.5 hours.

Contraindications

• Ketamine is contraindicated in patients with psychiatric disturbances, hypertension, or hypersensitivity to the drug. Ketamine should not be used in pregnant or lactating patients.

Adverse Reactions and Side Effects*

• CNS: <u>emergence reactions</u> • **EENT:** diplopia, nystagmus, increased intraocular pressure • **Resp:** respiratory depression and apnea (rapid IV administration of large doses), laryngospasm • **CV:** <u>hypertension</u>, <u>tachycardia</u>, hypotension, bradycardia, arrhythmias • **GI:** nausea, vomiting, excessive salivation • **Derm:** erythema, rash • **Local:** pain at injection site • **MS:** increased skeletal muscle tone.

---

*<u>Underlines</u> indicate most frequent; CAPITALS indicate life-threatening.

Ketorolac Tromethamine	Nonopioid analgesic, Nonsteroidal anti-inflammatory agent
Toradol	pH 6.9–7.9

≋ ADMINISTRATION CONSIDERATIONS

Usual Dose

ADULTS: 30 mg as a single dose or q 6 hr (not to exceed 120 mg/day).

ADULTS <50 kg OR GERIATRIC PATIENTS >65 yr: 15 mg as a single dose or q 6 hr (not to exceed 60 mg/day).

Dilution

• **Direct IV:** Administer **undiluted.**

Compatibility

• **Solution:** D5/0.9% NaCl ✦ D5W ✦ Ringer's injection ✦ lactated Ringer's injection ✦ 0.9% NaCl.

Incompatibility

• **Syringe:** diazepam ✦ hydroxyzine ✦ meperidine ✦ morphine ✦ nalbuphine ✦ prochlorperazine ✦ promethazine.

Rate of Administration

• **Direct IV:** Administer bolus doses over at least 15 seconds.

≋ CLINICAL PRECAUTIONS

• Assess pain (note type, location, and intensity) prior to and following administration. For breakthrough pain, supplement Ketorolac with low doses of opioids as needed unless contraindicated; do not increase the dose or frequency of Ketorolac. Coadministration with opioid analgesics may have additive analgesic effects and may permit lower opioid doses. Ketorolac may be administered on a routine or p.r.n. schedule depending on the type and severity of the pain.

• The combined duration of Ketorolac by any route (IM, IV, or PO) should not exceed 5 days.

• Use ketorolac cautiously in patients who have asthma,

aspirin-induced allergy, and nasal polyps. These patients are at increased risk for developing hypersensitivity reactions. Assess for rhinitis, asthma, and urticaria. Cross-sensitivity with other nonsteroidal anti-inflammatory agents or salicylates may occur.

- Use ketorolac cautiously in patients with a history of GI bleeding or cardiovascular disease. Dosage reduction may be necessary in patients with renal impairment (creatinine clearance ≤30 ml/min).
- Geriatric patients are more likely to experience GI bleeding and adverse CNS effects from ketorolac.
- Concurrent use with aspirin may decrease effectiveness. Additive adverse GI effects occur with aspirin, other nonsteroidal anti-inflammatory agents, potassium supplements, glucocorticoids, or alcohol. Chronic use with acetaminophen may increase the risk of adverse renal reactions. Ketorolac may decrease the effectiveness of diuretics or antihypertensive therapy. Ketorolac may increase serum lithium levels and increase the risk of toxicity. Concurrent use of ketorolac with methotrexate increases the risk of toxicity. Ketorolac increases the risk of bleeding with cefamandole, cefotetan, cefoperazone, valproic acid or plicamycin, thrombolytic agents, or anticoagulants. Concurrent use with antineoplastic agents or radiation therapy increases the risk of adverse hematologic reactions. Ketorolac may increase the risk of nephrotoxicity from cyclosporine.
- Safe use during pregnancy or lactation has not been established. Use of ketorolac during the second or third trimester may cause premature closure of the ductus arteriosus in the newborn. Since ketorolac crosses the placenta, use during labor may result in bleeding problems in the infant (Pregnancy Category C). Avoid during pregnancy, labor, delivery, and lactation.

Lab Test Considerations

- Liver function tests, especially AST (SGOT) and ALT (SGPT), should be evaluated periodically in patients receiving prolonged courses of ketorolac. Levels may be increased. • Ketorolac may cause prolonged bleeding time that may persist for 24–48 hours following discontinuation of therapy.

Patient/Family Teaching

• Instruct patient on how and when to ask for pain medication. • Ketorolac may cause drowsiness or dizziness. Advise patient to avoid driving or other activities requiring alertness until response to the medication is known. • Caution patient to avoid the concurrent use of alcohol, aspirin, ibuprofen, naproxen, acetaminophen, or other over-the-counter medications without consulting with physician or pharmacist. • Instruct patient to notify physician if rash, itching, visual disturbances, weight gain, edema, black stools, or persistent headache occurs. • Advise patients with hydrogel soft contact lenses that ketorolac may cause redness and burning.

☰ PHARMACOLOGIC PROFILE

Indications

• Ketorolac is indicated in the short-term management of moderately severe acute pain. The total course by any route should not exceed 5 days.

Action

• Ketorolac inhibits prostaglandin synthesis producing peripherally mediated analgesia. It also has antipyretic and anti-inflammatory properties.

Time/Action Profile (analgesic effect)

Onset	Peak	Duration
UK	UK	6–8 hr

Pharmacokinetics

• **Distribution:** Ketorolac enters breast milk and cerebrospinal fluid in low concentrations. Remainder of distribution is not known. • **Metabolism and Excretion:** Less than 50% of ketorolac is metabolized by the liver. Ketorolac and its metabolites are excreted primarily by the kidneys (92%). Six percent is excreted in feces. • **Half-life:** 4.5 hours (range 3.8–6.3 hours; increased in elderly patients and patients with impaired renal function).

Contraindications

• Ketorolac is contraindicated in patients with known hypersensitivity to it. Cross-sensitivity with other nonsteroidal anti-inflammatory agents may exist. Injectable dosage form contains alcohol and should be avoided in patients with known intolerance. • Ketorolac should not be used to prevent pain before or during major surgery. • Ketorolac should not be used during labor, delivery, or lactation. • Patients receiving aspirin, other nonsteroidal anti-inflammatory drugs, or probenecid should not receive Ketorolac.

Adverse Reactions and Side Effects*

• **CNS:** <u>drowsiness</u>, dizziness, headache, abnormal thinking, euphoria • **EENT:** abnormal vision • **Resp:** dyspnea, asthma • **CV:** edema, vasodilation, pallor • **GI:** abnormal taste, dry mouth, nausea, dyspepsia, GI pain, diarrhea, bleeding • **GU:** urinary frequency, oliguria, renal toxicity • **Hemat:** prolonged bleeding time • **Derm:** sweating, pruritus, urticaria, purpura • **Local:** injection site pain • **Neuro:** paresthesia.

Labetalol Hydrochloride	Antihypertensive (alpha- and beta-adrenergic blocker)
Normodyne, Trandate	pH 3–4

≋ ADMINISTRATION CONSIDERATIONS

Usual Dose

ADULTS: 20 mg; may give an additional 40–80 mg at 10-min intervals until desired response is obtained, or 2 mg/min infusion (cumulative dose should not exceed 300 mg).

Dilution

• **Direct IV:** Administer **undiluted**. • Solution ranges from clear, colorless to slight yellow in color. • **Continuous**

---

*<u>Underlines</u> indicate most frequent; CAPITALS indicate life-threatening.

Infusion: Add 200 mg to 160 ml of diluent (1 mg/1 ml solution) or 200 mg to 250 ml of diluent (2 mg/3 ml solution). • Compatible diluents include D5W, 0.9% NaCl, D5/0.25% NaCl, D5/0.9% NaCl, D5/Ringer's solution, D5/LR, Ringer's, and lactated Ringer's solution. • When diluted with 0.9% NaCl, solution is stable for 24 hours at room temperature or if refrigerated.

Compatibility

• **Y-site:** amikacin • aminophylline • ampicillin • butorphanol • calcium gluconate • cefazolin • ceftazidime • ceftizoxime • chloramphenicol • cimetidine • clindamycin • dopamine • enalaprilat • erythromycin lactobionate • famotidine • fentanyl • gentamicin • heparin • lidocaine • magnesium sulfate • meperidine • metronidazole • morphine • oxacillin • penicillin G potassium • piperacillin • potassium chloride • potassium phosphate • ranitidine • sodium acetate • tobramycin • trimethoprim/sulfamethoxazole • vancomycin.

Incompatibility

• **Y-site:** cefoperazone • nafcillin.
• **Additive:** sodium bicarbonate.

Rate of Administration

• **Direct IV:** Administer by injecting 20 mg over 2 minutes; increase dose to 40–80 mg every 10 minutes until desired response is achieved. • **Continuous Infusion:** Administer at a rate of 2 mg/min and titrate for desired response. Infuse via infusion pump to ensure accurate dosage of medication.

≋ CLINICAL PRECAUTIONS

• Patients receiving labetalol IV must be supine during and for 3 hours after administration. Vital signs should be monitored every 5–15 minutes during and for several hours after administration. Assess patient for bradycardia. Assess for orthostatic hypotension when assisting patient up from supine position.
• Monitor intake and output ratios and daily weight. Assess patient routinely for evidence of congestive heart

failure (peripheral edema, dyspnea, rales/crackles, fatigue, weight gain, jugular venous distention).

- Concurrent halothane anesthesia may produce severe myocardial depression. Additive bradycardia may occur with concurrent use of cardiac glycosides. Additive hypotension may occur with concurrent use of other antihypertensive agents, nitrates, and acute ingestion of alcohol. Concurrent thyroid administration may decrease effectiveness. Labetalol may antagonize beta-adrenergic bronchodilators. Cimetidine decreases metabolism and may increase toxicity of labetalol. Glutethimide may decrease the effects of labetalol. Labetalol may blunt tachycardia produced by nitroglycerin. Concurrent use of MAO inhibitor therapy and labetalol should be avoided. This combination may produce hypertension for up to 14 days following discontinuation of MAO inhibitor.
- Use with caution in patients with renal impairment. Dosage reduction is recommended.
- Use labetalol cautiously in patients with thyrotoxicosis or hypoglycemia, as symptoms may be masked.
- Geriatric patients may exhibit altered sensitivity to beta-adrenergic blockers. Dosage adjustments may be necessary.
- Pregnant or lactating patients should not receive labetalol because it may cause apnea, low Apgar scores, bradycardia, and hypoglycemia in the newborn (Pregnancy Category C). Safe use of labetalol in children has not been established.

Lab Test Considerations

- Hepatic and renal function and CBC should be monitored routinely in patients receiving prolonged therapy.
- Labetalol may cause elevations in serum potassium, uric acid, LDH, AST (SGOT), ALT (SGPT), alkaline phosphatase, ANA titer, BUN, serum lipoprotein, and triglyceride concentrations.

Patient/Family Teaching

- Caution patient to make position changes slowly to minimize orthostatic hypotension. Patient should also be instructed to call for assistance when ambulating during period of dose adjustment. • Reinforce need to continue additional therapies for hypertension (weight loss, restricted sodium intake, stress reduction, regular exercise, moderation of alcohol consumption, and cessation of smoking).

 PHARMACOLOGIC PROFILE

Indications
• Labetalol is used in the management of severe hypertension. • Labetalol is also used to produce controlled hypotension during surgery (unlabeled use).

Action
• Labetalol blocks stimulation of beta$_1$ (myocardial) and beta$_2$ (pulmonary and vascular) adrenergic receptor sites. It also has alpha-adrenergic blocking activity, which results in peripheral vasodilation and orthostatic hypotension. The overall effect is to decrease blood pressure and heart rate.

Time/Action Profile (antihypertensive effect)

Onset	Peak	Duration
2–5 min	5–15 min	2–4 hr (up to 24 hr)

Pharmacokinetics
• **Distribution:** Labetalol displays moderate penetration of the CNS. It also crosses the placenta and enters breast milk. • **Metabolism and Excretion:** Labetalol undergoes extensive hepatic metabolism. • **Half-life:** 3–8 hours.

Contraindications
• Labetalol is contraindicated in patients with hypersensitivity to it or to parabens and edetate. Labetalol should be avoided in patients with uncompensated congestive heart failure, pulmonary edema, cardiogenic shock, bradycardia, or heart block. Pregnant or lactating patients should not receive labetalol.

Adverse Reactions and Side Effects*
• **CNS:** <u>fatigue</u>, <u>weakness</u>, dizziness, depression, memory loss, mental changes, nightmares • **EENT:** dry eyes, blurred

---

*<u>Underlines</u> indicate most frequent; CAPITALS indicate life-threatening.

vision • **Resp:** bronchospasm, wheezing • **CV:** BRADYCARDIA, CONGESTIVE HEART FAILURE, PULMONARY EDEMA, orthstatic hypotension, peripheral vasoconstriction • **GI:** constipation, diarrhea, nausea, change in taste • **GU:** impotence, diminished libido, urinary retention • **Derm:** rash, itching • **Endo:** hyperglycemia, hypoglycemia • **MS:** joint pain, arthralgia.

Leucovorin Calcium	*Vitamin (folic acid analogue), Antidote (for methotrexate, fluorouracil, other folic acid antagonists)*
Wellcovorin, citrovorum factor, 5-formyl tetrahydrofolate, folinic acid	pH 7.7–8.1

≋ ADMINISTRATION CONSIDERATIONS

Usual Dose

Advanced Colorectal Cancer (in combination with fluorouracil)

ADULTS: leucovorin 200 mg/m² by slow injection followed by fluorouracil 370 mg/m² *or* leucovorin 20 mg/m² followed by 425 mg/m² fluorouracil. Regimen is repeated daily for 5 days at 4-wk intervals for two cycles. Entire process may be repeated at 4–5-wk intervals as tolerated. See *fluorouracil* monograph on page 440.

High-Dose Methotrexate-Leucovorin Rescue

ADULTS: 15 mg q 6 hr for 10 doses or until serum methotrexate level is less than 0.05 micromolar. If delayed early elimination or acute renal injury occurs, increase to 150 mg q 3 hr until methotrexate serum level is less than 1 micromolar then decrease to 15 mg q 3 hr until serum methotrexate level is less than 0.05 micromolar. See *methotrexate sodium* monograph on page 611.

Impaired Methotrexate Elimination or Inadvertent Overdose

Note: Must begin leucovorin within 24 hr of methotrexate.

ADULTS AND CHILDREN: 10 mg/m^2 followed by 10 mg/m^2 PO q 6 hr for 72 hr. If serum creatinine at 24 hr is 50% greater than premethotrexate level, dosage should be increased to 100 mg/m^2 q 3 hr until serum methotrexate level is less than 10^{-8} M. Many other rescue protocols are used.

Adjunct to Trimetrexate Therapy

ADULTS: 20 mg/m^2 q 6 hr for 24 days.

Megaloblastic Anemia

ADULTS AND CHILDREN: up to 1 mg/day.

Treatment of Hematologic Toxicity of Other Folic Acid Antagonists

ADULTS AND CHILDREN: 5–15 mg.

Prevention of Hematologic Toxicity of Other Folic Acid Antagonists

ADULTS AND CHILDREN: 0.4–5 mg with each dose of folic acid antagonist.

Dilution

• To **reconstitute** 50-mg vial of leucovorin calcium for injection, add 5 ml of bacteriostatic water or sterile water for injection, to yield a concentration of 10 mg/ml. Use 10 ml of diluent for 100-mg vial. The 350-mg vial should be reconstituted with 17 ml of diluent for a concentration of 20 mg/ml. • Do not use a diluent containing benzyl alcohol for doses greater than 10 mg/m^2. • Use immediately if reconstituted with sterile water for injection. Stable for 7 days when reconstituted with bacteriostatic water. • **Intermittent Infusion:** May be **diluted** in 100–500 ml of D5W, D10W, 0.9% NaCl, Ringer's, or lactated Ringer's solution. • Stable for 24 hours.

Compatibility

• **Syringe:** bleomycin • cisplatin • cyclophosphamide • doxorubicin • fluorouracil • furosemide • heparin • methotrexate • metoclopramide • mitomycin • vinblastine • vincristine.

• **Y-site:** bleomycin • cisplatin • cyclophosphamide • doxorubicin • filgrastim • fluconazole • fluorouracil • furo-

semide • heparin • methotrexate • metoclopramide • mitomycin • piperacillin/tazobactam • tacrolimus • vinblastine
• vincristine.

- **Additive:** cisplatin • floxuridine • fluorouracil.

Incompatibility

- **Syringe:** droperidol.
- **Y-site:** droperidol • foscarnet.

Rate of Administration

- **Direct IV:** Rate of direct IV infusion should not exceed
160 mg/min.

≋ CLINICAL PRECAUTIONS

- Make sure leucovorin calcium is available before administering high-dose methotrexate. Administration must be
initiated within 24 hours of methotrexate therapy. Coadministration with high-dose methotrexate requires cru-
cial timing of dosing and knowledge of methotrexate
levels.
- Administer as soon as possible after a toxic overdose
of folic acid antagonists (pyrimethamine and trimethoprim). Effectiveness of leucovorin therapy begins to decrease 1 hour after overdose.
- Monitor for development of allergic reactions (rash, urticaria, wheezing). Notify physician if these occur.
- Assess degree of weakness and fatigue in patients with
megaloblastic anemia.
- Leucovorin may decrease the anticonvulsant effect of
barbiturates, phenytoin, or primidone.
- Use leucovorin cautiously in patients with undiagnosed
anemia, as it may mask the progression of pernicious
anemia.
- Use cautiously in patients with ascites, renal failure, dehydration, or pleural effusions.
- Do not confuse with folic acid, which is ineffective for
folate antagonist overdosage (see *folic acid* monograph
on page 445).
- Although safe use in pregnancy is not established, leucovorin has been used safely to treat megaloblastic anemia
in pregnancy (Pregnancy Category C).

Lab Test Considerations

• *For Leucovorin Rescue:* Monitor serum methotrexate levels to determine dosage and effectiveness of therapy. Leucovorin calcium levels should be equal to or greater than methotrexate level. Rescue continues until serum methotrexate level is less than 5×10^{-8} M. • Monitor creatinine clearance and serum creatinine prior to and every 24 hours during therapy to detect methotrexate toxicity. An increase of more than 50% over the pretreatment concentration at 24 hours is associated with severe renal toxicity. Monitor urine pH every 6 hours throughout therapy. Urine pH should be maintained at more than 7 to decrease nephrotoxic effects of high-dose methotrexate. Sodium bicarbonate or acetazolamide may be ordered to alkalinize urine. • Monitor plasma folic acid levels, hemoglobin, hematocrit, and reticulocyte count prior to and periodically during course of therapy in patients with megaloblastic anemia.

Patient/Family Teaching

• Explain purpose of leucovorin rescue to the patient. Instruct the patient to drink at least 3 liters of fluid each day during leucovorin rescue. • Encourage patients with folic acid deficiency to eat a diet high in folic acid (meat proteins, bran, dried beans, and green leafy vegetables).

PHARMACOLOGIC PROFILE

Indications

• In combination with fluorouracil, leucovorin is used in the palliative management of advanced colorectal cancer to prolong survival. • Leucovorin is used to minimize the hematologic effects of high-dose methotrexate therapy ("leucovorin rescue"). • It is also used in the management of overdoses of folic acid antagonists (pyrimethamine or trimethoprim) and in the treatment of folic acid deficiency unresponsive to oral replacement.

Action

• Leucovorin is the reduced form of folic acid, which serves as a cofactor in the synthesis of DNA and RNA. Its administration brings about the reversal of toxic effects of folic acid antagonists, such as methotrexate and trimethoprim. It also serves to reverse deficiency states.

Time/Action Profile (serum folate levels)

Onset	Peak	Duration
<5 min	UK	3–6 hr

Pharmacokinetics
• **Distribution:** Leucovorin is widely distributed and concentrates in the CNS and liver. • **Metabolism and Excretion:** Leucovorin is extensively converted to tetrahydrofolic derivatives, including 5-methyltetrahydrofolate, a major storage form. • **Half-life:** 3.5 hours.

Contraindications
• Leucovorin is contraindicated in patients who had previous hypersensitivity to it. Some products contain benzyl alcohol and should be avoided in infants or other patients with known intolerance.

Adverse Reactions and Side Effects*
• **Misc:** allergic reactions (rash, urticaria, wheezing).

Levorphanol Tartrate
Opioid analgesic (agonist)

Levo-Dromoran   pH 4.3

Schedule II

ADMINISTRATION CONSIDERATIONS

Usual Dose
ADULTS ≥50 kg: 2 mg q 6–8 hr. Larger doses may be required in patients with severe chronic or escalating pain.
ADULTS <50 kg AND CHILDREN: 0.02 mg/kg q 6–8 hr.

Dilution
• **Direct IV:** May be administered **undiluted**.

---

*Underlines indicate most frequent; CAPITALS indicate life-threatening.

Compatibility
- **Syringe:** glycopyrrolate.

Incompatibility
- **Additive:** aminophylline • ammonium chloride • amo-barbital • chlorothiazide • heparin • methicillin • pentobarbital • phenobarbital • phenytoin • secobarbital • sodium bicarbonate • thiopental.

Rate of Administration
- **Direct IV:** Administer slowly, over 3–5 minutes. Rapid administration may lead to increased respiratory depression, hypotension, and circulatory collapse.

≋ CLINICAL PRECAUTIONS

- Assess type, location, and intensity of pain prior to and 20 minutes (peak) following administration. Regularly administered doses may be more effective than p.r.n. administration. Analgesic is more effective if given before pain becomes severe. Coadministration with nonopioid analgesics may have additive analgesic effects and permit lower opioid doses.
- An equianalgesic chart (Appendix B, page 1045) should be used when changing routes or when changing from one opioid to another.
- Assess blood pressure, pulse, and respiratory rate before and periodically during administration. If respiratory rate is less than 10 ml/minute, assess level of sedation. Physical stimulation may be sufficient to prevent significant hypoventilation. Dose may need to be decreased by 25–50%.
- Assess bowel function routinely. Prevention of constipation should be instituted with increased intake of fluids and bulk, stool softeners, and laxatives to minimize constipating effects. Stimulant laxatives should be administered routinely if opioid use exceeds 2–3 days, unless contraindicated.
- Prolonged use may lead to physical and psychological dependence and tolerance. This should not prevent patient from receiving adequate analgesia. Most patients who receive levorphanol for medical reasons do not develop psychological dependency. Progressively higher

doses may be required to relieve pain with long-term therapy. Medication should be gradually discontinued after long-term use to prevent withdrawal symptoms.

- Use levorphanol with extreme caution in patients receiving MAO inhibitors, as this combination may result in unpredictable, severe reactions. Decrease initial dose of levorphanol to 25% of usual dose.

- Assess level of sedation. Initial drowsiness will diminish with continued use. Additive CNS depression may occur with concurrent use of alcohol, antihistamines, antidepressants, or sedative/hypnotics.

- Administration of partial-antagonist opioid analgesics may precipitate opioid withdrawal in physically dependent patients. Nalbuphine or pentazocine may decrease analgesic effect.

- Levorphanol should be used with caution in patients with head trauma; increased intracranial pressure; severe renal, hepatic, or pulmonary disease; hypothyroidism; adrenal insufficiency; alcoholism; undiagnosed abdominal pain; prostatic hypertrophy; in elderly or debilitated patients (dosage reduction suggested); and patients who may have been addicted to opioids previously.

- Safe use in pregnancy, lactation, or children has not been established. Use of levorphanol during labor may cause respiratory depression in the newborn.

Toxicity and Overdose Alert

- If an opioid antagonist is required to reverse respiratory depression or coma, naloxone (Narcan) is the antidote. Dilute the 0.4-mg ampule of naloxone in 10 ml of 0.9% NaCl and administer 0.5 ml (0.02 mg) by direct IV push every 2 minutes. For children and patients weighing <40 kg, dilute 0.1 mg of naloxone in 10 ml of 0.9% NaCl for a concentration of 10 mcg/ml and administer 0.5 mcg every 1–2 minutes. Titrate the dose to avoid withdrawal, seizures, and severe pain. Monitor patient closely; dose may need to be repeated or naloxone infusion administered.

Lab Test Considerations

- Levorphanol may increase plasma amylase and lipase levels.

Patient/Family Teaching

• Instruct patient on how and when to ask for pain medication. • Medication may cause drowsiness or dizziness. Advise patient to call for assistance when ambulating or smoking. Caution patient to avoid activities that require alertness until response to the medication is known. • Advise patient to make position changes slowly to minimize orthostatic hypotension. • Instruct patient to avoid concurrent use of alcohol or other CNS depressants. • Advise ambulatory patients that nausea and vomiting may be decreased by lying down. • Encourage patient to turn, cough, and breathe deeply every 2 hours to prevent atelectasis.

 PHARMACOLOGIC PROFILE

Indications

• Levorphanol is used in the management of moderate to severe pain.

Action

• Levorphanol binds to opiate receptors in the CNS, altering the perception of and response to pain. It also produces generalized CNS depression.

Time/Action Profile (analgesic effect)

Onset	Peak	Duration
UK	within 20 min	4–5 hr†

†Duration increases to 6–8 hr after 2–3 days because of drug accumulation.

Pharmacokinetics

• **Distribution:** UK. • **Metabolism and Excretion:** Levorphanol is mostly metabolized by the liver. • **Half-life:** 12–16 hours (accumulation occurs after 2–3 days of dosing).

Contraindications

• Levorphanol is contraindicated in patients with previous hypersensitivity to it or to phenol. Avoid chronic use during pregnancy or lactation.

Adverse Reactions and Side Effects*

• **CNS:** <u>sedation</u>, <u>confusion</u>, headache, euphoria, floating feeling, unusual dreams, hallucinations, dysphoria • **EENT:** miosis, diplopia, blurred vision • **Resp:** RESPIRATORY DEPRESSION • **CV:** <u>hypotension</u>, bradycardia • **GI:** nausea, vomiting, <u>constipation</u>, dry mouth • **GU:** urinary retention • **Derm:** sweating, flushing • **Misc:** tolerance, physical dependence, psychological dependence.

Levothyroxine Sodium	Thyroid hormone
Levothyroid, Levoxyl, Synthroid	pH 7.5

≋ ADMINISTRATION CONSIDERATIONS

Usual Dose

Hypothyroidism

ADULTS: 50–100 mcg (0.05–0.1 mg)/day as a single dose.

CHILDREN >10 yr: 1.5–2.25 mcg (0.0015–0.00225 mg)/kg/day *or* up to 150–200 mcg (0.15–0.2 mg)/day given once daily.

CHILDREN 6–10 yr: 3–3.75 mcg (0.003–0.00375 mg)/kg/day *or* 75–112 mcg (0.075–0.112 mg)/day given once daily.

CHILDREN 1–5 yr: 2.25–3.75 mcg (0.00225–0.00375 mg)/kg/day *or* 56–75 mcg (0.056–0.075 mg)/day given once daily.

CHILDREN 6–12 mo: 3.75–4.5 mcg (0.00375–0.0045 mg)/kg/day *or* 37.5–56 mcg (0.0375–0.056 mg)/day given once daily.

INFANTS 0–6 mo: 3.75–4.5 mcg (0.00375–0.0045 mg)/kg/day *or* 18.7–37.5 mcg (0.0187–0.0375 mg)/day given as a single dose.

PREMATURE INFANTS OR INFANTS AT RISK FOR HEART FAILURE: 18.75 mcg (0.01875 mg)/day. At 4–6 wk may be increased to 37.5 mcg (0.0375 mg)/day given as a single dose.

*Underlines indicate most frequent; CAPITALS indicate life-threatening.

Myxedema Coma

ADULTS: 200–500 mcg; if no response in 24 hr, may give additional 100–300 mcg (0.1–0.3 mg); then daily administration of 50–200 mcg (0.05–0.2 mg).

Dilution

• **Direct IV: Dilute** the 50-, 200-, or 500-mcg vial with 0.5, 2, or 5 ml, respectively, of 0.9% NaCl without preservatives (diluent usually provided), for a concentration of 100 mcg/ml. Shake well to dissolve completely. • Administer solution immediately after preparation; discard unused portion.

Incompatibility

• Information unavailable. Do not admix with other medications or solutions.

Rate of Administration

• **Direct IV:** Administer at a rate of 100 mcg over 1 minute. Do not add to IV infusions; may be administered through Y-tubing or a 3-way stopcock.

≋ CLINICAL PRECAUTIONS

• Assess apical pulse and blood pressure prior to and periodically during therapy. Assess for tachyarrhythmias and chest pain.
• Use levothyroxine cautiously in patients with cardiovascular disease, severe renal insufficiency, or uncorrected adrenocortical disorders (dosage reduction may be required).
• Elderly and myxedematous patients are extremely sensitive to thyroid hormones; initial dosage should be markedly reduced.
• IV phenytoin causes the release of thyroid hormone. Thyroid hormones increase the effect of oral anticoagulants. Levothyroxine may cause an increase in the requirement for insulin or oral hypoglycemic agents in diabetics. Additive CNS and cardiac stimulation with concurrent use of sympathomimetic agents (amphetamines, vasopressors, decongestants). Levothyroxine may decrease some effects of beta-adrenergic blockers.
• When changing from oral to IV levothyroxine, in adults

the IV dose is ½ of the oral dose; in children, the IV dose is ¾ of the oral dose.
• Levothyroxine has been used safely in pregnancy (Pregnancy Category A).

Toxicity and Overdose Alert

• Overdose is manifested as hyperthyroidism (tachycardia, chest pain, nervousness, insomnia, diaphoresis, tremors, weight loss). Usual treatment is to withhold dose for 2–6 days. Sympathetic overstimulation may be controlled by beta-adrenergic blocking agents, such as propranolol. Oxygen and supportive measures to control symptoms such as fever are also used.

Lab Test Considerations

• Thyroid function studies should be monitored prior to and throughout course of therapy. • Monitor blood and urine glucose in diabetic patients. Insulin or oral hypoglycemic dose may need to be increased.

Patient/Family Teaching

• Explain to patient that levothyroxine does not cure hypothyroidism, it provides a thyroid hormone; therapy is lifelong. • Advise patient to notify physician if headache, nervousness, diarrhea, excessive sweating, heat intolerance, chest pain, increased pulse rate, palpitations, weight loss more than 2 lb/wk, or any unusual symptoms occur. • Emphasize importance of follow-up examinations to monitor effectiveness of therapy. Thyroid function tests are performed at least once yearly. • For children, discuss with parents need for routine follow-up studies to ensure correct development. Inform parent that partial hair loss may be experienced by children on thyroid therapy.

≋ PHARMACOLOGIC PROFILE

Indications

• Levothyroxine is used as a replacement or substitution therapy in diminished or absent thyroid function of many causes.

Action

• Principal effect of levothyroxine is increasing metabolic rate of body tissues. Thyroid hormones promote gluconeogenesis, increase utilization and mobilization of glycogen stores, and stimulate protein synthesis. They also promote cell growth and differentiation and aid in the development of the brain and CNS.

Time/Action Profile (effects on thyroid hormone levels)

	Onset	Peak†	Duration‡
T_4	6–8 hr	3–4 wk	UK
T_3	UK	48–72 hr	up to 72 hr

†With chronic dosing.
‡After discontinuation of chronic therapy.

Pharmacokinetics

• **Distribution:** Levothyroxine is distributed into most body tissues. It does not readily cross the placenta. Small amounts enter breast milk. • **Metabolism and Excretion:** Levothyroxine is metabolized by the liver, undergoes enterohepatic recirculation, and is excreted in feces via bile. • **Half-life:** 6–7 days.

Contraindications

• Levothyroxine is contraindicated in patients with hypersensitivity to it or mannitol. It should be avoided in patients with recent myocardial infarction, or thyrotoxicosis.

Adverse Reactions and Side Effects*

• **CNS:** <u>irritability</u>, <u>insomnia</u>, <u>nervousness</u>, headache • **CV:** <u>tachycardia</u>, <u>arrhythmias</u>, increased cardiac output, angina pectoris, increased blood pressure, CARDIOVASCULAR COLLAPSE, hypotension • **GI:** diarrhea, cramps, vomiting • **Derm:** increased sweating, hair loss (children only) • **Endo:** menstrual irregularities • **Metab:** <u>weight loss</u>, heat intolerance • **MS:** accelerated bone maturation in children.

---

*<u>Underlines</u> indicate most frequent; CAPITALS indicate life-threatening.

Lidocaine Hydrochloride	*Antiarrhythmic* *(group IB)*
Xylocaine HCl, lignocaine HCl	**pH 5−7** **(premixed 3.5−6)**

 ADMINISTRATION CONSIDERATIONS

Usual Dose

ADULTS: 50−100-mg bolus (or 1−1.5 mg/kg, may repeat bolus or portion of bolus dose in 5 min), then 1−4-mg/min (20−50 mcg/kg/min) infusion (not to exceed 200−300 mg in 1 hr).

CHILDREN: 0.5−1-mg/kg bolus, repeat as needed (not to exceed 3−5 mg/kg total dose), 10−50 mcg/kg/min infusion.

Dilution

• **Direct IV:** Administer IV loading dose of 1 mg/kg **undiluted**. May follow with second loading dose of ½−⅓ of original dose after 5 minutes. Follow by IV infusion. • Available in 1%, 2%, 4%, 10%, and 20% solutions. Only 1% and 2% solutions are used for direct IV injection. Do not use lidocaine with preservatives or other medications, such as epinephrine, for IV injection. • **Continuous Infusion:** To prepare for IV infusion, add 1 g lidocaine to 250, 500, or 1000 ml of D5W. Solution is stable for 24 hours. Other compatible solutions include D5/LR, D5/0.45% NaCl, D5/0.9% NaCl, 0.45% NaCl, 0.9% NaCl, and lactated Ringer's solution.

Compatibility

• **Y-site:** alteplase ◆ amrinone ◆ cefazolin ◆ ciprofloxacin ◆ diltiazem ◆ dobutamine ◆ enalaprilat ◆ famotidine ◆ haloperidol ◆ labetalol ◆ meperidine ◆ morphine ◆ nitroglycerin ◆ nitroprusside ◆ potassium chloride ◆ streptokinase ◆ vitamin B complex with C.

• **Additive:** aminophylline ◆ atracurium ◆ bretylium ◆ calcium chloride ◆ calcium glucepate ◆ calcium gluconate ◆ chloramphenicol ◆ chlorothiazide ◆ cimetidine ◆ dexamethasone ◆ diphenhydramine ◆ dobutamine ◆ dopamine ◆ ephedrine ◆ erythromycin lactobionate ◆ furosemide ◆ heparin ◆ hydrocortisone sodium succinate ◆ hydroxyzine ◆ insulin ◆ metaraminol ◆ nitroglycerin ◆ penicillin G potassium

♦ pentobarbital ♦ phenylephrine ♦ potassium chloride ♦ procainamide ♦ prochlorperazine ♦ promazine ♦ ranitidine ♦ sodium bicarbonate ♦ sodium lactate ♦ verapamil ♦ vitamin B complex with C.

Incompatibility

• **Additive:** methohexital ♦ phenytoin. • Do not admix with blood transfusions.

Rate of Administration

• **Direct IV:** Administer IV loading dose of 1 mg/kg at a rate of 25–50 mg over 1 minute. • **Continuous Infusion:** Administer via infusion pump for accurate dose at a rate of 1–4 mg/min (see Infusion Rate Table below).

LIDOCAINE (Xylocaine) INFUSION RATE TABLE

Dilution: May be prepared as 1 g/1000 ml = 1 mg/ml
1 g/500 ml = 2 mg/ml
1 g/250 ml = 4 mg/ml
4 g/500 ml = 8 mg/ml
Loading dose: 50–100 mg at 25–50 mg/min

LIDOCAINE INFUSION RATES (ml/hr)

Dose (mg/min)	1 mg/ml Concentration	2 mg/ml Concentration	4 mg/ml Concentration	8 mg/ml Concentration
1 mg/min	60 ml/hr	30 ml/hr	15 ml/hr	7.5 ml/hr
2 mg/min	120 ml/hr	60 ml/hr	30 ml/hr	15 ml/hr
3 mg/min	180 ml/hr	90 ml/hr	45 ml/hr	22.5 ml/hr
4 mg/min	240 ml/hr	120 ml/hr	60 ml/hr	30 ml/hr

≋ CLINICAL PRECAUTIONS

• Monitor ECG continuously and blood pressure and respiratory status frequently throughout administration.
• Additive cardiac depression and toxicity may occur with phenytoin, quinidine, procainamide, or propranolol. Cimetidine and beta-adrenergic blockers may decrease metabolism and increase risk of toxicity.
• If arrhythmias recur, a small bolus (0.5 mg/kg) may be given and the infusion rate increased. If only the infusion rate is increased, the full effect will not occur for 5–8 hours.

- Use cautiously in patients with liver disease or congestive heart failure; in patients weighing less than 50 kg or geriatric patients (smaller loading dose and/or lower infusion rates may be necessary). Geriatric patients are more sensitive to cardiac and CNS effects of lidocaine.
- Safe use in pregnancy or lactation has not been established (Pregnancy Category B).

Toxicity and Overdose Alert

- Serum lidocaine levels should be monitored periodically throughout prolonged or high-dose therapy. Therapeutic serum lidocaine levels range from 1.5–5 mcg/ml.
- Signs and symptoms of toxicity include confusion, excitation, blurred or double vision, nausea, vomiting, ringing in ears, tremors, twitching, convulsions, difficulty breathing, severe dizziness or fainting, and unusually slow heart rate. If symptoms of toxicity occur, stop infusion and monitor patient closely.

Lab Test Considerations

- Electrolytes should be monitored periodically during prolonged therapy.

Patient/Family Teaching

- Lidocaine may cause drowsiness and dizziness. Advise patient to call for assistance during ambulation and transfer.

≋ PHARMACOLOGIC PROFILE

Indications

- Lidocaine is used in the acute treatment of ventricular arrhythmias.

Action

- Lidocaine suppresses automaticity of conduction tissue and spontaneous depolarization of the ventricles during diastole by altering the flux of sodium ions across cell membranes. It has little or no effect on heart rate.

Time/Action Profile (antiarrhythmic effect)

Onset	Peak	Duration
immediate	immediate	10–20 min

Pharmacokinetics

• **Distribution:** Lidocaine is widely distributed. It concentrates in adipose tissue, crosses the blood–brain barrier and placenta. • **Metabolism and Excretion:** Most metabolism of lidocaine occurs in the liver. • **Half-life:** The half-life of lidocaine is biphasic, with an initial phase of 7–30 minutes and a terminal phase of 90–120 minutes.

Contraindications

• Lidocaine is contraindicated in patients with previous hypersensitivity to it. Patients with advanced AV block should not receive lidocaine.

Adverse Reactions and Side Effects*

• **CNS:** <u>drowsiness</u>, dizziness, lethargy, <u>confusion</u>, nervousness, SEIZURES, tremor • **CV:** hypotension, arrhythmias, bradycardia, CARDIAC ARREST • **GI:** nausea, vomiting.

Liothyronine Sodium	*Thyroid hormone*
Triostat, T_3	pH 10.5

ADMINISTRATION CONSIDERATIONS

Usual Dose

ADULTS: 25–50 mcg, to be repeated at 4–12-hr intervals. Initial daily doses of at least 65 mcg are associated with decreased mortality. In general, doses of greater than 100 mcg/day are not recommended. Patients with cardiovascular disease should receive initial doses of 10–20 mcg.

Dilution

• **Direct IV:** May be administered **undiluted**.

Incompatibility

• Information unavailable. Do not admix with other medications or solutions.

Rate of Administration

• **Direct IV:** Administer as a bolus.

---

*<u>Underlines</u> indicate most frequent; CAPITALS indicate life-threatening.

≋ CLINICAL PRECAUTIONS

- Assess apical pulse and blood pressure prior to and continuously throughout therapy. Assess for tachyarrhythmias and chest pain.
- Geriatric patients are more sensitive to the cardiovascular effects of thyroid hormones.
- Oral therapy should be initiated as soon as patient's condition is stabilized and patient is able to take oral medication. When changing to oral therapy, discontinue injections and begin oral therapy at a low dose, increasing gradually according to response.
- Liothyronine has been used safely during pregnancy (Pregnancy Category A). Use cautiously during lactation. Safe use in children has not been established.

Toxicity and Overdose Alert

- Overdose is manifested as hyperthyroidism (tachycardia, chest pain, nervousness, insomnia, diaphoresis, tremors, weight loss). Usual treatment is to withhold dose for 2–6 days.

Lab Test Considerations

- Thyroid function studies should be monitored prior to and throughout course of therapy. • Monitor blood and urine glucose in diabetic patients; insulin or oral hypoglycemic dose may need to be increased.

Patient/Family Teaching

- Advise patient to notify physician if headache, nervousness, diarrhea, excessive sweating, heat intolerance, chest pain, increased pulse rate, palpitations, weight loss of greater than 2 lb/wk, or any unusual symptoms occur.
- Emphasize importance of follow-up examinations to monitor effectiveness of therapy. Thyroid function tests are performed at least once yearly.

≋ PHARMACOLOGIC PROFILE

Indications

- Liothyronine is used as thyroid replacement therapy in myxedema coma.

Action

• The principal effect of thyroid hormones is to increase the metabolic rate of body tissues. They promote gluconeogenesis, increase utilization and mobilization of glycogen stores, and stimulate protein synthesis. In addition, they promote cell growth and aid in the development of the brain and CNS.

Time/Action Profile

Onset	Peak†	Duration‡
unknown	24–72 hr	72 hr

†After chronic dosing.
‡After discontinuation of chronic therapy.

Pharmacokinetics

• **Distribution:** Liothyronine is distributed into many body tissues. Thyroid hormones do not readily cross the placenta; minimal amounts enter breast milk. • **Metabolism and Excretion:** Metabolism of liothyronine occurs in the liver and other tissues. • **Half-life:** 1–2 days (increased in hypothyroidism).

Contraindications

• Liothyronine sodium is contraindicated in patients with hypersensitivity to it. Injectable product contains alcohol and ammonium hydroxide. Avoid use in patients with intolerance to these additives.

Adverse Reactions and Side Effects*

• **CNS:** <u>irritability</u>, <u>nervousness</u>, <u>insomnia</u>, headache • **CV:** <u>tachycardia</u>, <u>arrhythmias</u>, increased cardiac output, angina pectoris, increased blood pressure, cardiovascular collapse, hypotension • **GI:** diarrhea, cramps, vomiting • **Derm:** increased sweating.

---

*<u>Underlines</u> indicate most frequent; CAPITALS indicate life-threatening.

Lorazepam	Sedative/hypnotic (benzodiazepine)
Ativan	pH UK

Schedule IV

≋ ADMINISTRATION CONSIDERATIONS

Usual Dose

Preoperative Sedation
ADULTS: 44 mcg (0.044 mg)/kg (not to exceed 2 mg).

Operative Amnesia
ADULTS: up to 50 mcg (0.05 mg)/kg (not to exceed 4 mg), given 15–20 min before procedure.

Status Epilepticus (unlabeled use)
ADULTS: 0.05 mg/kg (not to exceed 4 mg), may repeat in 10–15 min (up to 8 mg/12 hr).

INFANTS AND CHILDREN: 0.03–0.1 mg/kg, may be followed in 10–15 min by 0.05 mg/kg for 2 additional doses (unlabeled).

Antiemetic during Chemotherapy
ADULTS: 2 mg 30 min prior to emetogenic chemotherapy, then 2 mg q 4 hr as needed (unlabeled).

Dilution
• **Direct IV:** Dilute immediately before use with an equal amount of sterile water, D5W, or 0.9% NaCl for injection.
• Do not use if solution is colored or contains a precipitate.

Compatibility
• **Syringe:** cimetidine.
• **Y-site:** acyclovir ◆ allopurinol sodium ◆ atracurium ◆ cisplatin ◆ cyclophosphamide ◆ cytarabine ◆ diltiazem ◆ doxorubicin ◆ filgrastim ◆ fludarabine ◆ melphalan ◆ methotrexate ◆ paclitaxel ◆ pancuronium ◆ piperacillin/tazobactam ◆ tacrolimus ◆ vecuronium ◆ vinorelbine ◆ zidovudine.

Incompatibility
• **Y-site:** buprenorphine ◆ ondansetron ◆ sargramostim.

Rate of Administration

• **Direct IV:** Administer directly into vein, or through Y-site injection or via 3-way stopcock of a running IV infusion at a rate of 2 mg over 1 minute. Rapid IV administration may result in apnea, hypotension, bradycardia, or cardiac arrest.

≋ CLINICAL PRECAUTIONS

• Assess level of consciousness and sedation frequently during operative use. Monitor vital signs routinely.
• Following parenteral administration, keep patient supine for at least 8 hours and observe closely.
• Use lorazepam with caution in patients with severe hepatic or renal impairment.
• Dosage reduction may be necessary for elderly or debilitated patients. Because lorazepam has a relatively short duration of action and no active metabolite, it may be easier to use in geriatric patients.
• Additive CNS depression may occur with concurrent use of other CNS depressants, including alcohol, antihistamines, antidepressants, opioid analgesics, and other sedative/hypnotics. Lorazepam may decrease the efficacy of levodopa. Smoking may increase metabolism and decrease effectiveness of lorazepam. Probenecid may decrease metabolism of lorazepam, enhancing its actions.
• Lorazepam should be avoided during pregnancy or lactation (Pregnancy Category D). Use cautiously in patients with childbearing potential. Safe use in children under 18 years is not established.

Patient/Family Teaching

• Lorazepam causes drowsiness and may cause dizziness. Advise patient to avoid driving or other activities requiring alertness until response to medication is known. • Caution patient to avoid taking alcohol or other CNS depressants within 24 hours of the administration of this medication. • Instruct patient to inform physician if pregnancy is suspected.

≋ PHARMACOLOGIC PROFILE

Indications

• Lorazepam provides preoperative sedation, relieves pre-operative anxiety, and provides operative amnesia. • **Unlabeled Uses:** Lorazepam has been used in the management of status epilepticus and prophylactically during emetogenic chemotherapy.

Action

• Lorazepam depresses the CNS, probably by potentiating gamma-aminobutyric acid (GABA), an inhibitory neurotransmitter.

Time/Action Profile (sedation)

Onset	Peak	Duration
5–15 min	UK	up to 48 hr

Pharmacokinetics

• **Distribution:** Lorazepam is widely distributed. It crosses the blood–brain barrier and the placenta and enters breast milk. • **Metabolism and Excretion:** Lorazepam is highly metabolized by the liver. • **Half-life:** 10–20 hours.

Contraindications

• Lorazepam is contraindicated in patients with hypersensitivity to it. Cross-sensitivity with other benzodiazepines may exist. Parenteral product contains benzyl alcohol and propylene glycol and should be avoided in patients with known intolerance to these additives. Lorazepam should be avoided in comatose patients or those with pre-existing CNS depression, uncontrolled severe pain, narrow-angle glaucoma, pregnancy, or lactation (Pregnancy Category D).

Adverse Reactions and Side Effects*

• **CNS:** <u>dizziness</u>, <u>drowsiness</u>, <u>lethargy</u>, hangover, paradoxical excitation, headache, mental depression • **EENT:** blurred vision • **Resp:** respiratory depression • **GI:** nausea, vomiting, diarrhea, constipation • **Derm:** rashes • **Misc:** tolerance, psychological dependence, physical dependence.

---

*<u>Underlines</u> indicate most frequent; CAPITALS indicate life-threatening.

Magnesium Sulfate

Electrolyte, Anticonvulsant

pH 5.5–7

ADMINISTRATION CONSIDERATIONS

Usual Dose

Each g magnesium sulfate contains 8 mEq magnesium. Dose should not exceed 30–40 g in adults.

Magnesium Deficiency

ADULTS: up to 5 g.

Eclampsia, Pre-eclampsia

ADULTS: 4 g IV initially, followed by 1–2-g/hr infusion or 1–2 g q 2 hr. Supplemental IM doses may also be given.

Dietary Supplement (part of parenteral nutrition)

ADULTS: 8–24 mEq/day.
CHILDREN: 2–10 mEq/day or 0.25–0.5 mEq/kg/day (up to 16 mEq).

Anticonvulsant

ADULTS: 4–5 g.

Dilution

• **Direct IV:** Administer 10% solution **undiluted**. • **Continuous Infusion:** When given as an anticonvulsant, dilute 4 g in 250 ml of D5W or 0.9% NaCl. • When given for hypomagnesemia, may dilute 5 g in 1 liter of D5W, 0.9% NaCl, Ringer's or lactated Ringer's solution.

Compatibility

Syringe: metoclopramide.

• **Y-site:** acyclovir • amikacin • ampicillin • cefamandole • cefazolin • cefoperazone • cefotaxime • cefoxitin • cephalothin • cephapirin • chloramphenicol • clindamycin • dobutamine • doxycycline • enalaprilat • erythromycin lactobionate • esmolol • famotidine • fludarabine • gallium nitrate • gentamicin • heparin • hydrocortisone sodium succinate • idarubicin • insulin • kanamycin • labetalol • meperidine • metronidazole • minocycline • morphine • nafcillin • ondansetron • oxacillin • paclitaxel • penicillin G potassium • piperacillin • piperacillin/tazobactam • potassium chloride

• sargramostim • ticarcillin • tobramycin • trimethoprim/sulfamethoxazole • vancomycin • vitamin B complex with C.

• **Additive:** calcium gluconate • cephalothin • chloramphenicol • cisplatin • hydrocortisone sodium succinate • isoproterenol • methyldopate • norepinephrine • penicillin G potassium • potassium phosphate • verapamil • vitamin B complex with C.

Incompatibility

• **Additive:** amphotericin B • calcium gluceptate • clindamycin • cyclosporine • dobutamine • polymyxin • procaine • sodium bicarbonate • tobramycin.

Rate of Administration

• **Direct IV:** Administer at a rate of 1.5 ml of a 10% solution (or its equivalent) over 1 minute. • **Continuous Infusion:** When given as an anticonvulsant, administer at a rate not to exceed 3 ml/min. • When given for hypomagnesemia, administer slowly over 3 hours. • Use infusion pump to regulate rate accurately.

≋ CLINICAL PRECAUTIONS

- Monitor pulse, blood pressure, respirations, and ECG frequently throughout administration of parenteral magnesium sulfate. Respirations should be at least 16/min prior to each dose.
- Monitor intake and output ratios. Urine output should be maintained at a level of at least 100 ml every 4 hours.
- Monitor neurologic status prior to and throughout course of therapy. Institute seizure precautions. Patellar reflex (knee jerk) should be tested before each parenteral dose of magnesium sulfate. If response is absent, no additional doses should be administered until positive response is obtained.
- Magnesium potentiates neuromuscular blocking agents.
- Use cautiously in patients with renal insufficiency (dosage reduction may be necessary if creatinine clearance is <30 ml/min).
- Geriatric patients are more likely to develop hypomagnesemia, but are also more likely to develop hypermagnesemia following administration of magnesium.
- If mother has received magnesium sulfate for eclamp-

sia, monitor newborn for hypotension, hyporeflexia, and other signs of magnesium toxicity, including neuromuscular and respiratory depression. If possible, magnesium sulfate should not be administered in the 2 hours prior to birth (Pregnancy Category A).

Toxicity and Overdose Alert

• Magnesium toxicity is manifested by a prolonged P-Q and widened QRS interval, loss of deep tendon reflexes, heart block, respiratory paralysis, and cardiac arrest. Treatment includes IV calcium gluconate to antagonize the effects of magnesium.

Lab Test Considerations

• Serum magnesium levels and renal function should be monitored periodically throughout administration of parenteral magnesium sulfate. Normal average serum magnesium levels are 1.5–2.5 mEq/liter.

Patient/Family Teaching

• Explain purpose of therapy to patient.

≋ PHARMACOLOGIC PROFILE

Indications

• Magnesium sulfate is used to replace magnesium in deficiency states. • It is also used in the management of eclampsia and pre-eclampsia, and as an anticonvulsant.

Action

• Magnesium is essential for the activity of many enzymes and plays an important role in neurotransmission and muscular excitability.

Time/Action Profile (anticonvulsant effect)

Onset	Peak	Duration
immediate	UK	30 min

Pharmacokinetics

• **Distribution:** Magnesium is widely distributed. It readily crosses the placenta and is present in breast milk. • **Me-**

tabolism and Excretion: Excretion of magnesium occurs primarily by the kidneys. • **Half-life:** UK.

Contraindications

• Magnesium sulfate should not be given to patients with hypermagnesemia, hypocalcemia, anuria, or heart block, or to patients in active labor.

Adverse Reactions and Side Effects*

• **CNS:** drowsiness • **Resp:** decreased respiratory rate • **CV:** bradycardia, arrhythmias, hypotension • **GI:** diar-rhea • **Derm:** flushing, sweating • **F and E:** hypocalcemia • **Metab:** hypothermia • **Neuro:** decreased deep-tendon reflexes, PARALYSIS.

Mannitol	*Osmotic diuretic*
Osmitrol	pH 4.5–7

≋ ADMINISTRATION CONSIDERATIONS

Usual Dose

Edema, Oliguric Renal Failure
Precede with a test dose of 0.2 g/kg over 3–5 min.
ADULTS: 50–100 g as a 5–25% solution.
CHILDREN: 0.25–2 g/kg (60 mg/m^2) as a 15–20% solution.

Reduction of Intracranial or Intraocular Pressure
ADULTS: 0.25–2 g/kg as 15–25% solution.
CHILDREN: 2 g/kg (30–60 mg/m^2) as a 15–20% solution (500 mg/kg may be sufficient in small or debilitated patients).

Diuresis in Drug Intoxications
ADULTS: 50–200 g as a 5–25% solution titrated to maintain urine flow of 100–500 ml/hr.
CHILDREN: 2 g/kg (60 mg/m^2) as a 5–10% solution.

---

*Underlines indicate most frequent; CAPITALS indicate life-threatening.

Dilution

• **Intermittent Infusion:** Administer by IV infusion **undiluted.** • If solution contains crystals, warm bottle in hot water and shake vigorously. Do not administer solution in which crystals remain undissolved. Cool to body temperature. Use an in-line filter for 15%, 20%, and 25% infusions.

Compatibility

• **Y-site:** allopurinol sodium • fludarabine • fluorouracil • gallium nitrate • idarubicin • melphalan • ondansetron • paclitaxel • piperacillin/tazobactam • sargramostim • vinorelbine.

• **Additive:** amikacin • bretylium • cefamandole • cefoxitin • cimetidine • cisplatin • dopamine • gentamicin • metoclopramide • netilmicin • ofloxacin • ondansetron • tobramycin • verapamil.

Incompatibility

• **Y-site:** filgrastim.
• **Additive:** blood products • imipenem/cilastatin.

Rate of Administration

• **Intermittent Infusion:** *Test Dose:* Administer over 3–5 minutes for adults or children to produce a urine output of 30–50 ml/hr. If urine flow does not increase, administer second test dose. If urine output is not at least 30–50 ml/hr for 2–3 hours after second test dose, patient should be re-evaluated. • *Oliguria:* Administration rate should be titrated to produce a urine output of 30–50 ml/hr for adults. Administer children's dose over 2–6 hours. • *Increased Intracranial Pressure or Intraocular Pressure:* Administer dose over 30–60 minutes in adults or children. • *Diuresis in Drug Intoxication:* Titrate rate to maintain a urine flow of 100–500 ml/hr.

≋ CLINICAL PRECAUTIONS

• Monitor vital signs, urine output, central venous pressure (CVP), and pulmonary artery pressures (PAP) prior to and hourly throughout administration. Assess patient for signs and symptoms of dehydration (decreased skin turgor, fever, dry skin and mucous membranes, thirst) or signs of fluid overload (increased CVP, dyspnea, rales/crackles, edema).

- Observe infusion site frequently for infiltration. Extravasation may cause tissue irritation and necrosis.
- Assess patient for anorexia, muscle weakness, numbness, tingling, paresthesia, confusion, and excessive thirst. Notify physician promptly if these signs of electrolyte imbalance occur.
- In patients receiving mannitol for increased intracranial pressure, monitor neurologic status and intracranial pressure readings.
- In patients receiving mannitol for increased intraocular pressure, monitor for persistent or increased eye pain or decreased visual acuity.
- Do not administer electrolyte-free mannitol solution with blood. If blood must be administered simultaneously with mannitol, add at least 20 mEq NaCl to each liter of mannitol.
- Mannitol enhances lithium excretion and may decrease its effectiveness. Concurrent use with other diuretics potentiates diuresis and lowering of intraocular pressure.
- Safe use during pregnancy or lactation has not been established (Pregnancy Category B).

Lab Test Consideration

- Renal function and serum electrolytes should be monitored routinely throughout course of therapy.

Patient/Family Teaching

- Explain purpose of therapy to patient.

≋ PHARMACOLOGIC PROFILE

Indications

- Mannitol is used as an adjunct in the treatment of acute oliguric renal failure, in the treatment of edema, and to reduce intracranial or intraocular pressure. It is also used to promote the excretion of certain toxic substances.

Action

- Mannitol increases the osmotic pressure of the glomerular filtrate, thereby inhibiting reabsorption of water and electrolytes. By doing so it causes excretion of water, sodium, potassium, chloride, calcium, phosphorus, magnesium, urea, and uric acid.

Time/Action Profile (diuresis)

	Onset	Peak	Duration
diuresis	30–60 min	1 hr	6–8 hr
intraocular pressure	within 15 min	30–60 min	4–8 hr
CSF pressure	within 15 min	UK	3–8 hr

Pharmacokinetics

• **Distribution:** Distribution of mannitol is confined to the extracellular space. It does not usually cross the blood–brain barrier or eye. • **Metabolism and Excretion:** Mannitol is excreted by the kidneys, with minimal metabolism by the liver. • **Half-life:** 100 minutes.

Contraindications

• Mannitol is contraindicated in patients with hypersensitivity to it, and in patients with anuria, dehydration, or active intracranial bleeding.

Adverse Reactions and Side Effects*

• **CNS:** headache, confusion • **EENT:** blurred vision, rhinitis • **CV:** transient volume expansion, tachycardia, chest pain, congestive heart failure, pulmonary edema • **GI:** thirst, nausea, vomiting • **GU:** renal failure, urinary retention • **F and E:** hyponatremia, hypernatremia, hypokalemia, hyperkalemia, dehydration • **Local:** phlebitis at IV site.

Mechlorethamine Hydrochloride	*Antineoplastic (alkylating agent)*
Mustargen, mustine HCl, nitrogen mustard	pH 3–5

≋ ADMINISTRATION CONSIDERATIONS

Usual Dose

ADULTS AND CHILDREN: 400 mcg (0.4 mg)/kg as single dose or 2–4 divided doses over 2 or 4 days repeated q 3–6 wk. If

---

*Underlines indicate most frequent; CAPITALS indicate life-threatening.

patient has had recent chemotherapy or radiation, dose should not exceed 200–300 mcg (0.2–0.3 mg)/kg.

Dilution

• **Direct IV:** Discard vial if droplets of water appear to be present prior to reconstitution. **Dilute** each 10 mg with 10 ml of 0.9% NaCl or sterile water for injection. Do not remove the needle from the vial stopper prior to agitating the solution. Allow the solution to dissolve completely. Reconstituted solution decomposes in 15 minutes. Administer immediately. • Do not use a discolored solution or one that contains precipitates. • Solution should be prepared in a biologic cabinet. Wear gloves, gown, and mask while handling medication. All equipment in contact with this medication must be decontaminated prior to disposal. Soak gloves, IV tubing, and syringes in a solution of 5% sodium thiosulfate and 5% sodium bicarbonate for 45 minutes. Unused portions of the drug must be mixed with equal amounts of this solution. Discard all contaminated equipment in specially designated containers. • If medication comes in contact with skin, flush with a large volume of water for 15 minutes, followed by a 2% sodium thiosulfate solution. If eye contact occurs, flush eye with 0.9% NaCl and notify physician immediately (see Appendix F).

Compatibility

• **Y-site:** filgrastim • fludarabine • melphalan • ondansetron • sargramostim • vinorelbine.

Incompatibility

• **Y-site:** allopurinol sodium.
• **Additive:** methohexital.

Rate of Administration

• **Direct IV:** Withdraw desired amount of drug and administer over 3–5 minutes via Y-tubing or 3-way stopcock into a free-flowing solution of 0.9% NaCl.

≋ CLINICAL PRECAUTIONS

• Monitor blood pressure, pulse, and respiratory rate frequently during administration. In obese or edematous patients, dosage should be based on ideal body weight.
• Assess injection site frequently for redness, irritation, or

inflammation. Mechlorethamine is a vesicant. If extravasation occurs, infusion must be stopped and restarted elsewhere to avoid damage to subcutaneous tissue. Infiltrate affected area promptly with isotonic sodium thiosulfate (mix 4 ml of 10% sodium thiosulfate with 6 ml of sterile water for injection or 1.6 ml of 25% sodium thiosulfate with 8.4 ml of sterile water for injection) or 1% lidocaine and apply ice compresses for 6–12 hours. If administering sodium thiosulfate, which neutralizes mechlorethamine, inject 1–4 ml, 1 ml for each ml extravasated, through existing IV cannula or SC if needle has been removed.

- Monitor intake and output, appetite, and nutritional intake. Nausea and vomiting may occur 1–3 hours after therapy. Vomiting may persist for 8 hours; nausea may last 24 hours. Parenteral antiemetic agents should be administered 30–45 minutes prior to therapy and routinely around the clock for the next 24 hours as indicated. Adjust diet as tolerated to help maintain fluid and electrolyte balance and nutritional status.

- Monitor for bone marrow depression. Assess for fever, chills, sore throat, and signs of infection. Assess for bleeding (bleeding gums, bruising, petechiae; guaiac test stools, urine, and emesis). Avoid giving IM injections and taking rectal temperatures. Apply pressure to venipuncture sites for 10 minutes. Anemia may occur. Monitor for increased fatigue and dyspnea. Mechlorethamine may cause additive myelosuppression with other antineoplastic agents or radiation therapy. It may also decrease the antibody response to live virus vaccines and increase the risk of adverse reactions.

- Monitor for symptoms of gout (increased uric acid, joint pain, edema). Encourage patient to drink at least 2 liters of fluid each day. Allopurinol may be given to decrease uric acid levels. Alkalinization of urine may be ordered to increase excretion of uric acid.

- Mechlorethamine should be used cautiously in patients with infections, decreased bone marrow reserve, or other chronic debilitating illnesses. Patients who have received prior radiotherapy require dosage reduction.

- Use with caution in patients with childbearing potential. Mechlorethamine should be avoided during pregnancy or lactation (Pregnancy Category D).

Lab Test Considerations

• Monitor CBC and differential prior to and periodically throughout therapy. The nadir of leukopenia occurs in 7–14 days. Notify physician if leukocyte count is less than 1000/mm³. The nadir of thrombocytopenia occurs in 9–16 days. Notify physician if platelet count is less than 75,000/mm³. Recovery of leukopenia and thrombocytopenia occurs in 20 days. • Monitor liver function studies (AST [SGOT], ALT [SGPT], LDH, bilirubin) and renal function studies (BUN, creatinine) prior to and periodically throughout therapy to detect hepatotoxicity and nephrotoxicity. • May cause increased uric acid levels.

Patient/Family Teaching

• Advise patient to notify physician in case of fever, chills, sore throat, signs of infection, bleeding gums, bruising, petechiae, or blood in urine, stool, or emesis. Caution patient to avoid crowds and persons with known infections. Instruct patient to use soft toothbrush and electric razor. Caution patient not to drink alcoholic beverages or take products containing aspirin, ibuprofen, or naproxen. • Patients with childbearing potential should use a nonhormonal method of birth control during and for at least 4 months after therapy. • Discuss with patient the possibility of hair loss. Explore methods of coping. • Instruct patient not to receive any vaccinations without advice of physician. • Instruct patient to notify physician if skin rash occurs. Rash may occur spontaneously or may be a reactivation of herpes zoster.

≋ PHARMACOLOGIC PROFILE

Indications

• Mechlorethamine is used as part of combination therapy of Hodgkin's disease and malignant lymphomas. It is also used palliatively in bronchogenic carcinoma, breast carcinoma, ovarian carcinoma, and leukemias.

Action

• Mechlorethamine interferes with DNA and RNA synthesis by cross-linking strands (cell cycle–phase nonspecific). This results in death of rapidly replicating cells, particularly malignant ones.

Time/Action Profile (effects on blood counts)

	Onset	Peak	Duration
WBCs	24 hr	7–14 days	10–21 days
platelets	UK	9–16 days	20 days

Pharmacokinetics

• **Distribution:** UK. • **Metabolism and Excretion:** Mechlorethamine is rapidly degraded in body tissues and fluids. • **Half-life:** UK.

Contraindications

• Mechlorethamine is contraindicated in patients who have hypersensitivity to it. Pregnant or lactating patients should not receive mechlorethamine.

Adverse Reactions and Side Effects*

• **CNS:** weakness, headache, drowsiness, vertigo, SEIZURES • **GI:** nausea, vomiting, diarrhea, anorexia • **GU:** gonadal suppression • **Hemat:** anemia, leukopenia, thrombocytopenia • **Derm:** rashes, alopecia • **Local:** phlebitis, tissue necrosis • **Metab:** hyperuricemia • **Misc:** reactivation of herpes zoster.

Melphalan	Antineoplastic agent (alkylating agent)
Alkeran, L-PAM, L-Sarcolysin, Phenylalanine mustard	pH UK

ADMINISTRATION CONSIDERATIONS

Usual Dose

ADULTS: 16 mg/m^2 q 2 wk for 4 doses, then q 4 wk.

Dilution

• **Intermittent Infusion: Reconstitute** with 10 ml of diluent supplied by manufacturer for a concentration of 5 mg/ml and shake vigorously until solution is clear. **Dilute** dose im-

---

*Underlines indicate most frequent; CAPITALS indicate life-threatening.

mediately with 0.9% NaCl for a concentration not to exceed 0.45 mg/ml. • Administer within 60 minutes of reconstitution. • Solution should be prepared in a biologic cabinet. Wear gloves, gown, and mask while handling medication. Discard IV equipment in specially designated container (see Appendix F). If solution contacts skin or mucosa, immediately wash skin or mucosa with soap and water.

Compatibility

• **Y-site:** acyclovir • amikacin • aminophylline • ampicillin • aztreonam • bleomycin • bumetanide • buprenorphine • butorphanol • calcium gluconate • carboplatin • carmustine • cefazolin • cefoperazone • cefotaxime • cefotetan • ceftazidime • ceftizoxime • ceftriaxone • cefuroxime • cimetidine • cisplatin • clindamycin • cyclophosphamide • cytarabine • dacarbazine • dactinomycin • daunorubicin • dexamethasone • diphenhydramine • doxorubicin • doxycycline • droperidol • enalaprilat • etoposide • famotidine • floxuridine • fluconazole • fludarabine • fluorouracil • furosemide • gallium nitrate • ganciclovir • gentamicin • haloperidol • heparin • hydrocortisone • hydromorphone • hydroxyzine • idarubicin • ifosfamide • imipenem/cilastatin • lorazepam • mannitol • mechlorethamine • meperidine • mesna • methotrexate • methylprednisolone • metoclopramide • metronidazole • minocycline • mitomycin • mitoxantrone • morphine • nalbuphine • netilmicin • ondansetron • pentostatin • piperacillin • plicamycin • potassium chloride • prochlorperazine • promethazine • ranitidine • sodium bicarbonate • streptozocin • thiotepa • ticarcillin • ticarcillin/clavulanate • tobramycin • trimethoprim/sulfamethoxazole • vancomycin • vinblastine • vincristine • vinorelbine • zidovudine.

Incompatibility

• **Y-site:** amphotericin B • chlorpromazine.
• **Intermittent Infusion:** Administer over 15–20 minutes.

≋ CLINICAL PRECAUTIONS

• Assess patient for allergy to chlorambucil. Patients may have cross-sensitivity.
• Melphalan may cause nausea and vomiting. Monitor in-

take and output, appetite, and nutritional intake. Antiemetics may be used prophylactically. Adjust diet as tolerated.

• Monitor for symptoms of gout (increased uric acid, joint pain, edema). Encourage patient to drink at least 2 liters of fluid per day. Allopurinol may be given to decrease uric acid levels.

• Monitor for bone marrow depression. Assess for fever, sore throat, and signs of infection. Assess for bleeding (bleeding gums; bruising; petechiae; guaiac stools, urine, and emesis). Avoid IM injections and rectal temperatures. Apply pressure to venipuncture sites for 10 minutes. Anemia may occur. Monitor for increased fatigue and dyspnea. Concurrent use of other antineoplastic agents or radiation therapy increases the risk of bone marrow depression.

• The risk of pulmonary toxicity is increased with concurrent use of carmustine. Concurrent IV use with cyclosporine may increase the risk of renal failure.

• Melphalan should be used with caution in patients with active infections, decreased bone marrow reserve, other chronic debilitating illnesses, impaired renal function (dose reduction recommended if BUN >30 mg/dl), or geriatric patients.

• Use cautiously in patients with childbearing potential. Avoid using melphalan during pregnancy or lactation (Pregnancy Category D). Safe use in children has not been established.

Lab Test Considerations

• Monitor CBC and differential weekly throughout therapy. The nadir of leukopenia and thrombocytopenia occur in 2–3 weeks. If leukocyte count is <3000/mm^3 or platelet count is <100,000/mm^3, melphalan therapy may need to be discontinued. Therapy may be resumed at a lower dose when counts return to normal. Recovery of leukopenia and thrombocytopenia occurs in 5–6 weeks. Monitor patients with leukopenia and neutropenia closely for infection; antibiotic support may be required. Geriatric patients may not develop fever when infection is present. • Monitor liver function studies (AST [SGOT], ALT [SGPT], LDH, bilirubin) and renal function studies (BUN, creatinine) prior to and periodically throughout therapy to detect hepatotoxicity and nephrotoxicity. • Melphalan may cause increased uric acid. Monitor periodically during therapy. • Elevated 5-hydroxyindoleacetic acid (5-HIAA) concentrations may occur as a result of tumor breakdown.

Patient/Family Teaching

• Advise patient to notify physician if fever, chills, dyspnea, persistent cough, sore throat, signs of infection, bleeding gums, bruising, petechiae, or blood in urine, stool, or emesis occurs. Caution patient to avoid crowds and persons with known infections. Instruct patient to use soft toothbrush and electric razor. Caution patient not to drink alcoholic beverages or take products containing aspirin, ibuprofen, or naproxen. • Instruct patient to notify physician if rash, itching, joint pain, or swelling occurs. • Instruct patient to inspect oral mucosa for redness and ulceration. If ulceration occurs, advise patient to use sponge brush and to rinse mouth with water after eating and drinking. Consult physician if pain interferes with eating. • Advise patient that although fertility may be decreased, contraception should be used during melphalan therapy because of potential teratogenic effects on the fetus. • Instruct patient not to receive any vaccinations without advise of physician. Melphalan may decrease antibody response to live virus vaccines and increase the risk of adverse reactions. • Emphasize need for periodic lab tests to monitor for side effects.

☰ PHARMACOLOGIC PROFILE

Indications

• Melphalan is used alone or with other treatment modalities in the management of ovarian cancer. • **Unlabeled Uses:** breast cancer, prostate cancer, testicular carcinoma, chronic myelogenous leukemia, and osteogenic sarcoma.

Action

• Melphalan inhibits DNA and RNA synthesis by alkylation (cell cycle–phase nonspecific), causing death of rapidly replicating cells, particularly malignant ones. Melphalan also has immunosuppressive properties.

Time/Action Profile (effect on blood counts)

Onset	Peak	Duration
5 days	2–3 wk	5–6 wk

Pharmacokinetics

• **Distribution:** Melphalan is rapidly distributed throughout total body water. • **Metabolism and Excretion:** Melphalan is rapidly metabolized in the bloodstream. Small amounts (10%) are excreted unchanged by the kidneys. • **Half-life:** 1.5 hours.

Contraindications

• Melphalan should not be used in patients with hypersensitivity to it or to chlorambucil. Diluent for injection contains alcohol; avoid using in patients with known alcohol intolerance. Pregnant or lactating patients should not receive melphalan.

Adverse Reactions and Side Effects*

• **Resp:** PULMONARY FIBROSIS, bronchopulmonary dysplasia • **GI:** nausea, vomiting, stomatitis, diarrhea • **GU:** gonadal suppression • **Derm:** rashes, pruritus, alopecia • **Endo:** menstrual irregularities • **Hemat:** leukopenia, thrombocytopenia, anemia • **Metab:** hyperuricemia • **Misc:** allergic reactions, including ANAPHYLAXIS.

Meperidine Hydrochloride	*Opioid analgesic (agonist)*
Demerol Hydrochloride, pethidine	pH 3.5–6

Schedule II

☰ ADMINISTRATION CONSIDERATIONS

Usual Dose

ADULTS: 100 mg q 3 hr as a constant infusion of 15–35 mg/hr or 0.3 mg/kg/hr.

---

*Underlines indicate most frequent; CAPITALS indicate life-threatening.

CHILDREN: 0.75 mg/kg q 2–3 hr *or* as a constant infusion of 0.35 mg/kg/hr (may be preceded by a loading dose of 1 mg/kg). *Preoperative sedation*—0.25–1 mg/kg.

Dilution

• **Direct IV:** Dilute for IV administraion to a concentration of 10 mg/ml with sterile water or 0.9% NaCl for injection. • **Continuous Infusion:** Dilute to a concentration of 1 mg/ml with D5W, D10W, dextrose/saline combinations, dextrose/Ringer's or lactated Ringer's injection combinations, 0.45% NaCl, 0.9% NaCl, Ringer's or lactated Ringer's solution.

Compatibility

• **Syringe:** atropine ◆ benzquinamide ◆ chlorpromazine ◆ cimetidine ◆ dimenhydrinate ◆ diphenhydramine ◆ droperidol ◆ fentanyl ◆ glycopyrrolate ◆ hydroxyzine ◆ metoclopramide ◆ midazolam ◆ perphenazine ◆ prochorperazine ◆ promazine ◆ promethazine ◆ ranitidine ◆ scopolamine.

• **Y-site:** amikacin ◆ ampicillin ◆ ampicillin/sulbactam ◆ aztreonam ◆ bumetanide ◆ cefamandole ◆ cefazolin ◆ cefotaxime ◆ cefotetan ◆ cefoxitin ◆ ceftizoxime ◆ ceftriaxone ◆ cefuroxime ◆ cephalothin ◆ cephapirin ◆ chloramphenicol ◆ clindamycin ◆ dexamethasone ◆ diltiazem ◆ diphenhydramine ◆ dobutamine ◆ dopamine ◆ doxycycline ◆ droperidol ◆ erythromycin lactobionate ◆ famotidine ◆ filgrastim ◆ fluconazole ◆ fludarabine ◆ gallium nitrate ◆ gentamicin ◆ heparin ◆ hydrocortisone sodium succinate ◆ insulin ◆ kanamycin ◆ labetalol ◆ lidocaine ◆ magnesium sulfate ◆ melphalan ◆ methyldopa ◆ methylprednisolone ◆ metoclopramide ◆ metoprolol ◆ metronidazole ◆ ondansetron ◆ oxacillin ◆ oxytocin ◆ paclitaxel ◆ penicillin G potassium ◆ piperacillin ◆ piperacillin/tazobactam ◆ potassium chloride ◆ propranolol ◆ ranitidine ◆ sargramostim ◆ ticarcillin ◆ ticarcillin/clavulanate ◆ tobramycin ◆ trimethoprim/sulfamethoxazole ◆ vancomycin ◆ verapamil ◆ vinorelbine.

• **Additive:** dobutamine ◆ scopolamine ◆ succinylcholine ◆ verapamil.

Incompatibility

• **Syringe:** heparin ◆ morphine ◆ pentobarbital.

• **Y-site:** allopurinol sodium ◆ cefoperazone ◆ idarubicin ◆ imipenem/cilastatin ◆ mezlocillin ◆ minocycline.

- **Additive:** aminophylline ✦ amobarbital ✦ furosemide ✦ heparin ✦ methicillin ✦ morphine ✦ phenobarbital ✦ phenytoin ✦ thiopental.

Rate of Administration

- **Direct IV:** Administer slowly. Rapid administration may lead to increased respiratory depression, hypotension, and circulatory collapse. • **Continuous Infusion:** Administer via infusion pump. Titrate according to patient needs.

≋ CLINICAL PRECAUTIONS

- Assess type, location, and intensity of pain prior to and 5–10 minutes (peak) following administration. When titrating opioid doses, increases of 25–50% should be administered until there is either a 50% reduction in the patient's pain rating on a numerical or visual analog scale or the patient reports satisfactory pain relief. Subsequent doses can be safely administered at the time of the peak if the previous dose is ineffective and side effects are minimal. Regularly administered doses may be more effective than p.r.n. administration. Analgesic is more effective if given before pain becomes severe. Coadministration with nonopioid analgesics may have additive analgesic effects and permit lower opioid doses.
- An equianalgesic chart (Appendix B, page 1045) should be used when changing routes or when changing from one opioid to another.
- Assess blood pressure, pulse, and respiratory rate before and periodically during administration. If respiratory rate is less than 10/min, assess level of sedation. Physical stimulation may be sufficient to prevent significant hypoventilation. Dose may need to be decreased by 25–50%.
- Chronic (more than 2 days) or high-dose therapy (more than 600 mg/day) should be undertaken with caution due to accumulation of the metabolite normeperidine. Monitor patient for CNS stimulatory effects (restlessness, irritability, seizures). Patients who are on large doses of meperidine or patients with hepatic and/or renal impair-

ment, patients with extensive burns, metastatic cancer, or sickle-cell disease are at greatest risk. Geriatric patients are also at risk for adverse CNS reactions and should not receive more than 1–2 doses for the management of acute pain.

- Assess bowel function routinely. Prevention of constipation should be instituted with increased intake of fluids and bulk, stool softeners, and laxatives to minimize constipating effects. Stimulant laxatives should be administered routinely if opioid use exceeds 2–3 days, unless contraindicated.

- Prolonged use may lead to physical and psychological dependence and tolerance. This should not prevent patient from receiving adequate analgesia. Most patients who receive meperidine for medical reasons do not develop psychological dependence. Progressively higher doses may be required to relieve pain with long-term therapy. Meperidine should be discontinued gradually after long-term use to prevent withdrawal symptoms.

- Assess level of sedation. Initial drowsiness will diminish with continued use. Additive CNS depression occurs with concurrent use of alcohol, antihistamines, and sedatives/hypnotics.

- Use with extreme caution in patients receiving MAO inhibitors or procarbazine. Combined use may result in unpredictable fatal reaction. Avoid concurrent use with amphetamines.

- Meperidine should be used cautiously in patients with head trauma; increased intracranial pressure; severe renal, hepatic, or pulmonary disease; hypothyroidism; adrenal insufficiency; alcoholism; undiagnosed abdominal pain; or prostatic hypertrophy. Elderly or debilitated patients should receive lower initial doses.

- Administration of partial-antagonist opioid analgesics may precipitate opioid withdrawal in physically dependent patients.

- Nalbuphine or pentazocine may decrease analgesia.

- Safe use during pregnancy has not been established (Pregnancy Category C). Although meperidine has been used during labor, respiratory depression may occur in the newborn.

Toxicity and Overdose Alert

• If an opioid antagonist is required to reverse respiratory depression or coma, naloxone (Narcan) is the antidote. Dilute the 0.4-mg ampule of naloxone in 10 ml of 0.9% NaCl and administer 0.5 ml (0.02 mg) by direct IV push every 2 minutes. For children and patients weighing <40 kg, dilute 0.1 mg of naloxone in 10 ml of 0.9% NaCl for a concentration of 10 mcg/ml and administer 0.5 mcg every 1–2 minutes. Titrate the dose to avoid withdrawal, seizures, and severe pain. In patients receiving meperidine chronically, naloxone may precipitate seizures by eliminating the effects of meperidine, allowing the convulsant activity of normeperidine to predominate. Monitor patient closely; dose may need to be repeated or naloxone infusion administered.

Lab Test Considerations

• Meperidine may increase plasma amylase and lipase concentrations.

Patient/Family Teaching

• Instruct patient on how and when to ask for pain medication. • Meperidine may cause drowsiness or dizziness. Advise patient to call for assistance when ambulating or smoking and to avoid activities requiring alertness until response to medication is known. • Advise patient to make position changes slowly to minimize orthostatic hypotension. • Instruct patient to avoid concurrent use of alcohol or other CNS depressants. • Encourage patient to turn, cough, and breathe deeply every 2 hours to prevent atelectasis.

 PHARMACOLOGIC PROFILE

Indications

• Meperidine is used alone and in combination with non-opioid analgesics in the management of moderate to severe pain. It is also used as an adjunct to anesthesia.

Action

• Meperidine binds to opiate receptors in the CNS, altering the perception of and response to painful stimuli, while producing generalized CNS depression.

Time/Action Profile (analgesia)

Onset	Peak	Duration
immediate	5–7 min	2–4 hr

Pharmacokinetics

• **Distribution:** Meperidine is widely distributed. It rapidly crosses the placenta and enters breast milk. • **Metabolism and Excretion:** Most metabolism of meperidine occurs in the liver. Some is converted to normeperidine, which has a long half-life (15–20 hours), and CNS stimulatory effects. Five percent is excreted unchanged by the kidneys. • **Half-life:** 3–8 hours (prolonged in impaired renal or hepatic function).

Contraindications

• Meperidine use is contraindicated in patients with hypersensitivity to it. Meperidine is also contraindicated within 14–21 days of MAO inhibitor therapy. Chronic use of meperidine should be avoided during pregnancy or lactation.

Adverse Reactions and Side Effects*

• **CNS:** <u>sedation</u>, <u>confusion</u>, headache, euphoria, floating feeling, unusual dreams, hallucinations, dysphoria • **EENT:** miosis, diplopia, blurred vision • **CV:** <u>hypotension</u>, bradycardia • **GI:** <u>nausea</u>, <u>vomiting</u>, <u>constipation</u> • **GU:** urinary retention • **Derm:** sweating, flushing • **Resp:** respiratory depression • **Misc:** tolerance, physical dependence, psychological dependence.

---

*<u>Underlines</u> indicate most frequent; CAPITALS indicate life-threatening.

Mesna	*Antidote for ifosfamide*
Mesnex, {Uromitexan}	pH 6.5–8.5

≋ ADMINISTRATION CONSIDERATIONS

Usual Dose
ADULTS: Give a dose of mesna equal to 20% of the ifosfamide dose at the same time as ifosfamide and 4 and 8 hr later. This regimen should follow each dose of ifosfamide.

Dilution
• **Direct IV:** Available in 2-, 4-, and 10-ml ampules, each containing a concentration of 100 mg/ml. **Dilute** in 8 ml, 16 ml, or 50 ml, respectively, of D5W, 0.9% NaCl, D5/0.9% NaCl, or lactated Ringer's solution, to yield a final concentration of 20 mg/ml. • Solution is clear and colorless. Must be stored under refrigeration. Use within 6 hours.

Compatibility
• **Syringe:** ifosfamide.
• **Y-site:** allopurinol sodium ✦ filgrastim ✦ fludarabine ✦ gallium nitrate ✦ melphalan ✦ ondansetron ✦ paclitaxel ✦ piperacillin/tazobactam ✦ sargramostim ✦ vinorelbine.
• **Additive:** cyclophosphamide ✦ hydroxyzine ✦ ifosfamide.

Incompatibility
• **Additive:** carboplatin ✦ cisplatin.

Rate of Administration
• **Direct IV:** Administer via rapid IV injection.

≋ CLINICAL PRECAUTIONS
• Monitor for the development of hemorrhagic cystitis in patients receiving ifosfamide.
• If dosage alterations are made for ifosfamide, similar alterations should be made for mesna.

{} = Available in Canada only.

- Safe use in pregnancy, lactation, or children has not been established (Pregnancy Category B).

Lab Test Considerations

  - Examination of the urine for microscopic hematuria is recommended prior to each dose of ifosfamide or cyclophosphamide and mesna. • Mesna causes a false-positive result when testing urinary ketones.

Patient/Family Teaching

  - Inform patient that unpleasant taste may occur during administration. • Advise patient to notify physician if nausea, vomiting, or diarrhea persists or is severe.

 PHARMACOLOGIC PROFILE

Indications

  - Mesna is used in the prevention of ifosfamide-induced hemorrhagic cystitis. • **Unlabeled Use:** Prevention of cyclophosphamide-induced hemorrhagic cystitis.

Action

  - Mesna binds to toxic metabolites of ifosfamide in the kidneys, thereby preventing hemorrhagic cystitis.

Time/Action Profile (protective effect)

Onset	Peak	Duration
rapid	UK	4 hr

Pharmacokinetics

  - **Distribution:** UK. • **Metabolism and Excretion:** Mesna is rapidly converted to mesna disulfide, then converted back to mesna in the kidneys, where it is able to bind to the toxic metabolites of ifosfamide. • **Half-life:** Mesna 0.36 hours; mesna disulfide 1.17 hours.

Contraindications

  - Mesna is contraindicated in patients with hypersensitivity to it or other thiol (rubber) compounds.

Adverse Reactions and Side Effects*

- **GI:** nausea, vomiting, diarrhea, unpleasant taste.

Metaraminol Bitartrate	*Vasopressor*
Aramine	pH 3.2–4.5

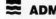 **ADMINISTRATION CONSIDERATIONS**

Usual Dose

Acute Treatment of Hypotension

ADULTS: 15–100 mg in 500 ml of solution infused at rate necessary to maintain desired blood pressure.

CHILDREN: 400 mcg (0.4 mg)/kg or 12 mg/m² infused at a rate necessary to maintain desired blood pressure.

Treatment of Severe Shock

ADULTS: 500 mcg (0.5 mg)–5 mg followed by IV infusion at rate necessary to maintain blood pressure.

CHILDREN: 10 mcg (0.01 mg)/kg *or* 300 mcg (0.3 mg)/m² followed by IV infusion at rate necessary to maintain blood pressure.

Dilution

- **Direct IV:** Direct IV injections may be administered **undiluted** and should be followed by a continuous infusion.
- **Continuous Infusion:** For adults, **dilute** 15–500 mg in 500 ml of 0.9% NaCl, D5W, D10W, D20W, D5/LR, D5/0.9% NaCl, or Ringer's solution. **Dilution** for pediatric patients may contain 1 mg/25 ml. • Solution is stable for 24 hours.

Compatibility

- **Y-site:** amrinone.
- **Additive:** amikacin • cephalothin • cephapirin • chloramphenicol • cimetidine • cyanocobalamin • dobutamine • ephedrine • epinephrine • hydrocortisone sodium phosphate • lidocaine • oxytocin • potassium chloride • promazine • sodium bicarbonate • verapamil.

---

*Underlines indicate most frequent; CAPITALS indicate life-threatening.

Incompatibility

- **Additive:** amphotericin B • barbiturates • dexamethasone • erythromycin lactobionate • fibrinogen • methicillin
• methylprednisolone • penicillin G potassium • phenytoin
• prednisolone sodium phosphate • ranitidine • thiopental.

Rate of Administration

- **Direct IV:** In severe shock, metaraminol may be administered via direct IV slowly, each 0.5 mg over at least 1 minute. • **Continuous Infusion:** Titrate rate of administration
to maintain the desired blood pressure. Infusion should be
administered via infusion pump to ensure precise amount
delivered.

≋ CLINICAL PRECAUTIONS

- Monitor blood pressure, pulse, respiration, ECG, and
  hemodynamic parameters every 5–15 minutes during
  and after administration until stable for at least 1 hour.
  Follow parameters (pulse, blood pressure, or ECG
  changes) for adjusting dosage or discontinuing medication. Monitor urinary output hourly; may decrease initially and then increase as blood pressure normalizes.
  Hypovolemia and electrolyte imbalances should be corrected prior to administration of metaraminol. Concurrent acidosis may decrease effectiveness.
- Allow at least 10 minutes before increasing the dose by
  any route, since the maximum effect is not immediately
  evident.
- Assess IV administration site frequently. Extravasation
  may cause necrosis and sloughing of tissue. If extravasation occurs, discontinue metaraminol and infiltrate affected area with 10–15 ml of 0.9% NaCl containing 5–
  10 mg of phentolamine. Infiltration within 12 hours of
  extravasation produces the most noticeable results.
- Administer metaraminol via a large vein; avoid veins in
  the ankle or dorsum of hand.
- Discontinue metaraminol gradually to prevent recurrent
  hypotension. Monitor patient closely following discontinuation, in the event that further metaraminol therapy
  is necessary. Therapy should be reinstated if systolic
  blood pressure falls below 70–80 mm Hg.

- Use cautiously in patients with hyperthyroidism, hypertension, heart disease, diabetes mellitus, severe liver disease, peripheral vascular disease, or history of malaria.
- Pressor effect may be partially antagonized by alpha-adrenergic blocking agents (labetalol, phenoxybenzamine, phentolamine, prazosin, or tolazoline) or agents with alpha-adrenergic blocking properties (haloperidol, loxapine, phenothiazines, thioxanthenes). Concurrent use with beta blockers may result in adverse cardiovascular effects (bradycardia, excessive hypertension). Use with cyclopropane or other halogenated hydrocarbon anesthetics, tricyclic antidepressants, maprotiline, or cardiac glycosides increases the risk of arrhythmias. Risk of hypertension and cardiac arrhythmias is increased with concurrent use of guanethidine, guanadrel, and MAO inhibitors. Pressor response may be enhanced by atropine. Diuretics may decrease arterial responsiveness to metaraminol. Additive vasoconstriction may occur with concurrent use of ergotamine, ergonovine, methylergonovine, methysergide, or oxytocin.
- Safe use in pregnancy or lactation has not been established (Pregnancy Category C).

Toxicity and Overdose Alert

- Symptoms of overdose include convulsions, severe hypertension, and arrhythmias. For excessive hypertension, rate of infusion should be decreased or temporarily discontinued until blood pressure is decreased. Although additional measures are usually not necessary because of the short duration of metaraminol, phentolamine may be administered IV if hypertension continues.

Patient/Family Teaching

- Instruct patient to inform nurse immediately of pain or discomfort at site of administration or if coldness of extremities or paresthesia occurs.

≋ PHARMACOLOGIC PROFILE
Indications
- Metaraminol is used in the management of hypotension and circulatory shock unresponsive to fluid volume replace-

ment, which may occur as a consequence of hemorrhage, drug reactions, or anesthesia.

Action

• Metaraminol stimulates alpha- and beta-adrenergic receptors, producing vasoconstriction and cardiac stimulation (inotropic effect). It releases norepinephrine from storage sites; prolonged use may lead to depletion and tachyphylaxis (tolerance developing over a short period of time).

Time/Action Profile (pressor response)

Onset	Peak	Duration
1–2 min	UK	20 min

Pharmacokinetics

• **Distribution:** Metaraminol does not cross the blood–brain barrier; remainder of distribution is not known. • **Metabolism and Excretion:** Metabolism of metaraminol occurs by tissue uptake. • **Half-life:** UK.

Contraindications

• Metaraminol is contraindicated in patients with hypersensitivity to it or to bisulfites. Use of metaraminol should be avoided in patients with peripheral or mesenteric vascular thrombosis, hypoxia, or hypercapnia and in patients undergoing cyclopropane or halogenated hydrocarbon anesthesia.

Adverse Reactions and Side Effects*

• **CNS:** apprehension, anxiety, restlessness, dizziness, faintness, headache, nervousness • **Resp:** respiratory distress • **CV:** arrhythmias, bradycardia, peripheral and visceral vasoconstriction, precordial pain • **Derm:** flushing, pallor, sweating • **GI:** nausea • **GU:** decreased urine output • **Local:** irritation, sloughing, tissue necrosis at IV site • **Misc:** tachyphylaxis.

---

*Underlines indicate most frequent; CAPITALS indicate life-threatening.

Methicillin	*Anti-infective*
Sodium	*(penicillinase-resistant penicillin)*
Staphcillin	**pH 6–8.5**
	2.6–3.1 mEq Na/g

 ADMINISTRATION CONSIDERATIONS

Usual Dose

ADULTS AND CHILDREN >**40 kg:** 1–2 g q 4 hr (up to 24 g/day).

CHILDREN <**40 kg:** 16.7–33.3 mg/kg q 4 hr or 25–50 mg/kg q 6 hr (up to 300 mg/kg/day in divided doses).

Meningitis

NEONATES ≥**2 kg:** 50 mg/kg q 8 hr during first 7 days of life, then 50 mg/kg q 6 hr.

NEONATES <**2 kg:** 25–50 mg/kg q 12 hr during first 7 days of life, then 50 mg/kg q 8 hr.

Dilution

• To **reconstitute,** add 1.5 ml of sterile water or 0.9% NaCl for injection to each 1-g vial, 5.7 ml to each 4-g vial, and 8.6 ml to each 6-g vial for a concentration of 500 mg/ml. • Solution is straw-colored. • **Direct IV:** Each ml (500 mg) of reconstituted solution should be **further diluted** in 25 ml of 0.9% NaCl for injection. • **Intermittent Infusion: Dilute** in 0.9% NaCl, D5W, D10W, D5/0.9% NaCl, D5/LR, Ringer's or lactated Ringer's solution for a concentration of 2–20 mg/ml. • Diluted concentrations of 2–20 mg/ml are stable for 8 hours at room temperature.

Compatibility

• **Syringe:** chloramphenicol ✦ colistimethate ✦ erythromycin lactobionate ✦ gentamicin ✦ lidocaine ✦ polymyxin B ✦ procaine.

• **Y-site:** heparin ✦ hydrocortisone sodium succinate ✦ potassium chloride ✦ verapamil ✦ vitamin B complex with C. • If aminoglycosides and penicillins or cephalosporins must be given concurrently, administer in separate sites.

• **Additive:** aminophylline ✦ ascorbic acid ✦ calcium chloride ✦ calcium gluconate ✦ cephalothin ✦ chloramphenicol ✦ colistimethate ✦ corticotropin ✦ dimenhydrinate ✦ diphenhydramine ✦ erythromycin ✦ gentamicin ✦ penicillin G

• polymyxin B • potassium chloride • prednisolone • procaine • verapamil.

Incompatibility

• **Syringe:** heparin • kanamycin.

• **Additive:** amikacin • chlorpromazine • codeine • levorphanol • meperidine • metaraminol • methadone • methohexital • morphine • promethazine • vancomycin. Manufacturer recommends that methicillin not be admixed with other drugs.

Rate of Administration

• **Direct IV:** Administer at a rate of 10 ml over 1 minute.
• **Intermittent Infusion:** Infuse over 20–30 minutes. May be infused up to 8 hours.

≋ CLINICAL PRECAUTIONS

- Assess patient for infection (vital signs; appearance of wound, sputum, urine, and stool; WBC) at beginning and throughout course of therapy.
- Obtain a history before initiating therapy to determine previous use of and reactions to penicillins or cephalosporins. Persons with a negative history of penicillin sensitivity may still have an allergic response. Observe patient for signs and symptoms of anaphylaxis (rash, pruritus, laryngeal edema, wheezing). Discontinue the drug immediately if these occur. Keep epinephrine, an antihistamine, and resuscitation equipment close by in the event of an anaphylactic reaction.
- Obtain specimens for culture and sensitivity prior to initiating therapy. First dose may be given before receiving results.
- Assess vein for signs of irritation and phlebitis. Change IV site every 48 hours to prevent phlebitis.
- Use methicillin cautiously in patients with severe renal impairment. Dosage reduction or increased dosing interval is recommended if creatinine clearance is <10 ml/min. Patients with a history of previous hypersensitivity reactions should be given methicillin cautiously.
- Probenecid decreases renal excretion and increases blood levels of methicillin. Methicillin may alter the effect of oral anticoagulants.

- Safe use in pregnancy or lactation has not been established (Pregnancy Category B).

Lab Test Considerations

- Renal function tests should be monitored periodically during prolonged therapy. • Methicillin may cause positive direct Coombs' test.

Patient/Family Teaching

- Advise patient to report signs of superinfection (black, furry overgrowth on the tongue, vaginal itching or discharge, loose or foul-smelling stools) and allergy promptly.
- Instruct patient to notify physician if fever and diarrhea develop, especially if stool contains blood, pus, or mucus. Advise patient not to treat diarrhea without consulting physician or pharmacist.

PHARMACOLOGIC PROFILE

Indications

- Methicillin is used in the treatment of the following infections due to susceptible strains of penicillinase-producing staphylococci: respiratory tract infections, skin and skin structure infections, bone and joint infections, urinary tract infections, endocarditis, septicemia, and meningitis.

Action

- Methicillin binds to the bacterial cell wall, leading to cell death. It resists the action of penicillinase, an enzyme capable of inactivating penicillin, resulting in bactericidal action against susceptible bacteria. Its spectrum includes activity against most Gram-positive aerobic cocci, but less so than that of penicillin. Spectrum is notable for activity against penicillinase-producing strains of *Staphylococcus aureus* and *S. epidermidis*.

Time/Action Profile (blood levels)

Onset	Peak
rapid	end of infusion

Pharmacokinetics

• **Distribution:** Methicillin is widely distributed. Penetration into CSF is minimal but sufficient in the presence of inflamed meninges. It crosses the placenta and enters breast milk. • **Metabolism and Excretion:** Methicillin is excreted unchanged by the kidneys. • **Half-life:** 20–30 minutes (increased in renal impairment).

Contraindications

• Methicillin is contraindicated in patients with hypersensitivity to penicillins. Cross-sensitivity with cephalosporins may occur.

Adverse Reactions and Side Effects*

• **CNS:** SEIZURES (high doses) • **Derm:** <u>rashes</u>, urticaria • **GI:** <u>nausea</u>, <u>vomiting</u>, <u>diarrhea</u>, hepatitis • **GU:** interstitial nephritis • **Hemat:** blood dyscrasias • **Local:** phlebitis at IV site • **Misc:** superinfection, <u>allergic reactions</u>, including ANAPHYLAXIS and serum sickness.

Methocarbamol	Skeletal muscle relaxant (centrally acting)
Carbacot, Robaxin Injection, Skelax	pH 4–5

ADMINISTRATION CONSIDERATIONS

Usual Dose

Muscle Spasm

ADULTS: 1 g. If oral route of administration does not become feasible, up to 1 g q 8 hr for up to 3 days can be given. May be repeated after a 48-hr rest period.

Tetanus

ADULTS: 1–2 g; additional 1–2 g may be given (total initial dose not to exceed 3 g); repeat 1–2 g q 6 hr until nasogastric tube is inserted, then change to oral.
CHILDREN: 15 mg/kg; may be repeated q 6 hr.

---

*<u>Underlines</u> indicate most frequent; CAPITALS indicate life-threatening.

Dilution

• **Direct IV:** May be administered **undiluted**. • **Intermittent Infusion: Dilute** each dose in no more than 250 ml of 0.9% NaCl or D5W for injection. • Do not refrigerate after dilution.

Rate of Administration

• **Direct IV:** Administer at a rate of 3 ml (300 mg) over 1 minute.

≋ CLINICAL PRECAUTIONS

- Monitor pulse and blood pressure every 15 minutes during administration. Provide safety measures as indicated. Supervise ambulation and transfer of patients.
- Have patient remain recumbent during and for at least 10–15 minutes following infusion to avoid orthostatic hypotension.
- Assess patient for allergic reactions (skin rash, asthma, hives, wheezing, hypotension) following parenteral administration. Keep epinephrine and oxygen on hand in the event of a reaction.
- Assess patient for pain, muscle stiffness, and range of motion prior to and periodically throughout therapy.
- Monitor IV site. Injection is hypertonic and may cause thrombophlebitis. Avoid extravasation.
- Use methocarbamol cautiously in patients with a history of seizure disorders.
- Geriatric patients may require lower doses.
- Additive CNS depression may occur with other CNS depressants, including alcohol, antihistamines, opioid analgesics, and sedative/hypnotics.
- Safe use in pregnancy, lactation, or children has not been established.

Lab Test Considerations

• Monitor renal function periodically during prolonged therapy, as polyethylene glycol 300 vehicle is nephrotoxic. • May cause falsely increased urinary 5-hydroxyindoleacetic acid (5-HIAA) and vanillylmandelic acid (VMA) determinations.

Patient/Family Teaching

• Instruct patient to make position changes slowly to minimize orthostatic hypotension. • Methocarbamol may cause dizziness, drowsiness, and blurred vision. Advise patient to avoid driving and other activities requiring alertness until response to drug is known. Advise patient to avoid concurrent use of alcohol and other CNS depressants while taking this medication. • Encourage patient to comply with additional therapies prescribed for muscle spasm (rest, physical therapy, heat). • Inform patient that urine may turn black, brown, or green, especially if left standing. • Instruct patient to notify physician if skin rash, itching, fever, or nasal congestion occurs. • Emphasize the importance of routine follow-up examinations to monitor progress.

≋ PHARMACOLOGIC PROFILE

Indications

• Methocarbamol is used as an adjunct to rest and physical therapy in the treatment of muscle spasm associated with acute painful musculoskeletal conditions and as an adjunct in the management of tetanus.

Action

• Methocarbamol produces skeletal muscle relaxation, probably due to CNS depression.

Time/Action Profile (skeletal muscle relaxation)

Onset	Peak	Duration
immediate	end of infusion	UK

Pharmacokinetics

• **Distribution:** Methocarbamol is widely distributed and crosses the placenta. • **Metabolism and Excretion:** Metabolism of methocarbamol occurs in the liver. • **Half-life:** 1–2 hours.

Contraindications

• Methocarbamol is contraindicated in patients with hypersensitivity to it or to polyethylene glycol. It should be avoided in patients with renal impairment.

Adverse Reactions and Side Effects*

• **CNS:** SEIZURES, drowsiness, <u>dizziness</u>, <u>light-headedness</u> • **EENT:** blurred vision, nasal congestion • **CV:** hypotension, bradycardia • **GI:** <u>nausea</u>, <u>anorexia</u>, <u>GI upset</u> • **GU:** brown, black, or green urine • **Derm:** urticaria, pruritus, rashes, flushing • **Local:** phlebitis at IV site • **Misc:** fever, allergic reactions including ANAPHYLAXIS.

Methohexital Sodium	*Barbiturate anesthetic (ultra-short acting)*
Brevital, {Brietal}	**pH 9.5–11**

Schedule IV

 ADMINISTRATION CONSIDERATIONS

Usual Dose

All doses must be individualized.

Induction

ADULTS AND CHILDREN: 1–2 mg/kg.

Maintenance

ADULTS: 250 mcg (0.25 mg)–1 mg/kg (20–40 mg) q 4–7 min as needed or continuous infusion of 0.2% solution, usually at rate of 3 ml/min (6 mg/min).

Dilution

• **Direct IV: Dilute** 500 mg of methohexital with 50 ml of sterile water for injection, D5W, or 0.9% NaCl. • Solution should be freshly prepared and used within 24 hours of reconstitution. Refrigerate and keep sealed. Do not administer solutions containing a precipitate. • **Continuous Infusion:** To prepare a 1% (10 mg/ml) solution, **reconstitute** each 2.5-g vial with 15 ml or each 5-g vial with 30 ml of sterile water, D5W, or 0.9% NaCl. Initial solution will be yellow. **Further**

---

*Underlines indicate most frequent; CAPITALS indicate life-threatening.

{} = Available in Canada only.

dilute the 2.5-g vial in 250 ml or the 5-g vial in 500 ml. • Solution should be used only if clear and colorless. • To prepare a 0.2% solution, dilute 500 mg in 250 ml of D5W or 0.9% NaCl. Do not dilute with sterile water to avoid hypotonicity. • Solution is stable for 24 hours.

Incompatibility

• **Syringe:** glycopyrrolate.
• **Additive:** atropine ◆ chlorpromazine ◆ cimetidine ◆ clindamycin ◆ droperidol ◆ fentanyl ◆ hydralazine ◆ kanamycin ◆ lidocaine ◆ mechlorethamine ◆ metaraminol ◆ methicillin ◆ methyldopate ◆ metocurine ◆ oxytetracycline ◆ pancuronium ◆ penicillin G potassium ◆ pentazocine ◆ prochlorperazine ◆ promazine ◆ promethazine ◆ propiomazine ◆ scopolamine ◆ succinylcholine ◆ streptomycin ◆ tubocurarine.

Rate of Administration

• **Direct IV:** Induction dose is administered at a rate not to exceed 1 ml (10 mg) over 5 seconds. Anesthesia is maintained by intermittent injections every 4–7 minutes or by **continuous infusion** of a 0.2% solution at an average of 3 ml/min (1 drop/sec).

≋ CLINICAL PRECAUTIONS

• Assess blood pressure, ECG, heart rate, and respiratory status continuously throughout methohexital therapy. Methohexital should be used only by individuals qualified to administer anesthesia and experienced in endotracheal intubation. Equipment for this procedure should be immediately available. Apnea may occur immediately after IV injection, especially in the presence of opioid premedication.

• Dose is individualized according to depth of anesthesia desired; concurrent use of other medications and/or nitrous oxide; patient's condition, age, weight, and sex. Middle-aged or elderly patients may require smaller doses than young patients. Tolerance may develop with repeated use, such as in burn patients. Individuals tolerant to alcohol or barbiturates may require higher doses.

• Repeated doses or continuous infusion of methohexital may cause prolonged somnolence and respiratory and circulatory depression. If the patient requires a second anesthetic in the same day, reduction in the dose of methohexital may be required.

- Methohexital may be given in doses sufficient to produce deep surgical anesthesia, but such doses may cause dangerous respiratory and circulatory depression.
- Premedication with anticholinergics (atropine, glycopyrrolate) may be used to decrease mucous secretions. Opioid analgesics may be administered preoperatively to enhance the poor analgesic effects of methohexital. Preoperative medications should be given so that peak effect is attained shortly before induction of anesthesia. Muscle relaxants, if required, should be administered separately.
- Monitor IV site carefully. Extravasation may cause pain, swelling, ulceration, and necrosis. Intra-arterial injection may cause arteritis, vasospasm, edema, thrombosis, and gangrene of the extremity.
- Additive CNS depression occurs with alcohol, antihistamines, opioid analgesics, and sedative/hypnotics.
- Use cautiously in Addison's disease, severe anemia, severe cardiovascular or hepatic disease, myxedema, shock or hypotension, or pulmonary disease and in elderly, debilitated, or obese patients.
- Safe use in pregnancy has not been established (Pregnancy Category B).

Toxicity and Overdose Alert

- Overdose may occur from rapid injection (drop in blood pressure, possibly to shock levels) or excessive or repeated injections (respiratory distress, laryngospasm, apnea).

Patient/Family Teaching

- Methohexital may cause psychomotor impairment for 24 hours following administration. Caution patient to avoid driving or other activities requiring alertness for 24 hours. • Advise patient to avoid use of alcohol or other CNS depressants for 24 hours following anesthesia, unless directed by physician or dentist.

☰ PHARMACOLOGIC PROFILE

Indications

- Methohexital is used for induction of general anesthesia. It is also used as sole anesthesia in short (<15 minutes), minimally painful procedures; as a supplement to other anesthetic agents; or to produce unconsciousness during balanced anesthesia.

Action

• Methohexital produces CNS depression probably by potentiating gamma-aminobutyric acid (GABA), an inhibitory neurotransmitter, resulting in unconsciousness and general anesthesia. It has no analgesic properties.

Time/Action Profile (anesthesia)

Onset	Peak	Duration
within 60 sec	UK	5–7 min

Pharmacokinetics

• **Distribution:** Methohexital accumulates and may be slowly re-released from lipoid tissues. Small amounts are excreted in breast milk following large doses to the mother.
• **Metabolism and Excretion:** Methohexital is mostly metabolized by the liver with some metabolism in kidneys and brain. • **Half-life:** 4 hours (increased in elderly patients).

Contraindications

• Methohexital is contraindicated in patients with hypersensitivity to it and in patients with porphyria. It should be avoided during lactation.

Adverse Reactions and Side Effects*

• **CNS:** SEIZURES, restlessness, anxiety, headache, emergence delirium • **EENT:** rhinitis • **Resp:** coughing, LARYNGO-SPASM, apnea, respiratory depression, dyspnea, bronchospasm • **CV:** CARDIORESPIRATORY ARREST, hypotension • **GI:** hiccups, salivation, nausea, vomiting, abdominal pain • **Derm:** erythema, pruritus, urticaria • **MS:** muscle twitching • **Local:** phlebitis at IV site • **Misc:** shivering, allergic reactions.

---

*<u>Underlines</u> indicate most frequent; CAPITALS indicate life-threatening.

Methotrexate Sodium	*Antineoplastic (antimetabolite), Immunosuppressant*
amethopterin, Folex PFS, Methotrexate LPF	pH 8.5

≋ ADMINISTRATION CONSIDERATIONS

Usual Dose

Acute Lymphatic Leukemia Induction
ADULTS AND CHILDREN: *Induction* 3.3 mg/m^2/day IM with prednisone followed by *maintenance* of 2.5 mg/kg IV q 14 days.

Osteosarcoma
ADULTS AND CHILDREN: 12 g/m^2 as a 4-hr infusion followed by leucovorin rescue (15 mg leucovorin q 6 hr for 10 doses starting 24 hr after methotrexate is started), usually as part of a combination chemotherapeutic regimen (dose may be increased to 15 g/m^2 to achieve a peak serum methotrexate level of 1×10^{-3} M).

Psoriasis
ADULTS: 10 mg once weekly; may be increased up to 25 mg weekly. Therapy should be preceded by a 5–10-mg test dose.

Dilution
• **Direct IV:** Injectable forms are available as a powder or preservative-free solution. Reconstitute immediately before use. Discard unused portion. • **Reconstitute** each vial of powder with 2–10 ml of sterile water for injection, 0.9% NaCl, or bacteriostatic water for injection with benzyl alcohol or parabens (for *Mexate*) or 2–25 ml of 0.9% NaCl (for *Folex*), for a concentration no greater than 25 mg/ml. Use sterile preservative-free diluents for high-dose regimens to prevent complications from large amounts of benzyl alcohol. Do not use preparations that are discolored or that contain a precipitate. • Solution for injection should be prepared in a biologic cabinet. Wear gloves, gown, and mask while handling medication. Discard equipment in specially designated containers (see Appendix F). • **Intermittent/Continuous**

Infusion: May be **diluted** in D5W, D5/0.9% NaCl, or 0.9% NaCl and infused as intermittent or continuous infusion.

Compatibility

- **Syringe:** bleomycin ✦ cisplatin ✦ cyclophosphamide ✦ doxapram ✦ doxorubicin ✦ fluorouracil ✦ furosemide ✦ heparin ✦ leucovorin ✦ mitomycin ✦ vinblastine ✦ vincristine.

- **Y-site:** allopurinol sodium ✦ bleomycin ✦ cimetidine ✦ cisplatin ✦ cyclophosphamide ✦ dexamethasone ✦ diphenhydramine ✦ doxorubicin ✦ famotidine ✦ filgrastim ✦ fludarabine ✦ fluorouracil ✦ furosemide ✦ gallium nitrate ✦ ganciclovir ✦ heparin ✦ hydromorphone ✦ leucovorin ✦ lorazepam ✦ melphalan ✦ methylprednisolone ✦ metoclopramide ✦ mitomycin ✦ morphine ✦ ondansetron ✦ paclitaxel ✦ piperacillin/tazobactam ✦ prochlorperazine ✦ ranitidine ✦ sargramostim ✦ vancomycin ✦ vinblastine ✦ vincristine ✦ vinorelbine.

- **Additive:** cephalothin ✦ cyclophosphamide ✦ cytarabine ✦ fluorouracil ✦ hydroxyzine ✦ mercaptopurine ✦ sodium bicarbonate ✦ vincristine.

Incompatibility

- **Syringe:** droperidol.
- **Y-site:** chlorperazine ✦ idarubicin ✦ promethazine.
- **Additive:** bleomycin ✦ prednisolone.

Rate of Administration

- **Direct IV:** Has been administered at a rate of 10 mg/min into a Y-site or 3-way stopcock of a free-flowing IV. ✦ **Intermittent/Continuous Infusion:** Administration rates of 4–20 hours have been used.

≋ CLINICAL PRECAUTIONS

- Monitor blood pressure, pulse, and respiratory rate periodically during administration.
- Monitor for abdominal pain, diarrhea, or stomatitis. If these occur, therapy may need to be discontinued.
- Monitor for bone marrow depression. Assess for fever, sore throat, and signs of infection. Assess for bleeding (bleeding gums, bruising, petechiae, guaiac test stools, urine, emesis). Avoid giving IM injections and taking rectal temperatures. Hold pressure on all venipuncture sites for at least 10 minutes. Anemia may occur. Monitor for increased fatigue, dyspnea, and orthostatic hypoten-

sion. Concurrent use of other antineoplastic agents or radiation therapy increases the risk of bone marrow depression.

- Monitor intake and output ratios and daily weights. Use cautiously in patients with renal impairment as dosage reduction is required.
- Monitor for symptoms of pulmonary toxicity, which may manifest early as a dry nonproductive cough.
- Monitor for symptoms of gout (increased uric acid, joint pain, edema). Encourage patient to drink at least 2 liters of fluid each day. Allopurinol and alkalinization of urine may be used to decrease uric acid levels.
- Assess patient's nutritional status. Administering an antiemetic prior to and periodically throughout therapy and adjusting diet as tolerated may help maintain fluid and electrolyte balance and nutritional status.
- The following drugs may increase the toxicity of methotrexate: high-dose salicylates, nonsteroidal anti-inflammatory agents, sulfonylureas (oral hypoglycemic agents), phenytoin, phenylbutazone, tetracyclines, probenecid, and chloramphenicol. Asparaginase may decrease the effects of methotrexate.
- The risk of hepatotoxicity is increased by concurrent use of other hepatotoxic agents. Use cautiously in patients with hepatic impairment. If bilirubin is 3–5 mg/dl or AST (SGOT) is more than 180 U/ml, decrease dose by 25%. If bilirubin is greater than 5 mg/dl, omit dose.
- Use methotrexate cautiously in geriatric patients due to decreased metabolism and excretion and increased risk of interactions from concurrent medications.
- The risk of nephrotoxicity is increased by concurrent use of other nephrotoxic agents. Assure adequate hydration and renal function prior to each dose. Creatinine clearance should be more than 60 ml/min.
- Use cautiously in patients with active infections, decreased bone marrow reserve, or other chronic debilitating illnesses.
- If methotrexate is to be given intrathecally, only preservative-free (LPF or PFS) products should be used.
- Methotrexate should be used with extreme caution in patients with childbearing potential because it may cause fetal anomalies or death (Pregnancy Category X). Avoid use during pregnancy or lactation.

Toxicity and Overdose Alert

• With high-dose therapy, patient must receive folinic acid or citrovorum factor (leucovorin rescue) exactly when ordered to prevent fatal toxicity.

Lab Test Considerations

• Monitor CBC and differential prior to and frequently throughout therapy. The nadir of leukopenia and thrombocytopenia occurs in 7–14 days. Leukocyte and thrombocyte counts usually recover 7 days after the nadir.
• Renal (BUN and creatinine) and hepatic function (AST [SGOT], ALT [SGPT], bilirubin, and LDH) should be monitored prior to and routinely throughout course of therapy.
• Urine pH should be monitored prior to high-dose methotrexate therapy and every 6 hours during leucovorin rescue. Urine pH should be kept above 7.0 to prevent renal damage. • Serum methotrexate levels should be monitored every 12–24 hours during high-dose therapy until levels are less than 5×10^{-8} M. This monitoring is essential to plan correct leucovorin dose and determine duration of rescue therapy. • Methotrexate may cause elevated serum uric acid concentrations, especially during initial treatment of leukemia and lymphoma.

Patient/Family Teaching

• Caution patient to avoid crowds and persons with known infections. Physician should be informed immediately if symptoms of infection occur. • Instruct patient to report unusual bleeding or bruising. Advise patient of thrombocytopenia precautions (use soft toothbrush and electric razor; avoid falls; do not drink alcoholic beverages or take medication containing aspirin, ibuprofen, or naproxen, as these may precipitate gastric bleeding). • Instruct patient to inspect oral mucosa for erythema and ulceration. If ulceration occurs, advise patient to use sponge brush and to rinse mouth with water after eating and drinking. Local therapies may be used if mouth pain interferes with eating. • Instruct patient to avoid the use of over-the-counter drugs without first consulting physician or pharmacist. • Advise patient that this medication may have teratogenic effects. A nonhormonal method of contraception should be used during therapy and for at least 12 weeks after completion of therapy by both male and female patients. • Discuss the possibility of hair loss with patient. Explore methods of coping. • Instruct patient not to receive any vaccinations without advice of physician. Methotrexate may decrease the antibody response to live virus vaccines and increase the risk of adverse reactions. • Caution patient to use sunscreen and protective clothing to prevent photosensitivity reactions. • Emphasize the need for periodic lab tests to monitor for side effects.

≋ PHARMACOLOGIC PROFILE

Indications

• Methotrexate is used alone or in combination with other treatment modalities (other antineoplastic agents, surgery, or radiation therapy) in the treatment of leukemias, osteosarcoma, and other tumors. It is also used as an immunosuppressant in the treatment of severe psoriasis.

Action

• Methotrexate interferes with folic acid metabolism. This results in inhibition of DNA synthesis and cell reproduction (cell cycle–S phase specific) and subsequent death of rapidly replicating cells, particularly malignant ones. It also has immunosuppressive activity.

Time/Action Profile (effects on blood counts)

Onset	Peak	Duration
4–7 days	7–14 days	21 days

Pharmacokinetics

• **Distribution:** Methotrexate is actively transported across cell membranes and is widely distributed. It does not reach therapeutic concentrations in the CSF. It crosses the placenta and enters breast milk in low concentrations. • **Metabolism and Excretion:** Excretion of methotrexate occurs mostly as unchanged drug by the kidneys. • **Half-life:** 2–4 hours (increased in renal impairment).

Contraindications

• Methotrexate is contraindicated in patients with hypersensitivity to it. Some products contain benzyl alcohol and should be avoided in patients with known intolerance. • Pregnant or lactating females should not receive methotrexate.

Adverse Reactions and Side Effects*

• **CNS:** headaches, blurred vision, drowsiness, malaise, dizziness • **Resp:** PULMONARY TOXICITY • **GI:** <u>stomatitis</u>, <u>anorexia</u>, <u>nausea</u>, <u>vomiting</u>, hepatotoxicity, diarrhea, HEMORRHAGIC ENTERITIS • **GU:** gonadal suppression • **Derm:** rashes, urticaria, photosensitivity, pruritus, alopecia • **Hemat:** <u>anemia</u>, <u>leukopenia</u>, <u>thrombocytopenia</u> • **Metab:** hyperuricemia • **Misc:** <u>nephropathy</u>, chills, fever.

Methoxamine Hydrochloride	Vasopressor
Vasoxyl	pH 3–5

 ADMINISTRATION CONSIDERATIONS

Usual Dose

Vasopressor

ADULTS: 3–5 mg direct IV or continuous infusion at 5 mcg/min.

Antiarrhythmic

ADULTS: 10 mg (range 5–15 mg).

Dilution

• **Direct IV:** May be administered **undiluted**. • **Continuous Infusion:** Dilute 35–40 mg of methoxamine in 250 ml of D5W.

---

*<u>Underlines</u> indicate most frequent; CAPITALS indicate life-threatening.

Compatibility

• **Y-site:** heparin ♦ hydrocortisone sodium succinate ♦ potassium chloride ♦ vitamin B complex with C.

Rate of Administration

• **Direct IV:** Administer at a rate of 5 mg over 1 minute when the systolic blood pressure is less than 60 mm Hg, or when an emergency situation occurs. • Rapid administration may cause added stress on the myocardium by increasing peripheral vascular resistance during decreased stroke volume and cardiac output. • In paroxysmal supraventricular tachycardia, the 10-mg dose is administered slowly over 3–5 minutes. • **Continuous Infusion:** Infuse slowly. Titrate according to patient's response.

≋ CLINICAL PRECAUTIONS

- Monitor blood pressure, pulse, and hemodynamic parameters prior to and frequently throughout therapy. Blood pressure should be maintained at slightly less than normal. Correct hypovolemia and any electrolyte disturbances prior to administration.
- Observe IV site frequently. Extravasation may cause necrosis and sloughing.
- Methoxamine should be used cautiously in patients with hypoxia, cardiovascular disease, severe hypertension, thrombosis, hyperthyroidism, pheochromocytoma, bradycardia, or heart block.
- The risk of arrhythmias is increased by concurrent use of bretylium, cardiac glycosides, or halogenated hydrocarbon anesthetics.
- The following agents may increase the pressor response to methoxamine: guanethidine, doxapram, oxytocic agents, and tricyclic antidepressants.
- Decreased pressor response or possible hypotension may occur with agents having alpha-adrenergic blocking properties (labetalol, phenoxybenzamine, phentolamine, prazosin, terazosin, doxazosin, tolazoline, phenothiazines, or haloperidol).
- When used during pregnancy, methoxamine may cause uterine contractions or fetal bradycardia (Pregnancy Cat-

egory C). Safe use during lactation or in children has not been established.

Toxicity and Overdose Alert

• Excessive bradycardia may be treated with IV atropine. An alpha-adrenergic blocking agent (phentolamine) may be used to treat severe hypotension.

Patient/Family Teaching

• Advise patient to notify nurse or physician immediately if pain at the IV site occurs.

≋ PHARMACOLOGIC PROFILE

Indications

• Methoxamine is used to maintain blood pressure during general anesthesia with agents capable of sensitizing the myocardium to arrhythmias (cyclopropane). It has also been used during spinal anesthesia and to terminate paroxysmal supraventricular tachyarrhythmias (SVT).

Action

• Methoxamine is a direct-acting alpha-adrenergic amine that causes peripheral vasoconstriction, which results in increased systolic and diastolic pressure. Heart rate is slowed as a result of vagal stimulation.

Time/Action Profile (pressor response)

Onset	Peak	Duration
immediate	UK	5–15 min

Pharmacokinetics

• **Distribution:** UK. • **Metabolism and Excretion:** UK. • **Half-life:** UK.

Contraindications

• Methoxamine is contraindicated in patients with hypersensitivity to it or to bisulfites.

Adverse Reactions and Side Effects*

• **CNS:** headache, anxiety • **CV:** bradycardia, hypertension, premature ventricular contractions • **GI:** vomiting, nausea • **GU:** urinary urgency • **Derm:** sweating, piloerection.

Methyldopate Hydrochloride	Antihypertensive (centrally acting alpha-adrenergic agonist)
Aldomet Ester Hydrochloride	pH 3–4.2

≋ ADMINISTRATION CONSIDERATIONS

Usual Dose

ADULTS: 250–500 mg q 6 hr (up to 1 g q 6–12 hr).
CHILDREN: 5–10 mg/kg q 6 hr (not to exceed 3000 mg/24 hr or 65 mg/kg/24 hr, whichever is less).

Dilution

• **Intermittent Infusion: Dilute** in 100 ml of D5W, 0.9% NaCl, D5/0.9% NaCl, 5% sodium bicarbonate, or Ringer's solution.

Compatibility

• **Y-site:** esmolol ◆ meperidine ◆ morphine.
• **Additive:** aminophylline ◆ ascorbic acid ◆ chloramphenicol ◆ diphenhydramine ◆ heparin ◆ magnesium sulfate ◆ multivitamins ◆ netilmicin ◆ potassium chloride ◆ promazine ◆ sodium bicarbonate ◆ succinylcholine ◆ verapamil ◆ vitamin B complex with C.

Incompatibility

• **Additive:** amphotericin B ◆ barbiturates ◆ sulfonamides.

Rate of Administration

• **Intermittent Infusion:** Infuse slowly over 30–60 minutes for adults or children.

---

*Underlines indicate most frequent; CAPITALS indicate life-threatening.

≋ CLINICAL PRECAUTIONS

- Monitor blood pressure and pulse frequently during initial dosage adjustment and periodically throughout course of therapy for significant changes. Due to its delayed onset, methyldopate should *not* be used in emergency situations.
- Monitor intake and output ratios and weight and assess for edema daily, especially at beginning of therapy. If weight gain or edema occurs, sodium and water retention may be treated with diuretics.
- When changing from IV to oral forms, dosage should remain consistent.
- Additive hypotension may occur with other antihypertensive agents, acute ingestion of alcohol, and nitrates. Amphetamines, tricyclic antidepressants, nonsteroidal anti-inflammatory agents, and phenothiazines may decrease antihypertensive effect of methyldopate. Methyldopate may increase lithium toxicity. Additive hypotension and CNS toxicity may occur with concurrent use of levodopa.
- Use methyldopate cautiously in patients with a previous history of liver disease. Geriatric patients may be more likely to experience adverse CNS reactions.
- Methyldopate has been used safely during pregnancy (Pregnancy Category B). Safe use during lactation has not been established, but no adverse effects on the infant have been noted.

Toxicity and Overdose Alert

• If overdose occurs, monitor blood pressure frequently. Treatment includes elevation of legs, replacement of volume with IV fluids, and administration of vasopressors if hypotension is severe.

Lab Test Considerations

• Renal and hepatic function and CBC should be monitored prior to and periodically throughout therapy. • Methyldopate may cause a positive direct Coombs' test, which may be associated rarely with hemolytic anemia. • BUN, serum potassium, sodium, prolactin, uric acid, AST

(SGOT), ALT (SGPT), alkaline phosphatase, and bilirubin may be increased by methyldopate. • Methyldopate may interfere with serum creatinine and AST (SGOT) measurements.

Patient/Family Teaching

• Methyldopate controls but does not cure hypertension. Encourage patient to comply with additional interventions for hypertension (weight reduction, low-sodium diet, discontinuation of smoking, moderation of alcohol consumption, regular exercise, and stress management). Instruct patient and family on proper technique for monitoring blood pressure. • Inform patient that urine may darken or turn red-black when left standing. • Methyldopate may cause drowsiness. Advise patient to avoid activities requiring alertness until response to medication is known. Drowsiness usually subsides after 7–10 days of continuous use. • Caution patient to avoid sudden changes in position to decrease orthostatic hypotension. • Advise patient that frequent mouth rinses, good oral hygiene, and sugarless gum or candy may minimize dry mouth. • Instruct patient to notify physician if fever, muscle aches, or flu-like syndrome occurs.

≋ PHARMACOLOGIC PROFILE

Indications

• Methyldopate is used in combination with other antihypertensives in the management of moderate to severe hypertension.

Action

• Methyldopate stimulates central alpha-adrenergic receptors, resulting in decreased sympathetic outflow. Result is inhibition of cardioacceleration and vasoconstrictor center. Overall effect is decrease in total peripheral resistance, with little change in heart rate or cardiac output. As a result, blood pressure is lowered.

Time/Action Profile (antihypertensive effect)

Onset	Peak	Duration
4–6 hr	UK	10–16 hr

Pharmacokinetics

• **Distribution:** Methyldopate crosses the blood–brain barrier and the placenta. Small amounts enter breast milk.
• **Metabolism and Excretion:** Methyldopate hydrochloride is slowly converted to methyldopa. It is then partially metabolized by the liver, partially excreted unchanged by the kidneys. • **Half-life:** 1.7 hours.

Contraindications

• Methyldopate is contraindicated in patients with hypersensitivity to it or to bisulfites. Methyldopate should be avoided in patients with active liver disease.

Adverse Reactions and Side Effects*

• **CNS:** <u>sedation</u>, depression, decreased mental acuity • **EENT:** nasal stuffiness • **CV:** orthostatic hypotension, bradycardia, MYOCARDITIS, edema • **GI:** diarrhea, dry mouth, HEPATITIS • **GU:** <u>impotence</u> • **Hemat:** hemolytic anemia • **Misc:** fever.

Methylergonovine Maleate	*Oxytocic*
Methergine	pH 2.7–3.5

 ADMINISTRATION CONSIDERATIONS

Usual Dose

ADULTS: 200 mcg (0.2 mg) q 2–4 hr for up to 5 doses; if necessary may then change to oral form.

Dilution

• **Direct IV:** May be given **undiluted** or **diluted** in 5 ml of 0.9% NaCl and administered through Y-site or 3-way stopcock. Do not add to IV solution. Refrigerate; stable for storage at room temperature for 60 days; deteriorates over time. Use only solutions that are clear and colorless and that contain no precipitate.

---

*<u>Underlines</u> indicate most frequent; CAPITALS indicate life-threatening.

Compatibility

- **Y-site:** heparin ◆ hydrocortisone sodium succinate ◆ potassium chloride ◆ vitamin B complex with C.

Incompatibility

- **Syringe:** Do not mix in syringe with any other drug.

Rate of Administration

- **Direct IV:** Administer at a rate of 0.2 mg over 1 minute.

≋ CLINICAL PRECAUTIONS

- Monitor blood pressure, heart rate, and uterine response (contractility, vaginal bleeding) frequently during medication administration.
- Assess patient for signs of ergotism (cold, numb fingers and toes; chest pain; nausea; vomiting; headache; muscle pain; weakness). Excessive vasoconstriction may result when used with other vasopressors such as dopamine, or in heavy cigarette smokers.
- Use cautiously in hypertensive or eclamptic patients, as they are more susceptible to hypertensive and arrhythmogenic side effects. Use with caution in patients with severe hepatic or renal disease or sepsis.
- Avoid using methylergonovine during pregnancy or labor (Pregnancy Category C). With usual doses, no adverse effects have been noted on lactation.

Lab Test Considerations

- If no response occurs to methylergonovine, calcium levels may need to be assessed. Effectiveness of medication is decreased in hypocalcemic patients. • Methylergonovine may cause decreased serum prolactin levels.

Patient/Family Teaching

- Advise patient that medication may cause menstrual-like cramping. • Caution patient to avoid smoking, as nicotine constricts blood vessels. • Instruct patient to notify physician if infection develops, since this may cause increased sensitivity to the methylergonovine.

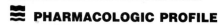

≋ PHARMACOLOGIC PROFILE

Indications
• Methylergonovine is used in the prevention and treatment of postpartum or postabortion hemorrhage caused by uterine atony or subinvolution.

Action
• Methylergonovine directly stimulates uterine and vascular smooth muscle.

Time/Action Profile (effect on uterine contractions)

Onset	Peak	Duration
immediate	UK	45 min–3 hr

Pharmacokinetics
• **Distribution:** Distribution of methylergonovine is not known. Small amounts enter breast milk. • **Metabolism and Excretion:** The metabolic fate of methylergonovine is unknown, although it is probably metabolized by the liver. • **Half-life:** 30–120 minutes.

Contraindications
• Methylergonovine is contraindicated in patients with hypersensitivity to it. • Methylergonovine should not be used during pregnancy or to induce labor.

Adverse Reactions and Side Effects*
• **CNS:** dizziness, headache • **EENT:** tinnitus • **Resp:** dyspnea • **CV:** palpitations, hypotension, chest pain, hypertension, arrhythmias • **GI:** nausea, vomiting • **GU:** cramps • **Derm:** diaphoresis • **Misc:** allergic reactions.

---

*Underlines indicate most frequent; CAPITALS indicate life-threatening.

Methylprednisolone Sodium Succinate	*Glucocorticoid* *(intermediate acting)*
A-methaPred, Solu-Medrol	pH 7–8

≋ ADMINISTRATION CONSIDERATIONS

Usual Dose

ADULTS: *Most indications*—10–40 mg repeated as needed; *high-dose "pulse" therapy*—30 mg/kg q 4–6 hr as needed; *acute exacerbations of multiple sclerosis*—160 mg/day for 7 days, then 64 mg every other day for one month; *acute spinal cord injury*—30 mg/kg followed 45 minutes later by 5.4 mg/kg/hr continuous infusion for 23 hours (unlabeled); *adjunct in the management of* P. carinii *pneumonia in HIV-positive patients*—30 mg twice daily for 5 days, then 30 mg once daily for 5 days, then 15 mg once daily for 11 days (unlabeled).

CHILDREN: *Status asthmaticus*—1–2 mg/kg, followed by 0.5–1 mg/kg q 6 hr (unlabeled); *high-dose "pulse" therapy*—30 mg/kg, followed by 10 mg/kg/day for 6 days, then 15–30 mg/kg/day for 3 days or 600 mg/m^2 for 3 days; *acute spinal cord injury*—30 mg/kg followed 45 minutes later by 5.4 mg/kg/hr continuous infusion for 23 hours (unlabeled); *adjunct in the management of* P. carinii *pneumonia in HIV-positive patients* ≥13 yr—30 mg twice daily for 5 days, then 30 mg once daily for 5 days, then 15 mg once daily for 7–11 days (unlabeled); *adjunct in the management of* P. carinii *pneumonia in HIV-positive patients* <13 yr—4–8 mg/kg/day in divided doses q 6–12 hr for 5 days, then change to oral prednisone (unlabeled).

Dilution

• **Direct IV: Reconstitute** with provided solution (Act-O-Vials) or 2 ml of bacteriostatic water (with benzyl alcohol) for injection. • **Intermittent/Continuous Infusion:** May be **diluted further** in D5W, 0.9% NaCl, or D5/0.9% NaCl. • Solution may form a haze upon dilution.

Compatibility

• **Syringe:** metoclopramide.

• **Y-site:** acyclovir • amrinone • cisplatin • cyclophosphamide • cytarabine • doxorubicin • enalaprilat • famotidine

• fludarabine • melphalan • meperidine • methotrexate • morphine • potassium chloride.

• **Additive:** chloramphenicol • cimetidine • clindamycin • dopamine • heparin • norepinephrine • penicillin G potassium • theophylline • verapamil.

Incompatibility

• **Y-site:** allopurinol sodium • ciprofloxacin • filgrastim • ondansetron • paclitaxel • sargramostim • vinorelbine.

• **Additive:** calcium gluconate • glycopyrrolate • metaraminol • nafcillin • penicillin G sodium.

Rate of Administration

• **Direct IV:** May be administered direct IV push over 1–several minutes. • **Intermittent/Continuous Infusion:** Administer as an intermittent or continuous infusion at the prescribed rate. Has been infused over 24–48 hours.

≋ CLINICAL PRECAUTIONS

• Methylprednisolone is indicated for many conditions. Assess the involved systems prior to and periodically throughout course of therapy.

• Assess patient for signs of adrenal insufficiency (hypotension, weight loss, weakness, nausea, vomiting, anorexia, lethargy, confusion, restlessness) prior to and periodically throughout course of therapy.

• Monitor intake and output ratios and daily weights. Observe patient for the appearance of peripheral edema, steady weight gain, rales/crackles, or dyspnea.

• Chronic treatment will lead to adrenal suppression and therefore should never be abruptly discontinued. During periods of stress (surgery, infection) supplemental doses will be needed.

• If dose is ordered daily or every other day, administer in the morning to coincide with the body's normal secretion of cortisol.

• Signs of infections (fever, inflammation) may be masked during treatment.

• Children receiving chronic therapy should also have periodic evaluations of growth.

• Safe use during pregnancy or lactation has not been established. Chronic use during pregnancy may result in adrenal suppression in the newborn. Chronic high-dose therapy is not recommended during lactation.

Lab Test Considerations

• Patients on prolonged courses of therapy should routinely have hematologic values, serum electrolytes, serum and urine glucose evaluated. Methylprednisolone may cause decreased WBC counts and decreased serum potassium, calcium, protein-bound iodine, and thyroxine concentrations. Additive hypokalemia may occur with concurrent use of diuretics, amphotericin B, mezlocillin, piperacillin, or ticarcillin and may increase the risk of cardiac glycoside toxicity. • Methylprednisolone may cause increased blood glucose, especially in persons with diabetes. • Requirements for insulin or oral hypoglycemic agents may be increased. Serum sodium, serum cholesterol, and serum lipid values may also be increased. • Guaiac-test stools. • Periodic adrenal function tests may be ordered to assess degree of hypothalamic-pituitary-adrenal (HPA) axis suppression during chronic therapy. • Methylprednisolone may suppress reactions to allergy skin tests.

Patient/Family Teaching

• Instruct patient to notify physician immediately if signs of adrenal insufficiency (anorexia, nausea, fatigue, weakness, hypotension, dyspnea, and hypoglycemia) appear after chronic therapy. This condition can be life-threatening. • Encourage patient on long-term therapy to eat a diet high in protein, calcium, and potassium and low in sodium and carbohydrates (see Appendix H for foods included). • This drug causes immunosuppression and may mask symptoms of infection. Instruct patient to avoid people with known contagious illnesses and to report possible infections. • Review side effects with patient. Instruct patient to inform physician promptly if severe abdominal pain or tarry stools occur. Patient should also report unusual swelling, weight gain, tiredness, bone pain, bruising, nonhealing sores, visual disturbances, or behavior changes. • Instruct patient to inform physician if symptoms of underlying disease return or worsen. • Advise patient to carry appropriate identification in the event of an emergency in which patient cannot relate medical history.

• Caution patient to avoid vaccinations without consulting physician. Methylprednisolone may decrease antibody response to live virus vaccines and increase the risk of adverse reactions. • Emphasize the importance of follow-up examinations to monitor progress and side effects.

 PHARMACOLOGIC PROFILE

Indications

• Methylprednisolone is used in a wide variety of situations including chronic inflammatory diseases, allergic diseases, hematologic diseases, neoplastic diseases, and autoimmune diseases. It is suitable for alternate-day dosing.

Action

• Methylprednisolone suppresses inflammation and the normal immune response. In addition, it has numerous intense metabolic effects. Adrenal suppression occurs at chronic doses of 4 mg/day or more. Mineralocorticoid (sodium-retaining) activity is minimal. Major therapeutic benefits include suppression of inflammation and modification of the normal immune response.

Time/Action Profile (anti-inflammatory activity)

Onset	Peak	Duration
rapid	UK	UK

Pharmacokinetics

• **Distribution:** Methylprednisolone is widely distributed. It crosses the placenta, and small amounts enter breast milk. • **Metabolism and Excretion:** Most of methylprednisolone is metabolized by the liver; small amounts are excreted unchanged by the kidneys. • **Half-life:** 80–190 minutes. Adrenal suppression lasts 1.25–1.5 days.

Contraindications

• Methylprednisolone is contraindicated in patients with active untreated infections, except for some forms of meningitis. Chronic use should be avoided during lactation. Parenteral methylprednisolone contains benzyl alcohol and should not be given to patients with known intolerance or newborns.

Adverse Reactions and Side Effects*

These reactions are more likely to occur in patients on high-dose, long-term therapy.

• **CNS:** headache, restlessness, psychoses, <u>depression</u>, <u>euphoria</u>, personality changes, increased intracranial pressure (children only) • **EENT:** cataracts, increased intraocular pressure • **CV:** <u>hypertension</u> • **GI:** <u>nausea</u>, vomiting, <u>anorexia</u>, peptic ulceration • **Hemat:** thromboembolism, thrombophlebitis • **Derm:** <u>decreased wound healing</u>, <u>petechiae</u>, <u>ecchymoses</u>, <u>fragility</u>, <u>hirsutism</u>, <u>acne</u> • **Endo:** <u>adrenal suppression</u>, hyperglycemia • **F and E:** hypokalemia, hypokalemic alkalosis, fluid retention • **Metab:** weight loss, weight gain • **MS:** <u>muscle wasting</u>, muscle pain, aseptic necrosis of joints, <u>osteoporosis</u>; <u>cushingoid appearance (moon face, buffalo hump)</u>.

Metoclopramide Hydrochloride	Antiemetic, GI stimulant
{Maxeran}, Octamide PFS, Reglan	pH 3–6.5

ADMINISTRATION CONSIDERATIONS

Usual Dose

Prevention of Nausea and Vomiting Associated with Chemotherapy

ADULTS: 1–2 mg/kg starting 30 min before chemotherapy, then q 2 hr for 2 doses, then q 3 hr for 3 doses; may also be given as an infusion at 0.5 mg/kg/hr for 8 hr preceded by an initial dose of 3 mg/kg.

CHILDREN: 1 mg/kg, may be repeated after 60 min, or 1–3 mg/kg 30 min before chemotherapy.

Facilitation of Small-Bowel Intubation or Upper GI Radiography

ADULTS AND CHILDREN >14 yr: 10 mg.

CHILDREN 6–14 yr: 2.5–5 mg (dose should not exceed 0.5 mg/kg).

CHILDREN <6 yr: 0.1 mg/kg.

---

*<u>Underlines</u> indicate most frequent; CAPITALS indicate life-threatening.

{} = Available in Canada only.

Peristaltic Stimulant

ADULTS: 10 mg.

CHILDREN: 1 mg/kg, may repeat after 60 min.

Dilution

• **Direct IV:** May be administered **undiluted.** • **Intermittent Infusion:** Doses exceeding 50 mg should be diluted for IV infusion in 50 ml of D5W, 0.9% NaCl, D5/0.45% NaCl, Ringer's solution, or lactated Ringer's solution. • Diluted solution is stable for 48 hours if protected from light, or 24 hours under normal light. Discard unused portions.

Compatibility

• **Syringe:** aminophylline • ascorbic acid • atropine • benztropine • bleomycin • butorphanol • chlorpromazine • cisplatin • cyclophosphamide • cytarabine • dexamethasone • dimenhydrinate • diphenhydramine • doxorubicin • droperidol • fentanyl • fluorouracil • heparin • hydrocortisone • hydroxyzine • regular insulin • leucovorin • lidocaine • magnesium sulfate • meperidine • methotrimeprazine • methylprednisolone sodium succinate • midazolam • mitomycin • morphine • pentazocine • perphenazine • prochlorperazine • promazine • promethazine • ranitidine • scopolamine • vinblastine • vincristine • vitamin B complex with C.

• **Y-site:** acyclovir • bleomycin • ciprofloxacin • cisplatin • cyclophosphamide • diltiazem • doxorubicin • droperidol • famotidine • filgrastim • fluconazole • fludarabine • fluorouracil • foscarnet • gallium nitrate • heparin • idarubicin • leucovorin • melphalan • meperidine • methotrexate • mitomycin • morphine • ondansetron • paclitaxel • piperacillin/tazobactam • sargramostim • tacrolimus • vinblastine • vincristine • vinorelbine • zidovudine.

• **Additive:** clindamycin • multivitamins • potassium acetate • potassium chloride • potassium phosphate • verapamil.

Incompatibility

• **Syringe:** ampicillin • calcium gluconate • cephalothin • chloramphenicol • furosemide • penicillin G potassium • sodium bicarbonate.

• **Y-site:** allopurinol sodium • furosemide.

• **Additive:** calcium gluconate • cisplatin • erythromycin lactobionate • furosemide • methotrexate • penicillin G potassium • sodium bicarbonate.

Rate of Administration

- **Direct IV:** Doses may be given slowly over at least 1–2 minutes. Rapid administration causes a transient but intense feeling of anxiety and restlessness followed by drowsiness.
- **Intermittent Infusion:** Infuse slowly over at least 15 minutes.

≋ CLINICAL PRECAUTIONS

- Administer IV dose 30 minutes prior to administration of chemotherapeutic agent.
- Assess patient for nausea, vomiting, abdominal distention, and bowel sounds prior to and following administration. Assess nutritional status, and fluid and electrolyte status.
- Assess patient for extrapyramidal effects (involuntary movements, facial grimacing, rigidity, shuffling walk, trembling of hands) periodically throughout course of therapy. Extrapyramidal effects are more common in children and the elderly and may be prevented or treated with diphenhydramine 1 mg/kg given 15 minutes before metoclopramide (see *diphenhydramine hydrochloride* monograph, page 332). The risk of extrapyramidal (dystonic) reactions is increased with concurrent use of haloperidol or phenothiazines and with doses >2 mg/kg.
- Metoclopramide may cause additive CNS depression with other CNS depressants, including alcohol, antidepressants, antihistamines, opioid analgesics, and sedative/hypnotics. Diabetics may require adjustments in insulin dosing during metoclopramide therapy. Metoclopramide may also affect the GI absorption of orally administered drugs as a result of effect on GI motility. Opioid analgesics and anticholinergics may decrease the beneficial GI effects of metoclopramide. Metoclopramide may increase the neuromuscular blocking effects of succinylcholine. Concurrent use with MAO inhibitors may result in hypertension.
- Metoclopramide may exaggerate hypotension during general anesthesia.
- Safe use during pregnancy and lactation has not been established (Pregnancy Category B).

Toxicity and Overdose Alert

• Symptoms of toxicity include drowsiness, disorientation, and extrapyramidal symptoms, all of which are self-limiting and usually subside within 24 hours. Muscle hypertonia, irritability, and agitation are common. Treatment may include anticholinergic agents, antiparkinsonian drugs, or antihistamines with anticholinergic properties such as diphenhydramine.

Patient/Family Teaching

• Metoclopramide may cause drowsiness. Caution patient to avoid driving or other activities requiring alertness until response to medication is known. • Advise patient to avoid concurrent use of alcohol and other CNS depressants while taking this medication. • Advise patient to notify physician immediately if involuntary movement of eyes, face, or limbs occurs.

≋ PHARMACOLOGIC PROFILE

Indications

• Metoclopramide is used to prevent chemotherapy-induced emesis and in the treatment of diabetic gastric stasis. Metoclopramide is also used to facilitate small-bowel intubation in radiographic procedures.

Action

• Metoclopramide blocks dopamine receptors in chemoreceptor trigger zone of the CNS. It stimulates motility of the upper GI tract and accelerates gastric emptying, resulting in decreased nausea and vomiting and decreased symptoms of gastric stasis.

Time/Action Profile (effects on peristalsis)

Onset	Peak	Duration
1–3 min	immediate	1–2 hr

Pharmacokinetics

• **Distribution:** Metoclopramide is widely distributed into body tissues and fluids. It crosses the blood–brain barrier and placenta and enters breast milk in concentrations greater than that of plasma. • **Metabolism and Excretion:** Metoclopramide is partially metabolized by the liver. Twenty-five percent is eliminated unchanged in the urine. • **Half-life:** 2.5–5 hours.

Contraindications

• Metoclopramide is contraindicated in patients with hypersensitivity to it. Its use should be avoided in patients with possible GI obstruction or hemorrhage, pheochromocytoma, or a history of seizure disorders. Avoid concurrent use with levodopa, due to variable effects of drugs on each other's activity.

Adverse Reactions and Side Effects*

• **CNS:** <u>restlessness</u>, <u>drowsiness</u>, <u>fatigue</u>, <u>extrapyramidal reactions</u>, depression, irritability, anxiety • **CV:** arrhythmias • **GI:** constipation, diarrhea, nausea, dry mouth • **Endo:** gynecomastia.

Metocurine Iodide	*Neuromuscular blocking agent (nondepolarizing)*
Metubine	pH 4–4.3

≋ ADMINISTRATION CONSIDERATIONS

Usual Dose

Surgery
ADULTS: 150–400 mcg (0.15–0.4 mg)/kg initially; additional doses of 0.5–1 mg may be given q 30–90 min.

Adjunct to Electroconvulsive Therapy
ADULTS: 2–3 mg (range 1.75–5.5 mg).

Dilution
• **Direct IV:** May be administered **undiluted**.

Incompatibility
• **Syringe:** barbiturates • meperidine • morphine • sodium bicarbonate.

---

*<u>Underlines</u> indicate most frequent; CAPITALS indicate life-threatening.

Rate of Administration

- **Direct IV:** Administer over 30–60 seconds. Relaxation from initial dose lasts 25–90 minutes (average 60 minutes); administer supplemental doses of 0.5–1 mg as needed. Dose is titrated to patient response.

≋ CLINICAL PRECAUTIONS

- Assess respiratory status continuously throughout metocurine therapy. Metocurine should be used only by individuals experienced in endotracheal intubation, and equipment for this procedure should be immediately available.
- Neuromuscular response to metocurine should be monitored with a peripheral nerve stimulator. Paralysis is initially selective and usually occurs consecutively in the following muscles: levator muscles of eyelids, muscles of mastication, limb muscles, abdominal muscles, muscles of the glottis, intercostal muscles, and the diaphragm. Recovery of muscle function usually occurs in reverse order. Observe the patient for residual muscle weakness and respiratory distress during the recovery period.
- Metocurine has no analgesic or sedative properties. Adequate anesthesia/analgesia should *always* be used when metocurine is used as an adjunct to surgical procedures. When used concurrently with opioid analgesics, the risk of bradycardia, hypotension, and effects of histamine release may be increased.
- Use cautiously in patients with a history of pulmonary disease, or of renal or hepatic impairment. Elderly patients may have increased recovery time, and dosage requirements may vary in this group of patients. Prolonged respiratory paralysis may occur in patients with myasthenia gravis or myasthenic syndromes.
- Intensity and duration of paralysis may be prolonged by pretreatment with succinylcholine, general anesthesia, amingolycoside antibiotics, polymyxin B, colistin, clindamycin, lidocaine, quinidine, procainamide, beta-adrenergic blocking agents, potassium-losing diuretics, and magnesium. Ether, methoxyflurane, halothane, enflurane, or isoflurane increases intensity and

duration of action (doses of metocurine should be decreased by approximately ⅓–½). Doxapram masks residual effects of metocurine.

- Safe use in pregnancy or lactation has not been established (Pregnancy Category C).

Toxicity and Overdose Alert

- If overdose occurs, use peripheral nerve stimulator to determine the degree of neuromuscular blockade. Maintain airway patency and ventilation until recovery of normal respirations occurs. Administration of anticholinesterase agents (edrophonium, neostigmine, pyridostigmine) may be used to antagonize the action of metocurine. Atropine is usually administered prior to or concurrently with anticholinesterase agents to counteract their muscarinic effects. Administration of fluids and vasopressors may be necessary to treat severe hypotension or shock.

Patient/Family Teaching

- Explain all procedures to patient receiving metocurine therapy without anesthesia, as consciousness is not affected by metocurine alone. Reassure patient that communication abilities will return as the medication wears off.

PHARMACOLOGIC PROFILE

Indications

- Metocurine produces skeletal muscle paralysis after induction of anesthesia in surgical procedures. It is also used as an adjunct to electroconvulsive therapy.

Action

- Metocurine prevents neuromuscular transmission by blocking the effect of acetylcholine at the myoneural junction, which results in skeletal muscle paralysis. It has no anxiolytic or analgesic properties.

Time/Action Profile (skeletal muscle paralysis)

Onset	Peak	Duration
within 1–4 min	3–5 min	35–60 min†

†Total recovery of function may take several hours.

Pharmacokinetics

• **Distribution:** Metocurine is extensively distributed and crosses the placenta. • **Metabolism and Excretion:** Fifty percent is excreted unchanged in urine. • **Half-life:** 3.6 hours.

Contraindications

• Metocurine is contraindicated in patients with hypersensitivity to it or to iodides or phenol.

Adverse Reactions and Side Effects*

• **EENT:** excess salivation • **Resp:** bronchospasm, APNEA • **CV:** hypotension, arrhythmias • **GI:** decreased GI tone, decreased GI motility • **MS:** muscle weakness • **Misc:** allergic reactions.

Metoprolol Tartrate	Beta-adrenergic blocker (cardioselective)
{Betaloc}, Lopressor	pH 7.5

≋ ADMINISTRATION CONSIDERATIONS

Usual Dose

Myocardial Infarction Prophylaxis—Acute Treatment

ADULTS: 5 mg q 2 min for 3 doses, then change to oral metoprolol (25–50 mg q 6 hr for 48 hr, then 100 mg twice daily) 15 min after last IV dose.

Dilution

• **Direct IV:** May be administered **undiluted**.

Compatibility

• **Y-site:** alteplase ◆ meperidine ◆ morphine.
• **Solution:** D5W ◆ 0.9% NaCl.

---

*Underlines indicate most frequent; CAPITALS indicate life-threatening.

{} = Available in Canada only.

Rate of Administration
- **Direct IV:** May be administered by injecting 5 mg slowly over 2 minutes.

≋ CLINICAL PRECAUTIONS

- Vital signs and ECG should be monitored every 5–15 minutes during and for several hours after parenteral administration.
- Assess frequency and duration of episodes of chest pain throughout therapy.
- Monitor intake and output ratios and daily weights. Assess patient routinely for evidence of fluid overload (peripheral edema, dyspnea, rales/crackles, fatigue, weight gain, jugular venous distention).
- When changing from IV to oral metoprolol, oral doses are much larger due to extensive first-pass hepatic metabolism following oral administration. IV doses of metoprolol avoid first-pass metabolism and are therefore much smaller.
- General anesthesia, IV phenytoin, and verapamil may cause additive myocardial depression. Additive bradycardia may occur with concurrent use of cardiac glycosides. Additive hypotension may occur with other antihypertensive agents, acute ingestion of alcohol, or nitrates.
- Concurrent use with amphetamines, cocaine, ephedrine, epinephrine, norepinephrine, phenylephrine, or pseudoephedrine may result in excess alpha-adrenergic stimulation, hypertension, and bradycardia. Metoprolol may produce hypertension within 14 days of MAO inhibitor therapy. Metoprolol may negate the beneficial beta₁ cardiac effects of dopamine or dobutamine. Concurrent thyroid administration may decrease effectiveness of metoprolol.
- Use with caution in patients with hyperthyroidism (may mask symptoms) or diabetes mellitus (may mask signs of hypoglycemia). Geriatric patients may have altered sensitivity to beta-adrenergic blocking agents.
- Use cautiously during pregnancy. Metoprolol may cause apnea, low Apgar scores, bradycardia, and hypoglycemia

in the newborn (Pregnancy Category B). Safe use during lactation or in children has not been established.

Lab Test Considerations

• Metoprolol may occasionally cause elevations in serum potassium, uric acid, lipoprotein levels, and BUN.
• Hepatic and renal function and CBC should be monitored periodically in patients receiving prolonged therapy.

Patient/Family Teaching

• Instruct patient to notify physician if slow pulse rate, dizziness, light-headedness, or depression occurs. Metoprolol should not be abruptly discontinued.

PHARMACOLOGIC PROFILE

Indications

• Metoprolol is used in the prevention of myocardial re-infarction.

Action

• Metoprolol blocks stimulation of beta$_1$ (myocardial) adrenergic receptors with less effect on beta$_2$ (pulmonary, vascular, or uterine) receptor sites. The overall beneficial effect is that of decreased blood pressure and heart rate.

Time/Action Profile (beta-adrenergic blockade)

Onset	Peak	Duration
immediate	20 min	5–8 hr

Pharmacokinetics

• **Distribution:** Metoprolol crosses the blood–brain barrier and the placenta. Small amounts enter breast milk. • **Metabolism and Excretion:** Metoprolol is mostly metabolized by the liver. • **Half-life:** 3–7 hours.

Contraindications

• Metoprolol is contraindicated in patients with uncompensated congestive heart failure, pulmonary edema, cardiogenic shock, bradycardia, or heart block.

Adverse Reactions and Side Effects*

• **CNS:** <u>fatigue</u>, <u>weakness</u>, dizziness, <u>depression</u>, memory loss, mental changes, nightmares • **EENT:** blurred vision • **Resp:** bronchospasm, wheezing • **CV:** BRADYCARDIA, PULMONARY EDEMA, CONGESTIVE HEART FAILURE, peripheral vasoconstriction • **GI:** constipation, diarrhea, nausea • **GU:** impotence, diminished libido.

Metronidazole/ Metronidazole Hydrochloride	Anti-infective (miscellaneous)
Flagyl IV RTU, Flagyl IV, Metronidazole Redi-Infusion, Metro IV	pH 5–7 pH 0.5–2 before diluting and neutralizing pH 6–7 after diluting and neutralizing

ADMINISTRATION CONSIDERATIONS

Usual Dose

Anaerobic Infections

ADULTS AND CHILDREN >7 days: Initial dose 15 mg/kg, then 7.5 mg/kg q 6 hr (not to exceed 4 g/day).

INFANTS <7 days: 15 mg/kg initially, then 7.5 mg/kg q 12 hr, starting 24 hr after first dose.

PREMATURE INFANTS: 15 mg/kg initially, then 7.5 mg/kg q 12 hr starting 48 hr after first dose.

Amebiasis

ADULTS: 500–750 mg q 8 hr (unlabeled).

Dilution

• **Intermittent Infusion:** Ready-to-use products are **pre-diluted** and ready to use (5 mg/ml). • Prefilled plastic mini-bags should not be used in serial connections, as air embolism may result. Crystals may form during refrigeration but will

---

*<u>Underlines</u> indicate most frequent; CAPITALS indicate life-threatening.

dissolve when warmed to room temperature. • Preparation of lyophilized powder *Flagyl IV* requires a specific process. Do not use aluminum needles or hubs; color will turn orange/rust. • **Add** 4.4 ml of sterile or bacteriostatic sterile water, or 0.9% or bacteriostatic 0.9% NaCl for injection (100 mg/ml). Solution should be clear, pale yellow-green. Do not use cloudy or precipitated solution. **Dilute further** to a concentration not to exceed 8 mg/ml with 0.9% NaCl, D5W, or lactated Ringer's solution. Neutralize solution with 5 mEq sodium bicarbonate for each 500 mg. Mix thoroughly. Carbon dioxide gas will be generated and may require venting. • Do not refrigerate. Stable for 24 hours at room temperature.

Compatibility

• **Y-site:** acyclovir • allopurinol sodium • cyclophosphamide • diltiazem • enalaprilat • esmolol • fluconazole • foscarnet • hydromorphone • labetalol • magnesium sulfate • melphalan • meperidine • morphine • perphenazine • piperacillin/tazobactam • sargramostim • tacrolimus • vinorelbine. • Manufacturer recommends discontinuing primary IV during metronidazole infusion.

• **Additive:** amikacin • aminophylline • cefazolin • cefotaxime • ceftazidime • cefuroxime • chloramphenicol • ciprofloxacin • clindamycin • fluconazole • gentamicin • heparin • multivitamins • netilmicin • tobramycin. • Manufacturer recommends not admixing with other medications.

Incompatibility

• **Additive:** amino acids • aztreonam • dopamine.

Rate of Administration

• **Intermittent Infusion:** Administer IV doses as a slow infusion, each single dose over 1 hour.

≋ CLINICAL PRECAUTIONS

- Assess patient for infection (vital signs; appearance of wound, sputum, urine, and stool; WBC) at beginning and throughout course of therapy.
- Obtain specimens for culture and sensitivity prior to initiating therapy. First dose may be given before receiving results.
- Monitor neurologic status during and after IV infusions

for numbness, paresthesia, weakness, ataxia, or convulsions.

- Monitor intake and output and daily weights, especially for patients on sodium restriction. Each 500 mg of lyophilized powder Flagyl IV for dilution contains 5 mEq of sodium; each 500 mg of metronidazole ready-to-use contains 14 mEq of sodium.

- Cimetidine may decrease the metabolism of metronidazole. Phenobarbital increases metabolism and may decrease effectiveness. A disulfiram-like reaction may occur with alcohol ingestion. Metronidazole may cause acute psychosis and confusion with disulfiram. There is increased risk of leukopenia with concurrent use of fluorouracil or azathioprine. The anticoagulant effect of warfarin may be enhanced by metronidazole. The effects of phenytoin and lithium may be increased by metronidazole.

- Use metronidazole cautiously in patients with a history of blood dyscrasias, seizures, or neurologic problems. Patients with severe hepatic impairment or geriatric patients may require reduced dosage.

- Although safe use of IV metronidazole in pregnancy has not been established, the oral form has been used to treat trichomoniasis in the second and third trimester, but not as single-dose regimen (Pregnancy Category B). Safe use in children has not been established (use is unlabeled).

Lab Test Considerations

- Metronidazole may cause low serum AST (SGOT) levels.

Patient/Family Teaching

- Caution patients to avoid intake of alcoholic beverages or alcohol-containing preparations during and for at least 1 day following treatment with metronidazole; a disulfiram-like reaction (flushing, nausea, vomiting, headache, abdominal cramps) may occur. • Metronidazole may cause dizziness or light-headedness. Caution patient to avoid activities requiring alertness until response to medication is known. • Advise patient that frequent mouth rinses, good oral hygiene, and sugarless gum or candy may minimize dry mouth. • Advise patient to inform physician if pregnancy is suspected prior to taking this medication. • Inform patient that medication may cause urine to turn dark. • Advise patient to consult physician if there is no improvement in a few days or if signs and symptoms of superinfection (black, furry overgrowth on tongue; vaginal itching or discharge; loose or foul-smelling stools) or allergy develop.

≋ PHARMACOLOGIC PROFILE

Indications

• Metronidazole is used in the treatment of the following anaerobic infections: intra-abdominal infections, gynecologic infections, skin and skin structure infections, lower respiratory tract infections, bone and joint infections, CNS infections, septicemia, and endocarditis. It is also used as a perioperative prophylactic agent in colorectal surgery.

Action

• Metronidazole disrupts DNA and protein synthesis in susceptible organisms, resulting in bactericidal, trichomonacidal, or amebicidal action. Metronidazole is most notable for activity against anaerobic bacteria, including *Bacteroides* and *Clostridium*. In addition, it is active against *Trichomonas vaginalis, Entamoeba histolytica,* and *Giardia lamblia.*

Time/Action Profile (blood levels)

Onset	Peak
rapid	end of infusion

Pharmacokinetics

• **Distribution:** Metronidazole is widely distributed into most tissues and fluids, including CSF. It crosses the placenta and enters breast milk in concentrations equal to plasma levels. • **Metabolism and Excretion:** Metronidazole is partially metabolized by the liver (30–60%), partially excreted unchanged in the urine, with 6–15% eliminated in the feces. • **Half-life:** 6–8 hours.

Contraindications

• Metronidazole is contraindicated in patients with hypersensitivity to it. It should not be used in the first trimester of pregnancy or during lactation. Lyophilized powder contains mannitol and should be avoided in patients with known intolerance.

Adverse Reactions and Side Effects*

• **CNS:** <u>headache</u>, vertigo, SEIZURES, <u>dizziness</u> • **GI:** <u>nausea</u>, <u>vomiting</u>, <u>abdominal pain</u>, <u>anorexia</u>, dry mouth, <u>diarrhea</u>, unpleasant taste, furry tongue, glossitis • **Derm:** urticaria, rashes • **Hemat:** leukopenia • **Local:** phlebitis at IV site • **Neuro:** peripheral neuropathy • **Misc:** superinfection.

Mezlocillin Sodium	*Anti-infective*
	(extended-spectrum penicillin)
Mezlin	pH 4.5–8 (depends on concentration)
	Na 1.85 mEq/g

≋ ADMINISTRATION CONSIDERATIONS

Usual Dose

ADULTS: *Most infections*—3–4 g q 4–6 hr (33.3–58.3 mg/kg q 4 hr or 50–87.5 mg/kg q 6 hr; not to exceed 24 g/day). *Acute uncomplicated gonococcal urethritis:* 1–2 g single dose preceded by 1 g probenecid orally 30 min before.

CHILDREN 1 mo–12 yr: 50 mg/kg q 4 hr.

NEONATES >2 kg: 50 mg/kg q 8 hr during first 7 days of life, then 50 mg/kg q 6 hr.

NEONATES <2 kg: 50 mg/kg q 12 hr during first 7 days of life, then 50 mg/kg q 8 hr.

Dilution

• **Direct IV:** The initial **reconstitution** is made with at least 10 ml of sterile water for injection, 0.9% NaCl, or D5W. Shake vigorously. • Reconstituted solution is stable for 48 hours at room temperature and 72 hours if refrigerated. Solution is colorless to pale yellow; darkened solution does not affect potency. • **Intermittent Infusion:** Dilute in 50–100 ml of 0.9% NaCl, D5W, D10W, D5/0.25% NaCl, D5/0.45% NaCl, Ringer's or lactated Ringer's solution.

---

*Underlines indicate most frequent; CAPITALS indicate life-threatening.

Compatibility

- **Syringe:** heparin.
- **Y-site:** cyclophosphamide ◆ famotidine ◆ fludarabine ◆ hydromorphone ◆ morphine ◆ perphenazine ◆ sargramostim ◆ tacrolimus.

Incompatibility

- **Y-site:** ciprofloxacin ◆ filgrastim ◆ idarubicin ◆ meperidine ◆ ondansetron ◆ verapamil. • If aminoglycosides and penicillins or cephalosporins must be given concurrently, administer in separate sites at least 1 hour apart.
- **Additive:** ciprofloxacin.

Rate of Administration

- **Direct IV:** Inject slowly, 1 g over 3–5 minutes to minimize vein irritation. • **Intermittent Infusion:** Administer over 30 minutes.

≋ CLINICAL PRECAUTIONS

- Change IV sites every 48 hours to prevent phlebitis.
- Assess patient for infection (vital signs; appearance of wound, sputum, urine, and stool; WBC) at beginning and throughout course of therapy.
- Obtain specimens for culture and sensitivity prior to initiating therapy. First dose may be given before receiving results.
- Obtain a history before initiating therapy to determine previous use of and reactions to penicillins or cephalosporins. Persons with a negative history of penicillin sensitivity may still have an allergic response. Observe patient for signs and symptoms of anaphylaxis (rash, pruritus, laryngeal edema, wheezing). Discontinue the drug and notify the physician immediately if these occur. Keep epinephrine, an antihistamine, and resuscitation equipment close by in the event of an anaphylactic reaction.
- Use cautiously in patients with renal impairment. Dosage reduction is suggested if creatinine clearance is 30 ml/min or less. Use cautiously in patients with pre-existing hepatic disease.
- Probenecid decreases renal excretion and increases blood levels of mezlocillin. Mezlocillin may alter excre-

tion of lithium. Concurrent use of diuretics may increase the risk of hypokalemia. Hypokalemia increases the risk of cardiac glycoside toxicity. The risk of hepatotoxicity is increased when used with other hepatotoxic drugs.
• Safe use in pregnancy or lactation has not been established (Pregnancy Category B).

Lab Test Considerations

• Renal and hepatic function, CBC, and serum potassium should be evaluated prior to and routinely throughout course of therapy. • Mezlocillin may cause false-positive urine protein test results and may cause elevated serum creatinine, AST (SGOT), ALT (SGPT), bilirubin, and alkaline phosphatase. In addition, it may elevate serum sodium and decrease serum potassium levels.

Patient/Family Teaching

• Advise patient to report the signs of superinfection (black, furry overgrowth on the tongue; vaginal itching or discharge; loose or foul-smelling stools) and allergy. • Advise patient to notify physician if fever and diarrhea develop, especially if stool contains blood, pus, or mucus. Instruct patient not to treat diarrhea without consulting physician or pharmacist.

≋ PHARMACOLOGIC PROFILE

Indications

• Mezlocillin is used in the treatment of serious infections due to susceptible organisms, including skin and skin structure infections, bone and joint infections, septicemia, respiratory tract infections, intra-abdominal infections, gynecologic infections, and urinary tract infections. The combination with an aminoglycoside or agent with similar spectrum is recommended for infections suspected to be caused by *Pseudomonas aeruginosa,* other Gram-negative organisms or mixed infections. Mezlocillin has been combined with other antibiotics in the treatment of infections in immunosuppressed patients.

Action

• Mezlocillin binds to the bacterial cell wall membrane, causing cell death in susceptible bacteria. Its spectrum is similar to penicillin but greatly extended to include several important Gram-negative aerobic pathogens, notably *Pseudomonas aeruginosa, Escherichia coli, Proteus mirabilis,* and *Providencia rettgeri* (combination therapy recommended). It is also active against some anaerobic bacteria, including *Bacteroides,* but it is not active against penicillinase-producing staphylococci or beta-lactamase producing Enterobacteriaceae.

Time/Action Profile (blood levels)

Onset	Peak
rapid	end of infusion

Pharmacokinetics

• **Distribution:** Mezlocillin is widely distributed. It enters CSF well only when meninges are inflamed, and crosses the placenta and enters breast milk in low concentrations. • **Metabolism and Excretion:** 55–60% of mezlocillin is excreted unchanged by the kidneys. Small amounts are metabolized by the liver; 15–30% is excreted in the bile. • **Half-life:** 0.7–1.3 hours (increased in renal impairment).

Contraindications

• Mezlocillin is contraindicated in patients with hypersensitivity to penicillins or cephalosporins.

Adverse Reactions and Side Effects*

• **CNS:** confusion, lethargy, SEIZURES (high doses) • **CV:** congestive heart failure, arrhythmias • **GI:** nausea, diarrhea, abnormal liver function tests • **GU:** hematuria (children only) • **Derm:** rashes, urticaria • **F and E:** hypokalemia, hypernatremia • **Hemat:** bleeding, blood dyscrasias, increased bleeding time • **Local:** phlebitis at IV site • **Metab:** metabolic alkalosis • **Misc:** superinfection, hypersensitivity reactions, including ANAPHYLAXIS and serum sickness.

---

*Underlines indicate most frequent; CAPITALS indicate life-threatening.

Miconazole	*Antifungal*
Monistat IV	pH 3.7–5.7

ADMINISTRATION CONSIDERATIONS

Usual Dose
ADULTS: 67–1200 mg q 8 hr.
CHILDREN **1–12 yr:** 6.7–13.3 mg/kg q 8 hr (not to exceed 15-mg/kg dose).
CHILDREN **<1 yr:** 5–10 mg/kg q 8 hr.

Dilution
• **Intermittent Infusion: Dilute** each dose in at least 200 ml of 0.9% NaCl or D5W. • Solution is stable at room temperature for 48 hours. Darkened color of solution shows deterioration; discard.

Compatibility
• **Y-site:** allopurinol sodium • filgrastim • foscarnet • melphalan • ondansetron • sargramostim • vinorelbine.
• **Additive:** Manufacturer does not recommend admixing miconazole with other medications.

Incompatibility
• **Y-site:** fludarabine • piperacillin/tazobactam.

Rate of Administration
• **Intermittent Infusion:** Administer over 30–60 minutes. • Rapid administration may cause transient tachycardia, arrhythmias, cardiorespiratory arrest, or anaphylaxis.

CLINICAL PRECAUTIONS

- Initial dose of 200 mg should be administered under physician's supervision to determine hypersensitivity.
- Assess patient for infection prior to and throughout course of therapy.
- Obtain specimens for culture prior to treatment. First dose may be given before receiving results.
- Monitor IV site closely for phlebitis.
- Nausea and vomiting may be minimized by reducing dose, slowing the infusion rate, avoiding administration

at mealtime, or by using prophylactic antiemetics or antihistamines.
- Treatment of fungal meningitis requires concurrent intrathecal miconazole (20 mg q 3–7 days).
- Treatment of bladder mycoses requires concurrent irrigation with miconazole (200 mg 2–4 times daily or continuously).
- Miconazole enhances the anticoagulant effect of warfarin. Concurrent use with rifampin or isoniazid decreases blood levels and effectiveness of miconazole. Miconazole may enhance the effect of oral hypoglycemic agents.
- Safe use in pregnancy, lactation, or children <1 year has not been established (Pregnancy Category C).

Lab Test Considerations

- Hemoglobin, hematocrit, serum electrolytes, and lipids should be monitored periodically throughout therapy. Miconazole may cause abnormalities in tests of serum lipid concentrations.

Patient/Family Teaching

- Instruct patient to notify nurse or physician if signs of hypersensitivity reaction (fever, chills, skin rash, itching) or phlebitis (redness, swelling, pain at the injection site) occur.

≋ PHARMACOLOGIC PROFILE

Indications

- Miconazole is used intravenously in the treatment of severe systemic fungal infections, including fungal pneumonia and disseminated infections.

Action

- Miconazole alters permeability of fungal cell membrane and function of fungal enzymes, resulting in a fungistatic or fungicidal action. It is active against all pathogenic fungi and Gram-positive bacteria including *Aspergillus, Coccidioides, Cryptococcus, Candida albicans, Histoplasma,* and dermatophytes.

Time/Action Profile (blood levels)

Onset	Peak
rapid	end of infusion

Pharmacokinetics

• **Distribution:** Following administration, miconazole is widely distributed. CSF penetration is poor, necessitating intrathecal administration in the treatment of meningitis. • **Metabolism and Excretion:** Miconazole is mostly metabolized by the liver. • **Half-life:** 24 hours.

Contraindications

• Miconazole is contraindicated in patients with hypersensitivity to it or to castor oil.

Adverse Reactions and Side Effects*

• **CNS:** drowsiness, dizziness, anxiety, headache • **EENT:** blurred vision, dry eyes • **CV:** arrhythmias • **GI:** <u>nausea</u>, <u>vomiting</u>, diarrhea, bitter taste • **F and E:** hyponatremia • **Hemat:** anemia • **Local:** <u>phlebitis</u>, <u>pruritus</u> • **Misc:** hyperlipidemia, fever, increased libido, allergic reaction, including ANAPHYLAXIS.

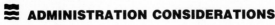

Midazolam Hydrochloride	*Sedative/hypnotic (benzodiazepine)*
Versed	pH 3

Schedule IV

≋ ADMINISTRATION CONSIDERATIONS

Usual Dose

Dosage must be individualized, taking caution to reduce dosage in elderly patients and those who are already sedated.

---

*<u>Underlines</u> indicate most frequent; CAPITALS indicate life-threatening.

Conscious Sedation for Short Procedures (endoscopy or cardiovascular procedures)

ADULTS: 1–2.5 mg initially; dosage may be increased further as needed, waiting at least 2 min between increments; total doses >5 mg are rarely needed. If additional doses are required to maintain sedation, 25% of the initial dose required for sedation may be used.

GERIATRIC (>60 YR) OR DEBILITATED PATIENTS: Initial dose should not exceed 1.5 mg; dosage may be increased further as needed, waiting at least 2 min between increments. Total doses >3.5 mg are rarely needed. If additional doses are required to maintain sedation, 25% of the initial dose required for sedation may be used.

Adjunct to Induction of Anesthesia (without premedication)

ADULTS UP TO 55 YR: 200–350 mcg/kg initially. May give additional dose of 25% of initial dose, if needed, up to 600 mcg/kg total.

GERIATRIC (≥55 YR BUT GENRALLY HEALTHY): initial dose 150–300 mcg/kg.

GERIATRIC (≥55 YR AND SERIOUSLY ILL OR DEBILITATED PATIENTS): initial dose 150–250 mcg/kg.

CHILDREN: 50–200 mcg/kg (decreased if used with premedication).

Adjunct to Induction of Anesthesia (with opioid or sedative premedication)

ADULTS UP TO 55 YR: 150–350 mcg/kg initially (generally not more than 250 mcg/kg). May give additional doses in increments of 25% of induction dose.

GERIATRIC (≥55 YR BUT GENERALLY HEALTHY): initial dose 200 mcg/kg.

GERIATRIC (≥55 YR AND SERIOUSLY ILL OR DEBILITATED PATIENTS): initial dose 150 mcg/kg.

Adjunct to Local Anesthesia (unlabeled use)

ADULTS: 30–60 mcg/kg; may require further adjustment.

Dilution

• **Direct IV:** Administer **undiluted or diluted** with D5W, 0.9% NaCl, or lactated Ringer's injection through Y-site or 3-way stopcock. • Solution is stable for 24 hours if diluted with D5W or 0.9% NaCl, or 4 hours if diluted with lactated Ringer's injection. • Solution is colorless to light yellow.

Compatibility

*   **Syringe:** atracurium ✦ atropine ✦ benzquinamide ✦ buprenorphine ✦ butorphanol ✦ chlorpromazine ✦ cimetidine ✦ diphenhydramine ✦ droperidol ✦ fentanyl ✦ glycopyrrolate ✦ hydromorphone ✦ hydroxyzine ✦ meperidine ✦ metoclopramide ✦ morphine ✦ nalbuphine ✦ promazine ✦ promethazine ✦ scopolamine ✦ thiethylperazine ✦ trimethobenzamide.
*   **Y-site:** atracurium ✦ famotidine ✦ fluconazole ✦ pancuronium ✦ vecuronium.

Incompatibility

*   **Syringe:** dimenhydrinate ✦ pentobarbital ✦ perphenazine ✦ prochlorperazine ✦ ranitidine.
*   **Y-site:** foscarnet.

Rate of Administration

*   **Direct IV:** Administer each dose slowly over at least 2 minutes. Monitor IV site closely to avoid extravasation. Titrate dose to patient response. In patients who are over 60 years or debilitated, give no more than 1.5 mg over at least 2 minutes. Wait at least 2 minutes then give no more than 1 mg over 2 minutes, then wait at least 2 minutes before giving more.

☰ CLINICAL PRECAUTIONS

*   Assess level of sedation and level of consciousness throughout and for 2–6 hours following administration. Dosage must be individualized, taking caution to reduce dosage and injection rate in elderly patients and those who are already sedated. Range of titration from sedation to unconsciousness with midazolam is relatively narrow.
*   Monitor blood pressure, pulse, and respiration continuously throughout administration. Oxygen and resuscitative equipment should be immediately available.
*   Use cautiously in patients with pulmonary disease, congestive heart failure, renal impairment, or severe hepatic impairment. Elderly or debilitated patients are more susceptible to depressant effects; dosage reduction is required. Safe use in children has not been established.
*   Additive CNS depression may occur with alcohol, antihistamines, opioid analgesics, and other sedative/hypnotics; midazolam dose should be decreased by 30% if used concurrently (50% in geriatric patients). Concur-

rent use with antihypertensives, acute ingestion of alcohol, or nitrates increases the risk of hypotension.
• Use cautiously in patients with childbearing potential. Avoid using midazolam during pregnancy or lactation (Pregnancy Category D).

Toxicity and Overdose Alert

• If overdose occurs, flumazenil (Mazicon) (see *flumazenil* monograph, page 437) is the antidote. • Monitor pulse, respiration, and blood pressure continuously until stable. Maintain patent airway and assist ventilation as needed. If hypotension occurs, treatment includes IV fluids, repositioning, and vasopressors.

Patient/Family Teaching

• Inform patient that this medication will decrease mental recall of the procedure. • Midazolam may cause drowsiness or dizziness. Advise patient to request assistance prior to ambulation and transfer, and to avoid driving or other activities requiring alertness for 24 hours following administration. • Instruct patient to inform physician prior to administration if pregnancy is suspected. • Advise patient to avoid alcohol or other CNS depressants for 24 hours following administration of midazolam.

 PHARMACOLOGIC PROFILE

Indications

• Midazolam is used to produce anterograde amnesia postoperatively and to aid in the induction of anesthesia. • It also provides conscious sedation before diagnostic or radiographic procedures. • Midazolam may also be used to provide conscious sedation during dental and minor surgical procedures (unlabeled use).

Action

• Midazolam acts at many levels of the CNS to produce short-term, generalized CNS depression. These effects may be mediated by gamma-aminobutyric acid (GABA), an inhibitory neurotransmitter. It has no analgesic properties.

Time/Action Profile (sedation)

Onset	Peak	Duration
1.5–5 min	rapid	2–6 hr

Pharmacokinetics

• **Distribution:** Midazolam crosses the blood–brain barrier and placenta. • **Metabolism and Excretion:** It is almost exclusively metabolized by the liver. • **Half-life:** 1–12 hours (increased in renal impairment or congestive heart failure).

Contraindications

• Midazolam is contraindicated in patients with hypersensitivity to it. Cross-sensitivity with other benzodiazepines may occur. Avoid using midazolam in patients who are in shock or in comatose patients or those with pre-existing CNS depression. Midazolam should not be used in patients who have uncontrolled severe pain. Injection contains benzyl alcohol and should be avoided in patients with known intolerance. Pregnant or lactating patients should not receive midazolam.

Adverse Reactions and Side Effects*

• **CNS:** headache, excess sedation, drowsiness, agitation • **EENT:** blurred vision • **Resp:** coughing, LARYNGOSPASM, bronchospasm, RESPIRATORY DEPRESSION, APNEA • **CV:** arrhythmias, CARDIAC ARREST • **GI:** hiccups, nausea, vomiting • **Derm:** rashes • **Local:** phlebitis at IV site.

Milrinone Lactate	Inotropic agent
Primacor	pH 3.2–4.0

 ADMINISTRATION CONSIDERATIONS

Usual Dose

ADULTS: Loading dose—50 mcg/kg followed by infusion at 0.50 mcg/kg/min (range 0.375–0.75 mcg/kg/min).

---

*Underlines indicate most frequent; CAPITALS indicate life-threatening.

Dilution

• **Direct IV:** Loading dose may be administered **undiluted**. • **Continuous Infusion:** The 20-mg vial may be **diluted** with 180 ml of diluent for a concentration of 100 mcg/ml, with 113 ml of diluent for a concentration of 150 mcg/ml, or with 80 ml of diluent for a concentration of 200 mcg/ml. Compatible diluents include 0.45% NaCl, 0.9% NaCl, and D5W. • Solution is colorless to pale yellow. Do not use solutions that are discolored or contain particulate matter.

Compatibility

• **Syringe:** atropine ✦ calcium chloride ✦ digoxin ✦ epinephrine ✦ lidocaine ✦ morphine ✦ propranolol ✦ sodium bicarbonate ✦ verapamil.

• **Y-site:** digoxin ✦ propranolol ✦ quinidine gluconate.

• **Additive:** quinidine gluconate.

Incompatibility

• **Syringe:** bumetanide ✦ furosemide.

• **Y-site:** furosemide ✦ procainamide.

• **Additive:** procainamide.

Rate of Administration

• **Direct IV:** Administer the loading dose over 10 minutes. • **Continuous Infusion:** See Infusion Rate Table below.

**MILRINONE (Primacor) INFUSION RATE TABLE
(at various concentrations)**

Milrinone loading dose: 50 mcg/kg over 10 min (may be given as undiluted drug)

Milrinone Infusion Rates (mcg/kg/min)	100 mcg/ml Concentration	200 mcg/ml Concentration	300 mcg/ml Concentration
0.375 (mcg/kg/min)	0.22 ml/kg/hr	0.15 ml/kg/hr	0.11 ml/kg/hr
0.400 (mcg/kg/min)	0.24 ml/kg/hr	0.16 ml/kg/hr	0.12 ml/kg/hr
0.500 (mcg/kg/min)	0.30 ml/kg/hr	0.20 ml/kg/hr	0.15 ml/kg/hr
0.600 (mcg/kg/min)	0.36 ml/kg/hr	0.24 ml/kg/hr	0.18 ml/kg/hr
0.700 (mcg/kg/min)	0.42 ml/kg/hr	0.28 ml/kg/hr	0.21 ml/kg/hr
0.750 (mcg/kg/min)	0.45 ml/kg/hr	0.30 ml/kg/hr	0.22 ml/kg/hr

≋ CLINICAL PRECAUTIONS

• Monitor heart rate and blood pressure continuously during administration. Milrinone should be slowed or discontinued if blood pressure drops excessively.

- Monitor fluid and electrolyte status and daily weight. Cardiac index, central venous pressure (CVP), and pulmonary capillary wedge pressure (PCWP) measurements should be used to determine efficacy of milrinone. The effects of previous aggressive diuretic therapy should be corrected to allow for optimal filling pressure. Electrolyte abnormalities should also be corrected to decrease the risk of arrhythmias.
- Monitor ECG continuously during infusion. Arrhythmias are common and may be life-threatening. The risk of ventricular arrhythmias is increased in patients with a history of arrhythmias, electrolyte abnormalities, abnormal digoxin levels, or patients who have undergone insertion of vascular catheters.
- Patients with atrial fibrillation or flutter may require pretreatment with digoxin since milrinone may increase ventricular response rates.
- Monitor infusion site closely to prevent extravasation.
- Use cautiously in patients with renal impairment. Infusion rates should be decreased if creatinine clearance is 50 ml/min/1.73 m^2 or less.
- Safe use in pregnancy, lactation, or children has not been established (Pregnancy Category C).

Toxicity and Overdose Alert

- Overdose manifests as hypotension. Dose should be decreased or discontinued. Supportive measures may be necessary.

Lab Test Considerations

- Monitor electrolytes and renal function frequently during administration. Hypokalemia should be corrected prior to administration. • If creatinine clearance is less than 50 ml/min, reduction of infusion rate is recommended. • Monitor platelet count during therapy.

Patient/Family Teaching

- Inform patient and family of reasons for administration. Milrinone is not a cure but a temporary measure to control the symptoms of congestive heart failure.

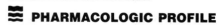

PHARMACOLOGIC PROFILE

Indications
• Short-term treatment of congestive heart failure unresponsive to conventional therapy with cardiac glycosides, diuretics, and vasodilators.

Action
• Increases myocardial contractility. • Decrease preload and afterload by a direct dilating effect on vascular smooth muscle. Net hemodynamic effect is increased cardiac output (inotropic effect).

Time/Action Profile (hemodynamic effects)

Onset	Peak	Duration
5–15 min	UK	UK

Pharmacokinetics
• **Distribution:** UK. • **Metabolism and Excretion:** 80–90% of milrinone is excreted unchanged by the kidneys. • **Half-life:** 2.3 hours (increased in renal impairment).

Contraindications
• Milrinone should be avoided in patients with severe aortic or pulmonic valvular heart disease. It may increase outflow tract obstruction in patients with hypertrophic subaortic stenosis.

Adverse Reactions and Side Effects*
• **CNS:** headache, tremor • **CV:** <u>VENTRICULAR ARRHYTHMIAS</u>, <u>supraventricular arrhythmias</u>, hypotension, angina pectoris, chest pain • **F and E:** hypokalemia • **Hemat:** thrombocytopenia.

---

*<u>Underlines</u> indicate most frequent; CAPITALS indicate life-threatening.

Minocycline Hydrochloride	*Anti-infective (tetracycline)*
Minocin	pH 2–2.8

≋ ADMINISTRATION CONSIDERATIONS

Usual Dose

ADULTS: 200 mg initially, then 100 mg q 12 hr.
CHILDREN ≥8 YR: 4 mg/kg initially, then 2 mg/kg q 12 hr.

Dilution

• **Intermittent Infusion: Dilute** each 100 mg with 5 ml of sterile water for injection for a concentration of 20 mg/ml. **Dilute further** to concentration of 100–200 mcg/ml in 500–1000 ml of 0.9% NaCl, D5W, D5/0.9% NaCl, Ringer's or lactated Ringer's solution. • Solution is stable for 24 hours at room temperature.

Compatibility

• **Y-site:** allopurinol sodium ◆ cyclophosphamide ◆ filgrastim ◆ fludarabine ◆ heparin ◆ hydrocortisone sodium succinate ◆ magnesium sulfate ◆ melphalan ◆ perphenazine ◆ potassium chloride ◆ sargramostim ◆ vinorelbine ◆ vitamin B complex with C.

Incompatibility

• **Y-site:** hydromorphone ◆ meperidine ◆ morphine ◆ piperacillin/tazobactam.

Rate of Administration

• **Intermittent Infusion:** Administer at prescribed rate, usually over 6 hours, immediately following dilution. Avoid rapid infusions. May cause thrombophlebitis; avoid extravasation.

≋ CLINICAL PRECAUTIONS

• Assess patient for infection (vital signs; appearance of wound, sputum, urine, and stool; WBC) at beginning and throughout course of therapy.
• Obtain specimens for culture and sensitivity prior to initiating therapy. First dose may be given before receiving results.

- Minocycline should be used cautiously in cachectic or debilitated patients or patients who have hepatic or renal disease. Geriatric patients may be more sensitive to the CNS effects of minocycline.
- Minocycline may enhance the effect of oral anticoagulants and decrease the effectiveness of oral contraceptives.
- Because of its effects on teeth and bones, minocycline should not be used during pregnancy or lactation or in children under 8 years (Pregnancy Category D).

Lab Test Considerations

- Minocycline may cause increased AST (SGOT), ALT (SGPT), serum alkaline phosphatase, bilirubin, and amylase concentrations.

Patient/Family Teaching

- Minocycline commonly causes dizziness, light-headedness, or unsteadiness. Caution patient to avoid activities requiring alertness until response to medication is known. • Caution patient to use sunscreen and protective clothing to prevent photosensitivity reactions. • Advise patient to use a nonhormonal method of contraception while taking minocycline. • Advise patient to report the signs of superinfection (black, furry overgrowth on the tongue; vaginal itching or discharge; loose or foul-smelling stools). Skin rash, pruritus, and urticaria should also be reported. • Instruct the patient to notify the physician if symptoms do not improve.

≋ PHARMACOLOGIC PROFILE

Indications

- Minocycline is used most commonly in the treatment of infections due to unusual (atypical) organisms, including *Mycoplasma, Chlamydia,* and *Rickettsia.* It may be used in the treatment of gonorrhea in patients who cannot tolerate conventional therapy.

Action

- Minocycline inhibits bacterial protein synthesis at the level of the 30S ribosome, resulting in bacteriostatic action against susceptible bacteria. It is active against a wide variety of Gram-positive, Gram-negative, and atypical organisms, including *Neisseria meningitidis, N. gonorrhoeae, Treponema pallidum, Chlamydia trachomatis, Ureaplasma urealyticum, Mycoplasma pneumoniae,* and *Nocardia.*

Time/Action Profile (blood levels)

Onset	Peak
rapid	end of infusion

Pharmacokinetics

• **Distribution:** Minocycline is widely distributed, with some penetration into CSF. It crosses the placenta and enters breast milk. • **Metabolism and Excretion:** 5–20% of minocycline is excreted unchanged by the urine. Some metabolism occurs in the liver with enterohepatic circulation and excretion in bile and feces. • **Half-life:** 11–26 hours.

Contraindications

• Minocycline is contraindicated in patients with hypersensitivity to it, and in children younger than 8 years of age, as it may cause permanent yellow-brown discoloration and softening of teeth and bones. Pregnant or lactating patients should not receive minocycline.

Adverse Reactions and Side Effects*

• **CNS:** light-headedness, dizziness, vertigo • **EENT:** vestibular reactions • **GI:** nausea, vomiting, diarrhea, pancreatitis, hepatotoxicity • **Derm:** rashes, photosensitivity • **Hemat:** blood dyscrasias • **Local:** phlebitis at IV site • **Misc:** superinfection, hypersensitivity reactions.

Mitomycin	*Antineoplastic (antitumor antibiotic)*
Mutamycin	pH 6–8

≋ **ADMINISTRATION CONSIDERATIONS**

Usual Dose

ADULTS AND CHILDREN: 10–20 mg/m^2 q 6–8 wk.

---

*Underlines indicate most frequent; CAPITALS indicate life-threatening.

Dilution

• **Direct IV:** Reconstitute 5-mg vial with 10 ml, 10-mg vial with 40 ml, and 40-mg vial with 80 ml of sterile water for injection. Shake the vial; may need to stand at room temperature for additional time to dissolve. Final solution is blue-gray. • Solution should be prepared in a biologic cabinet. Wear gloves, gown, and mask while handling medication. Discard equipment in designated containers (see Appendix F). • Reconstituted solution is stable for 7 days at room temperature, 14 days if refrigerated.

Compatibility

• **Syringe:** bleomycin ◆ cisplatin ◆ cyclophosphamide ◆ doxorubicin ◆ droperidol ◆ fluorouracil ◆ furosemide ◆ heparin ◆ leucovorin ◆ methotrexate ◆ metoclopramide ◆ vinblastine ◆ vincristine.

• **Y-site:** allopurinol sodium ◆ bleomycin ◆ cisplatin ◆ cyclophosphamide ◆ doxorubicin ◆ droperidol ◆ fluorouracil ◆ furosemide ◆ heparin ◆ leucovorin ◆ melphalan ◆ methotrexate ◆ metoclopramide ◆ ondansetron ◆ vinblastine ◆ vincristine.

• **Solution:** lactated Ringer's injection ◆ 0.3% NaCl ◆ 0.5% NaCl ◆ 0.9% NaCl.

Incompatibility

• **Y-site:** filgrastim ◆ piperacillin/tazobactam ◆ sargramostim ◆ vinorelbine.
• **Additive:** bleomycin.
• **Solution:** D5W.

Rate of Administration

• **Direct IV:** May be administered IV push over 5–10 minutes through a free-flowing IV of 0.9% NaCl or D5W.

≋ CLINICAL PRECAUTIONS

• Monitor vital signs periodically during administration.
• Ensure patency of IV. Mitomycin is a vesicant. If patient complains of discomfort at IV site, discontinue immediately and restart infusion at another site. Extravasation may also occur painlessly, may cause delayed erythema and ulceration weeks or months after administration at

or distant from site of infusion, and may cause severe tissue necrosis. Surgical excision at the involved area may be necessary.

- Monitor intake and output, appetite, and nutritional intake. Nausea and vomiting usually occur within 1–2 hours. Vomiting may stop within 3–4 hours; nausea may persist for 2–3 days. Antiemetics may be used prophylactically. Adjust diet as tolerated to help maintain fluid and electrolyte balance and nutritional status.

- Monitor for bone marrow depression. Assess for fever, sore throat, and signs of infection due to leukopenia. Assess for bleeding (bleeding gums, bruising, petechiae; guaiac test stools, urine, and emesis) due to thrombocytopenia. Avoid giving IM injections and taking rectal temperatures. Apply pressure to venipuncture sites for 10 minutes. Additive bone marrow depression may occur with other antineoplastic agents or radiation therapy.

- Assess respiratory status and chest x-ray examination prior to and periodically throughout therapy. Cough, bronchospasm, hemoptysis, or dyspnea usually occurs after several doses and may be indicative of pulmonary toxicity, which may be life-threatening.

- Use cautiously in patients with renal impairment (use not recommended if serum creatinine is more than 1.7 mg/100 ml). Geriatric patients may be more sensitive to the effects of mitomycin due to age-related decrease in renal function.

- Monitor for potentially fatal hemolytic–uremic syndrome in patients receiving long-term therapy. Symptoms include microangiopathic hemolytic anemia, thrombocytopenia, renal failure, and hypertension.

- Use cautiously in patients with active untreated infections, decreased bone marrow reserve, other chronic debilitating illness, impaired liver function, or pulmonary disorders.

- Mitomycin should be used cautiously in patients with childbearing potential and avoided in pregnant or lactating patients (Pregnancy Category UK).

Lab Test Considerations

- Monitor CBC and differential prior to and periodically throughout course of therapy and for several months following therapy. Peripheral blood smears should be observed for fragmented RBCs. • The nadir of leukopenia occurs in 4 weeks. The nadir of thrombocytopenia occurs in 4–6 weeks. If leukocyte count is <3000/mm^3 or the platelet count is <75,000/mm^3 or is progressively declining, subsequent doses are reduced. Recovery of leukopenia and thrombocytopenia occurs within 10 weeks after cessation of therapy. • Myelosuppression may be irreversible. Repeat courses of therapy are held until leukocyte count is greater than 4000/mm^3 and platelet count is greater than 100,000/mm^3. • Monitor liver function studies (AST [SGOT], ALT [SGPT], lactate dehydrogenase, bilirubin) and renal function studies (BUN, creatinine) prior to and periodically throughout therapy to detect hepatotoxicity and nephrotoxicity. Dose is held if serum creatinine is greater than 1.7 mg/dl.

Patient/Family Teaching

• Advise patient to notify physician promptly if fever; chills; sore throat; signs of infection; bleeding gums; bruising; petechiae; or blood in urine, stool, or emesis occurs. Caution patient to avoid crowds and persons with known infections. Instruct patient to use soft toothbrush and electric razor. Patients should be cautioned not to drink alcoholic beverages or take products containing aspirin, ibuprofen, or naproxen. • Instruct patient to notify physician if decreased urine output, edema in lower extremities, shortness of breath, skin ulceration, or persistent nausea occurs. • Instruct patient to inspect oral mucosa for redness and ulceration. If ulceration occurs, advise patient to use sponge brush and rinse mouth with water after eating and drinking. Further treatment is required if pain interferes with eating. • Discuss with patient the possibility of hair loss. Explore coping strategies. • Advise patients of childbearing age to use a nonhormonal method of contraception. • Instruct patient not to receive any vaccinations without advice of physician. Mitomycin may decrease antibody response to live virus vaccines and increase the risk of adverse reactions. • Emphasize need for periodic lab tests to monitor for side effects.

≋ PHARMACOLOGIC PROFILE

Indications
- Mitomycin is used with other agents in the management of disseminated gastric carcinoma or pancreatic carcinoma.

Action
- Mitomycin primarily inhibits DNA synthesis by causing cross-linking. It also inhibits RNA and protein synthesis (cell cycle–phase nonspecific, but is most active in S and G phases), resulting in death of rapidly replicating cells, particularly malignant ones.

Time/Action Profile (effects on blood counts)

Onset	Peak	Duration
3–8 wk	4–8 wk	up to 3 mo

Pharmacokinetics
- **Distribution:** Mitomycin is widely distributed and concentrates in tumor tissue. It does not enter CSF. • **Metabolism and Excretion:** Mitomycin is mostly metabolized by the liver. Small amounts (less than 10%) are excreted unchanged by the kidneys and in bile. • **Half-life:** 50 minutes.

Contraindications
- Mitomycin is contraindicated in patients who have hypersensitivity to it or to mannitol. Mitomycin should not be used in pregnant or lactating patients.

Adverse Reactions and Side Effects*
- **Resp:** PULMONARY TOXICITY • **CV:** edema • **GI:** <u>nausea</u>, <u>vomiting</u>, anorexia, stomatitis • **GU:** renal failure, gonadal suppression • **Derm:** alopecia, desquamation • **Hemat:** anemia, <u>leukopenia</u>, <u>thrombocytopenia</u> • **Local:** <u>phlebitis</u> at IV site • **Misc:** prolonged malaise, fever, HEMOLYTIC UREMIC SYNDROME.

---

*<u>Underlines</u> indicate most frequent; CAPITALS indicate life-threatening.

Mitoxantrone Hydrochloride	*Antineoplastic (antitumor antibiotic)*
Novantrone	pH 3–4.5

≋ ADMINISTRATION CONSIDERATIONS

Usual Dose

Leukemias

ADULTS: *Initially*—12 mg/m^2/day for 3 days as IV infusion (usually given with cytosine arabinoside 100 mg/m^2/day for 7 days as continuous IV infusion); if incomplete remission occurs, a second induction may be given. *Maintenance*—12 mg/m^2/day for 2 days as IV infusion (usually given with cytosine arabinoside 100 mg/m^2/day for 5 days as continuous IV infusion), given 6 wk after induction, with another course 4 wk later. See *cytarabine* monograph on page 262.

Breast Carcinoma, Hepatic Carcinoma, Non-Hodgkin's Lymphoma (unlabeled)

ADULTS: 14 mg/m^2 q 21 days (12 mg/m^2 if bone marrow reserve is limited).

Dilution

• **Direct IV: Dilute** dark-blue mitoxantrone solution in at least 50 ml of 0.9% NaCl or D5W. Discard unused solution appropriately. • Solution should be prepared in a biologic cabinet. Wear gloves, gown, and mask while handling medication. Discard equipment in designated containers (see Appendix F, page 1068). Avoid contact with skin. Use Luer-Lock tubing to prevent accidental leakage. If contact with skin occurs, immediately wash skin with soap and water. • Clean all spills with an aqueous solution of calcium hypochlorite. Mix solution by adding 5.5 parts (per weight) of calcium hypochlorite to 13 parts water. • **Intermittent IV:** May be **further diluted** in D5W, 0.9% NaCl, or D5/0.9% NaCl and used immediately.

Compatibility

• **Y-site:** allopurinol sodium • filgrastim • fludarabine • melphalan • ondansetron • sargramostim • vinorelbine.

• **Additive:** cyclophosphamide • cytarabine • fluorouracil • hydrocortisone sodium succinate • potassium chloride.

Incompatibility

- **Y-site:** paclitaxel • piperacillin/tazobactam.
- **Additive:** heparin.

Rate of Administration

- **Direct IV:** Administer slowly over at least 3 minutes into the tubing of a free-flowing IV of 0.9% NaCl or D5W.

≋ CLINICAL PRECAUTIONS

- Monitor for hypersensitivity reaction (rash, urticaria, bronchospasm, tachycardia, hypotension). If these occur, stop infusion. Keep epinephrine, an antihistamine, and resuscitation equipment close by in the event of an anaphylactic reaction.
- Monitor IV site. If extravasation occurs, discontinue IV and restart at another site. Mitoxantrone is not a vesicant, but is an irritant.
- Monitor intake and output, appetite, and nutritional intake. Assess patient for nausea and vomiting. Antiemetics may be administered prophylactically. Adjust diet as tolerated to help maintain fluid and electrolyte balance and nutritional status.
- Monitor for bone marrow depression. Assess for fever, sore throat, and signs of infection caused by leukopenia. Assess for bleeding (bleeding gums, bruising, petechiae; guaiac test stools, urine, and emesis) caused by thrombocytopenia. Avoid IM injections and rectal temperatures. Apply pressure to venipuncture sites for 10 minutes. Additive bone marrow depression may occur with concurrent use of other antineoplastics or radiation therapy. Use cautiously in patients with underlying infections, depressed bone marrow reserve, hepatobiliary dysfunction, or other chronic debilitating illness. Dosage reduction in these patients may be necessary.
- Monitor chest x-ray, ECG, echocardiography, and radionuclide angiography to determine ejection fraction prior to and periodically during therapy. May cause cardiotoxicity, especially in patients who have received daunorubicin or doxorubicin. Assess for rales/crackles, dyspnea, edema, jugular vein distention, ECG changes, arrhythmias, and chest pain. Use cautiously in patients with

underlying cardiovascular disease or previous radiation therapy to the mediastinum.
- Monitor for symptoms of gout (increased uric acid levels and joint pain and swelling). Encourage patient to drink at least 2 liters of fluid per day.
- Use cautiously in patients with childbearing potential; avoid using during pregnancy or lactation (Pregnancy Category D). Safe use in children has not been established.

Lab Test Considerations

- Monitor CBC and differential prior to and periodically throughout therapy. The nadir of leukopenia usually occurs within 10 days, and recovery usually occurs within 21 days. • Monitor liver function studies (AST [SGOT], ALT [SGPT], lactate dehydrogenase, bilirubin) and renal function studies (BUN, creatinine) prior to and periodically throughout therapy to detect hepatotoxicity and nephrotoxicity. • Mitoxantrone may cause increased serum and urine uric acid concentrations. Monitor periodically during therapy. Allopurinol may be given to decrease serum uric acid levels.

Patient/Family Teaching

- Advise patient to notify physician promptly in the event of fever, chills, sore throat, signs of infection, bleeding gums, bruising, petechiae, or blood in urine, stool, or emesis. Caution patient to avoid crowds and persons with known infections. Instruct patient to use soft toothbrush and electric razor. • Patients should be cautioned not to drink alcoholic beverages or take products containing aspirin, ibuprofen, or naproxen. • Instruct patient to notify physician if abdominal pain, yellow skin, cough, diarrhea, or decreased urine output occurs. • Inform patient that medication may cause the urine and sclera to turn blue-green. • Instruct patient to inspect oral mucosa for redness and ulceration. If mouth sores occur, advise patient to use sponge brush and rinse mouth with water after eating and drinking. Further treatment is required if pain interferes with eating. • Discuss with patient the possibility of hair loss. Explore coping strategies. • Advise patients with childbearing potential to use a nonhormonal method of contraception during therapy because of possible teratogenic effects. • Instruct patient not to receive any vaccinations without advice of physician. Mitoxantrone may decrease antibody response to live virus vaccines and increase the risk of adverse reactions.

≋ PHARMACOLOGIC PROFILE

Indications
• Mitoxantrone is used in combination with other antineoplastic agents in the treatment of acute nonlymphocytic leukemia in adults. • **Unlabeled Uses:** Carcinoma of the breast, hepatic carcinoma, and non-Hodgkin's lymphoma.

Action
• Mitoxantrone inhibits DNA synthesis (cell cycle–phase nonspecific) resulting in death of rapidly replicating cells, particularly malignant ones.

Time/Action Profile (effect on WBC counts)

Onset	Peak	Duration
UK	10–14 days	21–28 days

Pharmacokinetics
• **Distribution:** Mitoxantrone is widely distributed but has limited penetration of CSF. • **Metabolism and Excretion:** Small amounts (<10%) are excreted unchanged by the kidneys. Mitoxantrone is mostly eliminated by hepatobiliary clearance. • **Half-life:** 5.8 days.

Contraindications
• Mitoxantrone is contraindicated in patients with hypersensitivity to it. Pregnant or lactating patients should not be given mitoxantrone.

Adverse Reactions and Side Effects*
• **CNS:** headache, SEIZURES • **EENT:** conjunctivitis, blue-green sclera • **Resp:** cough, dyspnea • **CV:** cardiotoxicity, ECG changes, arrhythmias • **GI:** nausea, vomiting, diarrhea, abdominal pain, stomatitis, hepatic toxicity • **GU:** renal fail-

---

*Underlines indicate most frequent; CAPITALS indicate life-threatening.

ure, gonadal suppression, blue-green urine • **Derm:** <u>alopecia</u>, rashes • **Hemat:** <u>anemia</u>, <u>leukopenia</u>, <u>thrombocytopenia</u> • **Metab:** hyperuricemia • **Misc:** <u>fever</u>, hypersensitivity reactions.

Mivacurium Chloride	*Neuromuscular blocking agent (nondepolarizing)*
Mivacron	pH 3.5–5

ADMINISTRATION CONSIDERATIONS

Usual Dose

Initial Intubation Dosage/Surgical Relaxation
ADULTS: 150–200 mcg (0.15–0.2 mg)/kg [not to exceed 250 mcg (0.25 mg)/kg].

PATIENTS WITH CARDIOVASCULAR DISEASE OR INCREASED SENSITIVITY TO HISTAMINE: 150 mcg (0.15 mg)/kg.

CHILDREN 2–12 yr: 200–250 mcg (0.2–0.25 mg)/kg.

Maintenance Dose
ADULTS: 100 mcg (0.1 mg)/kg as bolus doses q 15 min or as a continuous infusion at 9–10 mcg/kg/min for 15 min, then 6–7 mcg/kg/min. If infusion is begun simultaneously with initial dose, start with rate of 4 mcg/kg/min. Infusion rates may range from 1–15 mcg/kg/min.

CHILDREN 2–12 yr: 14 mcg/kg/min (range 5–31 mcg/kg/min).

Dilution
• **Direct IV:** May be administered **undiluted**. • **Continuous Infusion:** May be **diluted** to 500 mcg (0.5 mg/ml) in D5W, D5/0.9% NaCl, 0.9% NaCl, lactated Ringer's solution, or D5/LR. • Solution is stable for 24 hours at room temperature. Discard unused portion after each use. • Also available in premixed infusion of D5W.

Compatibility
• **Y-site:** alfentanil ✦ droperidol ✦ fentanyl ✦ midazolam ✦ sufentanil.

Incompatibility

- **Y-site:** barbiturates.
- **Additive:** Do not admix with other medications.

Rate of Administration

- **Direct IV:** Administer over 5–15 minutes. • **Continuous Infusion:** Titrate rate according to patient response and peripheral nerve stimulator.

⩶ CLINICAL PRECAUTIONS

- Assess respiratory status continuously throughout mivacurium therapy. Mivacurium should be used only by individuals experienced in endotracheal intubation, and equipment for this procedure should be readily available.
- Neuromuscular response to mivacurium should be monitored with a peripheral nerve stimulator. Paralysis is initially selective and usually occurs sequentially in the following muscles: levator muscles of eyelids, muscles of mastication, limb muscles, abdominal muscles, muscles of the glottis, intercostal muscles, and the diaphragm. Recovery of muscle function usually occurs in reverse order. Children may require larger doses at more frequent intervals than adults. Safe use in children younger than 2 years has not been established.
- Observe the patient for residual muscle weakness and respiratory distress during the recovery period. Monitor effects with peripheral nerve stimulator.
- Mivacurium has no effect on consciousness or the pain threshold. Adequate anesthesia/analgesia should *always* be used when mivacurium is used as an adjunct to surgical procedures.
- Use cautiously in patients with a history of pulmonary disease or renal or liver impairment, and in elderly or debilitated patients, as these patients may be very sensitive to drug effects. Smaller maintenance doses may be used.
- Patients with electrolyte disturbances and those who are receiving cardiac glycosides may experience more arrhythmias. Obese patients are more prone to hypotension. In obese patients, dosage should be based on ideal body weight.

- Using mivacurium in patients with myasthenia gravis or myasthenic syndromes should be undertaken with *extreme caution,* as prolonged respiratory paralysis may occur. The intensity and duration of paralysis may also be prolonged by pretreatment with succinylcholine, general anesthetics, aminoglycoside antibiotics, polymyxin B, colistin, clindamycin, lidocaine, quinidine, procainamide, beta-adrenergic blocking agents, potassium-losing diuretics, and magnesium. Initial dose should be decreased by at least 25% when given following enflurane or isoflurane. Some reduction is also required with desflurane. Infusion rates should be decreased by 25% when used with enflurane or isoflurane, and by 20% when used with halothane.
- Safe use in pregnant or lactating patients has not been established (Pregnancy Category C).

Toxicity and Overdose Alert

- If overdose occurs, use peripheral nerve stimulator to determine the degree of neuromuscular blockade. Maintain airway patency and ventilation until recovery of normal respirations occurs. • Administration of anticholinesterase agents (edrophonium, neostigmine, pyridostigmine) may be used to antagonize the action of mivacurium. Atropine is usually administered prior to or concurrently with anticholinesterase agents to counteract the muscarinic effects. Administration of fluids and vasopressors may be necessary to treat severe hypotension or shock.

Patient/Family Teaching

- Explain all procedures to patient receiving mivacurium therapy without anesthesia, as consciousness is not affected by mivacurium alone. • Reassure patient that communication abilities will return as the medication wears off.

≋ PHARMACOLOGIC PROFILE

Indications

- Mivacurium is used to produce skeletal muscle paralysis during surgical procedures in conjunction with general anesthesia. It has also been used to facilitate endotracheal intubation (succinylcholine is preferred because its onset is quicker) and to facilitate compliance during mechanical ventilation.

Action
• Mivacurium prevents neuromuscular transmission by blocking the effect of acetylcholine at the myoneural junction. It has no anxiolytic or analgesic properties.

Time/Action Profile (skeletal muscle paralysis)†

	Onset	Peak	Duration
adults	rapid	3.3 min	26 min
children	rapid	1.0 min	19 min

†When used in conjunction with general anesthesia.

Pharmacokinetics
• **Distribution:** Tissue distribution of mivacurium is limited. • **Metabolism and Excretion:** Mivacurium is rapidly metabolized by cholinesterases in plasma. • **Half-life:** 2 hours.

Contraindications
• Mivacurium is contraindicated in patients with hypersensitivity to it or to benzyl alcohol (multidose vials only). Cross-sensitivity with other similar agents may exist.

Adverse Reactions and Side Effects*
• **CNS:** dizziness • **Resp:** bronchospasm, wheezing, hypoxemia • **CV:** tachycardia, bradycardia, arrhythmias, hypotension • **Derm:** flushing, rash, urticaria, erythema • **Local:** phlebitis • **MS:** muscle spasms.

*Underlines indicate most frequent; CAPITALS indicate life-threatening.

Morphine Sulfate	Opioid analgesic (agonist)
Astramorph PF, Duramorph, MS, MSO$_4$	pH 2.5–6

Schedule II

≋ ADMINISTRATION CONSIDERATIONS

As tolerance to the analgesic effects of opioids develops, doses exceeding those usually recommended may be required.

Usual Dose

ADULTS: 2.5–15 mg q 3–4 hr or IV infusion initiated with a loading dose of 15 mg followed by infusion at 0.8–10 mg/hr, rate increased as needed. Doses of 20–150 mg/hr or more have been used.

CHILDREN: 50–100 mcg (0.05–0.1 mg)/kg. Continuous infusions of 25 mcg–2.6 mg (0.025–2.6 mg)/kg/hr have been used for chronic pain due to cancer; 10–40 mcg (0.01–0.04 mg)/kg/hr has been used postoperatively.

NEONATES: not more than 15–20 mcg (0.015–0.02 mg)/kg/hr.

Dilution

• **Direct IV: Dilute** with at least 5 ml of sterile water or 0.9% NaCl for injection. • Solution is colorless; do not administer discolored solutions. • **Continuous Infusion:** May be added to D5W, D10W, 0.9% NaCl, 0.45% NaCl, Ringer's or lactated Ringer's solution, dextrose/saline solutions, or dextrose/Ringer's or lactated Ringer's solutions in a concentration of 0.1–1 mg/ml or greater for continuous infusion.

Compatibility

• **Syringe:** atropine ♦ benzquinamide ♦ bupivacaine ♦ chlorpromazine ♦ cimetidine ♦ dimenhydrinate ♦ diphenhydramine ♦ droperidol ♦ glycopyrrolate ♦ hydroxyzine ♦ metoclopramide ♦ midazolam ♦ milrinone ♦ perphenazine ♦ promazine ♦ ranitidine ♦ scopolamine.

• **Y-site:** allopurinol sodium ♦ amikacin ♦ aminophylline ♦ ampicillin ♦ ampicillin/sulbactam ♦ atenolol ♦ atracurium ♦ aztreonam ♦ bumetanide ♦ calcium chloride ♦ cefamandole ♦ cefazolin ♦ cefoperazone ♦ ceforanide ♦ cefotaxime ♦ cefotetan ♦ cefoxitin ♦ ceftazidime ♦ ceftizoxime ♦ ceftriaxone

• cefuroxime • cephalothin • cephapirin • chloramphenicol • clindamycin • cyclophosphamide • cytarabine • dexamethasone • digoxin • diltiazem • dopamine • doxorubicin • doxycycline • enalaprilat • erythromycin lactobionate • esmolol • famotidine • filgrastim • fluconazole • fludarabine • foscarnet • gentamicin • heparin • hydrocortisone sodium succinate • insulin • kanamycin • labetalol • lidocaine • magnesium sulfate • melphalan • methotrexate • methyldopate • methylprednisolone • metoclopramide • metoprolol • metronidazole • mezlocillin • nafcillin • ondansetron • oxacillin • oxytocin • paclitaxel • pancuronium • penicillin G potassium • piperacillin • piperacillin/tazobactam • potassium chloride • propranolol • ranitidine • sodium bicarbonate • ticarcillin • ticarcillin/clavulanate • tobramycin • trimethoprim/sulfamethoxazole • vancomycin • vecuronium • vinorelbine • vitamin B complex with C • zidovudine.

• **Additive:** atracurium • dobutamine • fluconazole • furosemide • ondansetron • succinylcholine • verapamil.

Incompatibility

• **Syringe:** meperidine • thiopental.
• **Y-site:** furosemide • gallium nitrate • minocycline • sargramostim.
• **Additive:** aminophylline • amobarbital • chlorothiazide • heparin • meperidine • methicillin • phenobarbital • phenytoin • sodium bicarbonate • thiopental.

Rate of Administration

• **Direct IV:** Administer 2.5–15 mg over 4–5 minutes. Rapid administration may lead to increased respiratory depression, hypotension, and circulatory collapse. • **Continuous Infusion:** Administer via infusion pump to control the rate. Dose should be titrated to ensure adequate pain relief without excessive sedation, respiratory depression, or hypotension. Rapid administration may lead to increased respiratory depression, hypotension, and circulatory collapse. • May be administered via patient-controlled analgesia (PCA) pump.

≋ CLINICAL PRECAUTIONS

• Assess type, location, and intensity of pain prior to and 20 minutes (peak) following administration. When titrating opioid doses, increases of 25–50% should be administered until there is either a 50% reduction in the patient's pain rating on a numerical or visual analogue scale or the patient reports satisfactory pain relief. Subsequent doses may be safely administered at the time of the peak if the previous dose is ineffective and side effects are minimal. Regularly administered doses may be more effective than p.r.n. administration. Analgesic is more effective if given before pain becomes severe. Coadministration with nonopioid analgesics may have additive analgesic effects and may permit lower doses.

- Patients on a continuous infusion should have additional bolus dose provided every 15–30 minutes, as needed for breakthrough pain. The bolus dose is usually set to the amount of drug infused each hour by continuous infusion.

- An equianalgesic chart (Appendix B, page 1045) should be used when changing routes or when changing from one opioid to another. When transferring from IV morphine to extended-release oral tablets, administer a total daily dose of oral morphine equivalent to previous daily dose and divided every 8 hours (Roxanol SR) or every 12 hours (MS Contin, Oramorph SR).

- Patients taking sustained-release opioid preparations need to have short-acting supplementary opioids available for breakthrough pain. Breakthrough doses should be equivalent to one sixth of the 24-hour total dose (see Equianalgesic Chart, Appendix B, page 1045 for calculation), and should be given every 2 hours as needed. Patients should be instructed that breakthrough doses can be taken at any time, and can even be taken at the same time as the sustained-release preparation.

- Assess blood pressure, pulse, and respiratory rate before and periodically during administration. If respiratory rate is less than 10/min, assess level of sedation. Dose may need to be decreased by 25–50%. Physical stimulation may be sufficient to prevent significant hypoventilation.

- Assess bowel function routinely. Prevention of constipation should be instituted with increased intake of fluids and bulk, stool softeners, and laxatives to minimize constipating effects. Stimulant laxatives should be administered routinely if opioid use exceeds 2–3 days, unless contraindicated.

- Prolonged use may lead to physical and psychological dependence and tolerance. This should not prevent patient from receiving adequate analgesia. Most patients who receive morphine for medical reasons do not develop psychological dependence. Progressively higher doses may be required to relieve pain with long-term therapy. Medication should be discontinued gradually after long-term use, to prevent withdrawal symptoms.

- Administration of partial-antagonist opioid analgesics may precipitate opioid withdrawal in physically dependent patients. Nalbuphine or pentazocine may decrease analgesia.
- Assess level of sedation. Initial drowsiness will diminish with continued use. Additive CNS depression may occur with concurrent use of alcohol, sedative/hypnotics, and antihistamines.
- Use with *extreme caution* in patients receiving MAO inhibitors. Concurrent use may result in unpredictable, severe reactions. Initial dose of morphine should be decreased to 25% of usual dose.
- Use morphine cautiously in patients with head trauma; increased intracranial pressure; severe renal, hepatic, or pulmonary disease; hypothyroidism; adrenal insufficiency; or alcoholism. Geriatric or debilitated patients may be more sensitive to CNS and constipating effects of morphine. Use with caution in patients with undiagnosed abdominal pain.
- Morphine has been used safely during labor to relieve pain but may cause respiratory depression in the newborn (Pregnancy Category C).

Toxicity and Overdose Alert

- If an opioid antagonist is required to reverse respiratory depression or coma, naloxone (Narcan) is the antidote. Dilute the 0.4-mg ampule of naloxone in 10 ml of 0.9% NaCl and administer 0.5 ml (0.02 mg) by direct IV push every 2 minutes. For children and patients weighing <40 kg, dilute 0.1 mg of naloxone in 10 ml of 0.9% NaCl for a concentration of 10 mcg/ml and administer 0.5 mcg every 1–2 minutes. Titrate the dose to avoid withdrawal, seizures, and severe pain.

Lab Test Considerations

- Morphine may increase plasma levels of amylase and lipase.

Patient/Family Teaching

• Instruct patient on how and when to ask for pain medication. • Medication may cause drowsiness or dizziness. Caution patient to call for assistance when ambulating or smoking, and to avoid driving or other activities requiring alertness until response to medication is known. • Advise patient to make position changes slowly to minimize orthostatic hypotension. • Caution patient to avoid concurrent use of alcohol or other CNS depressants with this medication. • Encourage patient to turn, cough, and breathe deeply every 2 hours to prevent atelectasis.

• **Home Care Issues:** Explain to patient and family how and when to administer morphine and how to care for the equipment properly. • Emphasize the importance of aggressive prevention of constipation with the use of this drug.

 PHARMACOLOGIC PROFILE

Indications

• Morphine is used in the management of severe pain. It is also used in the management of pulmonary edema and the management of pain associated with myocardial infarction.

Action

• Morphine binds to opiate receptors in the CNS, where it alters the perception of and response to painful stimuli while producing generalized CNS depression.

Time/Action Profile (analgesia)

Onset	Peak	Duration
immediate	20 min	4–5 hr

Pharmacokinetics

• **Distribution:** Morphine is widely distributed. It crosses the placenta and enters breast milk in small amounts. • **Metabolism and Excretion:** Morphine is mostly metabolized by the liver. • **Half-life:** 2–3 hours.

Contraindications

• Morphine is contraindicated in patients with hypersensitivity to it. Avoid chronic use in pregnant or lactating patients.

Adverse Reactions and Side Effects*

• **CNS:** <u>sedation</u>, <u>confusion</u>, headache, euphoria, floating feeling, unusual dreams, hallucinations, dysphoria, dizziness • **EENT:** miosis, diplopia, blurred vision • **Resp:** respiratory depression • **CV:** <u>hypotension</u>, bradycardia • **GI:** nausea, vomiting, <u>constipation</u> • **GU:** urinary retention • **Derm:** sweating, flushing • **Misc:** tolerance, physical dependence, psychological dependence.

Multiple Vitamins	Vitamins
Multiple Vitamin Concentrate Injection, M.V.C. 9+3, M.V.I. -12, M.V.I. Pediatric	pH 4.5–8.5

ADMINISTRATION CONSIDERATIONS

Usual Dose

Amount sufficient to meet RDA (Recommended Daily Allowances—see Appendix I) for age group. Usually added to large volume of parenteral or total parenteral nutrition (hyperalimentation) solutions.

Dilution

• **Continuous Infusion:** Dilute each 5- or 10-ml ampule in 500–1000 ml of D5/LR, D5/0.9% NaCl, D5W, D10W, D20W, lactated Ringer's injection, 0.9% NaCl, 3% NaCl, or 1/6 M sodium lactate. • Do not administer solution that has crystallized. Solution is bright yellow and will color IV solution.

Compatibility

• **Y-site:** acyclovir ♦ ampicillin ♦ cefazolin ♦ cephalothin ♦ cephapirin ♦ diltiazem ♦ erythromycin lactobionate ♦ fludarabine ♦ gentamicin ♦ tacrolimus.
• **Additive:** cefoxitin ♦ isoproterenol ♦ methyldopa ♦ metoclopramide ♦ netilmicin ♦ norepinephrine ♦ sodium bicarbonate ♦ verapamil.

---

*<u>Underlines</u> indicate most frequent; CAPITALS indicate life-threatening.

Incompatibility

• **Additive:** Incompatible in solution with many antibiotics or bleomycin.

Rate of Administration

• **Continuous Infusion:** Administer multivitamin infusion by infusion only; do not use direct IV injection.

≋ CLINICAL PRECAUTIONS

• Assess patient for signs of nutritional deficiency prior to and throughout therapy. Patients at risk include those who are elderly, debilitated, burned, unable to take oral nutrition, and those with malabsorption syndromes or chronic alcoholism.
• Vitamins are usually given orally but may be given parenterally to patients in whom oral administration is not feasible.
• Large amounts of vitamin B_6 may interfere with the beneficial effect of levodopa.

Toxicity and Overdose Alert

• Toxicity rarely occurs with multivitamin preparations due to the small amounts per unit of fat-soluble vitamins. For symptoms, see individual vitamin entries.

Patient/Family Teaching

• Encourage patient to comply with physician's recommendations. Explain that the best source of vitamins is a well-balanced diet with foods from the four basic food groups.

≋ PHARMACOLOGIC PROFILE

Indications

• Multiple vitamins are used as replacement in patients who are unable to ingest oral feedings or vitamins, thereby treating or preventing deficiencies.

Action

• Multiple-vitamin formulations contain fat-soluble vitamins (A, D, and E) and water-soluble vitamins (B-complex vitamins B_1, B_2, B_3, B_5, B_6, B_{12}, vitamin C, biotin, and folic acid). These vitamins are a diverse group of compounds necessary for normal growth and development that act as coenzymes or catalysts in numerous metabolic processes. Parenteral multiple vitamins do not contain vitamin K.

Time/Action Profile

Onset	Peak	Duration
UK	UK	UK

Pharmacokinetics

• **Distribution:** Vitamins are widely distributed, cross the placenta, and enter breast milk. Fat-soluble vitamins (A, D, and E) are stored in fatty tissues and the liver. • **Metabolism and Excretion:** Vitamins are utilized in various biologic processes. Excess amounts of water-soluble vitamins (B vitamins, vitamin C, and folic acid) are excreted unchanged by the kidneys. • **Half-life:** UK.

Contraindications

• IV multivitamins should be avoided in patients with hypersensitivity to preservatives or additives, including polysorbates or propylene glycol.

Adverse Reactions and Side Effects*

In recommended doses, adverse reactions are extremely rare.

• **Misc:** allergic reactions to preservatives or additives.

---

*<u>Underlines</u> indicate most frequent; CAPITALS indicate life-threatening.

Muromonab-CD3	*Immunosuppressant* *(monoclonal antibody)*
Orthoclone OKT3	pH 7

≋ ADMINISTRATION CONSIDERATIONS

Usual Dose
ADULTS: 5 mg/day for 10–14 days.
CHILDREN <12 yr: 100 mcg (0.1 mg)/kg/day for 10–14 days.

Dilution
• **Direct IV:** Draw **undiluted** solution into syringe via low-protein-binding 0.2- or 0.22-micrometer filter to ensure removal of translucent protein particles that may be present. Discard filter and attach 20-gauge needle for IV administration. • Keep medication refrigerated at 2–8°C. Do not shake vial.

Compatibility
• Do not administer as an infusion; do not admix; do not administer in IV line containing other medications.

Rate of Administration
• **Direct IV:** Administer IV push over <1 minute.

≋ CLINICAL PRECAUTIONS

• Initial dose is administered during hospitalization; patient should be monitored closely for 48 hours. Subsequent doses may be administered on outpatient basis. Assess for cytokine release syndrome (CRS), usually manifested by fever and chills, nausea and vomiting, chest pain, shortness of breath, dizziness, diarrhea, and trembling of hands, but may occasionally cause a severe, life-threatening shocklike reaction. The severity of this reaction is greatest with the initial dose and diminishes with successive doses. Reaction occurs within 30–60 minutes and may persist for up to 6 hours. Acetaminophen and antihistamines may be used to treat early reactions. Patient temperature should be maintained below 37.8°C (100°F) at administration of each dose. Manifestations of CRS may be minimized or prevented by pre-treatment with methylprednisolone 8 mg/kg given 1–4 hours prior to first dose of muromonab-CD3. Hydrocortisone 100 mg IV may also be ordered 30 minutes after the first and possibly second dose to control respiratory side effects. Serious symptoms of CRS may require oxygen, IV fluids, glucocorticoids, vasopressors, antihistamines, and intubation.

- Dosage of glucocorticoids and azathioprine may be reduced and cyclosporine discontinued during 10–14-day course of muromonab-CD3 because of increased risk of infection and lymphoproliferative disorders. Cyclosporine may be resumed 3 days before the end of muromonab-CD3 therapy.
- Assess for fluid overload (monitor weight for 3% or more weight gain in the previous week and intake and output; assess for edema and rales/crackles). Chest x-ray should be obtained prior to beginning therapy. Fluid-overloaded patients are at high risk of developing pulmonary edema. Monitor vital signs and breath sounds closely.
- Monitor for infection (fever, chills, rash, sore throat, purulent discharge, dysuria). If these symptoms occur, they may necessitate discontinuation of therapy. Concurrent use of other immunosuppressants increases the risk of infection.
- Monitor for development of aseptic meningitis. Onset is usually within 3 days of beginning therapy. Assess for fever, headache, nuchal rigidity, and photophobia.
- Additive immunosuppression may occur with other immunosuppressive agents.
- Use muromonab-CD3 cautiously in patients with active infections, depressed bone marrow reserve, chronic debilitating illnesses, or congestive heart failure.
- Safe use in pregnancy or children younger than 2 years has not been established (Pregnancy Category C).

Lab Test Considerations

• Monitor CBC and differential prior to and periodically throughout therapy. • Monitor assays of T cell with CD3 antigen or plasma levels as determined by an ELISA (target should be >800 ng/ml) daily. • Monitor serum creatinine and hepatic enzymes (AST [SGOT], ALT [SGPT], alkaline phosphatase, bilirubin), especially during the first 1–3 days of therapy. May cause transient increases.

Patient/Family Teaching

• Explain the purpose of muromonab to patient and family. Inform patient of possible initial-dose side effects, which are markedly reduced in subsequent doses. Explain that patient will need to resume lifelong therapy with other immunosuppressive drugs after completion of muromonab course. • Instruct patient not to receive any vaccinations and to avoid contact with persons receiving oral polio vaccine without first obtaining advice of physician. • Instruct patient to continue to avoid crowds and persons with known infections, as this drug suppresses the immune system.

≋ PHARMACOLOGIC PROFILE

Indications

• Muromonab-CD3 is used in the treatment of acute renal allograft rejection reactions in transplant patients that have occurred despite conventional antirejection therapy. • It has also been used in the treatment of acute hepatic or cardiac allograft rejection reactions in transplant patients that have occurred despite conventional antirejection therapy (unlabeled use).

Action

• Muromonab-CD3 is a purified immunoglobulin antibody that acts as an immunosuppressant by interfering with normal T-cell function.

Time/Action Profile (noted as levels of circulating CD3-positive T cells)

Onset	Peak	Duration
minutes	4–7 days	1 wk

Pharmacokinetics

• **Distribution:** UK. • **Metabolism and Excretion:** UK. • **Half-life:** UK.

Contraindications

• Muromonab-CD3 is contraindicated in patients with hypersensitivity to muromonab-CD3, murine (mouse) proteins, or polysorbate. It should be avoided in patients with previous muromonab therapy, fluid overload, fever >37.8°C or 110°F, chickenpox or recent exposure to chickenpox, or herpes zoster. • Avoid use during lactation.

Adverse Reactions and Side Effects*

• **CNS:** <u>tremor</u>, aseptic meningitis, dizziness • **Resp:** <u>dyspnea</u>, <u>shortness of breath</u>, <u>wheezing</u>, PULMONARY EDEMA • **CV:** <u>chest pain</u> • **GI:** <u>vomiting</u>, <u>nausea</u>, <u>diarrhea</u> • **Misc:** <u>fever</u>, <u>chills</u>, infections, increased risk of lymphoma, <u>hypersensitivity reactions</u>.

Nafcillin Sodium	*Anti-infective*
	(penicillinase-resistant penicillin)
Nafcil, Nallpen, Unipen	pH 6–8.5
	2.9 mEq Na/g

≋ ADMINISTRATION CONSIDERATIONS

Usual Dose

ADULTS: 500–1500 mg q 4 hr (up to 20 g/day).

INFANTS AND CHILDREN: 10–20 mg/kg q 4 hr or 20–40 mg/kg q 8 hr (up to 200 mg/kg/day).

NEONATES ≥2 kg: *Meningitis*—50 mg/kg q 8 hr for first 7 days of life, then 50 mg/kg q 6 hr.

NEONATES <2 kg: *Meningitis*—25–50 mg/kg q 12 hr for first 7 days of life, then 50 mg/kg q 8 hr.

Dilution

• **Direct IV:** To **reconstitute**, add 1.7 ml of sterile water or bacteriostatic water for injection to each 500-mg vial, 3.4 ml to each 1-g vial, or 6.6–6.8 ml to each 2-g vial, for a concentration of 250 mg/ml. • Stable for 2–7 days if refrigerated.
• **Dilute** reconstituted solution with 15–30 ml of sterile water

---

*Underlines indicate most frequent; CAPITALS indicate life-threatening.

or 0.9% NaCl for injection. • **Intermittent Infusion:** Dilute
to a concentration of 2–40 mg/ml with sterile water for injection, 0.9% NaCl, D5W, D10W, D5/0.25% NaCl, D5/0.45%
NaCl, D5/0.9% NaCl, D5/LR, Ringer's or lactated Ringer's solution. • Stable for 24 hours at room temperature, 96 hours if
refrigerated.

Compatibility

- **Syringe:** cimetidine • heparin.
- **Y-site:** acyclovir • atropine • cyclophosphamide • diazepam • enalaprilat • esmolol • famotidine • fentanyl • fluconazole • foscarnet • hydromorphone • magnesium sulfate
• morphine • perphenazine • zidovudine.
- **Additive:** chloramphenicol • chlorothiazide • dexamethasone sodium phosphate • diphenhydramine • ephedrine • heparin • hydroxyzine • potassium chloride
• prochlorperazine • sodium bicarbonate • sodium lactate.

Incompatibility

- **Y-site:** droperidol • droperidol/fentanyl • insulin • labetalol • nalbuphine • pentazocine • verapamil.
- **Additive:** ascorbic acid • aztreonam • bleomycin • cytarabine • gentamicin • hydrocortisone sodium succinate
• methylprednisolone sodium succinate • promazine.

Rate of Administration

- **Direct IV:** Administer over 5–10 minutes. • **Intermittent Infusion:** Infuse over at least 30–60 minutes to avoid
vein irritation.

≋ CLINICAL PRECAUTIONS

- Assess patient for infection (vital signs; appearance of
wound, sputum, urine, and stool; WBC) at beginning
and throughout course of therapy.
- Obtain specimens for culture and sensitivity prior to initiating therapy. First dose may be given before receiving
results.
- Obtain a history before initiating therapy to determine
previous use of and reactions to penicillins or cephalosporins. Persons with a negative history of penicillin sensitivity may still have an allergic response. Observe patient for signs and symptoms of anaphylaxis (rash,

pruritus, laryngeal edema, wheezing). Discontinue nafcillin if these occur. Keep epinephrine, an antihistamine,
and resuscitation equipment close by in the event of an
anaphylactic reaction. Use with caution in patients with
a history of previous hypersensitivity reactions.

- Probenecid decreases renal excretion and increases
blood levels of nafcillin. Nafcillin may alter the effect of
oral anticoagulants.

- Nafcillin should be used cautiously in patients with severe renal impairment; dosage reduction may be required. Risk of nephrotoxicity may be increased with
other nephrotoxic agents.

- Safe use in pregnancy or lactation has not been established (Pregnancy Category B).

Lab Test Considerations

- Nafcillin may cause positive direct Coombs' test results.

Patient/Family Teaching

- Advise patient to report the signs of superinfection
(black, furry overgrowth on the tongue; vaginal itching or
discharge; loose or foul-smelling stools) and allergy to physician promptly. - Instruct patient to notify physician if
symptoms do not improve.

☰ PHARMACOLOGIC PROFILE

Indications

- Nafcillin is used in the treatment of the following infections due to susceptible strains of penicillinase-producing
staphylococci: respiratory tract infections, skin and skin
structure infections, bone and joint infections, urinary tract
infections, endocarditis, septicemia, and meningitis.

Action

- Nafcillin binds to bacterial cell wall, leading to cell death.
It resists the action of penicillinase, an enzyme capable of inactivating penicillin. The result is bactericidal action against
susceptible bacteria. - Nafcillin is active against most Gram-
positive aerobic cocci, but less so than penicillin. It is notable
for activity against penicillinase-producing strains of *Staphylo-*

coccus aureus and *S. epidermidis.* • It is not active against methicillin-resistant staphylococci.

Time/Action Profile (blood levels)

Onset	Peak
rapid	end of infusion

Pharmacokinetics

• **Distribution:** Nafcillin is widely distributed. Penetration into CSF is minimal but sufficient in the presence of inflamed meninges. It crosses the placenta and enters breast milk. • **Metabolism and Excretion:** Nafcillin is excreted unchanged by the kidneys. • **Half-life:** 30–90 minutes (increased in renal impairment).

Contraindications

• Nafcillin is contraindicated in patients with a history of hypersensitivity to penicillins.

Adverse Reactions and Side Effects*

• **CNS:** SEIZURES (high doses) • **GI:** <u>nausea</u>, <u>vomiting</u>, <u>diarrhea</u>, hepatitis • **GU:** interstitial nephritis • **Derm:** <u>rashes</u>, urticaria • **Hemat:** blood dyscrasias • **Local:** phlebitis at IV site • **Misc:** superinfection, <u>allergic reactions</u>, including ANAPHYLAXIS and serum sickness.

Nalbuphine Hydrochloride	Opioid analgesic (mixed agonist/antagonist)
Nubain	pH 3.5

 ADMINISTRATION CONSIDERATIONS

Usual Dose

Analgesia

ADULTS: Usual dose is 10 mg q 3–6 hr (0.14 mg/kg) in patients not physically dependent on opioid agonists (not to exceed 20 mg/single dose or 160 mg/24 hr).

---

*<u>Underlines</u> indicate most frequent; CAPITALS indicate life-threatening.

Supplement to Balanced Anesthesia

ADULTS: 300 mcg (0.3 mg)–3 mg/kg over 10–15 min initially. Maintenance dose 250–500 mcg (0.25–0.5 mg)/kg as needed.

Dilution

- **Direct IV:** May give IV **undiluted**.

Compatibility

- **Syringe:** atropine ◆ cimetidine ◆ diphenhydramine ◆ droperidol ◆ glycopyrrolate ◆ hydroxyzine ◆ lidocaine ◆ midazolam ◆ prochlorperazine ◆ ranitidine ◆ scopolamine ◆ trimethobenzamide.
- **Y-site:** filgrastim ◆ fludarabine ◆ melphalan ◆ paclitaxel ◆ vinorelbine.

Incompatibility

- **Syringe:** diazepam ◆ ketorolac ◆ pentobarbital.
- **Y-site:** allopurinol sodium ◆ nafcillin ◆ piperacillin/tazobactam ◆ sargramostim.

Rate of Administration

- **Direct IV:** Administer slowly, each 10 mg over 3–5 minutes.

≋ CLINICAL PRECAUTIONS

- Assess type, location, and intensity of pain prior to and 30 minutes (peak) following administration. When titrating opioid doses, increases of 25–50% should be administered until there is either a 50% reduction in the patient's pain rating on a numerical or visual analogue scale or the patient reports satisfactory pain relief. Subsequent doses may be safely administered at the time of the peak if the previous dose is ineffective and side effects are minimal. Patients requiring higher doses should be converted to an opioid agonist. Nalbuphine is not recommended for prolonged use or as first-line therapy for acute or cancer pain. Regularly administered doses may be more effective than p.r.n. administration. Analgesic is more effective if administered before pain becomes severe. Coadministration with nonopioid analgesics may have additive effects and permit lower opioid doses.
- An equianalgesic chart (Appendix B, page 1045) should be used when changing routes or when changing from one opioid to another.

- Assess blood pressure, pulse, and respirations before and periodically during administration. Nalbuphine produces respiratory depression, but this does not markedly increase with increased doses. If respiratory rate is <10/min, assess level of sedation. Physical stimulation may be sufficient to prevent significant hypoventilation. Dose may need to be decreased by 25–50%.

- Although this drug has a low potential for dependence, prolonged use may lead to physical and psychological dependence and tolerance. This should not prevent patient from receiving adequate analgesia. Most patients who receive nalbuphine for medical reasons do not develop psychological dependence.

- Assess prior analgesic history. Antagonistic properties may induce withdrawal symptoms (vomiting, restlessness, abdominal cramps, increased blood pressure, and temperature) in patients who are physically dependent on opioid agents.

- Use with extreme caution in patients receiving MAO inhibitors, as this combination may result in unpredictable, severe reactions. Reduce initial dose of nalbuphine to 25% of usual dose. Additive CNS depression occurs with concurrent use of alcohol, antihistamines, and sedative/hypnotics. Avoid concurrent use with agonist opioid analgesics, as this combination may diminish analgesic effect.

- Use nalbuphine cautiously in patients with head trauma; increased intracranial pressure; severe renal, hepatic, or pulmonary disease; hypothyroidism; adrenal insufficiency; alcoholism; undiagnosed abdominal pain; or prostatic hypertrophy. Elderly or debilitated patients may require dosage reduction.

- Nalbuphine has been used during labor but may cause respiratory depression in the newborn (Pregnancy Category C). Safe use during lactation or in children has not been established.

Toxicity and Overdose Alert

- If an opioid antagonist is required to reverse respiratory depression or coma, naloxone (Narcan) is the antidote. Dilute the 0.4-mg ampule of naloxone in 10 ml of 0.9% NaCl and administer 0.5 ml (0.02 mg) by direct IV push every 2 minutes. For children and patients weighing

<40 kg, dilute 0.1 mg of naloxone in 10 ml of 0.9% NaCl for a concentration of 10 mcg/ml and administer 0.5 mcg every 1–2 minutes. Titrate the dose to avoid withdrawal, seizures, and severe pain.

Lab Test Considerations

• Nalbuphine may cause elevated serum amylase and lipase levels.

Patient/Family Teaching

• Instruct patient on how and when to ask for pain medication. • Nalbuphine may cause drowsiness or dizziness. Advise patient to call for assistance when ambulating and to avoid activities requiring alertness until response to the medication is known. • Caution patient to make position changes slowly to minimize orthostatic hypotension. • Advise patient that frequent mouth rinses, good oral hygiene, and sugarless gum or candy may decrease dry mouth. • Encourage patient to turn, cough, and breathe deeply every 2 hours to prevent atelectasis. • Advise patient to avoid concurrent use of alcohol or other CNS depressants with this medication.

▤ PHARMACOLOGIC PROFILE

Indications

• Nalbuphine is used in the management of moderate to severe pain. It is also used as an analgesic during labor, as a sedative prior to surgery, and as a supplement in balanced anesthesia.

Action

• Nalbuphine binds to opiate receptors in the CNS, where it alters the perception of and response to painful stimuli while producing generalized CNS depression. In addition, it has partial antagonist properties, which may result in opioid withdrawal in physically dependent patients.

Time/Action Profile (analgesia)

Onset	Peak	Duration
2–3 min	30 min	3–6 hr

Pharmacokinetics

• **Distribution:** Nalbuphine probably crosses the placenta and enters breast milk. • **Metabolism and Excretion:** Nalbuphine is mostly metabolized by the liver and eliminated in the feces via biliary excretion. Minimal amounts are excreted unchanged by the kidneys. • **Half-life:** 5 hours.

Contraindications

• Nalbuphine is contraindicated in patients with hypersensitivity to it or to parabens or bisulfites. It should be avoided in patients who are physically dependent on opioid agonists.

Adverse Reactions and Side Effects*

• **CNS:** <u>sedation</u>, confusion, <u>headache</u>, euphoria, floating feeling, unusual dreams, hallucinations, dysphoria, <u>dizziness</u>, <u>vertigo</u> • **EENT:** miosis (high doses), blurred vision, diplopia • **Resp:** respiratory depression • **CV:** orthostatic hypotension, hypertension, palpitations • **GI:** <u>nausea</u>, <u>vomiting</u>, constipation, ileus, <u>dry mouth</u> • **GU:** urinary urgency • **Derm:** <u>sweating</u>, <u>clammy feeling</u> • **Misc:** tolerance, physical dependence, psychological dependence.

Naloxone Hydrochloride	Antidote (opioid antagonist)
Narcan	pH 3–4

☰ ADMINISTRATION CONSIDERATIONS

Usual Dose

Postoperative Opioid-Induced Respiratory Depression

ADULTS: 0.1–0.2 mg q 2–3 min until response obtained; may repeat q 1–2 hr if needed or continuous infusion of 3.7 mcg/kg/hr.

---

*<u>Underlines</u> indicate most frequent; CAPITALS indicate life-threatening.

CHILDREN: 5–10 mcg; may repeat q 2–3 min until response obtained. Additional doses may be given q 2–3 hr later if needed.

Opioid-Induced Respiratory Depression during Chronic (>1 wk) Opioid Use

ADULTS >40 kg: 20–40 mcg (0.02–0.04 mg) as small, frequent (q min) boluses or as an infusion titrated to improve respiratory function while not reversing analgesia.

ADULTS AND CHILDREN <40 kg: 0.5–2 mcg (0.0005–0.002 mg)/kg as small, frequent (q min) boluses titrated to improve respiratory function while not reversing analgesia.

Overdose of Opioids

ADULTS: 0.4 mg or 10 mcg/kg; may repeat q 2–3 min. Some patients may require up to 2 mg. If patient is suspected of being physically dependent on opioids, initial dose should be decreased to 0.1–0.2 mg. May also be given by continuous infusion at rate adjusted to patient's response.

CHILDREN: 0.01 mg/kg. If response is inadequate, increase to 0.1 mg/kg; may repeat IV dose q 2–3 min as needed.

NEONATES: 10 mg/kg, may repeat q 2–3 min as needed initially, then q 2–3 hr as needed.

Dilution

• Available in concentrations of 0.02 mg/ml (neonatal), 0.4 mg/ml, and 1 mg/ml. • **Direct IV:** Administer 0.4 mg/ml **undiluted** for suspected opioid overdose or **dilute** 0.4 mg of naloxone in 10 ml of sterile water or 0.9% NaCl for injection for patients with opioid-induced respiratory depression. For children or patients weighing <40 kg, **dilute** 0.1 mg of naloxone in 10 ml of sterile water or 0.9% NaCl for injection for a concentration of 10 mcg/ml. • **Continuous Infusion:** Dilute in D5W or 0.9% NaCl for injection. • Naloxone 2 mg in 500 ml equals a concentration of 4 mcg/ml. Mixture is stable for 24 hours; discard unused solution.

Compatibility

• **Syringe:** benzquinamide • heparin.
• **Additive:** verapamil.

Incompatibility

• **Additive:** Incompatible with preparations containing bisulfite, sulfite, and solutions with an alkaline pH.

Rate of Administration

- **Direct IV:** Administer at a rate of 0.1–0.4 mg or less over 15 seconds in patients with suspected opioid overdose. For patients with pain who develop opioid-induced respiratory depression, administer dilute solution of 0.4 mg/10 ml at a rate of 0.5 ml (0.02 mg) every 2 minutes. For children and patients weighing <40 kg, administer 10 mcg/ml solution at a rate of 0.5 mcg every 2 minutes. Titrate to patient response to avoid withdrawal, seizures, and severe pain. • **Continuous Infusion:** Titrate dose according to patient response. Supplemental doses administered IM, or a continuous infusion may provide longer-lasting effects. • Doses should be titrated carefully in postoperative patients to avoid interference with control of pain.

≋ CLINICAL PRECAUTIONS

- Monitor rate, rhythm, and depth of respirations, level of sedation, pulse, ECG, and blood pressure frequently for 3–4 hours after the expected peak analgesic blood concentrations. Following a moderate overdose of a short half-life opioid, physical stimulation may be enough to prevent significant hypoventilation. The effects of some opioids may last longer than the effects of naloxone, and repeat doses may be necessary. Resuscitation equipment, oxygen, vasopressors, and mechanical ventilation should be available to supplement naloxone therapy as needed.
- Patients who have been receiving opioids for more than 1 week are extremely sensitive to the effects of naloxone. Dilute and administer carefully.
- Assess patient for level of pain following administration when used to treat postoperative respiratory depression. Naloxone decreases respiratory depression but also reverses analgesia. Subsequent opioid doses may need to be decreased by 25–50%.
- Use cautiously in patients physically dependent on opioid analgesics (may precipitate severe withdrawal). Assess patient for signs and symptoms of opioid withdrawal (vomiting, restlessness, abdominal cramps, increased blood pressure, and temperature). Symptoms may occur within a few minutes to 2 hours. Severity depends on dose of naloxone, opioid involved, and degree

of physical dependence. Lack of significant improvement indicates that symptoms are due to a disease process or to other nonopioid CNS depressants not affected by naloxone.

- In patients receiving meperidine chronically, naloxone may precipitate seizures by eliminating the effects of meperidine, allowing the convulsant activity of the metabolite normeperidine to predominate (see *meperidine hydrochloride* monograph on page 589).
- Larger doses of naloxone may be necessary when used to antagonize the effects of buprenorphine, butorphanol, nalbuphine, pentazocine, and propoxyphene.
- Use cautiously in patients with cardiovascular disease.
- Use of naloxone in pregnancy may cause withdrawal in mother and fetus if mother is physically dependent on opioids (Pregnancy Category B). Safe use during lactation has not been established. Use with caution in neonates born to mothers who are physically dependent on opioids (may precipitate opioid withdrawal).

Toxicity and Overdose Alert

- Naloxone is a pure antagonist with no agonist (opioid-like) properties and minimal toxicity.

Patient/Family Teaching

- As naloxone becomes effective, explain the purpose and effects of naloxone to patient.

≋ PHARMACOLOGIC PROFILE

Indications

- Naloxone is used to reverse CNS depression and respiratory depression due to suspected opioid overdosage.

Action

- Naloxone competitively blocks the effects of opioids, including CNS depression, respiratory depression, and analgesia, without producing any agonist effects.

Time/Action Profile (reversal of opioid effects)

Onset	Peak	Duration
1–2 min	UK	45 min

Pharmacokinetics

• **Distribution:** Naloxone is rapidly distributed to tissues. It crosses the placenta. • **Metabolism and Excretion:** Naloxone is metabolized by the liver. • **Half-life:** 60–90 minutes (up to 3 hours in neonates).

Contraindications

• Naloxone is contraindicated in patients with hypersensitivity to it or to parabens (not present in all products).

Adverse Reactions and Side Effects*

• **CV:** ventricular tachycardia, ventricular fibrillation, hypotension, hypertension • **GI:** nausea, vomiting • **Misc:** opioid withdrawal, return of pain.

Neostigmine Methylsulfate	*Cholinergic (cholinesterase inhibitor)*
Prostigmin	**pH 5.9**

ADMINISTRATION CONSIDERATIONS

Usual Dose

Myasthenia Gravis

ADULTS: 0.5–7 mg initially, additional doses based on response q 1–3 hr.

CHILDREN: 10–40 mcg (0.01–0.04 mg)/kg q 2–3 hr.

Antidote for Nondepolarizing Neuromuscular Blockers

ADULTS: 0.5–2 mg slowly; may be repeated up to 2 total doses of 5 mg; pretreat with 0.6–1.2 mg atropine IV. Additional doses may be less than 0.5 mg.

CHILDREN: 40 mcg (0.04 mg)/kg given with 20 mcg (0.02 mg/kg) atropine.

Dilution

• **Direct IV:** Administer doses **undiluted**. Do not add to IV solutions. May be given through Y-site or 3-way stopcock

---

*Underlines indicate most frequent; CAPITALS indicate life-threatening.

of an IV of D5W, 0.9% NaCl, Ringer's solution, or lactated Ringer's solution.

Compatibility

- **Syringe:** glycopyrrolate ◆ heparin ◆ pentobarbital ◆ thiopental.
- **Y-site:** heparin ◆ hydrocortisone sodium succinate ◆ potassium chloride ◆ vitamin B complex with C.
- **Additive:** netilmicin.

Rate of Administration

- **Direct IV:** Administer each 0.5 mg over 1 minute.

≋ CLINICAL PRECAUTIONS

- Assess pulse, respiratory rate, and blood pressure prior to administration. Monitor for significant changes in heart rate.
- When neostigmine is used in myasthenia gravis, assess neuromuscular status, including vital capacity, ptosis, diplopia, chewing, swallowing, hand grasp, and gait, prior to administering and at peak effect. Patients with myasthenia gravis may be advised to keep a daily record of their condition and the effects of this medication. Assess patient for overdosage and underdosage or resistance. Both have similar symptoms (muscle weakness, dyspnea, dysphagia), but symptoms of overdosage usually occur within 1 hour of administration, whereas underdosage symptoms occur 3 or more hours after administration. Overdosage (cholinergic crisis) symptoms may also include increased respiratory secretions and saliva, bradycardia, nausea, vomiting, cramping, diarrhea, and diaphoresis. A Tensilon test (edrophonium chloride [see *edrophonium chloride* monograph on page 372]) may be used to distinguish between overdosage and underdosage. When changing over to oral therapy, oral and parenteral doses are not interchangeable due to poor oral absorption.
- When used as an antidote to nondepolarizing neuromuscular blocking agents, atropine may be ordered prior to or concurrently with neostigmine to prevent or treat bradycardia (see *atropine sulfate* monograph on page 97). Monitor reversal of effects of neuromuscular blocking

agents with a peripheral nerve stimulator. Recovery usually occurs consecutively in the following muscles: diaphragm, intercostal muscles, muscles of the glottis, abdominal muscles, limb muscles, muscles of mastication, and levator muscles of the eyelids. Closely observe the patient for residual muscle weakness and respiratory distress throughout the recovery period. Maintain airway patency and ventilation until recovery of normal respirations occurs.

- The action of neostigmine may be antagonized by drugs possessing anticholinergic properties, including antihistamines, antidepressants, atropine, haloperidol, phenothiazines, quinidine, and disopyramide. Neostigmine prolongs the action of depolarizing muscle-relaxing agents (succinylcholine, decamethonium).
- Use neostigmine cautiously in patients with a history of asthma, ulcer disease, cardiovascular disease, epilepsy, or hyperthyroidism.
- Using neostigmine during pregnancy may cause uterine irritability near term; newborns may display muscle weakness (Pregnancy Category C). Safe use during lactation has not been established.

Toxicity and Overdose Alert

- If overdose occurs, atropine is the antidote.

Patient/Family Teaching

- Patients with myasthenia gravis must continue regimen with such agents as a lifelong therapy. Instruct patient with myasthenia gravis to space activities to avoid fatigue.
- Advise patient to carry identification describing disease and medication regimen at all times.

☰ PHARMACOLOGIC PROFILE

Indications

- Neostigmine is used to increase muscle strength in the symptomatic treatment of myasthenia gravis and to reverse nondepolarizing neuromuscular blockers.

Action

- Neostigmine inhibits the breakdown of acetylcholine (by inhibiting cholinesterase) so that it accumulates and has a prolonged action. Effects include miosis, increased intestinal and skeletal muscle tone, bronchial and ureteral constriction, bradycardia, increased salivation, lacrimation, and sweating.

Time/Action Profile (cholinergic effects, increased muscle tone)

Onset	Peak	Duration
10–30 min	20–30 min	2–4 hr

Pharmacokinetics

• **Distribution:** Neostigmine does not appear to cross the placenta or enter breast milk. • **Metabolism and Excretion:** Neostigmine is metabolized by plasma cholinesterases and the liver. • **Half-life:** 40–60 minutes.

Contraindications

• Neostigmine is contraindicated in patients with hypersensitivity to it or to phenol (vials only). It should be avoided in patients with mechanical obstruction of the GI or GU tract.

Adverse Reactions and Side Effects*

• **CNS:** dizziness, weakness, SEIZURES • **EENT:** miosis, lacrimation • **Resp:** excessive secretions, bronchospasm • **CV:** bradycardia, hypotension • **GI:** abdominal cramps, nausea, vomiting, diarrhea, excess salivation • **Derm:** rashes, sweating.

Netilmicin Sulfate	Aminoglycoside
Netromycin	pH 3.5–6

≋ ADMINISTRATION CONSIDERATIONS

Usual Dose

All doses after initial loading dose should be determined by renal function/blood level monitoring.

ADULTS: *Most serious infections*—1.3–2.2 mg/kg q 8 hr *or* 2–3.25 mg/kg q 12 hr (up to 7.5 mg/kg/day or 12 mg/kg/day

---

*Underlines indicate most frequent; CAPITALS indicate life-threatening.

in cystic fibrosis patients). *Urinary tract infections*—1.5–2 mg/kg q 12 hr.

CHILDREN 6 wk–12 yr: 1.83–2.67 mg/kg q 8 hr *or* 2.75–4 mg/kg q 12 hr.

NEONATES UP TO 6 wk: 2–3.25 mg/kg q 12 hr.

Dilution

• **Intermittent Infusion: Dilute** each dose in 50–200 ml of D5/LR, D5/0.9% NaCl, D5W, D10W, Ringer's or lactated Ringer's solution, 0.9% NaCl, 3% NaCl, or 5% NaCl. Dilute in a proportionately smaller volume for pediatric patients.
• Solution is clear and colorless to pale yellow. Stable for 72 hours at room temperature.

Compatibility

• **Y-site:** aminophylline • calcium gluconate • filgrastim • fludarabine • melphalan • sargramostim • vinorelbine.
• **Additive:** aminocaproic acid • atropine • cefuroxime • chlorpromazine • clindamycin • dexamethasone sodium phosphate • diazepam • diphenhydramine • edetate calcium disodium • hydrocortisone sodium succinate • iron dextran • isoproterenol • methyldopa • metronidazole • multivitamins • neostigmine • norepinephrine • oxytocin • phytonadione • potassium chloride • procainamide • promethazine • triflupromazine • vitamin B complex with C.

Incompatibility

• **Syringe:** heparin.
• **Y-site:** allopurinol sodium • furosemide • heparin.
• If aminoglycosides and penicillins or cephalosporins must be given concurrently, administer in separate sites at least 1 hour apart.
• **Additive:** Give aminoglycosides and penicillins at least 1 hour apart to prevent inactivation.

Rate of Administration

• **Intermittent Infusion:** Infuse slowly over 30 minutes– 2 hours.

≋ CLINICAL PRECAUTIONS

• Assess patient for infection (vital signs; wound appearance, sputum, urine, and stool; WBC) at beginning and throughout course of therapy.

- Obtain specimens for culture and sensitivity prior to initiating therapy. First dose may be given before receiving results.
- Evaluate eighth cranial nerve function by audiometry prior to and throughout course of therapy. Hearing loss is usually in the high-frequency range. Prompt recognition and intervention are essential in preventing permanent damage. Also monitor for vestibular dysfunction (vertigo, ataxia, nausea, vomiting). Eighth cranial nerve dysfunction is associated with persistently elevated peak netilmicin levels. Neonates and geriatric patients are more likely to develop ototoxicity because of age-related decrease in renal function and difficulty in assessing hearing status.
- Keep patient well hydrated (1500–2000 ml/day) during therapy. Monitor intake and output and daily weights to assess hydration status and renal function. In obese patients, dose should be based on ideal body weight.
- Assess patient for signs of superinfection (fever, upper respiratory infection, vaginal itching or discharge, increasing malaise, diarrhea).
- Netilmicin is inactivated by penicillins when coadministered to patients with renal insufficiency. Possible respiratory paralysis may occur after administration of general anesthetics or neuromuscular blockers (tubocurarine, succinylcholine, decamethonium). The risk of ototoxicity is increased by concurrent use of loop diuretics. The risk of nephrotoxicity may be increased by concurrent use of other potentially nephrotoxic agents.
- Use cautiously in patients with renal impairment. Dosage reduction is required for any degree of decreased renal function. Neonates and geriatric patients are more likely to develop nephrotoxicity.
- Use netilmicin with caution in patients with neuromuscular diseases, such as myasthenia gravis.
- Safe use in pregnancy or lactation has not been established (Pregnancy Category D).

Toxicity and Overdose Alert

- Blood levels should be monitored periodically during therapy. Timing of blood levels is important in interpreting results. Draw blood for peak level 30 minutes after a 30-minute IV infusion is completed. Samples for trough levels should be drawn just prior to next dose. • Acceptable peak level is 6–12 mcg/ml; trough level should not exceed 0.5–2 mcg/ml.

Lab Test Considerations

• Monitor renal function by urinalysis, specific gravity, BUN, creatinine, and creatinine clearance prior to and throughout therapy. • Netilmicin may cause increased serum BUN, AST (SGOT), ALT (SGPT), lactate dehydrogenase (LDH), alkaline phosphatase, bilirubin, and creatinine concentrations. • It may also cause decreased serum calcium, magnesium, potassium, and sodium concentrations.

Patient/Family Teaching

• Instruct patient to report signs of hypersensitivity, tinnitus, vertigo, or hearing loss.

 PHARMACOLOGIC PROFILE

Indications

• Netilmicin is useful in the treatment of Gram-negative bacillary infections and infections due to staphylococci when penicillins or other less toxic drugs are contraindicated or resistance to other aminoglycosides has occurred. • It has been used in the treatment of the following infections due to susceptible organisms: bone infections, respiratory tract infections, skin and soft tissue infections, abdominal infections, complicated urinary tract infections, and septicemia.

Action

• Netilmicin inhibits protein synthesis in bacteria at the level of the 30S ribosome, resulting in bactericidal action against susceptible bacteria. • It is active against *Pseudomonas aeruginosa* and many Enterobacteriaceae, including *Citrobacter diversus, C. freundii, Enterobacter aerogenes, E. cloacae, Escherichia coli, Klebsiella, Morganella morganii, Proteus, Providencia, Salmonella,* and *Shigella.* • It also has activity against *Staphylococcus aureus* and *S. epidermidis.* • Activity against *Enterococcus* usually requires synergy with a penicillin.

Time/Action Profile (blood levels)

Onset	Peak
rapid	end of infusion

Pharmacokinetics

• **Distribution:** Netilmicin is widely distributed in extracellular fluids. It crosses the placenta and enters breast milk. Penetration into CSF is poor. • **Metabolism and Excretion:** Excretion is mainly (more than 90%) renal. Dosage adjustments are required for any decrease in renal function. Minimal amounts are metabolized by the liver. • **Half-life:** 2–3.4 hours (increased in renal impairment).

Contraindications

• Netilmicin is contraindicated in patients with hypersensitivity to it or to sulfites. Injection contains benzyl alcohol and should be avoided in newborns or patients with known intolerance. Cross-sensitivity with other aminoglycosides may occur.

Adverse Reactions and Side Effects*

• **EENT:** <u>ototoxicity</u> (vestibular and cochlear) • **GU:** <u>nephrotoxicity</u> • **Neuro:** enhanced neuromuscular blockade • **Misc:** hypersensitivity reactions, superinfection.

Niacin	*Vitamin (water soluble)*
Nicotinic acid	pH UK

≋ ADMINISTRATION CONSIDERATIONS

Usual Dose

ADULTS: 25–100 mg 2 or more times daily.
CHILDREN: Up to 300 mg/day.

Dilution

• **Direct IV:** Dilute to a strength of 2 mg/ml. • **Intermittent/Continuous Infusion:** Add to 500 ml of 0.9% NaCl.

Compatibility

• **Additive:** TPN solution.

---

*<u>Underlines</u> indicate most frequent; CAPITALS indicate life-threatening.

Incompatibility

- **Additive:** erythromycin ✦ kanamycin ✦ streptomycin ✦ alkalis ✦ strong acids.

Rate of Administration

- **Direct IV:** Administer at a rate not to exceed 2 mg/min.
- **Intermittent Infusion:** Administer at a rate not to exceed 2 mg/min.

≋ CLINICAL PRECAUTIONS

- Assess patient for signs of niacin deficiency (pellagra), which include dermatitis, stomatitis, glossitis, anemia, nausea and vomiting, confusion, memory loss, and delirium, prior to and periodically throughout therapy.
- Because of infrequency of single B-vitamin deficiencies, combinations (multivitamins) are commonly administered.
- Additive hypotension may occur with ganglionic blocking agents (guanethidine, guanadrel). Large doses may decrease the uricosuric effects of probenecid or sulfinpyrazone.
- Use cautiously in patients with liver disease, arterial bleeding, history of peptic ulcer disease, gout, glaucoma, or diabetes mellitus.
- Niacin has been used safely during pregnancy and lactation in amounts meeting the RDA (Pregnancy Category C).

Lab Test Considerations

- Serum glucose and uric acid levels and hepatic function tests should be monitored periodically during prolonged high-dose therapy. Notify physician if AST (SGOT), ALT (SGPT), or lactate dehydrogenase (LDH) becomes elevated. • May increase prothrombin times and decrease serum albumin. • High-dose therapy may cause elevated serum glucose and uric acid levels. May also cause falsely elevated urine glucose when measured with copper sulfate method (Clinitest) and catecholamine levels during high-dose therapy. Use glucose enzymatic tests (Tes-Tape, Keto-diastix) to measure urine glucose.

Patient/Family Teaching

• Inform patient that cutaneous flushing and a sensation of warmth, especially in the face, neck, and ears, and itching or tingling and headache may occur immediately after IV doses. These effects are usually transient and subside with continued therapy. • Encourage patient to comply with diet recommendations of physician. Explain that the best source of vitamins is a well-balanced diet with foods from the four basic food groups. Foods high in niacin include meats, eggs, milk, and dairy products; little is lost during ordinary cooking. • Emphasize the importance of follow-up examinations to evaluate progress.

PHARMACOLOGIC PROFILE

Indications

• Niacin is used in the treatment and prevention of niacin deficiency (pellagra).

Action

• Niacin is required as a coenzyme (for lipid metabolism, glycogenolysis, and tissue respiration). • Large doses decrease lipoprotein and triglyceride synthesis by inhibiting the release of free fatty acids from adipose tissue and decreasing hepatic lipoprotein synthesis. • Niacin also causes peripheral vasodilation in large doses.

Time/Action Profile (effect on lipids)

Onset	Peak	Duration
hours–days	UK	UK

Pharmacokinetics

• **Distribution:** Niacin is widely distributed following conversion to niacinamide. It enters breast milk. • **Metabolism and Excretion:** Amounts required for metabolic processes are converted to niacinamide. Large doses of niacin are excreted unchanged in the urine. • **Half-life:** 45 minutes.

Contraindications

• Niacin should be avoided in patients with previous hypersensitivity to it.

Adverse Reactions and Side Effects*

• **CNS:** nervousness, panic • **CV:** orthostatic hypotension • **EENT:** toxic amblyopia, blurred vision, proptosis, loss of central vision • **GI:** metallic taste • **Derm:** <u>flushing of the face and neck</u>, <u>pruritus</u>, burning, stinging or tingling of skin, increased sebaceous gland activity, rashes, hyperpigmentation, dry skin • **Hemat:** activation of fibrinolysis • **Metab:** hyperuricemia, hyperglycemia, glycosuria • **Misc:** ANAPHYLACTIC SHOCK.

Nicardipine Hydrochloride	*Antihypertensive, Calcium channel blocker*
Cardene IV	pH 3.5

≋ ADMINISTRATION CONSIDERATIONS

Usual Dose

As a Substitute for Oral Nicardipine

ADULTS: If oral dose is 20 mg q 8 hr, infusion rate should be 0.5 mg/hr; if oral dose is 30 mg q 8 hr, infusion rate is 1.2 mg/hr; if oral dose is 40 mg q 8 hr, then infusion rate is 2.2 mg/hr.

Initial Therapy in Previously Untreated Patients

ADULTS: Initiate therapy at 5 mg/hr, may be increased by 2.5 mg/hr q 15 min, up to 15 mg/hr until desired response is obtained, then decrease to 3 mg/hr. Subsequent adjustments may be required.

Dilution

• **Continuous Infusion: Dilute** each ampule (25 mg) with 240 ml of D5W, D5/0.45% NaCl, D5/0.9% NaCl, D5/40 mEq potassium, 0.45% NaCl, or 0.9% NaCl for 250 ml of a concentration 0.1 mg/ml. • Solution is light yellow; discard solution that is discolored or contains particulate matter. Solution is stable for 24 hours at room temperature.

---

*<u>Underlines</u> indicate most frequent; CAPITALS indicate life-threatening.

Incompatibility

• **Y-site/Additive:** lactated Ringer's injection ◆ 5% sodium bicarbonate.

Rate of Administration

• **Continuous Infusion:** Administer as a slow continuous infusion titrated to desired blood pressure (see Usual Dose section).

☰ CLINICAL PRECAUTIONS

• Monitor blood pressure frequently during administration. If nicardipine is being used in patients who have recently sustained acute cerebral infarction or hemorrhage, hypotension should be avoided.

• As soon as feasible, IV nicardipine should be replaced by maintenance antihypertensive therapy with oral agents.

• Change infusion site every 12 hours to prevent peripheral venous irritation.

• Use nicardipine cautiously in patients with a history of CHF. In some patients with CHF, nicardipine, particularly when used with a beta-adrenergic blocker, may produce negative inotropic effects.

• Because nicardipine is metabolized by the liver, dosage reduction may be necessary in patients with hepatic impairment. Dosage reduction may also be required in patients with reduced renal function. Nicardipine should also be used with caution in patients with pheochromocytoma.

• The effects of nicardipine do not appear to be altered in the elderly.

• The hypotensive effect of nicardipine may be enhanced by other antihypertensive agents, diuretics, nitrates, or fentanyl.

• The effects of nicardipine may be increased by concurrent use of cimetidine. Nicardipine may increase plasma levels of cyclosporine.

• Nicardipine should be used cautiously in patients with angina pectoris. Exacerbation of angina may occur rarely.

• Nicardipine does not protect against cardiovascular sequelae of abrupt discontinuation of beta-blocker therapy.

- Safe use of nicardipine in pregnancy, lactation, or children under the age of 18 years is not established (Pregnancy Category C).

Patient/Family Teaching

- Caution patient to make position changes slowly to minimize orthostatic hypotension. • Nicardipine may cause dizziness. Advise patient to request assistance with ambulation and transfer and to avoid activities requiring alertness until response to medication is known.

PHARMACOLOGIC PROFILE

Indications

- IV nicardipine is used in the short-term management of hypertension.

Action

- Nicardipine inhibits the transport of calcium into myocardial and vascular smooth muscle cells, resulting in inhibition of excitation-contraction coupling and subsequent contraction. Acts primarily by producing systemic vasodilation.

Time/Action Profile (effect on blood pressure when given by slow continuous infusion)

Onset	50% decrease in BP	Duration
within minutes	45 min	50 hr†

†Following discontinuation.

Pharmacokinetics

- **Distribution:** Distribution of nicardipine is not known. • **Metabolism and Excretion:** Nicardipine is mostly metabolized by the liver. Negligible amounts are excreted by the kidneys. • **Half-life:** 45 minutes (intermediate phase); 14.4 hours (terminal phase).

Contraindications

- Nicardipine should not be used in patients with known hypersensitivity and should also be avoided in patients with advanced aortic stenosis (may worsen myocardial oxygen balance).

Adverse Reactions and Side Effects*
• **CNS:** <u>headache</u>, dizziness • **CV:** hypotension, tachycardia, ECG abnormalities, arrhythmias • **GI:** nausea, vomiting • **GU:** polyuria • **Derm:** sweating • **Local:** injection site reactions.

Nitroglycerin	Vasodilator (nitrate), Antianginal (coronary vasodilator)
Nitro-Bid, Nitroject, Nitrostat, Tridil	pH 3–6.5

≋ ADMINISTRATION CONSIDERATIONS

Usual Dose
ADULTS: 5 mcg/min; may be increased by 5 mcg/min q 3–5 min to 20 mcg/min, then increased by 10 mcg/min q 3–5 min and if necessary by 20 mcg/min (dosing determined by hemodynamic parameters).
CHILDREN: 0.1 mcg/kg/min initially, may increase every 5–60 min to 0.5–20 mcg/kg/min (unlabeled).

Dilution
• **Continuous Infusion: Dilute** in D5W or 0.9% NaCl in a concentration of 50–200 mcg/ml, depending on patient fluid tolerance (see Infusion Rate Table below). Do not exceed 400 mcg/ml. • Doses must be diluted and administered as an infusion. Standard infusion sets made of polyvinyl chloride plastic may absorb up to 80% of the nitroglycerin in the solution. Use glass bottles only and special tubing provided by manufacturer. • Solution is stable for 48 hours at room temperature. Solution is not explosive either before or after dilution.

*Underlines indicate most frequent; CAPITALS indicate life-threatening.

Compatibility

- **Syringe:** heparin.
- **Y-site:** amrinone • atracurium • diltiazem • dobutamine • dopamine • famotidine • haloperidol • lidocaine • nitroprusside • pancuronium • ranitidine • streptokinase • tacrolimus • vecuronium.

Incompatibility

- **Y-site:** alteplase.
- **Additive:** Manufacturer recommends that nitroglycerin not be admixed with other medications.

Rate of Administration

- **Continuous Infusion:** Administer via infusion pump, without a filter, to ensure accurate rate. Titrate rate according to patient response.

NITROGLYCERIN INFUSION RATE TABLE

Dilution may be prepared as:

5 mg/100 ml (25 mg/500 ml, 50 mg/1000 ml) = 50 mcg/ml.
25 mg/250 ml (50 mg/500 ml, 100 mg/1000 ml) = 100 mcg/ml.
50 mg/250 ml (100 mg/500 ml, 200 mg/1000 ml) = 200 mcg/ml.

Note that different products are available in different concentrated solutions and should be used with appropriate tubing. Changes in tubing may change response to a given dose.

Dose (mcg/min)	50 mcg/ml Concentration	100 mcg/ml Concentration	200 mcg/ml Concentration
2.5 mcg/min	3 ml/hr	1.5 ml/hr	0.75 ml/hr
5 mcg/min	6 ml/hr	3 ml/hr	1.5 ml/hr
10 mcg/min	12 ml/hr	6 ml/hr	3 ml/hr
15 mcg/min	18 ml/hr	9 ml/hr	4.5 ml/hr
20 mcg/min	24 ml/hr	12 ml/hr	6 ml/hr
30 mcg/min	36 ml/hr	18 ml/hr	9 ml/hr
40 mcg/min	48 ml/hr	24 ml/hr	12 ml/hr
50 mcg/min	60 ml/hr	30 ml/hr	15 ml/hr
60 mcg/min	72 ml/hr	36 ml/hr	18 ml/hr

≋ CLINICAL PRECAUTIONS

- Patients receiving IV nitroglycerin require continuous ECG and blood pressure monitoring. Additional hemodynamic parameters may be ordered.
- Assess location, duration, intensity, and precipitating factors of patient's anginal pain.
- Monitor blood pressure and pulse prior to and following

administration. Geriatric patients are more sensitive to the hypotensive effects of nitroglycerin.

- Hypotensive effects may be exaggerated by concurrent use of antihypertensives, acute ingestion of alcohol, beta-adrenergic blocking agents, calcium channel blockers, haloperidol, or phenothiazines.
- Nitroglycerin should be used cautiously in patients with head trauma or cerebral hemorrhage, glaucoma, hypertrophic cardiomyopathy, or severe liver impairment.
- Use of nitroglycerin in pregnant patients may compromise maternal/fetal circulation (Pregnancy Category C). Safe use in children or during lactation has not been established.

Toxicity and Overdose Alert

- Nitroglycerin is metabolized rapidly; reducing or discontinuing infusion is usually sufficient. If severe hypertension occurs, IV alpha-adrenergic agonists (methoxamine, phenylephrine) may be used. Avoid use of epinephrine; may aggravate shocklike reaction. • Monitor methemoglobin concentrations. Methemoglobinemia is treated with high-flow oxygen and IV methylene blue.

Lab Test Considerations

- May cause increased urine catecholamines and urine vanillylmandelic acid concentrations. • Excessive doses may cause increased methemoglobin concentrations. • May cause falsely elevated serum cholesterol levels.

Patient/Family Teaching

- Caution patient to make position changes slowly to minimize orthostatic hypotension. • Inform patient that headache is a common side effect that should decrease with continuing therapy. Aspirin or acetaminophen may be ordered to treat headache. Notify physician or nurse if headache is persistent or severe.

≋ PHARMACOLOGIC PROFILE

Indications

- Nitroglycerin is used in the adjunct treatment of congestive heart failure in patients with acute myocardial infarction and in the management of anginal pectoris unresponsive to conventional therapy with other forms of nitrates and beta blockers. • It is also used to produce controlled hypotension during surgical procedures.

Action

• Nitroglycerin increases coronary blood flow by dilating coronary arteries and improving collateral flow to ischemic regions. It produces vasodilation (venous greater than arterial), decreases left ventricular end-diastolic pressure and left ventricular end-diastolic volume (preload) while reducing myocardial oxygen consumption. This results in diminished angina, increased cardiac output, and decreased blood pressure.

Time/Action Profile (cardiovascular effects)

Onset	Peak	Duration
immediate	UK	several minutes†

†Dose dependent.

Pharmacokinetics

• **Distribution:** Distribution of nitroglycerin is not known. • **Metabolism and Excretion:** Nitroglycerin undergoes rapid and almost complete metabolism by the liver. It is also metabolized by enzymes in the bloodstream. • **Half-life:** 1–4 minutes.

Contraindications

• Nitroglycerin is contraindicated in patients with hypersensitivity to it, or in patients with severe anemia, pericardial tamponade, or constrictive pericarditis. Large doses should be avoided in patients with known alcohol intolerance.

Adverse Reactions and Side Effects*

• **CNS:** <u>headache</u>, apprehension, weakness, <u>dizziness</u>, light-headedness, restlessness • **EENT:** blurred vision • **CV:** <u>hypotension</u>, <u>tachycardia</u>, syncope • **GI:** nausea, vomiting, abdominal pain • **Misc:** flushing, tolerance, cross-tolerance, alcohol intoxication (large doses only).

---

*<u>Underlines</u> indicate most frequent; CAPITALS indicate life-threatening.

Nitroprusside Sodium   *Antihypertensive*
(vasodilator)

{Nipride}, Nitropress   **pH 3.5–6**

 ADMINISTRATION CONSIDERATIONS

Usual Dose
Adults and Children: 0.3–10 mcg/kg/min. Should not exceed 10 min of therapy at 10 mcg/kg/min infusion rate or 3.5 mg/kg total for short-term infusion. Prolonged infusion rates should not exceed 3 mcg/kg/min.

Dilution
• **Continuous Infusion: Reconstitute** each 50 mg with 2–3 ml of D5W or sterile water for injection without preservatives. **Dilute further** in 250–1000 ml of D5W for concentrations of 200 mcg/ml–50 mcg/ml. Do not use other diluents for reconstitution or infusion. • Wrap infusion bottle in aluminum foil to protect from light; administration set tubing need not be covered. Amber plastic bags do not offer sufficient protection from light; wrap must be opaque. • Freshly prepared solution has a slight brownish tint; discard if solution is dark brown, orange, blue, green, or dark red. Solution must be used within 24 hours of preparation.

Compatibility
• **Syringe:** heparin.
• **Y-site:** amrinone • atracurium • diltiazem • dobutamine • enalaprilat • famotidine • indomethacin • lidocaine • nitroglycerin • pancuronium • tacrolimus • vecuronium.

Incompatibility
• **Additive:** Do not admix with other medications.

Rate of Administration
• **Continuous Infusion:** Administer via infusion pump to ensure accurate dosage rate (see Infusion Rate Table).

{} = Available in Canada only.

NITROPRUSSIDE (Nipride, Nitropress)
INFUSION RATE TABLE

Dilution may be prepared as: 50 mg/1000 ml = 50 mcg/ml
                              100 mg/1000 ml = 100 mcg/ml
                              200 mg/1000 ml = 200 mcg/ml

Nitroprusside Infusion Rates (mcg/kg/min)	50 mcg/ml Concentration	100 mcg/ml Concentration	200 mcg/ml Concentration
0.3 mcg/kg/min	0.36 ml/kg/hr	0.18 ml/kg/hr	0.09 ml/kg/hr
0.6 mcg/kg/min	0.72 ml/kg/hr	0.36 ml/kg/hr	0.18 ml/kg/hr
1 mcg/kg/min	1.2 ml/kg/hr	0.6 ml/kg/hr	0.3 ml/kg/hr
2 mcg/kg/min	2.4 ml/kg/hr	1.2 ml/kg/hr	0.6 ml/kg/hr
3 mcg/kg/min	3.6 ml/kg/hr	1.8 ml/kg/hr	0.9 ml/kg/hr
4 mcg/kg/min	4.8 ml/kg/hr	2.4 ml/kg/hr	1.2 ml/kg/hr
5 mcg/kg/min	6 ml/kg/hr	3 ml/kg/hr	1.5 ml/kg/hr
6 mcg/kg/min	7.2 ml/kg/hr	3.6 ml/kg/hr	1.8 ml/kg/hr
7 mcg/kg/min	8.4 ml/kg/hr	4.2 ml/kg/hr	2.1 ml/kg/hr
8 mcg/kg/min	9.6 ml/kg/hr	4.8 ml/kg/hr	2.4 ml/kg/hr
9 mcg/kg/min	10.8 ml/kg/hr	5.4 ml/kg/hr	2.7 ml/kg/hr
10 mcg/kg/min	12 ml/kg/hr	6 ml/kg/hr	3 ml/kg/hr

≋ CLINICAL PRECAUTIONS

- Monitor blood pressure, heart rate, and ECG frequently throughout course of therapy; continuous monitoring is preferred. Monitor for rebound hypertension following discontinuation of nitroprusside. Pulmonary capillary wedge pressures and urine output may be monitored in patients with myocardial infarction or congestive heart failure.
- If infusion of 10 mcg/kg/min for 10 minutes does not produce adequate reduction in blood pressure, manufacturer recommends nitroprusside be discontinued.
- Nitroprusside has been administered in left ventricular congestive heart failure concurrently with an inotropic agent (dopamine, dobutamine) when effective doses of nitroprusside restore pump function but cause excessive hypotension.
- The hypotension effect of nitroprusside is increased by concurrent use of ganglionic blocking agents, general anesthetics, and other antihypertensives. Geriatric patients are more sensitive to the hypotensive effects of nitroprusside.

- Use nitroprusside cautiously in patients with renal disease, due to increased risk of thiocyanate accumulation. Patients with hepatic disease have an increased risk of cyanide accumulation. Use cautiously in patients with hypothyroidism, hyponatremia, or vitamin B_{12} deficiency. Anuric patients should not be given nitroprusside at infusion rates greater than 1 mcg/kg/min.
- Safe use in pregnancy or lactation has not been established (Pregnancy Category C).

Toxicity and Overdose Alert

- If severe hypotension occurs, drug effects are quickly reversed, within 1–10 minutes, by decreasing rate or temporarily discontinuing infusion. May place patient in Trendelenburg position to maximize venous return. • Plasma thiocyanate levels should be monitored daily in patients receiving prolonged nitroprusside infusions at a rate >3 mcg/kg/min or 1 mcg/kg/min in patients with anuria. Thiocyanate levels should not exceed 1 millimole/liter. • Signs and symptoms of thiocyanate toxicity include toxic psychoses, hyperreflexia, confusion, weakness, tinnitus, seizures, and coma. • Cyanide toxicity may manifest as lactic acidosis, hypoxemia, tachycardia, altered consciousness, seizures, and characteristic breath odor similar to almonds. • Acute treatment of cyanide toxicity includes 4–6 mg/kg *sodium nitrite* (as a 3% solution) over 2–4 minutes. This acts as a buffer for cyanide by converting 10% of hemoglobin to methemoglobin. If administration of sodium nitrite is delayed, inhalation of crushed ampule (Vaporole, Aspirols) of *amyl nitrite* for 15–30 seconds of every minute should be started until sodium nitrite is running. Following completion of sodium nitrite infusion, administer *sodium thiosulfate* 150–200 mcg/kg (available as 25% and 50% solutions). This will convert cyanide to thiocyanate, which may then be eliminated. If required, entire regimen may be repeated in 2 hours at 50% of the initial doses. • If significant methemoglobinemia occurs, treatment is methylene blue 1–2 mg/kg administered over several minutes.

Lab Test Considerations

- Nitroprusside may cause a decreased bicarbonate concentration, pCO_2, and pH. • It may also increase lactate concentrations, serum cyanide, and thiocyanate concentrations. • Monitor serum methemoglobin concentrations in patients who have received >10 mg/kg and who exhibit signs of impaired oxygen delivery despite adequate cardiac output and adequate arterial pO_2.

Patient/Family Teaching

• Advise patient to report the onset of tinnitus, dyspnea, dizziness, headache, or blurred vision immediately.

≋ PHARMACOLOGIC PROFILE

Indications

• Nitroprusside is used in the management of hypertensive crises and to produce controlled hypotension during anesthesia. • It has also been used in the treatment of cardiac pump failure or cardiogenic shock alone or with dopamine (unlabeled use).

Action

• Nitroprusside produces peripheral vasodilation by direct action on venous and arteriolar smooth muscle. This results in rapid lowering of blood pressure and decreased cardiac preload and afterload.

Time/Action Profile (hypotensive effect)

Onset	Peak	Duration
immediate	rapid	1–10 min

Pharmacokinetics

• **Distribution:** UK. • **Metabolism and Excretion:** Nitroprusside is rapidly metabolized in RBCs and tissues to cyanide and subsequently by the liver to thiocyanate. • **Half-life:** UK.

Contraindications

• Nitroprusside should not be used in patients with hypersensitivity to it and should also be avoided in patients with decreased cerebral perfusion.

Adverse Reactions and Side Effects*

• **CNS:** <u>headache</u>, <u>dizziness</u>, restlessness • **EENT:** tinnitus, blurred vision • **CV:** palpitations, dyspnea, excessive hy-

---

*<u>Underlines</u> indicate most frequent; CAPITALS indicate life-threatening.

potension • **GI:** <u>nausea</u>, vomiting, <u>abdominal pain</u> • **F and E:** acidosis • **Local:** phlebitis at IV site • **Misc:** thiocyanate toxicity, cyanide toxicity, methemoglobinemia.

Norepinephrine Bitartrate	*Vasopressor*
Levophed	pH 3–4.5

 ## ADMINISTRATION CONSIDERATIONS

Usual Dose
ADULTS: 8–12 mcg/min initially, then 2–4 mcg/min maintenance infusion rate, titrated by blood pressure response.
CHILDREN: 2 mcg/min or 2 mcg/m^2/min *or* 0.5–1 mcg/min initially, then adjust dose according to response. Infusion rate is titrated by blood pressure response. In severe hypotension during cardiac arrest, use initial dose of 0.1 mcg (0.0001 mg)/kg/min; maintenance infusion rate is titrated by blood pressure response.

Dilution
• **Continuous Infusion:** Dilute 4 mg in 1000 ml of D5W or D5/0.9% NaCl, for a concentration of 4 mcg/ml. Do not dilute in 0.9% NaCl without dextrose. • Do not use discolored solutions (pink, yellow, brown) or those containing a precipitate.

Compatibility
• **Syringe:** heparin.
• **Y-site:** amrinone • diltiazem • famotidine • haloperidol • heparin • hydrocortisone sodium succinate • potassium chloride • vitamin B complex with C.
• **Additive:** calcium chloride • calcium gluceptate • calcium gluconate • cimetidine • dobutamine • heparin • hydrocortisone sodium succinate • magnesium sulfate • methylprednisolone sodium succinate • multivitamins • potassium chloride • ranitidine • succinylcholine • verapamil • vitamin B complex with C.

Incompatibility
- **Additive:** blood or plasma • aminophylline • amobarbital • cephapirin • chlorothiazide • chlorpheniramine • lidocaine • pentobarbital • phenobarbital • phenytoin • secobarbital • sodium bicarbonate • streptomycin • thiopental.

Rate of Administration
- **Continuous Infusion:** Titrate infusion rate according to patient response, using slowest possible rate to correct hypotension (see Infusion Rate Table below). Administer via infusion pump to ensure accurate dosage.

NOREPINEPHRINE INFUSION RATE TABLE

Dilution: May be prepared as 1 mg/250 cc = 4 mcg/ml.
To calculate infusion rate (ml/hr), multiply infusion rate in ml/min × 60.

CONCENTRATION = 4 mcg/ml	
Dose (mcg/min)	**Dose (ml/hr)**
2 mcg/min	30 ml/hr
4 mcg/min	60 ml/hr
6 mcg/min	90 ml/hr
8 mcg/min	120 ml/hr
10 mcg/min	150 ml/hr
12 mcg/min	180 ml/hr

≋ CLINICAL PRECAUTIONS

- Monitor blood pressure every 2–3 minutes until stabilized and every 5 minutes thereafter. Systolic blood pressure is usually maintained at 80–100 mm Hg or 30–40 mm Hg below the previously existing systolic pressure in previously hypertensive patients. Continue to monitor blood pressure frequently for hypotension following discontinuation of norepinephrine. ECG should be monitored continuously. Central venous pressure, intra-arterial pressure, pulmonary artery diastolic pressure, pulmonary capillary wedge pressure, and cardiac output may also be monitored.

- Volume depletion and electrolyte abnormalities should be corrected, if possible, prior to initiation of norepinephrine. If used for prolonged periods, norepinephrine may deplete plasma volume and cause ischemia of vital organs, resulting in hypotension when discontinued. Prolonged or large doses may also decrease cardiac output. Infusion should be discontinued gradually to prevent hypotension. Do not resume therapy unless blood pressure falls to 70–80 mm Hg.
- Monitor urine output throughout therapy.
- Assess IV site frequently throughout infusion. The antecubital or other large vein should be used to minimize risk of extravasation, which may cause tissue necrosis. Phentolamine 5–10 mg may be added to each liter of solution to prevent sloughing of tissue in extravasation. If extravasation occurs, the site should be infiltrated promptly with 10–15 ml of 0.9% NaCl solution containing 5–10 mg of phentolamine to prevent necrosis and sloughing. If prolonged therapy is required or blanching along the course of the vein occurs, change injection sites to provide relief from vasoconstriction.
- Heparin 10 mg may be added to each 500 ml of solution to prevent thrombosis in the infused vein, perivenous reactions, and necrosis in patients with severe hypotension following myocardial infarction.
- Use cautiously in patients with hypertension, hyperthyroidism, or cardiovascular disease.
- Myocardial irritability may occur with concurrent use of cyclopropane or halothane anesthesia, cardiac glycosides, doxapram, or with local use of cocaine. Concurrent use with MAO inhibitors, guanethidine, methyldopate, doxapram, or tricyclic antidepressants may result in severe hypertension. The vasopressor response to norepinephrine will be diminished by alpha-adrenergic blockers. Beta-adrenergic blockers may exaggerate hypertension or block cardiac stimulation. Enhanced vasoconstriction may follow concurrent use with ergot alkaloids (ergotamine, ergonovine, methylergonovine, methysergide) or oxytocin.
- During pregnancy, norepinephrine reduces uterine blood flow and should not be used. Safe use during lactation has not been established (Pregnancy Category C).

Toxicity and Overdose Alert

• If overdose occurs, discontinue norepinephrine and administer fluid and electrolyte replacement therapy. An alpha-adrenergic blocking agent, that is, phentolamine 5–10 mg (see *phentolamine mesylate* monograph on page 789), may be administered intravenously to treat hypertension.

Patient/Family Teaching

• Instruct patient to promptly report headache, dizziness, dyspnea, chest pain, or pain at infusion site.

 PHARMACOLOGIC PROFILE

Indications

• Norepinephrine produces vasoconstriction and myocardial stimulation, which may be required after adequate fluid replacement in the treatment of shock.

Action

• Norepinephrine stimulates alpha-adrenergic receptors located mainly in blood vessels, causing constriction of both capacitance and resistance vessels. It also has minor beta$_1$-adrenergic activity (myocardial stimulation). The net result is increased blood pressure and cardiac output.

Time/Action Profile (effect on blood pressure)

Onset	Peak	Duration
immediate	rapid	1–2 min

Pharmacokinetics

• **Distribution:** Norepinephrine concentrates in sympathetic nervous tissue. It does not cross the blood–brain barrier but readily crosses the placenta. • **Metabolism and Excretion:** Norepinephrine is taken up and metabolized rapidly by sympathetic nerve endings. • **Half-life:** UK.

Contraindications

• Norepinephrine should be avoided in pregnant patients or patients with vascular, mesenteric, or peripheral thrombosis. Norepinephrine is contraindicated in patients with hypoxia, hypercarbia, or hypotension secondary to hypovolemia. Patients with hypersensitivity to bisulfites should not receive norepinephrine.

Adverse Reactions and Side Effects*

• **CNS:** headache, anxiety, dizziness, weakness, tremor, restlessness, insomnia • **Resp:** dyspnea • **CV:** bradycardia, hypertension, arrhythmias, chest pain • **GU:** decreased urine output, renal failure • **Endo:** hyperglycemia • **F and E:** metabolic acidosis • **Local:** phlebitis at IV site • **Misc:** fever.

Octreotide Acetate	*Gastrointestinal hormone, Antidiarrheal*
Sandostatin	pH 3.9–4.5

ADMINISTRATION CONSIDERATIONS

Usual Dose

Subcutaneous route is preferred.

Carcinoid Tumors

ADULTS: 100–600 mcg/day in 2–4 divided doses during first 2 wk of therapy (range 50–1500 mcg/day). Initial dose should be 50 mcg.

VIPomas

ADULTS: 200–300 mcg/day in 2–4 divided doses during first 2 wk of therapy (range 150–750 mcg/day). Initial dose should be 50 mcg.

CHILDREN: 1–10 mcg (0.001–0.01 mg)/kg/day (unlabeled).

HIV-Associated Diarrhea

ADULTS: 100–1800 mcg/day in divided doses (unlabeled).

Dilution

• **Direct IV:** Administer **undiluted** as a bolus. • Do not use solution that is discolored or contains particulate matter. Ampules should be refrigerated, but may be stored at room temperature for the day they will be used. • **Intermittent In-**

---

*Underlines indicate most frequent; CAPITALS indicate life-threatening.

fusion: May be **diluted** in 50–200 ml of sterile isotonic saline solutions or sterile solutions of D5W. • Solutions are stable for 24 hours.

Compatibility
• **Additive:** heparin.

Incompatibility
• **Additive:** Octreotide is not compatible in TPN solutions because of the formation of an inactive conjugate, which may decrease the efficacy of the product.

Rate of Administration
• **Direct IV:** Administer via IV push over 3 minutes. In emergency situations, octreotide may be given by rapid bolus.
• **Intermittent Infusion:** Infuse IV over 15–30 minutes.

≋ CLINICAL PRECAUTIONS

- Assess frequency and consistency of stools, and bowel sounds throughout therapy. Assess patient's fluid and electrolyte balance and skin turgor for dehydration.
- Monitor pulse and blood pressure prior to and periodically throughout therapy.
- Monitor diabetic patients for signs of hypoglycemia. Some patients may require reduction in requirements for insulin, sulfonureas, and diazoxide. Patients with other abnormalities of carbohydrate metabolism (hyperglycemia or hypoglycemia) should be monitored for changes in blood glucose.
- Assess patient for gallbladder disease; assess for pain and monitor ultrasound examinations of gallbladder and bile ducts prior to and periodically throughout prolonged therapy, due to increased risk of stone formation.
- Octreotide may reduce blood levels of cyclosporine.
- Patients with renal impairment may require reduced doses of octreotide.
- Safe use in children, pregnancy, or lactation has not been established (Pregnancy Category B).

Lab Test Considerations

• Monitor 5-HIAA (urinary 5-hydroxyindoleacetic acid), plasma serotonin, plasma substance P in patients with carcinoid tumors; VIP (plasma vasoactive intestinal peptide) in patients with VIPoma; and free T_4 and serum glucose concentrations prior to and periodically throughout therapy in all patients taking octreotide. • Monitor quantitative 72-hour fecal fat and serum carotene determinations periodically for possible drug-induced aggravations of fat malabsorption. • Octreotide may cause a slight increase in liver enzymes.

Patient/Family Teaching

• Octreotide may cause dizziness, drowsiness, or visual disturbances. Caution patient to avoid driving or other activities requiring alertness until response to medication is known. • Advise patient to make position changes slowly to minimize orthostatic hypotension.

☰ PHARMACOLOGIC PROFILE

Indications

• Octreotide is used in treatment of severe diarrhea and flushing episodes in patients with GI endocrine tumors, including metastatic carcinoid tumors and vasoactive intestinal peptide tumors (VIPomas). It is also used to relieve symptoms and suppress tumor growth in patients with pituitary tumors associated with acromegaly and in the management of diarrhea associated with HIV infection (unlabeled use).

Action

• Octreotide suppresses secretion of serotonin and gastroenterohepatic peptides, increases absorption of fluid and electrolytes from the GI tract, and increases GI transit time. It also decreases levels of serotonin metabolites and suppresses growth hormone, insulin, and glucagon.

Time/Action Profile (GI effects)

Onset	Peak	Duration
UK	UK	up to 12 hr

Pharmacokinetics

• **Distribution:** UK. • **Metabolism and Excretion:** 32% of octreotide is excreted unchanged in urine. • **Half-life:** 1.5 hours.

Contraindications
• Octreotide is contraindicated in patients with hypersensitivity to it.

Adverse Reactions and Side Effects*
• **CNS:** headache, dizziness, fatigue, weakness, drowsiness • **EENT:** visual disturbances • **CV:** edema, palpitations, orthostatic hypotension • **GI:** nausea, diarrhea, abdominal pain, vomiting, fat malabsorption, cholelithiasis • **Derm:** flushing • **Endo:** hyperglycemia, hypoglycemia.

Ofloxacin	Anti-infective (fluoroquinolone)
Floxin IV	pH 3.5–5.8

 ADMINISTRATION CONSIDERATIONS

Usual Dose
ADULTS: *Most infections*—300–400 mg q 12 hr. *Uncomplicated gonorrhea*—400-mg infusion single dose. *Urinary tract infections*—200 mg q 12 hr.

Dilution
• **Intermittent Infusion: Dilute** to a concentration of 4 mg/ml with 50–100 ml of 0.9% NaCl, D5W, D5/0.9% NaCl, D5/LR, 5% sodium bicarbonate, D5/*Plasmalyte 56,* or sodium lactate. • Also available in premixed bottles and flexible containers with D5W, which need no further dilution. • Solution is light yellow to amber. • Dilute solution is stable for 72 hours at room temperature or 14 days if refrigerated. Discard unused solution.

Compatibility
• **Additive:** ceftazidime • clindamycin • gentamicin • piperacillin • tobramycin • vancomycin.

---

*Underlines indicate most frequent; CAPITALS indicate life-threatening.

Rate of Administration

• **Intermittent Infusion:** Administer by infusion only over at least 60 minutes. Bolus injections or more rapid infusion may cause hypotension.

≋ CLINICAL PRECAUTIONS

- Assess patient for infection (vital signs, urinalysis, frequency, urgency, cloudy or foul-smelling urine; sputum, fever, WBC) at beginning and throughout therapy.
- Obtain specimens for culture and sensitivity prior to initiating therapy. First dose may be given before receiving results.
- Ofloxacin should be used cautiously in patients with underlying CNS pathology.
- Use cautiously in patients with renal impairment. Patients with severe renal impairment require reduced doses of ofloxacin. Dose should be decreased and/or dosing interval increased if creatinine clearance is 50 ml/min or less.
- Ofloxacin should be discontinued if tendon pain or inflammation occurs. The risk of tendon rupture is increased in geriatric patients, patients receiving concurrent glucocorticoid therapy, or patients receiving long-term dialysis.
- Children under 18 years and pregnant patients should not receive ofloxacin (Pregnancy Category C). Safe use during lactation has not been established; high milk concentrations are achieved.

Lab Test Considerations

• Ofloxacin may cause increased serum AST (SGOT), ALT (SGPT). • It may also cause decreased WBC; increased or decreased serum glucose; and glucosuria, hematuria, proteinuria, and albuminuria.

Patient/Family Teaching

• Encourage patient to maintain a fluid intake of at least 1200–1500 ml/day to prevent crystalluria. • Ofloxacin may cause dizziness and drowsiness. Caution patient to avoid driving or other activities requiring alertness until response to medication is known. • Advise patient to report tendon pain or inflammation, and to refrain from exercising if these occur. • Caution patient to use sunglasses and avoid prolonged exposure to bright light to prevent photophobia. • Advise patient that frequent mouth rinses, good oral hygiene, and sugarless gum or candy may minimize dry mouth.

≋ PHARMACOLOGIC PROFILE

Indications

• Ofloxacin is used in the treatment of the following infections due to susceptible organisms: lower respiratory infections, skin and skin structure infections, and genitourinary tract infections (including prostatitis, gonorrhea, cervicitis, and urethritis).

Action

• Ofloxacin inhibits bacterial DNA synthesis by inhibiting DNA gyrase, resulting in death of susceptible bacteria. • It is active against many Gram-positive pathogens including staphylococci (*Staphylococcus epidermidis* and methicillin-resistant strains of *Staphylococcus aureus, Streptococcus pyogenes,* and *Streptococcus pneumoniae.* • Its Gram-negative spectrum is notable for activity against *Escherichia coli, Klebsiella* species, *Enterobacter, Salmonella, Shigella, Proteus vulgaris, Providencia stuartii, P. rettgeri, Morganella morganii, Pseudomonas aeruginosa, Serratia, Haemophilus* species, *Acinetobacter, Neisseria gonorrhea* and *N. meningitidis, Branhamella catarrhalis, Yersinia, Vibrio, Brucella, Campylobacter,* and *Aeromonas* species. • In addition, it is active against some anaerobic pathogens: *Bacteroides fragilis* and *B. intermedius, Clostridium perfringens* and *C. welchii, Gardnerella vaginalis, Peptococcus niger,* and *Peptostreptococcus.* • Additional spectrum includes *Chlamydia, Legionella, Mycobacterium,* and *Mycoplasma pneumoniae.* • It is not active against *Treponema pallidum.*

Time/Action Profile (blood levels)

Onset	Peak
rapid	end of infusion

Pharmacokinetics

• **Distribution:** Ofloxacin is widely distributed to body tissue and fluids. • **Metabolism and Excretion:** 70–80% of ofloxacin is excreted unchanged by the kidneys. • **Half-life:** 5–7 hours (increased in renal disease impairment).

Contraindications

• Ofloxacin is contraindicated in patients with hypersensitivity to it or to other fluoroquinolones. • Ofloxacin should be avoided in children younger than 18 years old and pregnant patients.

Adverse Reactions and Side Effects*

• **CNS:** tremors, <u>restlessness</u>, confusion, sleep disorders, nervousness, drowsiness, hallucinations, SEIZURES, dizziness • **EENT:** photophobia • **CV:** chest pain • **GI:** <u>nausea</u>, <u>diarrhea</u>, <u>vomiting</u>, <u>abdominal pain</u>, unpleasant taste, decreased appetite, dry mouth • **GU:** crystalluria, cylindruria, hematuria, vaginal discharge, genital pruritus • **Derm:** rash.

Ondansetron Hydrochloride	Antiemetic (serotonin antagonist)
Zofran	pH 3.3–4

ADMINISTRATION CONSIDERATIONS

Usual Dose

Prevention of Nausea/Vomiting Associated with Chemotherapy

ADULTS: Three doses of 150 mcg (0.15 mg)/kg/dose. Administer first dose 30 min before chemotherapy. Administer second and third doses 4 and 8 hr after first dose or a single dose of 32 mg beginning 30 min prior to chemotherapy.

CHILDREN >4 yr: Three doses of 150 mg (0.15 mg)/kg/dose. Administer first dose 30 min prior to chemotherapy. Administer second and third doses 4 and 8 hr after first dose.

---

*<u>Underlines</u> indicate most frequent; CAPITALS indicate life-threatening.

Prevention of Postoperative Nausea/Vomiting
ADULTS: 4-mg single dose.

Dilution
• **Direct IV:** Doses for prevention of postoperative nausea and vomiting may be administered **undiluted.** • **Intermittent Infusion: Dilute** doses for prevention of nausea and vomiting associated with chemotherapy in 50 ml of D5W or 0.9% NaCl. May also be diluted with D5/0.9% NaCl, D5/0.45% NaCl, and 3% NaCl. • Solution is clear and colorless. Stable for 7 days at room temperature following dilution.

Compatibility
• **Y-site:** amikacin • aztreonam • bleomycin • carboplatin • carmustine • cefazolin • cefotaxime • cefoxitin • ceftazidime • ceftizoxime • cefuroxime • chlorpromazine • cimetidine • cisplatin • clindamycin • cyclophosphamide • cytarabine • dacarbazine • dactinomycin • daunorubicin • dexamethasone sodium phosphate • diphenhydramine • doxorubicin • doxycycline • droperidol • etoposide • famotidine • filgrastim • floxuridine • fluconazole • fludarabine • gallium nitrate • gentamicin • haloperidol • heparin • hydrocortisone • hydromorphone • hydroxyzine • ifosfamide • imipenem/cilastatin • magnesium sulfate • mannitol • mechlorethamine • melphalan • meperidine • mesna • methotrexate • metoclopramide • miconazole • mitomycin • mitoxantrone • morphine • paclitaxel • pentostatin • piperacillin/tazobactam • potassium chloride • prochlorperazine edisylate • ranitidine • sodium acetate • streptozocin • teniposide • ticarcillin • ticarcillin/clavulanate • vancomycin • vinblastine • vincristine • vinorelbine • zidovudine.

• **Additive:** dexamethasone sodium phosphate • hydromorphone • morphine.

Incompatibility
• **Y-site:** acyclovir • allopurinol sodium • aminophylline • amphotericin B • ampicillin • ampicillin/sulbactam • cefoperazone • furosemide • ganciclovir • lorazepam • methylprednisolone sodium succinate • mezlocillin • piperacillin • sargramostim • sodium bicarbonate.

Rate of Administration
• **Direct IV:** Administer over a minimum of 30 seconds, preferably over 2–5 minutes. • **Intermittent Infusion:** Administer each dose as an IV infusion over 15 minutes.

≋ CLINICAL PRECAUTIONS

- Assess patient for nausea, vomiting, abdominal distention, and bowel sounds prior to and following administration.
- Not recommended for routine prophylaxis in postoperative patients in whom nausea and vomiting are not expected. Administer immediately before induction of anesthesia in situations where nausea and vomiting must be avoided. May also be used in patients with nausea and vomiting to prevent further episodes.
- Assess patient for extrapyramidal effects (involuntary movements, facial grimacing, rigidity, shuffling walk, trembling of hands) throughout therapy.
- Use ondansetron cautiously in patients with hepatic impairment. In this population, a single 8-mg dose beginning 30 minutes prior to chemotherapy is recommended.
- Safe use during pregnancy, lactation, or in children younger than 3 years old has not been established (Pregnancy Category B).

Lab Test Considerations

- Ondansetron may cause transient elevations in AST (SGOT) and ALT (SGPT) levels.

Patient/Family Teaching

- Advise patient to notify physician immediately if involuntary movement of eyes, face, or limbs occurs.

≋ PHARMACOLOGIC PROFILE

Indications

- Ondansetron is used in the prevention of nausea and vomiting associated with chemotherapy.

Action

- Ondansetron blocks the effects of serotonin at 5-HT$_3$ receptor sites (selective antagonist) located in vagal nerve terminals and the chemoreceptor trigger zone in the CNS.

Time/Action Profile (antiemetic effect)

Onset	Peak	Duration
rapid	15–30 min	4 hr

Pharmacokinetics

• **Distribution:** UK. • **Metabolism and Excretion:** Ondansetron is extensively metabolized by the liver. Five percent is excreted unchanged by the kidneys. • **Half-life:** 3.5–5.5 hours.

Contraindications

• Ondansetron is contraindicated in patients with hypersensitivity to it or to parabens.

Adverse Reactions and Side Effects*

• **CNS:** <u>headache</u> • **GI:** <u>diarrhea</u> • **Neuro:** extrapyramidal reactions.

Orphenadrine Citrate	Skeletal muscle relaxant (centrally acting)
Banflex, Blanex, Flexagin, Flexain, Flexoject, Flexon, K-Flex, Marflex, Myolin, Myotrol, Neocyten, Norflex, O-Flex, Orfro, Orphenate, Tega-Flex	pH 5–6

≋ ADMINISTRATION CONSIDERATIONS

Usual Dose

ADULTS: 60 mg q 12 hr as needed.

Dilution

• **Direct IV:** May be administered **undiluted**.

Incompatibility

• Information unavailable. Do not admix with other solutions or medications.

---

*<u>Underlines</u> indicate most frequent; CAPITALS indicate life-threatening.

Rate of Administration
- **Direct IV:** Administer over 5 minutes.

≋ CLINICAL PRECAUTIONS

- Assess patient for pain, muscle stiffness, and range of motion prior to and throughout therapy.
- Monitor pulse and blood pressure every 15 minutes during parenteral administration.
- Have patient remain recumbent during and for at least 10–15 minutes following administration to avoid orthostatic hypotension. Provide safety measures as indicated. Supervise ambulation and transfer of patient.
- Orphenadrine should be used cautiously in patients with glaucoma, hyperthyroidism, hepatic or renal impairment, cardiovascular disease, asthma, autonomic neuropathy, and GI infections and in elderly patients, who are at increased risk of adverse reactions. Exposure to increased environmental temperature may result in hyperthermia in patients receiving orphenadrine.
- Additive CNS depression may occur with concurrent use of other CNS depressants including alcohol, antihistamines, opioid analgesics, and sedative/hypnotics.
- Additive anticholinergic effects may occur with concurrent use of other agents having anticholinergic properties (antidepressants, antihistamines, phenothiazines, haloperidol, or disopyramide).
- Safe use of orphenadrine in pregnancy, lactation, or children has not been established. Use only when clearly needed in pregnant patients (Pregnancy Category C). Orphenadrine is not recommended for use in children.

Patient/Family Teaching

- Encourage patient to comply with additional therapies prescribed for muscle spasm (rest, physical therapy, heat).
- Orphenadrine may cause dizziness, drowsiness, and blurred vision. Caution patient to avoid driving and other activities requiring alertness until response to medication is known. • Instruct patient to make position changes slowly to minimize orthostatic hypotension. • Advise patient that frequent mouth rinses, good oral hygiene, and sugarless gum or candy may decrease dry mouth. • Advise patient to

notify nurse or physician if urinary retention occurs or if constipation persists. Discuss methods of preventing constipation with patient, such as increasing bulk in the diet, increasing fluid intake, and increasing mobility.

 PHARMACOLOGIC PROFILE

Indications

• Orphenadrine is used as an adjunct to rest and physical therapy in the treatment of muscle spasm associated with acute painful musculoskeletal conditions.

Action

• Orphenadrine produces skeletal muscle relaxation, probably due to CNS depression.

Time/Action Profile (skeletal muscle relaxation)

Onset	Peak	Duration
immediate	UK	UK

Pharmacokinetics

• **Distribution:** UK. • **Metabolism and Excretion:** Orphenadrine is mostly metabolized by the liver. Small amounts are excreted unchanged by the kidneys. • **Half-life:** 14 hours.

Contraindications

• Orphenadrine is contraindicated in patients who have hypersensitivity to it or to bisulfites. Orphenadrine should not be given to patients with obstruction of the GI tract, obstructive uropathy, myasthenia gravis, or acute hemorrhage.

Adverse Reactions and Side Effects*

• **CNS:** fainting, confusion, dizziness, light-headedness, drowsiness, excitability, nervousness, restlessness, headache, hallucinations • **EENT:** blurred vision, visual disturbances, mydriasis • **CV:** tachycardia, palpitations, orthostatic hypotension • **GI:** <u>dry mouth</u>, constipation, nausea, vomiting, trembling, GI disturbances • **GU:** urinary hesitancy, urinary retention • **Derm:** rash, pruritus, urticaria • **MS:** muscle weakness • **Misc:** allergic reactions including ANAPHYLAXIS.

---

*<u>Underlines</u> indicate most frequent; CAPITALS indicate life-threatening.

Oxacillin Sodium

Anti-infective
(penicillinase-resistant penicillin)

Bactocill, Prostaphlin

pH 6–8.5
2.5–3.1 mEq Na/g

ADMINISTRATION CONSIDERATIONS

Usual Dose

ADULTS AND CHILDREN ≥**40 kg:** 1–2 g q 4 hr (up to 20 g/day).

CHILDREN UP TO **40 kg:** *Most infections*—12.5–25 mg/kg q 6 hr or 16.7 mg/kg q 4 hr (up to 300 mg/kg/day).

PREMATURE INFANTS AND NEONATES: *Most infections*—6.25 mg/kg q 6 hr.

NEONATES >**2 kg:** *Meningitis*—50 mg/kg for first 7 days of life, then 50 mg/kg q 6 hr.

NEONATES <**2 kg:** *Meningitis*—25–50 mg/kg q 12 hr for first 7 days of life, then 50 mg/kg q 8 hr.

Dilution

• **Direct IV:** To **reconstitute,** add 1.4 ml of sterile water for injection to each 250-mg vial, 2.7–2.8 ml to each 500-mg vial, 5.7 ml to each 1-g vial, 11.4–11.5 ml to each 2-g vial, and 21.8–23 ml to each 4-g vial, for a concentration of 250 mg/1.5 ml. • Stable for 3 days at room temperature or 7 days if refrigerated. • **Further dilute** each reconstituted 250-mg or 500-mg vial with 5 ml of sterile water or 0.9% NaCl for injection, 10 ml for each1-g vial, 20 ml for each 2-g vial, and 40 ml for each 4-g vial. • **Intermittent Infusion: Dilute** to a concentration of 0.5–40 mg/ml with 0.9% NaCl, D5W, D5/0.9% NaCl, or lactated Ringer's solution.

Compatibility

• **Y-site:** acyclovir ⬩ cyclophosphamide ⬩ diltiazem ⬩ famotidine ⬩ fluconazole ⬩ foscarnet ⬩ heparin ⬩ hydrocortisone sodium succinate ⬩ hydromorphone ⬩ labetalol ⬩ magnesium sulfate ⬩ meperidine ⬩ morphine ⬩ perphenazine ⬩ potassium chloride ⬩ tacrolimus ⬩ vitamin B complex with C ⬩ zidovudine.

• **Additive:** cephapirin ⬩ chloramphenicol ⬩ potassium chloride ⬩ sodium bicarbonate.

Incompatibility

- **Y-site:** verapamil. • If aminoglycosides and penicillins or cephalosporins must be given concurrently, administer in separate sites at least 1 hour apart.
- **Additive:** cytarabine.

Rate of Administration

- **Direct IV:** Administer slowly over 10 minutes. • **Intermittent Infusion:** May be infused for up to 6 hours.

≋ CLINICAL PRECAUTIONS

- Assess patient for infection (vital signs; appearance of wound, sputum, urine, and stool; WBC) at beginning and throughout course of therapy.
- Obtain specimens for culture and sensitivity prior to initiating therapy. First dose may be given before receiving results.
- Obtain a history before initiating therapy to determine previous use of and reactions to penicillins or cephalosporins. Persons with a negative history of penicillin sensitivity may still have an allergic response. Use cautiously in patients with a history of previous hypersensitivity reactions.
- Observe patient for signs and symptoms of anaphylaxis (rash, pruritus, laryngeal edema, wheezing). Discontinue the drug and notify physician immediately if these occur. Keep epinephrine, an antihistamine, and resuscitation equipment close by in the event of an anaphylactic reaction.
- Probenecid decreases renal excretion and increases blood levels of oxacillin. Oxacillin may alter the effects of oral anticoagulants.
- Oxacillin should be used cautiously in patients with severe hepatic impairment. Dosage reduction is recommended in this population. Neonates and infants may develop hematuria, albuminuria, and azotemia with large doses.
- Safe use in pregnancy or lactation has not been established (Pregnancy Category B). Oxacillin has been used during pregnancy without adverse effects.

Lab Test Considerations

• CBC, BUN, creatinine, urinalysis, and liver function tests should be monitored periodically during therapy. Oxacillin may cause elevations in AST (SGOT) and ALT (SGPT) and may cause positive direct Coombs' test results.

Patient/Family Teaching

• Advise patient to report signs of superinfection (black, furry overgrowth on the tongue; vaginal itching or discharge; loose or foul-smelling stools) and allergy promptly to physician. • Instruct patient to notify physician if symptoms do not improve.

 PHARMACOLOGIC PROFILE

Indications

• Oxacillin is used in the treatment of the following infections due to susceptible strains of penicillinase-producing staphylococci: respiratory tract infections, skin and skin structure infections, bone and joint infections, urinary tract infections, endocarditis, septicemia, and meningitis.

Action

• Oxacillin binds to bacterial cell walls, leading to cell death in susceptible bacteria. • It resists the action of penicillinase, an enzyme capable of inactivating penicillin. Its spectrum includes activity against most Gram-positive aerobic cocci, but less so than penicillin, and is notable for activity against penicillinase-producing strains of *Staphylococcus aureus* and *S. epidermidis*. • It is not active against methicillin-resistant staphylococci.

Time/Action Profile (blood levels)

Onset	Peak
rapid	end of infusion

Pharmacokinetics

• **Distribution:** Oxacillin is widely distributed. Penetration into CSF is minimal but sufficient in the presence of inflamed meninges. It crosses the placenta and enters breast milk. • **Metabolism and Excretion:** Oxacillin is partially metabolized by the liver (49%) and partially excreted unchanged by the kidneys. • **Half-life:** 20–50 minutes (increased in severe hepatic impairment).

Contraindications

• Oxacillin is contraindicated in patients with hypersensitivity to penicillins.

Adverse Reactions and Side Effects*

• **CNS:** SEIZURES (high doses) • **GI:** <u>nausea</u>, <u>vomiting</u>, <u>diarrhea</u>, hepatitis • **GU:** interstitial nephritis • **Derm:** <u>rashes</u>, urticaria • **Hemat:** blood dyscrasias • **Local:** phlebitis at IV site • **Misc:** superinfection, <u>allergic reactions</u>, including ANAPHYLAXIS and serum sickness.

Oxymorphone Hydrochloride	Opioid analgesic (agonist)
Numorphan	pH 2.7–4.5

Schedule II

ADMINISTRATION CONSIDERATIONS

Usual Dose

ADULTS: 500 mcg (0.5 mg)–1 mg q 3–4 hr as needed; increase as needed. As tolerance to the analgesic effects of oxymorphone develops, usual doses may have to be exceeded to maintain pain control.

Dilution

• **Direct IV:** Administer **undiluted**.

Compatibility

• **Y-site:** glycopyrrolate ◆ hydroxyzine ◆ ranitidine.

Rate of Administration

• **Direct IV:** Administer over 2–3 minutes.

---

*<u>Underlines</u> indicate most frequent; CAPITALS indicate life-threatening.

≋ CLINICAL PRECAUTIONS

- Assess type, location, and intensity of pain prior to and 15–30 minutes (peak) following administration. When titrating opioid doses, increases of 25–50% should be administered until there is either a 50% reduction in the patient's pain rating on a numerical or visual analogue scale or the patient reports satisfactory pain relief. Subsequent doses may be safely administered at the time of the peak if the previous dose is ineffective and side effects are minimal. Regularly administered doses may be more effective than p.r.n. administration. Analgesic is more effective if given before pain becomes severe. Coadministration with nonopioid analgesics may have additive analgesic effects and may permit lower opioid doses.
- An equianalgesic chart (Appendix B, page 1045) should be used when changing routes or when changing from one opioid to another.
- Assess blood pressure, pulse, and respiratory rate before and periodically during administration. If respiratory rate is less than 10/min, assess level of sedation. Physical stimulation may be sufficient to prevent significant hypoventilation. Dose may need to be decreased by 25–50%. Initial drowsiness will diminish with continued use. Additive CNS depression may occur with concurrent use of alcohol, antihistamines, and sedative/hypnotics.
- Assess bowel function routinely. Prevention of constipation should be instituted with increased intake of fluids and bulk, stool softeners, and laxatives to minimize constipating effects. Stimulant laxatives should be administered routinely if opioid use exceeds 2–3 days, unless contraindicated.
- Prolonged use may lead to physical and psychological dependence and tolerance. This should not prevent patient from receiving adequate analgesia. Most patients who receive oxymorphone for medical reasons do not develop psychological dependence. Progressively higher doses may be required to relieve pain with long-term therapy. To prevent withdrawal symptoms, oxymorphone should be discontinued gradually after long-term use.

- Administration of partial-antagonist opioid analgesics may precipitate opioid withdrawal in physically dependent patients. Nalbuphine or pentazocine may decrease analgesia.
- Use oxymorphone with caution in patients receiving MAO inhibitors, as concurrent use may result in unpredictable reactions. Initial dose of oxymorphone should be decreased to 25% of usual dose.
- Use oxymorphone cautiously in patients with head trauma; increased intracranial pressure; severe renal, hepatic, or pulmonary disease; hypothyroidism; adrenal insufficiency; undiagnosed abdominal pain; prostatic hypertrophy; or alcoholism. Elderly or debilitated patients should receive reduced doses initially.
- Safe use during pregnancy has not been established (Pregnancy Category C). Although oxymorphone has been used safely during labor, respiratory depression may occur in the newborn. Safe use in children has not been established.

Toxicity and Overdose Alert

- If an opioid antagonist is required to reverse respiratory depression or coma, naloxone (Narcan) is the antidote. Dilute the 0.4-mg ampule of naloxone in 10 ml of 0.9% NaCl and administer 0.5 ml (0.02 mg) by direct IV push every 2 minutes. For children and patients weighing <40 kg, dilute 0.1 mg of naloxone in 10 ml of 0.9% NaCl for a concentration of 10 mcg/ml and administer 0.5 mcg every 1–2 minutes. Titrate the dose to avoid withdrawal, seizures, and severe pain.

Lab Test Considerations

- Oxymorphone may increase plasma amylase and lipase levels.

Patient/Family Teaching

- Instruct patient on how and when to ask for pain medication. • Oxymorphone may cause drowsiness or dizziness. Advise patient to call for assistance when ambulating or smoking. Caution patient to avoid driving and other activities requiring alertness until response to medication is known. • Advise patient to make position changes slowly to minimize orthostatic hypotension. • Advise patient to avoid concurrent use of alcohol or other CNS depressants with this medication. • Encourage patient to turn, cough, and breathe deeply every 2 hours to prevent atelectasis.

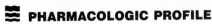 **PHARMACOLOGIC PROFILE**

Indications
• Oxymorphone is used in the management of moderate to severe pain, as a supplement in balanced anesthesia, and as an obstetrical analgesic. It is also used to decrease anxiety and dyspnea associated with pulmonary edema.

Action
• Oxymorphone binds to opiate receptors in the CNS, where it alters the perception of and response to painful stimuli, while producing generalized CNS depression.

Time/Action Profile (analgesic effect)

Onset	Peak	Duration
5–10 min	15–30 min	3–4 hr

Pharmacokinetics
• **Distribution:** Oxymorphone is widely distributed. It crosses the placenta and enters breast milk. • **Metabolism and Excretion:** Oxymorphone is mostly metabolized by the liver. • **Half-life:** 2.6–4 hours.

Contraindications
• Oxymorphone is contraindicated in patients with hypersensitivity to it. • Chronic use should be avoided in pregnant or lactating patients. • Oxymorphone should not be used in children younger than 12 years of age.

Adverse Reactions and Side Effects*
• **CNS:** <u>sedation</u>, <u>confusion</u>, headache, euphoria, floating feeling, unusual dreams, hallucinations, dysphoria, dizziness • **EENT:** miosis, diplopia, blurred vision • **Resp:** respiratory depression • **CV:** orthostatic hypotension • **GI:** nausea, vomiting, <u>constipation</u>, dry mouth • **GU:** urinary retention • **Derm:** sweating, flushing • **Misc:** tolerance, physical dependence, psychological dependence.

---

*<u>Underlines</u> indicate most frequent; CAPITALS indicate life-threatening.

Oxytocin	*Hormone*
	(oxytocic)
Pitocin, Syntocinon	**pH 2.5–4.5**

≋ ADMINISTRATION CONSIDERATIONS

Usual Dose
Note: 1 milliunit is equal to 1 mU.

Augmentation/Induction of Labor
ADULTS: 0.5–2 milliunits/min initially; increase by 1–2 milliunits q 15–60 minutes until pattern of contractions is established (maximum 20 milliunits/min). Usual rate required is 2–5 milliunits/min. Rate may be decreased once pattern is established.

Postpartum Control of Uterine Bleeding
ADULTS: 10 units at 20–40 milliunits/min following delivery of placenta(s).

Fetal Stress Test
ADULTS: 0.5 milliunits/min; may be increased (doubled) q 20 min until three moderate contractions occur in one 10-minute period, to a maximum of 20 milliunits/min (usual rate is 5–6 milliunits/min). Test should only be performed under maternal/fetal monitoring.

Incomplete/Inevitable/Therapeutic Abortion
ADULTS: 10 units infused at 20–40 milliunits/min. Not to exceed 30 units in a 12-hr period.

Control of Postabortion Bleeding
ADULTS: 10 units infused at 20–100 milliunits/min.

Dilution
• **Continuous Infusion:** *Induction of Labor*—**Dilute** 1 ml (10 units) in 1 liter of compatible infusion fluid for a concentration of 10 milliunits/ml. • *Postpartum Bleeding*—For control of postpartum bleeding, **dilute** 1–4 ml (10–40 units) in 1 liter of compatible infusion fluid (10–40 milliunits/ml). • *Incomplete or Inevitable Abortion*—**Dilute** 1 ml (10 units) in 500 ml of compatible infusion fluid, for a concentration of 20 milliunits/ml. • Rotate the infusion container to ensure

thorough mixing. Store this solution in the refrigerator, but do not freeze.

Compatibility

• **Y-site:** heparin • hydrocortisone sodium succinate • insulin • meperidine • morphine • potassium chloride.

• **Additive:** chloramphenicol • metaraminol • netilmicin • sodium bicarbonate • thiopental • verapamil • vitamin B complex with C.

• **Solution:** dextrose/Ringer's or lactated Ringer's combinations • dextrose/saline combinations • Ringer's or lactated Ringer's injection • D5W • D10W • 0.45% NaCl • 0.9% NaCl.

Incompatibility

• **Additive:** fibrinolysin.

Rate of Administration

• **Continuous Infusion:** *Induction of Labor*—Begin infusion at 1–2 milliunits/min (0.1–0.2 ml), increase in increments of 1–2 milliunits/min at 15–30-minute intervals until contractions simulate normal labor. • *Postpartum Bleeding*—Begin infusion at a rate of 20–40 milliunits/min to control uterine atony. Adjust the rate as indicated. • *Incomplete or Inevitable Abortion*—Infuse at a rate of 10–20 milliunits/min.

≋ CLINICAL PRECAUTIONS

• Fetal maturity, presentation, and pelvic adequacy should be assessed prior to administration of oxytocin for induction for labor.

• Assess character, frequency, and duration of uterine contractions; resting uterine tone; and fetal heart rate frequently throughout administration. If contractions occur <2 minutes apart and are >50–65 mm Hg on the monitor, if they last 60–90 seconds or longer, or if a significant change in fetal heart rate develops, stop infusion and turn patient on her left side to prevent fetal anoxia.

• Monitor maternal blood pressure and pulse frequently and fetal heart rate continuously throughout administration.

• Oxytocin occasionally causes water intoxication. Monitor patient for signs and symptoms (drowsiness, listlessness, confusion, headache, anuria, seizures) and notify physician if they occur.

- Severe hypertension may occur if oxytocin follows administration of vasopressors. Concurrent use with cyclopropane anesthesia may result in excessive hypotension.
- Use cautiously during first and second stages of labor. Sensitivity to oxytocin increases during the second stage. Oxytocin should not be used to augment labor in patients planning nonvaginal delivery.

Lab Test Considerations

- Monitor maternal electrolytes. Water retention may result in hypochloremia or hyponatremia.

Patient/Family Teaching

- Advise patient to expect contractions similar to menstrual cramps after administration has started.

≋ PHARMACOLOGIC PROFILE

Indications

- Oxytocin is used for the induction of labor at term, in the facilitation of uterine contractions at term, in the facilitation of threatened abortion, and for postpartum control of bleeding after expulsion of the placenta. • It is also used to evaluate fetal competence as part of a fetal stress test (unlabeled use).

Action

- Oxytocin stimulates uterine smooth muscle, producing uterine contractions similar to those in spontaneous labor. • It also stimulates mammary gland smooth muscle, thereby facilitating lactation, and has vasopressor and antidiuretic effects.

Time/Action Profile (uterine contractions)

Onset	Peak	Duration
immediate	UK	1 hr

Pharmacokinetics

- **Distribution:** Oxytocin is widely distributed in extracellular fluid. Small amounts reach fetal circulation. • **Metab-**

olism and Excretion: Oxytocin is rapidly metabolized by liver and kidneys. • **Half-life:** 3–9 minutes.

Contraindications

• Oxytocin is contraindicated in patients with hypersensitivity to it. Some products contain alcohol and should be avoided in patients with known intolerance. • It should not be used in patients anticipating a nonvaginal delivery.

Adverse Reactions and Side Effects*

Maternal

• **CNS:** SEIZURES, coma • **CV:** hypotension • **F and E:** water intoxication, hyponatremia, hypochloremia • **Hemat:** afibrinogenemia, thrombocytopenia • **Misc:** abruptio placentae, hypersensitivity, painful contractions, decreased uterine blood flow, increased uterine motility.

Fetal

• **CNS:** intracranial hemorrhage • **Resp:** hypoxia, asphyxia • **CV:** arrhythmias.

Paclitaxel	*Antineoplastic agent (antimicrotubule agent)*
Taxol	pH UK

≋ ADMINISTRATION CONSIDERATIONS

Usual Dose

ADULTS: *Ovarian cancer*—135 mg/m² over 24 hr q 3 wk (in Canada, recommended dose is 170 mg/m² q 3 wk). *Breast cancer*—175 mg/m² q 3 wk.

Dilution

• **Continuous Infusion:** Paclitaxel *must* be diluted prior to injection. **Dilute** contents of 5-ml (30-mg) vials to a concentration of 0.3–1.2 mg/ml with any of the following diluents: 0.9% NaCl; D5W, D5/0.9% NaCl, or dextrose in

---

*Underlines indicate most frequent; CAPITALS indicate life-threatening.

Ringer's solution. • Although haziness in the diluted solution is normal, inspect for particulate matter or discoloration before use. Use an in-line filter of not greater than 0.22-micron pore size. Solutions are stable for 27 hours at room temperature and lighting. Do not use PVC containers or administration sets because of the risk of exposure to potentially toxic components being leached from the plastic.

Compatibility

• **Y-site:** acyclovir • amikacin • aminophylline • ampicillin/sulbactam • bleomycin • butorphanol • calcium chloride • carboplatin • cefotetan • ceftazidime • ceftriaxone • cimetidine • cisplatin • cyclophosphamide • cytarabine • dacarbazine • dexamethasone sodium phosphate • diphenhydramine • doxorubicin • droperidol • etoposide • famotidine • floxuridine • fluconazole • fluorouracil • furosemide • ganciclovir • gentamicin • haloperidol • heparin • hydrocortisone • hydromorphone • ifosfamide • lorazepam • magnesium sulfate • mannitol • meperidine • mesna • methotrexate • metoclopramide • morphine • nalbuphine • ondansetron • pentostatin • potassium chloride • prochlorperazine • ranitidine • sodium bicarbonate • vancomycin • vinblastine • vincristine • zidovudine.

Incompatibility

• **Y-site:** amphotericin B • chlorpromazine • hydroxyzine • methylprednisolone • mitoxantrone.

Rate of Administration

• **Continuous Infusion:** Dose is administered as a 24-hour infusion for ovarian cancer and over 3 hours for breast cancer.

≋ CLINICAL PRECAUTIONS

- Monitor vital signs frequently, especially during first hour of 24-hour infusion.
- Monitor for hypersensitivity reactions continuously for the first 30 minutes of the infusion and frequently thereafter. These occur frequently (19%) during administration of paclitaxel. The most common manifestations are dyspnea, hypotension, and chest pain. Severe symptoms usually occur within the first 10 minutes of paclitaxel in-

fusion. If these occur, stop the infusion. Treatment may include bronchodilators, epinephrine, antihistamines, and glucocorticoids. Keep these agents and resuscitative equipment close by in the event of an anaphylactic reaction. Other manifestations of hypersensitivity reactions include flushing and rash. Pretreatment is recommended for *all* patients and should include a glucocorticoid (dexamethasone 20 mg orally or intravenously 12 and 6 hours prior to paclitaxel), diphenhydramine 50 mg intravenously 30–60 minutes prior to paclitaxel (or similar antihistamine), and an H_2 antagonist (cimetidine 300 mg IV, ranitidine 50 mg IV, or famotidine 20 mg IV 30–60 minutes prior to paclitaxel).

- Monitor cardiovascular status. Hypotension and bradycardia are common but usually do not require treatment. Continuous ECG monitoring is recommended only for patients with serious underlying cardiac conduction abnormalities.
- Monitor infusion site. Extravasation may cause phlebitis and cellulitus.
- Monitor for bone marrow depression. Anti-infective therapy may be required. Assess for fever, chills, sore throat, and signs of infection. Assess for bleeding (bleeding gums, bruising, petechiae; guaiac test stools, urine, and emesis). Avoid giving IM injections and taking rectal temperature. Apply pressure to venipuncture sites for 10 minutes. Additive bone marrow depression may occur with cisplatin or radiation therapy. Subsequent doses should be decreased by 20% in patients who develop severe neutropenia (WBC less than 500 cells/mm³ for a week or more).
- Assess for development of peripheral neuropathy. Early symptoms include numbness, tingling, or burning in hands or feet. Patients with pre-existing neuropathies are at greatest risk. If severe symptoms occur, subsequent dosage should be reduced by 20%.
- Assess patient for pain in joints and muscles, especially arms and legs. Arthralgias or myalgias usually begin 2–3 days after treatment and resolve within 5 days. Pain may be treated with nonopioid or opioid analgesics.
- Monitor intake and output, appetite, and nutritional intake. Paclitaxel causes nausea and vomiting in 60% of patients. Confer with physician regarding prophylactic

use of an antiemetic. Adjust diet as tolerated to help maintain fluid and electrolyte balance and nutritional status.

- Use cautiously in patients with severe hepatic impairment, active infections, decreased bone marrow reserve, or other chronic debilitating illnesses. Ketoconazole may inhibit the metabolism of paclitaxel and increase the risk of serious toxicity. Concurrent use should be undertaken with caution.
- Safe use in children has not been established. Use cautiously in patients with childbearing potential. Avoid paclitaxel during pregnancy or lactation.

Lab Test Considerations

- Monitor CBC and differential prior to and periodically throughout therapy. The nadir of leukopenia occurs in 11 days. Recovery usually occurs by days 15–21. The nadir of thrombocytopenia usually occurs at day 8 or 9 of paclitaxel therapy and usually does not fall below $100,000/mm^3$.
- Monitor liver function studies (AST [SGOT], ALT [SGPT], LDH, bilirubin) prior to and periodically throughout therapy to detect hepatotoxicity.

Patient/Family Teaching

- Advise patient to notify physician in the event of fever, chills, sore throat, signs of infection, bleeding gums, bruising, petechiae, or blood in urine, stool, or emesis. Caution patient to avoid crowds and persons with known infections. Instruct patient to use soft toothbrush and electric razor. • Patient should be cautioned not to drink alcoholic beverages or take products containing aspirin, ibuprofen, or naproxen. • Instruct patient to notify physician if abdominal pain, yellow skin, weakness, paresthesia, gait disturbances, or joint or muscle aches occur. • Instruct patient to inspect oral mucosa for redness and ulceration. If mouth sores occur, advise patient to use sponge brush and rinse mouth with water after eating and drinking. Oropharyngeal mucositis is dose-related and usually mild, resolving 5–7 days after therapy is discontinued. • Discuss with patient the possibility of hair loss. Complete loss of hair including scalp hair, eyebrows, eyelashes, and pubic hair occurs in almost all patients between days 14 and 21. Hair growth returns after therapy has ended. Explore coping strategies. • Advise patient to use a nonhormonal method of contraception. • Instruct patient not to receive any vaccinations without first obtaining advice of physician. • Emphasize the need for periodic lab tests to monitor for side effects.

 PHARMACOLOGIC PROFILE

Indications
• Paclitaxel is used in the management of ovarian cancer that has been unresponsive to first-line or other therapy and in the management of metastatic breast cancer.

Action
• Paclitaxel interferes with normal cellular microtubule function, which is required for interphase and mitosis, resulting in death of rapidly replicating cells, particularly malignant ones.

Time/Action Profile (effect on WBC counts)

Onset	Peak	Duration
UK	11 days	3 wk

Pharmacokinetics
• **Distribution:** UK. • **Metabolism and Excretion:** Although not extensively studied, paclitaxel appears to be highly metabolized by the liver. • **Half-life:** 5.3–17.4 hours.

Contraindications
• Paclitaxel is contraindicated in patients with hypersensitivity to it or to castor oil (vehicle contains polyoxethylated castor oil—Cremophor EL). • Patients with known alcohol intolerance should not receive paclitaxel (contains 50% dehydrated alcohol). • Use of paclitaxel should be avoided in pregnant or lactating patients. • Patients with WBCs <1500/mm³ should not be given paclitaxel.

Adverse Reactions and Side Effects*
• **CV:** <u>bradycardia</u>, <u>hypotension</u>, <u>abnormal ECG</u> • **GI:** <u>nausea</u>, <u>vomiting</u>, <u>diarrhea</u>, <u>stomatitis</u>, <u>abnormal liver func-</u>

---

*<u>Underlines</u> indicate most frequent; CAPITALS indicate life-threatening.

tion tests • **Derm:** <u>alopecia</u> • **Hemat:** <u>anemia</u>, <u>leukopenia</u>, <u>thrombocytopenia</u> • **MS:** <u>myalgia</u>, <u>arthralgia</u> • **Neuro:** <u>periph-eral neuropathy</u>. • **Misc:** <u>hypersensitivity reactions</u> including ANAPHYLAXIS.

Pamidronate Disodium	Electrolyte modifier (hypocalcemic)
Aredia	pH 6–7.4

≋ ADMINISTRATION CONSIDERATIONS

Usual Dose

ADULTS: *Hypercalcemia*—60 mg (range 30–90 mg). Course may be repeated after 7-day rest. *Paget's disease*—30 mg/day for 3 days.

Dilution

• **Continuous Infusion:** Reconstitute by adding 10 ml of sterile water for injection to each vial for a concentration of 30, 60, or 90 mg/10 ml. • Allow drug to dissolve before withdrawing. • {The Canadian product does not need to be reconstituted prior to dilution.} • **Dilute further** in 1000 ml of 0.45% NaCl, 0.9% NaCl, or D5W. • Solution is stable for 24 hours at room temperature.

Incompatibility

• **Additive:** calcium-containing solutions, such as Ringer's solution.

Rate of Administration

• **Continuous Infusion:** Administer 30 and 60 mg doses over at least 4 hours, and 90 mg dose over 24 hours.

≋ CLINICAL PRECAUTIONS

• Vigorous saline hydration, maintaining a urine output of 2000 ml/24 hr, should be undertaken concurrently with pamidronate therapy. Initiate saline hydration cautiously in patients with underlying cardiovascular disease, especially congestive heart failure. Monitor intake/output ra-

tios and blood pressure frequently during therapy. Assess for signs of fluid overload (edema, rales/crackles). Pamidronate may be used with loop diuretics.
- Patients with severe hypercalcemia (corrected serum calcium greater than 135 mg/dl) should be started at the 90-mg dose. Patients with mild hypercalcemia or renal impairment may be given 30 mg.
- Monitor symptoms of hypercalcemia (nausea, vomiting, anorexia, weakness, constipation, thirst, and cardiac arrhythmias).
- Observe for evidence of hypocalcemia (paresthesia, muscle twitching, laryngospasm, and Chvostek's or Trousseau's sign). Protect symptomatic patients by elevating and padding side rails; keep bed in low position.
- Hypokalemia and hypomagnesemia may increase the risk of cardiac glycoside toxicity. Electrolyte abnormalities should be corrected as they occur. Some patients require supplemental phosphates.
- Use cautiously in patients with renal impairment; lower doses or slower infusion rates may be necessary.
- Safe use in pregnancy, lactation, or children has not been established (Pregnancy Category C).

Lab Test Considerations
- Electrolytes (including calcium, phosphorus, and magnesium), hemoglobin, and creatinine should be monitored closely. CBC and platelet count should be monitored during the first 2 weeks of therapy.

Patient/Family Teaching
- Advise patient to report signs of hypercalcemic relapse (bone pain, anorexia, nausea, vomiting, thirst, lethargy) to the physician promptly. • Encourage patient to comply with dietary recommendations. Diet should contain adequate amounts of calcium and vitamin D. • Foods high in vitamin D include fish livers and oils and fortified milk, bread, and cereals. Food high in calcium include dairy products, canned salmon and sardines, broccoli, bok choy, tofu, molasses, and cream soups (see Appendix H). • Emphasize the need for keeping follow-up appointments to monitor progress, even after medication is discontinued, in order to detect possible relapse.

≋ PHARMACOLOGIC PROFILE

Indications

• Pamidronate is used in the management of moderate to severe hypercalcemia associated with malignancy. Paget's disease of bone may also be managed with pamidronate.

Action

• Pamidronate inhibits resorption of bone, resulting in decreased serum calcium.

Time/Action Profile (effect on serum calcium)

Onset	Peak	Duration
24 hr	7 days	UK

Pharmacokinetics

• **Distribution:** Pamidronate is rapidly adsorbed by bone, reaching high concentrations in bone, liver, spleen, teeth, and tracheal cartilage. Approximately 50% of a dose is retained by bone and then slowly released. • **Metabolism and Excretion:** 50% is excreted unchanged in the urine. • **Half-life:** Elimination half-life from plasma is biphasic—first phase 1.6 hours, second phase 27.2 hours. Elimination half-life from bone is 300 days.

Contraindications

• Pamidronate is contraindicated in patients who have hypersensitivity to it, to other biphosphonates, or to mannitol.

Adverse Reactions and Side Effects*

• **CNS:** fatigue • **EENT:** rhinitis • **CV:** fluid overload, hypertension, arrhythmias, tachycardia, syncope • **Resp:** rales • **GI:** anorexia, abdominal pain, constipation, nausea, vomiting • **F and E:** hypocalcemia, hypomagnesemia, hypokalemia, hypophosphatemia • **Hemat:** anemia • **Metab:** hypothyroidism • **MS:** bone pain • **Local:** phlebitis at injection site • **Misc:** fever, generalized pain.

---

*Underlines indicate most frequent; CAPITALS indicate life-threatening.

Pancuronium Bromide	*Neuromuscular blocking agent (nondepolarizing)*
Pavulon	pH 4

≋ ADMINISTRATION CONSIDERATIONS

Usual Dose

ADULTS AND CHILDREN >1 mo: 40–100 mcg (0.04–0.1 mg)/kg initially. Incremental doses of 10 mcg (0.01 mg)/kg may be given q 20–60 min to maintain paralysis. After anesthesia and/or intubation is performed, an initial dose of 40 mcg (0.04 mg)/kg may be used. Additional doses are titrated. A dose of 60–100 mcg/kg may be used to facilitate endotracheal intubation.

CHILDREN <1 mo: Dose requirements are determined following a test dose of 20 mcg (0.02 mg/kg).

Dilution

• **Direct IV:** May be administered **undiluted**. To prevent absorption by plastic, pancuronium should not be stored in plastic syringes, but may be administered in plastic syringes. • **Intermittent Infusion:** May be **diluted** in 0.9% NaCl, D5W, D5/0.9% NaCl, and lactated Ringer's injection. • Solution is stable for 48 hours.

Compatibility

• **Syringe:** heparin.
• **Y-site:** aminophylline ✦ cefazolin ✦ cefuroxime ✦ cimetidine ✦ dobutamine ✦ dopamine ✦ epinephrine ✦ esmolol ✦ fentanyl ✦ gentamicin ✦ heparin ✦ hydrocortisone sodium succinate ✦ isoproterenol ✦ lorazepam ✦ midazolam ✦ morphine ✦ nitroglycerin ✦ nitroprusside ✦ ranitidine ✦ trimethoprim/sulfamethoxazole ✦ vancomycin.
• **Additive:** verapamil.

Incompatibility

• **Y-site:** diazepam.

Rate of Administration

• **Direct IV:** Incremental doses may be administered every 20–60 minutes as needed. Dose is titrated to patient response. • **Intermittent Infusion:** Titrate rate according to patient response.

≋ CLINICAL PRECAUTIONS

- Assess respiratory status continuously throughout pancuronium therapy. Pancuronium should be used only for intubated patients. Assess patient for increased respiratory secretions; suction as necessary.

- Neuromuscular response to pancuronium should be monitored with a peripheral nerve stimulator intraoperatively. Monitor deep tendon reflexes during prolonged administration. Paralysis is initially selective and usually occurs consecutively in the following muscles: levator muscles of eyelids, muscles of mastication, limb muscles, abdominal muscles, muscles of the glottis, intercostal muscles, and diaphragm. Recovery of muscle function usually occurs in reverse order. Observe patient for residual muscle weakness and respiratory distress during the recovery period.

- Monitor heart rate, ECG, and blood pressure periodically throughout pancuronium therapy. Pancuronium may cause a slight increase in heart rate and blood pressure.

- Pancuronium has no effect on consciousness or the pain threshold. Adequate anesthesia/analgesia should *always* be used when pancuronium is used as an adjunct to surgical procedures or when painful procedures are performed. Benzodiazepines and/or analgesics should be administered concurrently when prolonged pancuronium therapy is used for ventilator patients, as patient is awake and able to feel all sensations. If eyes remain open throughout prolonged administration, protect corneas with artificial tears.

- Intensity and duration of paralysis may be prolonged by pretreatment with succinylcholine • general anesthesia • aminoglycoside antibiotics • polymyxin B • colistin • clindamycin • lidocaine • quinidine • procainamide • beta-adrenergic blocking agents • potassium-losing diuretics • magnesium.

- Use pancuronium cautiously in patients with any history of pulmonary disease or renal or liver impairment, in elderly or debilitated patients, and in patients with electrolyte disturbances or those receiving cardiac glycosides. Use with extreme caution in patients with myasthenia gravis or myasthenic syndromes.

- Although pancuronium has been safely used during cesarean section, use cautiously in pregnant patients (Pregnancy Category C). Neonates are very sensitive to the effects of pancuronium.

Toxicity and Overdose Alert

- If overdose occurs, use peripheral nerve stimulator to determine the degree of neuromuscular blockade. Maintain airway patency and ventilation until recovery of normal respirations occurs. Administration of anticholinesterase agents (edrophonium, neostigmine, pyridostigmine) may be used to antagonize the action of pancuronium. Atropine is usually administered prior to or concurrently with anticholinesterase agents.

Patient/Family Teaching

- Explain all procedures to patient receiving pancuronium therapy without anesthesia, as consciousness is not affected by pancuronium alone. Provide emotional support. • Reassure patient that communication abilities will return as the medication wears off.

≋ PHARMACOLOGIC PROFILE

Indications

- Pancuronium is used to produce skeletal muscle paralysis and facilitation of intubation after induction of anesthesia in surgical procedures. • It is also used during mechanical ventilation to increase pulmonary compliance.

Action

- Pancuronium prevents neuromuscular transmission by blocking the effect of acetylcholine at the myoneural junction. • It has no analgesic or anxiolytic effects.

Time/Action Profile (skeletal muscle paralysis)

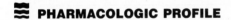

Onset	Peak	Duration
30–45 sec	3–4.5 min	35–45 min

Pharmacokinetics

- **Distribution:** Pancuronium rapidly distributes into extracellular fluid. Small amounts cross the placenta. • **Me-**

tabolism and Excretion: Pancuronium is excreted mostly unchanged by the kidneys; small amounts are eliminated in bile. • **Half-life:** 2 hours.

Contraindications

• Pancuronium is contraindicated in patients with hypersensitivity to it or to benzyl alcohol or bromides. Avoid use of benzyl alcohol–containing preparations in neonates.

Adverse Reactions and Side Effects*

Note: Almost all adverse reactions to pancuronium are extensions of pharmacologic effects.

• **CV:** mild tachycardia • **EENT:** excessive salivation (children) • **Resp:** apnea, wheezing • **Local:** burning sensation along vein • **MS:** muscle weakness • **Derm:** excessive sweating (children), rashes • **Misc:** allergic reactions.

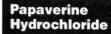

Papaverine Hydrochloride   *Vasodilator*

pH—not below 3

 ADMINISTRATION CONSIDERATIONS

Usual Dose

ADULTS: 30 mg initially; 30–120 mg may be repeated q 3 hr if necessary.

Dilution

• **Direct IV:** Administer **undiluted.** • Solution should be clear to light yellow. Do not refrigerate.

Compatibility

• **Syringe:** phentolamine.
• **Solution:** 0.9% NaCl ♦ 0.45% NaCl ♦ D5W ♦ D10W ♦ D5/0.9% NaCl ♦ D5/0.45% NaCl ♦ D5/0.25% NaCl ♦ Ringer's injection.

---

*Underlines indicate most frequent; CAPITALS indicate life-threatening.

Incompatibility
- **Additive:** aminophylline • alkaline solutions • bromides • iodides.
- **Solution:** lactated Ringer's injection.

Rate of Administration
- **Direct IV:** Administer over 1–2 minutes. Rapid administration may cause arrhythmias and apnea.

≋ CLINICAL PRECAUTIONS

- Monitor ECG, blood pressure, and pulse prior to and periodically throughout course of therapy. Withhold dose and notify physician if AV block is present.
- Monitor IV site for thrombosis (erythema, pain, edema).
- Use papaverine cautiously in patients with glaucoma, depressed cardiac conduction, priapism, sickle cell disease, impaired liver function, or coagulation defects.
- Papaverine may prevent desired response to levodopa in patients with Parkinson's disease. Alpha-adrenergic agonists (metaraminol, epinephrine, or phenylephrine) or cigarette smoking may reverse the vasodilating effects of papaverine.
- Safe use in pregnancy, lactation, or children has not been established (Pregnancy Category C).

Lab Test Considerations
- Monitor liver function studies. Papaverine may cause elevated AST (SGOT), ALT (SGPT), alkaline phosphatase, and bilirubin levels.

Patient/Family Teaching
- Encourage patient not to smoke, as nicotine will cause additional vasoconstriction. • Papaverine may cause dizziness or drowsiness. Advise patient to avoid driving or other activities requiring alertness until response to medication is known. • Caution patient to make position changes slowly to minimize orthostatic hypotension. • Instruct patient to notify physician if dizziness, drowsiness, jaundice, or vision changes occur.

≋ PHARMACOLOGIC PROFILE

Indications

- Although FDA-designated as ineffective for these indications, papaverine has been used in the following: management of cerebral and peripheral ischemia usually associated with arterial spasm; treatment of myocardial ischemia complicated by arrhythmias; improvement of collateral circulation in acute vascular occlusion; and management of ureteral, biliary, or GI colic.

Action

- Papaverine is claimed to dilate coronary, cerebral, pulmonary, and peripheral arteries by a direct spasmolytic action on vascular smooth muscle.

Time/Action Profile (vasodilating effects)

Onset	Peak	Duration
UK	UK	3 hr

Pharmacokinetics

- **Distribution:** UK. • **Metabolism and Excretion:** Papaverine is mainly metabolized by the liver. • **Half-life:** 0.5–2 hours (highly variable—may be as long as 24 hours).

Contraindications

- Papaverine is contraindicated in patients with hypersensitivity to it and in patients with complete AV block.

Adverse Reactions and Side Effects*

- **CNS:** depression, dizziness, vertigo, headache, drowsiness, sedation • **EENT:** dry throat, visual changes • **Resp:** APNEA • **CV:** arrhythmias, hypotension, slight hypertension • **GI:** dry mouth, constipation, nausea, diarrhea, abdominal distress, anorexia, hepatitis • **Derm:** flushing, sweating • **Local:** thrombosis at IV site.

---

*Underlines indicate most frequent; CAPITALS indicate life-threatening.

Pegaspargase	*Antineoplastic agent*
	(enzyme)
Oncaspar, PEG-ʟ-	
Asparaginase	**pH 7.3**

ADMINISTRATION CONSIDERATIONS

Usual Dose

ADULTS AND CHILDREN WITH BODY SURFACE AREA ≥ 0.6 m²:
2500 IU/m² q 14 days, usually in combination with other agents.

CHILDREN WITH BODY SURFACE AREA < 0.6 m²: 82.5 IU/kg q 14 days, usually in combination with other agents.

Dilution

• **Intermittent Infusion: Dilute** each dose in 100 ml of 0.9% NaCl or D5W. Do not shake or agitate. Do not use if solution is cloudy or has formed a precipitate. • Use only one dose per vial; do not re-enter the vial. Discard unused portions. • Solutions should be prepared in a biologic cabinet. Wear gloves, gown, and mask while handling medication. Discard equipment in specially designated containers (see Appendix F). • Keep refrigerated but do not freeze. Freezing destroys activity but does not change the appearance of pegaspargase.

Rate of Administration

• **Intermittent Infusion:** Administer over 1–2 hours via Y-site through an infusion that is already running.

CLINICAL PRECAUTIONS

• IM is the preferred route due to a lower incidence of adverse reactions.

• Assess patient for previous hypersensitivity reactions to native ʟ-asparaginase. Monitor for hypersensitivity reaction (urticaria, diaphoresis, facial swelling, joint pain, hypotension, bronchospasm). Epinephrine and resuscitation equipment should be readily available. Reaction may occur up to 2 hours after administration. Use cautiously in patients who have experienced previous hypersensitivity reactions to other drugs or agents.

- Monitor for the development of bone marrow depression. Assess for fever, sore throat, and signs of infection. Monitor platelet count throughout therapy. Assess for bleeding (bleeding gums, bruising, petechiae; guaiac test stools, urine, and emesis). Avoid giving IM injections and taking rectal temperatures. Apply pressure to venipuncture sites for 10 minutes. Anemia may occur. Monitor for increased fatigue, dyspnea, and orthostatic hypotension.
- Monitor patient frequently for signs of pancreatitis (nausea, vomiting, abdominal pain).
- Assess nausea, vomiting, and appetite. Weigh patient weekly. Confer with physician regarding an antiemetic prior to administration.
- Pegaspargase may alter the response to anticoagulants or antiplatelet agents. It may also alter the effectiveness of methotrexate. Other drugs that are metabolized by the liver may be affected by pegaspargase.
- Use cautiously in patients with childbearing potential. Safe use in pregnancy has not been established; use only if clearly needed.

Lab Test Considerations

• Monitor CBC prior to and periodically throughout therapy. May alter coagulation studies. Fibrinogen may be decreased; prothrombin time (PT) and partial thromboplastin time (PTT) may be increased. • Monitor serum amylase frequently to detect pancreatitis. Monitor blood glucose levels, may cause hyperglycemia. • May cause elevated BUN and serum creatinine levels. • Hepatotoxicity may be manifested by increased AST (SGOT), ALT (SGPT), or bilirubin levels. Liver function tests usually return to normal after therapy. • May cause decreased serum calcium levels. • May cause elevated serum and urine uric acid levels and hyponatremia.

Patient/Family Teaching

• Inform the patient of the possibility of hypersensitivity reactions, including anaphylaxis. • Advise the patient that concurrent use of other medications may increase the risk of bleeding and toxicity of pegaspargase. Consult physician or pharmacist before taking any other medications, including over-the-counter drugs. • Instruct patient to notify physician if abdominal pain, severe nausea and vomiting, jaundice, fever, chills, sore throat, bleeding or bruising, excess thirst or urination, or mouth sores occur. Caution patient to avoid crowds and persons with known infections. Instruct patient to use a soft toothbrush and electric razor and to be especially careful to avoid falls. Patients should also be cautioned not to drink alcoholic beverages or take medication containing aspirin, naproxen, or ibuprofen because these may precipitate gastric bleeding. • Instruct patient not to receive any vaccinations without advice of physician. Advise parents that this may alter child's immunization schedule. • Emphasize need for periodic lab tests to monitor for side effects.

PHARMACOLOGIC PROFILE

Indications

• Treatment (usually in combination with other agents) of acute lymphoblastic leukemia (ALL) in patients who have had previous hypersensitivity reactions to native L-asparaginase.

Action

• Pegaspargase is L-asparaginase bound to polyethylene glycol (PEG). It depletes asparagine, which leukemic cells cannot synthesize. Normal cells are able to produce their own asparagine and are less susceptible to the effects of asparaginase. Binding to PEG renders asparaginase less antigenic and therefore less likely to induce hypersensitivity reactions.

Time/Action Profile (hematologic effects)

Onset	Peak	Duration
rapid	UK	14 days

Pharmacokinetics

• **Distribution:** Distribution of pegaspargase is not known. • **Metabolism and Excretion:** Metabolism and excretion of pegaspargase are not known. • **Half-life:** 5.73 days (less in patients with previous hypersensitivity to native L-asparaginase).

Contraindications

• Pegaspargase is contraindicated in patients who have pancreatitis or a history of pancreatitis. It should not be used in patients who have experienced hemorrhagic adverse reactions from L-asparaginase. Pegaspargase is also contraindicated in patients who have had previous hypersensitivity reactions to it.

Adverse Reactions and Side Effects*

• **CNS:** malaise, SEIZURES, headache • **CV:** hypotension, tachycardia • **GI:** PANCREATITIS, nausea, vomiting, abdominal pain, lip edema, abnormal liver function tests, anorexia, diarrhea • **Derm:** jaundice • **Endo:** hyperglycemia (requiring insulin) • **F and E:** peripheral edema • **Hemat:** disseminated intravascular coagulation, decreased fibrinogen, hemolytic anemia, leukopenia, pancytopenia, thrombocytopenia, increased thromboplastin • **Local:** thrombosis, injection site hypersensitivity, injection site pain • **Metab:** hyperuricemia • **MS:** pain in extremities, myalgia, arthralgia • **Neuro:** paresthesia • **Misc:** HYPERSENSITIVITY REACTIONS, chills, night sweats.

Penicillin G Potassium	*Anti-infective* *(penicillin)*
Pfizerpen	pH 6–8.5 1.7 mEq K/million units 0.3 mEq Na/million units

ADMINISTRATION CONSIDERATIONS

Usual Dose

Note: 1 mg = 1600 units.

ADULTS: 1 million–5 million units q 4–6 hr.

CHILDREN: 8,333–16,667 units/kg q 4 hr or 12,500–25,000 units/kg q 6 hr (up to 400,000 units/kg/day).

**Underlines indicate most frequent; CAPITALS indicate life-threatening.

NEONATES: 30,000 units/kg q 12 hr (up to 1 million units/day for *Listeria* infections).

Dilution

• **Intermittent Infusion: Reconstitute** according to manufacturer's directions with sterile water for injection, D5W, or 0.9% NaCl. Add diluent slowly, directing stream against wall of vial. Shake vigorously. • Doses of 3 million units or less should be diluted in at least 50 ml; doses of more than 3 million units should be diluted with at least 100 ml of D5W, D10W, 0.45% NaCl, 0.9% NaCl, Ringer's or lactated Ringer's solution, dextrose/saline combinations, or dextrose/ Ringer's or lactated Ringer's combinations. • **Continuous Infusion:** Daily doses of 10 million units or more; may be diluted in 1–2 liters of compatible fluid.

Compatibility

• **Syringe:** heparin.

• **Y-site:** acyclovir • cyclophosphamide • diltiazem • enalaprilat • esmolol • fluconazole • foscarnet • hydromorphone • labetalol • magnesium sulfate • meperidine • morphine • perphenazine • potassium chloride • tacrolimus • verapamil • vitamin B complex with C. • If aminoglycosides and penicillins or cephalosporins must be given concurrently, administer at separate sites at least 1 hour apart.

• **Additive:** ascorbic acid • calcium chloride • calcium gluconate • cimetidine • corticotropin • dimenhydrinate • diphenhydramine • ephedrine • furosemide • hydrocortisone sodium succinate • lidocaine • magnesium sulfate • methylprednisolone sodium succinate • polymyxin B • potassium chloride • prednisolone sodium phosphate • procaine • prochlorperazine edisylate • ranitidine • verapamil.

Incompatibility

• **Syringe:** metoclopramide.

• **Additive:** aminophylline • amphotericin B • chlorpromazine • dopamine • hydroxyzine • metaraminol • pentobarbital • prochlorperazine mesylate • promazine • thiopental.

Rate of Administration

• **Intermittent Infusion:** Infuse over 1–2 hours in adults, 15–30 minutes in children. • **Continuous Infusion:** Doses greater than 10 million units/day should be administered by slow infusion. May be diluted and infused over 24 hours.

≋ CLINICAL PRECAUTIONS

- Assess patient for infection (vital signs; appearance of wound, sputum, urine, and stool; WBC) at beginning and throughout course of therapy.
- Obtain specimens for culture and sensitivity prior to initiating therapy. First dose may be given before receiving results.
- Obtain a history before initiating therapy to determine previous use of and reactions to penicillins or cephalosporins. Persons with a negative history of penicillin sensitivity may still have an allergic response. Observe patient for signs and symptoms of anaphylaxis (rash, pruritus, laryngeal edema, wheezing). Discontinue drug immediately if these occur. Keep epinephrine, an antihistamine, and resuscitation equipment close by in the event of an anaphylactic reaction.
- Change sites every 48 hours to prevent phlebitis.
- Use penicillin cautiously in patients with severe renal insufficiency. Dosage reduction is recommended.
- Probenecid decreases renal excretion and increases blood levels of penicillin. Therapy may be combined for this purpose. Effectiveness of penicillin may be decreased by concurrent use of chloramphenicol. The half-life of chloramphenicol may be increased by concurrent use of penicillin.
- Although safety is not established, penicillin has been used during pregnancy and lactation without adverse effects (Pregnancy Category B). Use cautiously during lactation.

Lab Test Considerations

- Patients receiving penicillin G may have false-positive results for urine glucose using the copper sulfate method (Clinitest). Use glucose enzymatic tests (Keto-Diastix, Tes-Tape) to test urine glucose. • Penicillin may cause positive direct Coombs' test results. • Hyperkalemia may develop following large doses of penicillin G potassium.

Patient/Family Teaching

- Advise patient to report the signs of superinfection (black, furry overgrowth on the tongue; vaginal itching or discharge; loose or foul-smelling stools) and allergy. • Instruct the patient to notify physician if symptoms do not improve. • Patients with an allergy to penicillin should be instructed to carry an identification card with this information at all times.

PHARMACOLOGIC PROFILE

Indications

• Penicillin is used in the treatment of a wide variety of infections, including pneumococcal pneumonia, streptococcal pharyngitis, syphilis, gonorrhea, and Lyme disease. • Treatment of enterococcal infections requires the addition of an aminoglycoside.

Action

• Penicillin binds to bacterial cell wall, resulting in cell death. It is active against most Gram-positive organisms, including streptococci (*Streptococcus pneumoniae,* group A beta-hemolytic streptococci), staphylococci (non-penicillinase-producing strains). It is also active against some Gram-negative organisms, such as *Neisseria meningitidis* and *N. gonorrhoeae.* Some anaerobic bacteria and spirochetes (including *Treponema pallidum* and *Borrelia burgdorferi*) are also susceptible.

Time/Action Profile (blood levels)

Onset	Peak
rapid	end of infusion

Pharmacokinetics

• **Distribution:** Penicillin is widely distributed, although CNS penetration is poor in the presence of uninflamed meninges. It crosses the placenta and enters breast milk. • **Metabolism and Excretion:** Penicillin is minimally metabolized by the liver and is excreted mainly unchanged by the kidneys. • **Half-life:** 30–60 minutes.

Contraindications

• Penicillin is contraindicated in patients with previous hypersensitivity to penicillins. Cross-sensitivity with cephalosporins may occur.

Adverse Reactions and Side Effects*

• **CNS:** SEIZURES (high doses) • **GI:** nausea, vomiting, diarrhea, epigastric distress • **GU:** interstitial nephritis • **Derm:** rashes, urticaria • **Hemat:** eosinophilia, hemolytic anemia, leukopenia • **Local:** phlebitis at IV site • **Misc:** superinfection, allergic reactions including ANAPHYLAXIS and serum sickness.

Penicillin G Sodium	*Anti-infective*
	(penicillin)
	pH 6–7.5
	2 mEq Na/million units

≋ ADMINISTRATION CONSIDERATIONS

Usual Dose

Note: 1 mg = 1600 units.

ADULTS: 1 million–5 million units q 4–6 hr.

CHILDREN: 8,333–16,667 units/kg q 4 hr or 12,500–25,000 units/kg q 6 hr (up to 400,000 units/kg/day).

NEONATES: 30,000 units/kg q 12 hr (up to 1 million units/day for *Listeria* infections).

Dilution

• **Intermittent Infusion:** Reconstitute according to manufacturer's directions with sterile water for injection, D5W, or 0.9% NaCl. Add diluent slowly, directing stream against wall of vial. Shake vigorously. • Doses of 3 million units or less should be **diluted** with at least 50 ml; doses of greater than 3 million units should be **diluted** with at least 100 ml of D5W or 0.9% NaCl. • **Continuous Infusion:** Daily doses of 10 million units or more; may be diluted in 1–2 liters of compatible fluid.

---

*Underlines indicate most frequent; CAPITALS indicate life-threatening.

Compatibility
- **Syringe:** cimetidine ✦ colistimethate ✦ heparin.
- **Additive:** calcium chloride ✦ calcium gluconate ✦ diphenhydramine ✦ furosemide ✦ hydrocortisone sodium succinate ✦ prednisolone sodium phosphate ✦ procaine ✦ ranitidine ✦ verapamil ✦ vitamin B complex with C.

Incompatibility
- **Y-site:** If aminoglycosides and penicillins or cephalosporins must be given concurrently, administer in separate sites at least 1 hour apart.
- **Additive:** amphotericin B ✦ bleomycin ✦ cephalothin ✦ chlorpromazine ✦ cytarabine ✦ hydroxyzine ✦ methylprednisolone sodium succinate ✦ prochlorperazine ✦ promethazine.

Rate of Administration
- **Intermittent Infusion:** Infuse over 1–2 hours in adults, 15–30 minutes in children. • **Continuous Infusion:** Doses greater than 10 million units/day should be administered by slow infusion. May be diluted and infused over 24 hours.

☰ CLINICAL PRECAUTIONS
- Assess patient for infection (vital signs; appearance of wound, sputum, urine, and stool; WBC) at beginning and throughout course of therapy.
- Obtain specimens for culture and sensitivity prior to initiating therapy. First dose may be given before receiving results.
- Obtain a history before initiating therapy to determine previous use of and reactions to penicillins or cephalosporins. Persons with a negative history of penicillin sensitivity may still have an allergic response. Observe patient for signs and symptoms of anaphylaxis (rash, pruritus, laryngeal edema, wheezing). Discontinue drug immediately if these occur. Keep epinephrine, an antihistamine, and resuscitation equipment close by in the event of an anaphylactic reaction.
- Change sites every 48 hours to prevent phlebitis.
- Use penicillin cautiously in patients with severe renal insufficiency. Dosage reduction is recommended.
- Probenecid decreases renal excretion and increases

blood levels of penicillin. Therapy may be combined for this purpose. Effectiveness of penicillin may be decreased by concurrent use of chloramphenicol. The half-life of chloramphenicol may be increased by concurrent use of penicillin.

- Although safety is not established, penicillin has been used during pregnancy and lactation without adverse effects (Pregnancy Category B). Use cautiously during lactation.

Lab Test Considerations

- Patients receiving penicillin G may have false-positive results for urine glucose using the copper sulfate method (Clinitest). Use glucose enzymatic tests (Keto-Diastix, Tes-Tape) to test urine glucose. • Penicillin may cause positive direct Coombs' test results.

Patient/Family Teaching

- Advise patient to report the signs of superinfection (black, furry overgrowth on the tongue; vaginal itching or discharge; loose or foul-smelling stools) and allergy. • Instruct the patient to notify physician if symptoms do not improve. • Patients with an allergy to penicillin should be instructed to carry an identification card with this information at all times.

☰ PHARMACOLOGIC PROFILE

Indications

- Penicillin is used in the treatment of a wide variety of infections, including pneumococcal pneumonia, streptococcal pharyngitis, syphilis, gonorrhea, and Lyme disease. • Treatment of enterococcal infections requires the addition of an aminoglycoside.

Action

- Penicillin binds to bacterial cell wall, resulting in cell death. It is active against most Gram-positive organisms, including streptococci (*Streptococcus pneumoniae,* group A beta-hemolytic streptococci), staphylococci (non-penicillinase-producing strains). It is also active against some Gram-negative organisms, such as *Neisseria meningitidis* and *N. gonorrhoeae*. Some anaerobic bacteria and spirochetes (including *Treponema pallidum* and *Borrelia burgdorferi*) are also susceptible.

Time/Action Profile (blood levels)

Onset	Peak
rapid	end of infusion

Pharmacokinetics

• **Distribution:** Penicillin is widely distributed, although CNS penetration is poor in the presence of uninflamed meninges. It crosses the placenta and enters breast milk. • **Metabolism and Excretion:** Penicillin is minimally metabolized by the liver and is excreted mainly unchanged by the kidneys. • **Half-life:** 30–60 minutes.

Contraindications

• Penicillin is contraindicated in patients with previous hypersensitivity to penicillins. Cross-sensitivity with cephalosporins may occur.

Adverse Reactions and Side Effects*

• **CNS:** SEIZURES (high doses) • **GI:** <u>nausea</u>, <u>vomiting</u>, <u>diarrhea</u>, <u>epigastric distress</u> • **GU:** interstitial nephritis • **Derm:** <u>rashes</u>, urticaria • **Hemat:** eosinophilia, hemolytic anemia, leukopenia • **Local:** <u>phlebitis</u> at IV site • **Misc:** superinfection, allergic reactions including ANAPHYLAXIS and serum sickness.

Pentamidine Isethionate	Anti-infective (antiprotozoal)
Pentacarinat, Pentam 300	pH 4.1–5.4

≋ ADMINISTRATION CONSIDERATIONS

Usual Dose

ADULTS AND CHILDREN: 4 mg/kg once daily for 14 days (treatment up to 21 days or longer may be required in AIDS

---

*<u>Underlines</u> indicate most frequent; CAPITALS indicate life-threatening.

patients). Some patients with mild infections may be managed with 3 mg/kg/day.

Dilution

• **Intermittent Infusion:** To **reconstitute**, add 3, 4, or 5 ml of sterile water for injection or D5W to each 300-mg vial for a concentration of 100, 75, or 60 mg/ml, respectively. Withdraw dose and **dilute further** in 50–250 ml of D5W.
• Solution is stable for 24 hours at room temperature. Discard unused portions.

Compatibility

• **Y-site:** diltiazem • zidovudine.

Incompatibility

• **Y-site:** fluconazole • foscarnet.

Rate of Administration

• **Intermittent Infusion:** Administer slowly over at least 60 minutes, preferably 1–2 hours.

≋ CLINICAL PRECAUTIONS

• Assess patient for infection (vital signs, sputum, WBC) and monitor respiratory status (rate, character, lung sounds, dyspnea, sputum) at beginning and throughout course of therapy.
• Obtain specimens prior to initiating therapy. First dose may be given before receiving results.
• Monitor blood pressure frequently during administration of pentamidine. Patient should be lying down during administration. Sudden, severe hypotension may occur following a single dose. Resuscitation equipment should be immediately available.
• Assess patient for signs of hypoglycemia (anxiety, chills, diaphoresis, cold pale skin, headache, increased hunger, nausea, nervousness, shakiness) and hyperglycemia (drowsiness, flushed dry skin, fruitlike breath odor, increased thirst, increased urination, loss of appetite), which may occur up to several months after therapy is discontinued.
• Pulse and ECG should be monitored prior to and periodically during course of therapy. Fatalities due to car-

diac arrhythmias, tachycardia, and cardiotoxicity have been reported.

- Assess for signs of electrolyte abnormalities. Correct as needed.
- Additive nephrotoxicity may occur with concurrent use of other nephrotoxic agents, including aminoglycosides, amphotericin B, and vancomycin. Patients with renal impairment require dosage reduction.
- Use pentamidine cautiously in patients with hypotension, hypertension, hypoglycemia, hyperglycemia, hypocalcemia, leukopenia, thrombocytopenia, anemia, cardiovascular disease, bone marrow depression, previous antineoplastic therapy or radiation therapy, diabetes mellitus, or liver impairment. Additive bone marrow depression may occur with antineoplastic agents or previous radiation therapy.
- Safe use during pregnancy or lactation has not been established (Pregnancy Category C). Avoid use during lactation.

Lab Test Considerations

• Blood glucose concentrations should be monitored prior to, daily during, and for several months following course of therapy. • Monitor BUN and serum creatinine prior to and daily during therapy to monitor for nephrotoxicity. • Monitor CBC, platelet count, and liver function tests prior to and every 3 days during course of therapy. Pentamidine may cause leukopenia, anemia, and thrombocytopenia and may cause elevated serum bilirubin, alkaline phosphatase, AST (SGOT), and ALT (SGPT) concentrations. • Serum calcium and magnesium concentrations should be monitored prior to and every 3 days during therapy, as pentamidine may cause hypocalcemia and hypomagnesemia. It may also cause elevated serum potassium concentrations.

Patient/Family Teaching

• Instruct patient to notify physician promptly if fever; sore throat; signs of infection; bleeding of gums; unusual bruising; petechiae; or blood in stool, urine, or emesis occurs. Caution patient to avoid crowds and persons with known infections. Instruct patient to use soft toothbrush and electric razor and to avoid falls. Patient should not be given IM injections or rectal thermometers. • Patient should also be cautioned not to drink alcoholic beverages or take medication containing aspirin, ibuprofen, or naproxen, as these may precipitate gastric bleeding. • Caution patient to make position changes slowly to minimize orthostatic hypotension. • Advise patient that an unpleasant metallic taste may occur with pentamidine administration but is not significant.

PHARMACOLOGIC PROFILE

Indications

• Pentamidine is used in the treatment of *Pneumocystis carinii* pneumonia (PCP).

Action

• Pentamidine appears to disrupt DNA or RNA synthesis in protozoa. It also has a direct toxic effect on pancreatic islet cells.

Time/Action Profile (blood levels)

Onset	Peak
rapid	end of infusion

Pharmacokinetics

• **Distribution:** Pentamidine is widely and extensively distributed. It does not appear to enter the CSF but concentrates in liver, kidneys, lungs, and spleen, with prolonged storage in some tissues. • **Metabolism and Excretion:** 1–30% is excreted unchanged by the kidneys. The remainder of its metabolic fate is unknown. • **Half-life:** 6.4–9.4 hours (increased in renal impairment).

Contraindications

• Pentamidine is contraindicated in patients with a history of previous anaphylactic reaction to pentamidine. It is not recommended during lactation.

Adverse Reactions and Side Effects*

• **CNS:** <u>anxiety</u>, <u>headache</u>, dizziness, confusion, hallucinations • **CV:** <u>HYPOTENSION</u>, ARRHYTHMIAS • **GI:** nausea, vomiting,

---

*<u>Underlines</u> indicate most frequent; CAPITALS indicate life-threatening.

abdominal pain, unpleasant metallic taste, anorexia, PANCREATI-
TIS, hepatitis • **GU:** acute renal failure • **Derm:** rash, pallor
• **Endo:** HYPOGLYCEMIA, hyperglycemia • **F and E:** hypocalcemia, hypomagnesemia, hyperkalemia • **Hemat:** leukopenia, thrombocytopenia, anemia • **Local:** phlebitis, pruritus,
urticaria at IV site • **Misc:** fever, chills, STEVENS-JOHNSON SYN-
DROME, allergic reactions including ANAPHYLAXIS.

Pentazocine Lactate	Opioid analgesic (mixed agonist/antagonist)
Talwin	pH 4–5

Schedule IV

≋ ADMINISTRATION CONSIDERATIONS

Usual Dose

Moderate to Severe Pain
ADULTS: 30 mg q 3–4 hr as needed (not to exceed 30 mg/dose
or 360 mg/day).

Obstetrical Use
ADULTS: 20 mg when contractions become regular; may be
repeated q 2–3 hr for 2–3 doses.

Dilution
• **Direct IV:** Manufacturer recommends diluting each 5
mg with at least 1 ml of sterile water for injection.

Compatibility
• **Syringe:** atropine • benzquinamide • chlorpromazine
• cimetidine • dimenhydrinate • diphenhydramine • droperidol • hydroxyzine • metoclopramide • perphenazine
• prochlorperazine edisylate • promazine • promethazine
• propiomazine • ranitidine • scopolamine.
• **Y-site:** heparin • hydrocortisone sodium succinate
• potassium chloride • vitamin B complex with C.

Incompatibility

- **Syringe:** glycopyrrolate ◆ heparin ◆ pentobarbital.
- **Y-site:** nafcillin.
- **Additive:** aminophylline ◆ amobarbital ◆ pentobarbital ◆ phenobarbital ◆ secobarbital ◆ sodium bicarbonate.

Rate of Administration

- **Direct IV:** Administer slowly, each 5 mg over at least 1 minute.

≋ CLINICAL PRECAUTIONS

- Assess type, location, and intensity of pain prior to and 15 minutes (peak) following administration. When titrating opioid doses, increases of 25–50% should be administered until there is either a 50% reduction in the patient's pain rating on a numerical or visual analogue scale, or the patient reports satisfactory pain relief. Subsequent doses may be safely administered at the time of the peak if the previous dose is ineffective and side effects are minimal. Patients requiring higher doses should be converted to an opioid agonist. Pentazocine is not recommended for prolonged use or as first-line therapy for acute or cancer pain. Regularly administered doses may be more effective than p.r.n. administration. Analgesic is more effective if administered before pain becomes severe. Coadministration with nonopioid analgesics may have additive effects and may permit lower opioid doses.
- An equianalgesic chart (Appendix B, page 1045) should be used when changing routes or when changing from one opioid to another.
- Assess blood pressure, pulse, and respirations before and periodically during administration. If respiratory rate is less than 10/min, assess level of sedation. Dose may need to be decreased by 25–50%. Pentazocine produces respiratory depression, but this does not markedly increase with increased doses. Additive CNS depression may occur with concurrent use of alcohol, antihistamines, and sedative/hypnotics.
- Assess prior analgesic history. Antagonistic properties of

pentozocine may induce withdrawal symptoms (vomiting, restlessness, abdominal cramps, increased blood pressure and temperature) in patients physically dependent on opioids.

- Although this drug has a low potential for dependence, prolonged use may lead to physical and psychological dependence and tolerance. This should not prevent patient from receiving adequate analgesia. Most patients receiving pentazocine for medical reasons do not develop psychological dependence.

- Use pentazocine with caution in patients receiving MAO inhibitors, as this combination may result in unpredictable reactions. Decrease initial dose of pentazocine to 25% of usual dose. Avoid concurrent use with agonist opioid analgesics, as this combination may diminish analgesic effect.

- Use pentazocine cautiously in patients with head trauma; increased intracranial pressure; severe renal, hepatic, or pulmonary disease; hypothyroidism; adrenal insufficiency; alcoholism; undiagnosed abdominal pain; or prostatic hypertrophy. Elderly, debilitated patients or patients with severe liver impairment require reduced dosage.

- Pentazocine has been used safely during labor, but may cause respiratory depression in the newborn (Pregnancy Category C). Safe use in lactation or children has not been established.

Toxicity and Overdose Alert

- If an opioid antagonist is required to reverse respiratory depression or coma, naloxone (Narcan) is the antidote. Dilute the 0.4-mg ampule of naloxone in 10 ml of 0.9% NaCl and administer 0.5 ml (0.02 mg) by direct IV push every 2 minutes. For children and patients weighing <40 kg, dilute 0.1 mg of naloxone in 10 ml of 0.9% NaCl for a concentration of 10 mcg/ml and administer 0.5 mcg every 1–2 minutes. Titrate the dose to avoid withdrawal, seizures, and severe pain.

Lab Test Considerations

- May cause elevated serum amylase and lipase levels.

Patient/Family Teaching

- Instruct patient on how and when to ask for pain medication. • Pentazocine may cause drowsiness, dizziness, or hallucinations. Advise patient to call for assistance when ambulating and to avoid driving or other activities requiring alertness until response to medication is known. • Encourage patient to turn, cough, and breathe deeply every 2 hours to prevent atelectasis. • Caution patient to make position changes slowly to minimize orthostatic hypotension. • Advise patient to avoid concurrent use of alcohol and other CNS depressants. • Advise patient that frequent mouth rinses, good oral hygiene, and sugarless gum or candy may decrease dry mouth.

 PHARMACOLOGIC PROFILE

Indications

- Pentazocine is used in the management of moderate to severe pain. • It has also been used as an analgesic during labor, as a sedative prior to surgery, and as a supplement in balanced anesthesia.

Action

- Pentazocine binds to opiate receptors in the CNS, altering the perception of and response to painful stimuli, while producing generalized CNS depression. • It also has partial antagonist properties, which may result in opioid withdrawal in physically dependent patients.

Time/Action Profile (time)

Onset	Peak	Duration
2–3 min	15 min	1 hr

Pharmacokinetics

- **Distribution:** Pentazocine is widely distributed and crosses the placenta. • **Metabolism and Excretion:** Pentazocine is mostly metabolized by the liver. Small amounts are excreted unchanged by the kidneys. • **Half-life:** 2–3 hours.

Contraindications

- Pentazocine is contraindicated in patients with hypersensitivity to it or to bisulfites. Avoid using pentazocine in patients who are physically dependent on opioids and who have not been detoxified, as this may precipitate withdrawal. Chronic use should be avoided during pregnancy or lactation.

Adverse Reactions and Side Effects*

• **CNS:** <u>sedation</u>, confusion, <u>headache</u>, <u>euphoria</u>, floating feeling, unusual dreams, <u>hallucinations</u>, dysphoria, <u>dizziness</u>, vertigo • **EENT:** miosis (high doses), blurred vision, diplopia • **Resp:** respiratory depression • **CV:** hypotension, hypertension, palpitations • **GI:** <u>nausea</u>, vomiting, constipation, ileus, dry mouth • **GU:** urinary retention • **Derm:** sweating, clammy feeling • **Misc:** tolerance, physical dependence, psychological dependence.

Pentobarbital Sodium	*Sedative/hypnotic (barbiturate)*
Nembutal	pH 9.5

Schedule II

 ADMINISTRATION CONSIDERATIONS

Usual Dose

Anticonvulsant/Hypnotic

ADULTS: 100 mg initially; additional doses may be given after at least 1 min between doses (up to a total of 500 mg).

CHILDREN: 50 mg initially; additional doses may be given after at least 1 min between doses.

Dilution

• **Direct IV:** Doses may be given **undiluted** or **diluted** with sterile water, 0.45% NaCl, 0.9% NaCl, D5W, D10W, Ringer's or lactated Ringer's solution, dextrose/saline combinations, or dextrose/Ringer's or lactated Ringer's combinations. • Do not use a solution that is discolored or that contains particulate matter.

---

*<u>Underlines</u> indicate most frequent; CAPITALS indicate life-threatening.

Compatibility

- **Syringe:** aminophylline ✦ ephedrine ✦ hyaluronidase ✦ hydromorphone ✦ neostigmine ✦ scopolamine ✦ sodium bicarbonate ✦ thiopental.
- **Y-site:** acyclovir ✦ regular insulin.
- **Additive:** amikacin ✦ aminophylline ✦ calcium chloride ✦ cephapirin ✦ chloramphenicol ✦ dimenhydrinate ✦ erythromycin lactobionate ✦ lidocaine ✦ thiopental ✦ verapamil.

Incompatibility

- **Syringe:** benzquinamide ✦ butorphanol ✦ chlorpromazine ✦ cimetidine ✦ dimenhydrinate ✦ diphenhydramine ✦ droperidol ✦ fentanyl ✦ glycopyrrolate ✦ hydroxyzine ✦ meperidine ✦ midazolam ✦ nalbuphine ✦ pentazocine ✦ perphenazine ✦ prochlorperazine edisylate ✦ promazine ✦ promethazine ✦ ranitidine.
- **Additive:** chlorpheniramine ✦ codeine ✦ ephedrine ✦ erythromycin gluceptate ✦ hydrocortisone ✦ hydroxyzine ✦ insulin ✦ levorphanol ✦ methadone ✦ norepinephrine ✦ penicillin G potassium ✦ pentazocine ✦ phenytoin ✦ promazine ✦ promethazine ✦ streptomycin ✦ triflupromazine ✦ vancomycin.

Rate of Administration

- **Direct IV:** Administer each 50 mg over at least 1 minute. Titrate slowly for desired response. Rapid administration may result in respiratory depression, apnea, laryngospasm, bronchospasm, or hypertension.

≋ CLINICAL PRECAUTIONS

- Assess location, duration, and characteristics of seizure activity when used as an anticonvulsant.
- Assess sleep patterns prior to and periodically throughout course of therapy. Hypnotic doses of pentobarbital suppress REM sleep. Patient may experience an increase in dreaming upon discontinuation of medication.
- Monitor respiratory status, pulse, and blood pressure frequently in patients receiving pentobarbital IV. Equipment for resuscitation and artificial ventilation should be readily available. Respiratory depression is dose dependent.
- Observe IV site for redness or irritation. Solution is highly alkaline; avoid extravasation, which may cause

tissue damage and necrosis. If extravasation occurs, may be treated with infiltration of 5% procaine solution into affected areas, and application of moist heat may be ordered.

- Prolonged therapy may lead to psychological and/or physical dependence.
- Assess postoperative patients for pain. Pentobarbital may increase responsiveness to painful stimuli.
- Monitor intracranial pressure and level of consciousness in patients in barbiturate coma.
- Supervise ambulation and transfer of patients following administration. Remove cigarettes. Side rails should be raised and call bell within reach at all times. Keep bed in low position.
- Additive CNS depression may occur with other CNS depressants, including alcohol, antihistamines, opioid analgesics, and other sedative/hypnotics. Pentobarbital may induce hepatic enzymes, which metabolize other drugs, decreasing their effectiveness, including oral contraceptives, oral anticoagulants, chloramphenicol, cyclosporine, dacarbazine, glucocorticoids, tricyclic antidepressants, and quinidine. It may also increase the risk of hepatic toxicity of acetaminophen. MAO inhibitors, valproic acid, or divalproex may decrease the metabolism of pentobarbital, increasing sedation.
- Use pentobarbital cautiously in patients with hepatic dysfunction or severe renal impairment. Geriatric or debilitated patients are more sensitive to the CNS effects (excitement, confusion, CNS depression) of pentobarbital and should receive reduced dosage.
- Use cautiously in patients with childbearing potential. Pentobarbital should not be used in pregnant or lactating patients (Pregnancy Category D).

Patient/Family Teaching

- Discuss the importance of preparing environment for sleep (dark room, quiet, avoidance of nicotine and caffeine). • Pentobarbital may cause daytime drowsiness. Caution patient to avoid activities requiring alertness until response to medication is known. • Caution patient to avoid taking alcohol or other CNS depressants concurrently with this medication. • Instruct patient to contact physician immediately if pregnancy is suspected.

≋ PHARMACOLOGIC PROFILE

Indications

• Pentobarbital is used as a hypnotic agent (short-term use). • It is also used in high doses to induce coma in selected patients with cerebral ischemia and in the management of increased intracranial pressure (unlabeled use).

Action

• Pentobarbital depresses the CNS, probably by potentiating gamma-aminobutyric acid (GABA), an inhibitory neurotransmitter. It produces all levels of CNS depression, including the sensory cortex, motor activity, and altered cerebellar function. • It may also decrease cerebral blood flow, cerebral edema, and intracranial pressure.

Time/Action Profile (hypnotic effect)

Onset	Peak	Duration
immediate	1 min	15 min

Pharmacokinetics

• **Distribution:** Pentobarbital is widely distributed, with highest concentrations in brain and liver. It crosses the placenta, and small amounts enter breast milk. • **Metabolism and Excretion:** Pentobarbital is metabolized by the liver, and minimal amounts are excreted unchanged by the kidneys. • **Half-life:** 35–50 hours.

Contraindications

• Pentobarbital is contraindicated in patients with hypersensitivity to it or to alcohol or propylene glycol. It should not be used in comatose patients, patients with pre-existing CNS depression (unless used to induce coma), pregnant or lactating patients, or patients with uncontrolled severe pain.

Adverse Reactions and Side Effects*

• **CNS:** drowsiness, lethargy, vertigo, depression, <u>hangover</u>, excitation, delirium • **Resp:** respiratory depression, LARYNGOSPASM, bronchospasm, hypotension (IV only) • **GI:** nausea, vomiting, diarrhea, constipation • **Derm:** rashes, urticaria • **Local:** phlebitis at IV site • **MS:** myalgia, arthralgia,

---

*<u>Underlines</u> indicate most frequent; CAPITALS indicate life-threatening.

neuralgia • **Misc:** hypersensitivity reactions, including ANGIO-EDEMA and serum sickness; psychological dependence, physical dependence.

Pentostatin	Antineoplastic (enzyme inhibitor)
Nipent	pH 7–8.5

≋ ADMINISTRATION CONSIDERATIONS

Usual Dose
ADULTS: 4 mg/m^2 q other wk.

Dilution
• **Reconstitute** by adding 5 ml of sterile water for injection to each 10-mg vial for a concentration of 2 mg/ml. Shake thoroughly to ensure complete dissolution of the drug. • Solution should be prepared in a biologic cabinet. Wear gloves, gown, and mask while handling medication. Discard equipment in specially designated containers (see Appendix F). Spills and wastes should be treated with 5% sodium hypochlorite solution prior to disposal. • **Direct IV:** May be administered **undiluted.** • **Intermittent Infusion:** Dilute in 25–50 ml of D5W or 0.9% NaCl. • Solutions are stable for 8 hours at room temperature. Discard unused solution.

Compatibility
• **Y-site:** fludarabine ✦ melphalan ✦ ondansetron ✦ paclitaxel ✦ sargramostim.

Rate of Administration
• **Direct IV:** Administer as a bolus injection over 5 minutes. • **Intermittent Infusion:** Administer over 20–30 minutes.

≋ CLINICAL PRECAUTIONS

• Monitor renal function and provide adequate hydration. Administer 500–1000 ml of D5/0.45% NaCl prior to administration and 500 ml of D5W or a similar solution after administration of pentostatin. Allopurinol and alkalinization of the urine may be required if serum uric acid concentrations are elevated.

- Monitor patient for CNS toxicity, which initially manifests as lethargy and may progress to seizures and coma. If these occur, pentostatin should be withheld.
- Monitor patient for allergic reactions including anaphylactic reactions and rash. Therapy may be discontinued if severe rash or anaphylaxis develops. Epinephrine, an antihistamine, and resuscitation equipment should be available during therapy.
- Assess patient for nausea and vomiting. Antiemetics should be administered regularly for 48–72 hours after pentostatin administration.
- Assess patient for signs of infection (vital signs, WBC) throughout therapy. Dose may be withheld if infection develops during therapy.
- The risk of fatal pulmonary toxicity is increased by concurrent use of fludarabine. Effects of vidarabine are increased by pentostatin, which may result in increased toxicity.
- If complete response occurs in less than 6 months, continue pentostatin for 2 more doses. If no response occurs in 6 months, pentostatin should be discontinued. If partial response occurs, pentostatin may be continued for 1 year.
- Use cautiously in patients with underlying cardiovascular disease; seizures; pre-existing renal, hepatic, or pulmonary disease; or other chronic debilitating illness.
- Use with caution in patients with childbearing potential (Pregnancy Category D). Safe use in pregnancy, lactation, or children is not established.

Lab Test Considerations

- Prior to initiating therapy, assess renal function by measuring serum creatinine or creatinine clearance. Serum creatinine should be measured prior to each dose. Dose may be withheld if serum creatinine is elevated. • Monitor CBC prior to each dose and periodically throughout therapy. Pentostatin should be temporarily withheld if the absolute neutrophil count (ANC) is less than 200 cells/mm^3 during treatment in a patient whose initial neutrophil count was greater than 500 cells/mm^3. Resume treatment when ANC returns to pretreatment levels. • May cause elevated liver function tests (AST [SGOT], ALT [SGPT], LDH, alkaline phosphatase). • May cause increased serum and urine uric acid concentrations. • Monitor peripheral blood for hairy cells periodically throughout therapy to determine response to treatment. • Bone marrow aspiration and biopsies may be required every 2–3 months to assess response to therapy.

Patient/Family Teaching

• Instruct patient to notify physician or nurse immediately if rash or signs of anaphylaxis develop. • Advise patient to notify physician promptly if fever, chills, sore throat, or signs of infection occur. Caution patient to avoid crowds and persons with known infections. • Advise patient to use sunscreen and protective clothing to prevent photosensitivity reactions.

PHARMACOLOGIC PROFILE

Indications

• Pentostatin is used in the treatment of hairy cell leukemia unresponsive to treatment with alfa-interferon.

Action

• Pentostatin inhibits adenine deaminase (ADA), an enzyme that blocks the synthesis of DNA, especially in T cells of the lymphoid system.

Time/Action Profile (clinical response)

Onset	Peak	Duration†
within 6 mo	UK	1 wk

†Inhibition of adenine deaminase.

Pharmacokinetics

• **Distribution:** UK. • **Metabolism and Excretion:** Pentostatin and its metabolites are renally excreted. • **Half-life:** 6 hours (increased in renal impairment).

Contraindications

• Pentostatin is contraindicated in patients with hypersensitivity to it or to mannitol.

Adverse Reactions and Side Effects*

• **CNS:** <u>central nervous system toxicity</u>, SEIZURES, <u>fatigue</u>, <u>headache</u>, anxiety, confusion, depression, dizziness, insomnia, nervousness, somnolence, weakness, malaise • **EENT:** abnormal vision, conjunctivitis, ear pain, eye pain • **Resp:** pulmonary toxicity, <u>cough</u>, <u>bronchitis</u>, dyspnea, pneumonia, pharyngitis, rhinitis, sinusitis • **CV:** chest pain, MYOCARDIAL INFARCTION, peripheral edema, arrhythmias, abnormal ECG • **GI:** <u>anorexia</u>, <u>nausea</u>, <u>vomiting</u>, <u>diarrhea</u>, <u>impaired hepatic function</u>, stomatitis, constipation, flatulence, abdominal pain • **GU:** nephrotoxicity, hematuria, dysuria • **Derm:** rashes, photosensitivity, herpes simplex, herpes zoster, pruritus, skin discoloration, seborrhea, sweating, dry skin, eczema, ecchymoses, petechiae • **Hemat:** <u>anemia</u>, <u>leukopenia</u>, <u>thrombocytopenia</u>, hemorrhage, thrombophlebitis • **Metab:** weight loss • **MS:** back pain, myalgia, arthralgia • **Neuro:** paresthesia • **Misc:** lymphadenopathy, infection, <u>generalized pain</u>, allergic reactions, chills, second neoplasms.

Perphenazine	*Antiemetic*
	(phenothiazine)
Trilafon	pH 4.2–5.6

ADMINISTRATION CONSIDERATIONS

Usual Dose

ADULTS: 1 mg q 1–2 min to a total of 5 mg or as an infusion at a rate not to exceed 1 mg/min.

Dilution

• **Direct IV: Dilute** to a concentration of 0.5 mg/ml with 0.9% NaCl. • **Intermittent Infusion:** May **dilute further** in 0.9% NaCl.

Compatibility

• **Syringe:** atropine ✦ butorphanol ✦ cimetidine ✦ dimenhydrinate ✦ diphenhydramine ✦ droperidol ✦ fentanyl ✦ me-

---

*<u>Underlines</u> indicate most frequent; CAPITALS indicate life-threatening.

peridine ✦ metoclopramide ✦ morphine ✦ pentazocine ✦ ranitidine ✦ scopolamine.

• **Y-site:** acyclovir ✦ amikacin ✦ ampicillin ✦ cefamandole ✦ cefazolin ✦ ceforanide ✦ cefotaxime ✦ cefoxitin ✦ cefuroxime ✦ cephalothin ✦ cephapirin ✦ chloramphenicol ✦ clindamycin ✦ doxycycline ✦ erythromycin lactobionate ✦ famotidine ✦ gentamicin ✦ kanamycin ✦ metronidazole ✦ mezlocillin ✦ minocycline ✦ nafcillin ✦ oxacillin ✦ penicillin G potassium ✦ piperacillin ✦ ticarcillin ✦ ticarcillin/clavulanate ✦ tobramycin ✦ trimethoprim/sulfamethoxazole ✦ vancomycin.

Incompatibility

• **Syringe:** midazolam ✦ pentobarbital ✦ thiethylperazine.
• **Y-site:** cefoperazone.

Rate of Administration

• **Direct IV:** Administer each 1 mg over at least 1 minute.
• **Intermittent Infusion:** Administer slowly at a rate not to exceed 1 mg/min.

≋ CLINICAL PRECAUTIONS

• To prevent contact dermatitis, avoid getting liquid preparations on hands, and wash hands thoroughly if spillage occurs.
• Administration should be limited to recumbent hospitalized patients.
• Assess nausea and vomiting prior to and following administration. Monitor intake and output. IV fluids and electrolytes may be required in addition to perphenazine.
• Monitor blood pressure (sitting, standing, lying), pulse, and respiratory rate prior to and frequently during the period of dosage adjustment. Excessive hypotension may be treated with IV norepinephrine.
• Observe patient for extrapyramidal symptoms (akathisia—restlessness; dystonia—muscle spasms and twisting motions; or pseudoparkinsonism—mask facies, pill-rolling motions, drooling, tremors, rigidity, shuffling gait, dysphagia). A reduction of dosage or discontinuation of medication may be necessary.
• Monitor for tardive dyskinesia (uncontrolled movements of face, mouth, tongue, or jaw and involuntary move-

ments of extremities). These side effects may be irreversible.

• Monitor for development of neuroleptic malignant syndrome (fever, respiratory distress, tachycardia, convulsions, diaphoresis, hypertension or hypotension, pallor, tiredness).

• Additive hypotension may occur with antihypertensive agents, acute ingestion of alcohol, or nitrates. Additive CNS depression may occur with concurrent use of MAO inhibitors or other CNS depressants, including alcohol, antihistamines, opioid analgesics, sedative/hypnotics, and general anesthetics. Additive anticholinergic effects may occur with concurrent use of other drugs possessing anticholinergic properties, including antihistamines, antidepressants, atropine, disopyramide, haloperidol, and other phenothiazines. Hypotension and tachycardia may occur with epinephrine. The risk of agranulocytosis is increased with antithyroid agents. The risk of extrapyramidal reactions is increased with lithium. Perphenazine may mask lithium toxicity. Perphenazine may decrease the antiparkinsonian effect of levodopa.

• Use cautiously in elderly or debilitated patients and in patients with diabetes mellitus, respiratory disease, prostatic hypertrophy, CNS tumors, or history of seizure disorder. Geriatric patients may require lower initial doses.

• Perphenazine is not recommended for use during pregnancy or lactation. Jaundice, hyporeflexia or hyperreflexia, and extrapyramidal reactions may occur in neonates. Safe use in pregnancy or lactation has not been established.

Lab Test Considerations

• Perphenazine may cause false-positive and false-negative pregnancy tests. • It may also cause blood dyscrasias; monitor CBC periodically throughout course of therapy. • Monitor liver function tests, urine bilirubin, and bile for evidence of hepatic toxicity periodically throughout course of therapy. Urine bilirubin may be falsely elevated.

Patient/Family Teaching

• Inform patient of possibility of extrapyramidal symptoms and tardive dyskinesia. Caution patient to report these symptoms immediately to physician or nurse. • Advise patient to make position changes slowly to minimize orthostatic hypotension. • Perphenazine may cause drowsiness. Caution patient to avoid activities requiring alertness until response to medication is known. • Caution patient to avoid taking alcohol or other CNS depressants concurrently with this medication. • Instruct patient to notify physician if urinary retention, uncontrolled movements, rash, fever, or yellow coloration of skin occurs, or if dry mouth or constipation persists. Sugarless candy or gum may diminish dry mouth, and an increase in fluid intake, bulk, or exercise may prevent constipation. • Inform patient that this medication may turn urine pink to reddish-brown.

PHARMACOLOGIC PROFILE

Indications

• Perphenazine is used in the management of severe nausea and vomiting. • It is also used in the management of intractable hiccups.

Action

• Perphenazine alters the effects of dopamine in the CNS. It possesses significant anticholinergic and alpha-adrenergic blocking activity. • It also blocks dopamine in the chemoreceptor trigger zone, resulting in decreased nausea and vomiting.

Time/Action Profile (antiemetic effect)

Onset	Peak	Duration
rapid	UK	UK

Pharmacokinetics

• **Distribution:** Perphenazine is widely distributed, achieving high concentrations in the CNS. It crosses the placenta and enters breast milk. • **Metabolism and Excretion:** Perphenazine is highly metabolized by the liver and GI mucosa, with some conversion to active compounds. • **Half-life:** UK.

Contraindications

• Perphenazine is contraindicated in patients with hypersensitivity to it or to bisulfites. Cross-sensitivity with other phenothiazines may occur. • Perphenazine should be avoided in patients with narrow-angle glaucoma, bone marrow depression, severe liver or cardiovascular disease, or intestinal obstruction. Pregnant or lactating patients should not be given perphenazine.

Adverse Reactions and Side Effects*

• **CNS:** sedation, <u>extrapyramidal reactions</u>, tardive dyskinesia, NEUROLEPTIC MALIGNANT SYNDROME • **CV:** hypotension, tachycardia • **EENT:** <u>dry eyes</u>, <u>blurred vision</u>, lens opacities • **GI:** <u>constipation</u>, dry mouth, ileus, anorexia, hepatitis • **GU:** urinary retention • **Derm:** rashes, <u>photosensitivity</u>, pigment changes • **Endo:** galactorrhea • **Hemat:** agranulocytosis, leukopenia • **Metab:** hyperthermia • **Misc:** allergic reactions.

Phenobarbital Sodium	*Sedative/hypnotic (barbiturate), Anticonvulsant (barbiturate)*
Luminal sodium	pH 8.5–10.5

Schedule IV

ADMINISTRATION CONSIDERATIONS

Usual Dose

Anticonvulsant
ADULTS: 100–320 mg (total of 600 mg/24-hr period).
CHILDREN: 10–20 mg/kg initially, followed by 1–6 mg/kg/day.

---

*<u>Underlines</u> indicate most frequent; CAPITALS indicate life-threatening.

Status Epilepticus
ADULTS: 10–20 mg/kg; may be repeated.
CHILDREN: 15–20 mg/kg.

Sedative
ADULTS: 15–60 mg twice daily or 10–40 mg three times daily.
CHILDREN: *Preoperative*—1–3 mg/kg 60–90 min before surgery.

Hypnotic
ADULTS: 100–325 mg at bedtime.

Dilution
• **Direct IV: Reconstitute** sterile powder for IV dose with 3 ml of sterile water for injection. **Dilute further** with 10 ml of sterile water. • Do not use solution that is not absolutely clear within 5 minutes after reconstitution or that contains a precipitate. Discard powder or solution that has been exposed to air for more than 30 minutes.

Compatibility
• **Syringe:** heparin.
• **Y-site:** enalaprilat.
• **Additive:** amikacin • aminophylline • calcium chloride • calcium gluconate • cephapirin • colistimethate • dimenhydrinate • polymyxin B • sodium bicarbonate • verapamil.
• **Solution:** D5W • D10W • 0.45% NaCl • 0.9% NaCl • Ringer's and lactated Ringer's solution • dextrose/saline combinations • dextrose/Ringer's or dextrose/lactated Ringer's combinations.

Incompatibility
• **Syringe:** benzquinamide • dimenhydrinate • diphenhydramine • erythromycin glucoptate • hydroxyzine • kanamycin • phenytoin • prochlorperazine • promazine • promethazine • ranitidine.
• **Y-site:** hydromorphone.
• **Additive:** cephalothin • chlorpromazine • codeine • ephedrine • hydralazine • hydrocortisone sodium succinate • hydroxyzine • insulin • levorphanol • meperidine • methadone • morphine • norepinephrine • pentazocine • procaine • prochlorperazine mesylate • promazine • promethazine • streptomycin • succinylcholine • vancomycin.

Rate of Administration

- **Direct IV:** Administer each 60 mg over at least 1 minute. Titrate slowly for desired response. Rapid administration may result in respiratory depression.

≋ CLINICAL PRECAUTIONS

- Assess location, duration, and characteristics of seizure activity when used as an anticonvulsant. When changing from phenobarbital to another anticonvulsant, gradually decrease phenobarbital dose while concurrently increasing dose of replacement medication to maintain anticonvulsant effects.
- Assess level of consciousness and anxiety when used as a sedative.
- Assess patients for pain. Phenobarbital may increase responsiveness to painful stimuli.
- Monitor respiratory status, pulse, and blood pressure frequently in patients receiving phenobarbital IV. Equipment for resuscitation and artificial ventilation should be readily available. Respiratory depression is dose dependent.
- Doses may require 15–30 minutes to reach peak concentrations in the brain. Administer minimal dose and wait for effectiveness before administering second dose to prevent cumulative barbiturate-induced depression.
- Phenobarbital is highly alkaline; avoid extravasation, which may cause tissue damage and necrosis. If extravasation occurs, may be treated with injection of 5% procaine solution into affected area and application of moist heat.
- Supervise ambulation and transfer of patients following administration. Remove cigarettes. Side rails should be raised and call bell within reach at all times. Keep bed in low position. Institute seizure precautions.
- Additive CNS depression may occur with concurrent use of other CNS depressants, including alcohol, antihistamines, opioid analgesics, and other sedative/hypnotics.
- Phenobarbital may induce (speed up) hepatic enzymes that metabolize other drugs, decreasing their effectiveness, including oral contraceptives, oral anticoagulants, chloramphenicol, cyclosporine, dacarbazine, glucocorti-

coids, tricyclic antidepressants, and quinidine. It may increase the risk of hepatic toxicity of acetaminophen. MAO inhibitors, valproic acid, or divalproex may decrease the metabolism of phenobarbital, increasing sedation. Phenobarbital may increase the risk of hematologic toxicity from cyclophosphamide. Use cautiously in patients with hepatic dysfunction or severe renal impairment. Elderly patients require dosage reduction.

- Use cautiously during pregnancy, as chronic use results in drug dependency in the infant and may result in coagulation defects and fetal malformation. Acute use at term may also result in respiratory depression in the newborn (Pregnancy Category D).

Toxicity and Overdose Alert

- Serum phenobarbital levels should be routinely monitored when used as an anticonvulsant. Therapeutic blood levels are 10–40 mcg/ml. Symptoms of toxicity include confusion, drowsiness, dyspnea, slurred speech, and staggering.

Patient/Family Teaching

- Medication may cause daytime drowsiness. Caution patient to avoid activities requiring alertness until response to medication is known. • Caution patient to avoid taking alcohol or other CNS depressants concurrently with this medication. • Instruct patient to contact physician immediately if pregnancy is suspected. • Advise patient to notify physician if fever, sore throat, mouth sores, unusual bleeding or bruising, nosebleeds, or petechiae occur.

≋ PHARMACOLOGIC PROFILE

Indications

- Phenobarbital is used as an anticonvulsant in tonic-clonic (grand mal), partial, and febrile seizures in children. • It is also used as a preoperative sedative and in other situations in which sedation may be required and as a hypnotic.

Action

- Phenobarbital produces all levels of CNS depression. It depresses the sensory cortex, decreases motor activity, and alters cerebellar function. • It also inhibits transmission in the nervous system and raises the seizure threshold. • Phenobarbital is capable of inducing (speeding up) enzymes in the liver that metabolize drugs, bilirubin, and other compounds.

Time/Action Profile (sedation)

Onset	Peak	Duration
5 min	30 min	4–6 hr

Pharmacokinetics

• **Distribution:** UK. • **Metabolism and Excretion:** 75% is metabolized by the liver, 25% is excreted unchanged by the kidneys. • **Half-life:** 2–6 days.

Contraindications

• Phenobarbital is contraindicated in patients with hypersensitivity to it or to alcohol or propylene glycol. Some products contain benzyl alcohol and should be avoided in patients with known intolerance. Lactating patients, comatose patients, or those with pre-existing CNS depression or uncontrolled severe pain should not receive phenobarbital.

Adverse Reactions and Side Effects*

• **CNS:** drowsiness, lethargy, vertigo, depression, <u>hangover</u>, excitation, delirium • **Resp:** respiratory depression, LARYNGOSPASM, bronchospasm • **CV:** hypotension • **GI:** nausea, vomiting, diarrhea, constipation • **Derm:** rashes, urticaria, photosensitivity • **Local:** phlebitis at IV site • **MS:** myalgia, arthralgia, neuralgia • **Misc:** hypersensitivity reactions, including ANGIOEDEMA and serum sickness; physical dependence, psychological dependence (prolonged use only).

---

*<u>Underlines</u> indicate most frequent; CAPITALS indicate life-threatening.

Phentolamine Mesylate	*Alpha-adrenergic blocking agent*
Regitine, {Rogitine}	pH 4.5–6.6

≋ ADMINISTRATION CONSIDERATIONS

Usual Dose

Diagnosis of Pheochromocytoma (phentolamine blocking test)
ADULTS: 2.5–5 mg.
CHILDREN: 1 mg or 3 mg/m^2 or 100 mcg (0.1 mg)/kg.

Hypertension Associated with Pheochromocytoma during Surgery
ADULTS: 5 mg given 1–2 hr preoperatively, repeated as necessary during the procedure or as an infusion of 500 mcg (0.5 mg)–1 mg/min.

CHILDREN: 1 mg or 100 mcg (0.1 mg)/kg or 3 mg/m^2 given 1–2 hr preoperatively, repeated as necessary during the procedure.

Prevention of Dermal Necrosis during Infusion of Norepinephrine
Add 10 mg phentolamine to each 1000 ml of fluid containing norepinephrine.

Dilution
• **Direct IV: Reconstitute** each 5 mg with 1 ml of sterile water for injection or 0.9% NaCl. • Discard unused solution.
• **Continuous Infusion: Dilute** 5–10 mg in 500 ml of D5W.
• May also add 10 mg to every 1000 ml of fluid containing norepinephrine for prevention of dermal necrosis and sloughing. Does not affect pressor effect of norepinephrine.

Compatibility
• **Syringe:** papaverine.
• **Additive:** dobutamine ◆ norepinephrine ◆ verapamil.

Rate of Administration
• **Direct IV:** Inject each 5 mg over 1 minute. • **Continuous Infusion:** Titrate infusion rate according to patient response.

{} = Available in Canada only.

☰ CLINICAL PRECAUTIONS

- Monitor blood pressure, pulse, and ECG every 2 minutes until stable during IV administration. If hypotensive crisis occurs, epinephrine is contraindicated and may cause paradoxical further decrease in blood pressure; norepinephrine may be used. Patient should remain supine throughout parenteral administration. Elderly patients are more susceptible to hypotensive effects; dosage reduction is recommended in this population.
- When phentolamine is used as a diagnostic agent, all nonessential medications should be discontinued 24–72 hours prior to test. Antihypertensive agents should be decreased or discontinued so that blood pressure returns to pretreatment levels. If patient is normotensive, the test should not be performed.
- To prevent dermal necrosis from extravasation associated with vasopressors, dilute 5–10 mg of phentolamine in 10 ml of 0.9% NaCl and infiltrate the site of extravasation promptly. Must be given within 12 hours of extravasation to be effective.
- Use cautiously in patients with peptic ulcer disease.
- Phentolamine antagonizes the effects of alpha-adrenergic stimulants and may decrease the pressor response to ephedrine, phenylephrine, or methoxamine. Hypotension, vasodilation, and tachycardia may be exaggerated by drugs that stimulate both alpha and beta receptors, such as epinephrine. Concurrent use with guanethidine or guanadrel may result in exaggerated hypotension and bradycardia. Phentolamine decreases peripheral vasoconstriction from high doses of dopamine.
- Safe use during pregnancy or lactation has not been established (Pregnancy Category C).

Patient/Family Teaching

- Advise patient to make position changes slowly to minimize orthostatic hypotension. - Instruct patient to notify physician or nurse if chest pain occurs during infusion.

PHARMACOLOGIC PROFILE

Indications

• Phentolamine is used in the treatment of hypertension associated with pheochromocytoma or adrenergic (sympathetic) excess, such as administration of phenylephrine, tyramine-containing foods in patients on MAO inhibitor therapy, or clonidine withdrawal. • It is also used to control blood pressure during surgical removal of a pheochromocytoma and to prevent dermal necrosis and sloughing following extravasation of norepinephrine, phenylephrine, or dopamine.

Action

• Phentolamine produces incomplete and short-lived blockade of alpha-adrenergic receptors located primarily in smooth muscle and exocrine glands. • It induces hypotension by direct relaxation of vascular smooth muscle and by alpha blockade. Phentolamine is able to reduce blood pressure in situations in which hypertension is due to adrenergic (sympathetic) excess. • When infiltrated locally, it reverses vasoconstriction caused by norepinephrine or dopamine.

Time/Action Profile (alpha-adrenergic blockade)

Onset	Peak	Duration
immediate	2 min	15–30 min

Pharmacokinetics

• **Distribution:** UK. • **Metabolism and Excretion:** 10% is excreted unchanged by kidneys. • **Half-life:** UK.

Contraindications

• Phentolamine is contraindicated in patients with hypersensitivity to it or to mannitol. It should be avoided in patients with coronary or cerebral arteriosclerosis or renal impairment.

Adverse Reactions and Side Effects*

• **CNS:** CEREBROVASCULAR SPASM, weakness, dizziness • **EENT:** nasal stuffiness • **CV:** <u>hypotension</u>, tachycardia, <u>arrhythmias</u>,

---

*<u>Underlines</u> indicate most frequent; CAPITALS indicate life-threatening.

angina, myocardial infarction • **Derm:** flushing • **GI:** <u>abdominal pain</u>, <u>nausea</u>, <u>vomiting</u>, diarrhea, aggravation of peptic ulcer.

Phenylephrine	*Vasopressor*
Neo-Synephrine Hydrochloride	pH 3–6.5

 ADMINISTRATION CONSIDERATIONS

Usual Dose
ADULTS: *Severe hypotension and shock*—100–180 mcg (0.1–0.18 mg)/min initially, 40–60 mcg (0.04–0.06 mg)/min maintenance. *Mild to moderate hypotension*—200 mcg (0.2 mg) not more often than q 10–15 min. *Hypotensive emergencies during spinal anesthesia*—200 mcg (0.2 mg) may be given; dose may be repeated and increased by not more than 200 mcg (0.2 mg), up to a total dose of 500 mcg (0.5 mg).

Dilution
• **Direct IV:** Dilute each 1 mg with 9 ml of sterile water for injection for a concentration of 1 mg/ml. • Phenylephrine is available in several concentrations. Carefully check the label for percentage of solution prior to administration. • **Continuous Infusion: Dilute** 10 mg in 500 ml of dextrose/Ringer's or lactated Ringer's combination, dextrose/saline combinations, D5W, D10W, Ringer's or lactated Ringer's solution, 0.45% NaCl, or 0.9% NaCl to provide a 1:50,000 solution.

Compatibility
• **Y-site:** amrinone • famotidine • haloperidol • zidovudine.
• **Additive:** chloramphenicol • dobutamine • lidocaine • potassium chloride • sodium bicarbonate.

Rate of Administration
• **Direct IV:** Administer each single dose over 1 minute.
• **Continuous Infusion:** Initial rate of infusion is 100–180 mcg/min. Maintenance rate is usually 40–60 mcg/min. Ti-

trate rate according to patient response. Infuse via infusion pump to ensure accurate dosage rate.

PHENYLEPHRINE INFUSION RATE TABLE

Dilution: 10 mg/500 ml = 20 mcg/ml.

Dose (mg/min)	Dose (ml/hr)
PHENYLEPHRINE INFUSION RATES (ml/hr) *CONCENTRATION = 20 mcg (0.02 mg)/ml*	
40 mcg (0.04 mg)/min	120 ml/hr
60 mcg (0.06 mg)/min	180 ml/hr
80 mcg (0.08 mg)/min	240 ml/hr
100 mcg (0.10 mg)/min	300 ml/hr
120 mcg (0.12 mg)/min	360 ml/hr
140 mcg (0.14 mg)/min	420 ml/hr
160 mcg (0.16 mg)/min	480 ml/hr
180 mcg (0.18 mg)/min	540 ml/hr

≋ CLINICAL PRECAUTIONS

- Monitor blood pressure every 2–3 minutes until stabilized and every 5 minutes thereafter during IV administration. Monitor ECG continuously for arrhythmias.
- Volume depletion and electrolyte disturbances should be corrected, if possible, prior to initiation of phenylephrine.
- Assess IV site frequently throughout infusion. Antecubital or other large vein should be used to minimize risk of extravasation, which may cause tissue necrosis. If extravasation occurs, the site should be infiltrated promptly with 10–15 ml of 0.9% NaCl solution containing 5–10 mg of phentolamine to prevent necrosis and sloughing.
- Concurrent use with MAO inhibitors, ergot alkaloids (ergonovine, methylergonovine), or oxytocics results in severe hypertension. Pressor response may also be increased by tricyclic antidepressants, trimethophan, doxapram, or methyldopa. Concurrent use with general anesthetics, cocaine, or cardiac glycosides may result in myocardial irritability. Risk of arrhythmias is increased by alpha-adrenergic blockers (labetalol, prazosin, tolazoline, haloperidol, loxapine, phenothiazines, phen-

oxybenzamine, phentolamine), which may antagonize vasopressor effects. Atropine blocks bradycardia from phenylephrine and enhances pressor effects. Concurrent use with beta-adrenergic blockers may result in hypertension and bradycardia.

- Use phenylephrine with caution in patients with occlusive vascular disease, cardiovascular disease, hyperthyroidism, or diabetes mellitus. Geriatric patients may be more sensitive to the vasopressor effects of phenylephrine.

- Safe use in pregnancy and lactation has not been established (Pregnancy Category C). Concurrent use with oxytocics during labor or delivery may cause hypertension.

Patient/Family Teaching

- Instruct patient to report headaches, dizziness, dyspnea, or pain at infusion site promptly.

≋ PHARMACOLOGIC PROFILE

Indications

- Phenylephrine is used as an adjunct in the management of shock to correct hypotension that may persist after adequate fluid replacement.

Action

- Phenylephrine constricts blood vessels by stimulating alpha-adrenergic receptors.

Time/Action Profile (vasopressor effects)

Onset	Peak	Duration
immediate	UK	15–20 min

Pharmacokinetics

- **Distribution:** UK. • **Metabolism and Excretion:** Phenylephrine is metabolized by the liver and other tissues. • **Half-life:** UK.

Contraindications

- Phenylephrine should not be used in patients with uncorrected fluid volume deficits, tachyarrhythmias, pheochromocytoma, angle-closure glaucoma, or hypersensitivity to bisulfites. Phenylephrine should not be used within 14 days of MAO inhibitors. • Some products contain bisulfites and should be avoided in patients with known hypersensitivity.

Adverse Reactions and Side Effects*

• **CNS:** dizziness, trembling, restlessness, anxiety, nervousness, weakness, dizziness, tremor, insomnia, headache • **Resp:** respiratory distress, dyspnea • **CV:** tachycardia, ARRHYTHMIAS, hypertension, chest pain, bradycardia, vasoconstriction • **Derm:** blanching, piloerection, pallor, sweating • **Local:** phlebitis, sloughing at IV sites.

Phenytoin Sodium	Anticonvulsant (hydantoin), Antiarrhythmic (group IB)
Dilantin	pH 10–12.3

≋ ADMINISTRATION CONSIDERATIONS

Usual Dose

Status Epilepticus
ADULTS: 15–20 mg/kg (rate not to exceed 25–50 mg/min) initially; may be followed 12–24 hr later with 100 mg q 6–8 hr for maintenance.
CHILDREN: 250 mg/m^2 or up to 15–20 mg/kg (at a rate of 0.5–3 mg/kg/min).

Antiarrhythmic
ADULTS: 100 mg q 5 min or 50–100 mg q 10–15 min until arrhythmia is abolished, 1000 mg (15 mg/kg) has been given, or toxicity occurs.

Dilution
• **Direct IV:** May be administered **undiluted**. • Slight yellow color will not alter solution potency. If refrigerated, may

---
*Underlines indicate most frequent; CAPITALS indicate life-threatening.

form precipitate, which dissolves after warming to room temperature. Discard solution that is not clear. • **Intermittent Infusion:** Administer by mixing with 0.9% NaCl in a concentration of 1–10 mg/ml. Administer immediately following admixture. Use tubing with a 0.22-micron in-line filter.

Compatibility

• **Y-site:** esmolol • famotidine • fluconazole • foscarnet • tacrolimus.

Incompatibility

• **Y-site:** ciprofloxacin • diltiazem • enalaprilat • hydromorphone • potassium chloride • vitamin B complex with C.

• **Additive:** Do not admix with other solutions or medications, especially dextrose, as precipitation will occur.

Rate of Administration

• **Direct IV:** Administer at a rate not to exceed 50 mg over 1 minute (25 mg/min in elderly patients; some patients may only tolerate rates of 5–10 mg/min; 1–3 mg/kg/min in neonates). Rapid administration may result in severe hypotension or CNS depression. • **Intermittent Infusion:** Complete infusion within 4 hours at a rate not to exceed 50 mg/min. Monitor cardiac function and blood pressure throughout infusion.

≋ CLINICAL PRECAUTIONS

- Assess location, duration, and characteristics of seizure activity. Implement seizure precautions.
- To prevent precipitation and minimize local venous irritation, follow infusion with 0.9% NaCl. Avoid extravasation; phenytoin is caustic to tissues.
- Monitor cardiac function and blood pressure throughout infusion. Monitor ECG continuously during treatment of arrhythmias.
- Initial dose should be based on ideal body weight + 1.33 (excess weight over ideal body weight in kg). This calculation takes into account preferential distribution into fat.
- Use cautiously in patients with severe liver disease; dosage reduction is recommended. Due to increased risk of serious adverse reactions, use with caution in elderly patients or those with severe cardiac or respiratory disease.

Total dose should be decreased and rate of injection slowed to 5–25 mg/min in geriatric or debilitated patients or patients with impaired liver function.

- Assess oral hygiene. Vigorous cleaning beginning within 10 days of initiation of phenytoin therapy may help control gingival hyperplasia.
- Phenylbutazone, disulfiram, isoniazid, chloramphenicol, and cimetidine may decrease phenytoin metabolism and increase blood levels of phenytoin. Barbiturates, alcohol, and warfarin may stimulate phenytoin metabolism and decrease blood levels. Phenytoin may stimulate the metabolism and decrease the effectiveness of digitoxin, methadone, lidocaine, and oral contraceptives. Phenytoin and dopamine may cause additive hypotension. Additive CNS depression may occur with other CNS depressants, including alcohol, antihistamines, antidepressants, opioid analgesics, and sedative/hypnotics. Additive myocardial depression may occur when phenytoin is used with lidocaine or beta-adrenergic blockers. Phenytoin may alter the effect of oral anticoagulants. Phenytoin may decrease absorption of folic acid.
- Chronic use of phenytoin during pregnancy may result in fetal hydantoin syndrome. If used at term, hemorrhage in the newborn may occur. Safe use during pregnancy or lactation has not been established (Pregnancy Category C).

Toxicity and Overdose Alert

- Serum phenytoin levels should be routinely monitored. Therapeutic blood levels are 10–20 mcg/ml. Free serum hydantoin concentrations should be monitored in patients with altered protein binding of phenytoin (neonates, patients with renal failure, hypoalbuminemia, or acute trauma). Therapeutic concentrations of free phenytoin are 0.8–2 mcg/ml. • Progressive signs and symptoms of phenytoin toxicity include nystagmus, ataxia, confusion, nausea, slurred speech, and dizziness.

Lab Test Considerations

- CBC and platelet count, serum calcium and albumin, urinalysis, and hepatic and thyroid function tests should be monitored prior to and monthly for the first several months, then periodically throughout course of therapy. Phenytoin may cause increased serum alkaline phosphatase and glucose levels. • Serum folate levels should be monitored periodically during therapy because of increased folate requirements of patients on long-term phenytoin therapy.

Patient/Family Teaching

• Phenytoin may cause drowsiness or dizziness. Caution patient to avoid driving or other activities requiring alertness until response to medication is known. Do not resume driving until physician gives clearance based on control of seizure disorder. • Instruct patient on importance of maintaining good dental hygiene during chronic therapy and seeing dentist every 3 months for teeth cleaning to prevent tenderness, bleeding, and gingival hyperplasia. Institution of oral hygiene program within 10 days of initiation of phenytoin therapy may minimize growth rate and severity of gingival enlargement. Patients younger than 23 years of age and those taking doses more than 500 mg/day are at increased risk for gingival hyperplasia. • Inform patient that phenytoin may color urine pink, red, or reddish brown, but that color change is not significant. • Advise diabetic patients to monitor urine glucose carefully and to notify physician of significant changes. • Advise patient to carry identification describing disease process and medication regimen at all times. • Advise patient to notify physician or nurse if skin rash, severe nausea or vomiting, drowsiness, slurred speech, unsteady gait, swollen glands, bleeding or tender gums, yellow skin or eyes, joint pain, fever, sore throat, unusual bleeding or bruising, persistent headache, or pregnancy occurs. • Emphasize the importance of routine examinations to monitor progress. Patient should have regular physical examinations, especially monitoring skin and lymph nodes, and EEG testing.

≋ PHARMACOLOGIC PROFILE

Indications

• Phenytoin is used in the treatment and prevention of tonic-clonic (grand mal) seizures and complex partial seizures. • It is also used as an antiarrhythmic, particularly for arrhythmias associated with cardiac glycoside toxicity (unlabeled use).

Action

• Phenytoin limits seizure propagation by altering ion transport and decreasing synaptic transmission. • Its antiarrhythmic properties are a result of improvement in AV conduction.

Time/Action Profile (anticonvulsant effect)

Onset	Peak	Duration
erratic	erratic	12–24 hr

Pharmacokinetics

• **Distribution:** Phenytoin preferentially distributes into adipose tissue. It crosses the placenta and enters breast milk. • **Metabolism and Excretion:** Phenytoin is mostly metabolized by the liver; minimal amounts excreted in the urine. • **Half-life:** 22 hours.

Contraindications

• Phenytoin is contraindicated in patients with hypersensitivity to it or to propylene glycol. Avoid use in patients with known alcohol intolerance. Phenytoin should not be used in patients with sinus bradycardia or heart block.

Adverse Reactions and Side Effects*

• **CNS:** <u>nystagmus</u>, <u>ataxia</u>, <u>diplopia</u>, drowsiness, lethargy, coma, dizziness, headache, nervousness, dyskinesia • **EENT:** <u>gingival hyperplasia</u> • **CV:** hypotension • **GI:** <u>nausea</u>, vomiting, anorexia, weight loss, constipation, hepatitis • **GU:** pink, red, reddish-brown discoloration of urine • **Derm:** hypertrichosis, <u>rashes</u>, exfoliative dermatitis • **F and E:** hypocalcemia • **Hemat:** APLASTIC ANEMIA, AGRANULOCYTOSIS, leukopenia, thrombocytopenia, megaloblastic anemia • **MS:** osteomalacia • **Misc:** lymphadenopathy, fever, allergic reactions, including STEVENS-JOHNSON SYNDROME.

---

*<u>Underlines</u> indicate most frequent; CAPITALS indicate life-threatening.

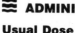

Physostigmine Salicylate   *Cholinergic (anticholinesterase agent)*

Antilirium   pH 3.5–5

≋ ADMINISTRATION CONSIDERATIONS

Usual Dose
Adults: 500 mcg (0.5 mg)–2 mg initially; subsequent doses of 1–4 mg q 20–30 min may be given as symptoms recur.
Children: 20 mcg/kg; may be repeated q 5–10 min, as needed, up to a total of 2 mg.

Dilution
• **Direct IV:** Administer **undiluted**.

Incompatibility
• Information unavailable; do not mix with other drugs or solutions.

Rate of Administration
• **Direct IV:** May be given through Y-site or 3-way stopcock at a rate not to exceed 1 mg/min (0.5 mg over 1 minute for children). Rapid administration may cause bradycardia; increased salivation, which can lead to respiratory distress; or seizures.

≋ CLINICAL PRECAUTIONS

• Monitor ECG, pulse, respiratory rate, and blood pressure frequently throughout administration.
• Because the duration of action of physostigmine is usually brief, repeated doses may be needed.
• Monitor neurologic status frequently. Institute seizure precautions and protect patient from self-injury due to CNS effects of overdose.
• Cholinergic effects of physostigmine may be antagonized by other drugs possessing anticholinergic properties, including antihistamines, antidepressants, atropine, haloperidol, phenothiazines, quinidine, and disopyramide. Physostigmine prolongs the action of depolarizing muscle-relaxing agents (succinylcholine, decamethonium).

- Physostigmine should be used cautiously in patients with any history of asthma, ulcer disease, cardiovascular disease, epilepsy, or hyperthyroidism.
- Avoid using physostigmine during pregnancy or lactation. Muscle weakness may occur in neonates.

Toxicity and Overdose Alert

- Overdose of physostigmine is manifested by bradycardia, respiratory distress, seizures, weakness, nausea, vomiting, stomach cramps, diarrhea, diaphoresis, and increased salivation and tearing. Atropine is the antidote. Treatment of overdose includes establishing an airway and supporting ventilation, atropine sulfate 2–4 mg in adults and 1 mg in children (may be repeated every 3–10 minutes to control muscarinic effects), pralidoxime chloride 50–100 mg/min (to control neurologic and skeletal muscle effects), and supportive therapy. See *atropine sulfate* monograph on page 97 and *pralidoxime chloride* monograph on page 834.

Patient/Family Teaching

- Instruct patient to report signs of systemic side effects (sweating, increased salivation, nausea, vomiting, diarrhea, bradycardia, weakness, and respiratory distress).

≋ PHARMACOLOGIC PROFILE

Indications

- Physostigmine is used to reverse life-threatening CNS effects that result from overdose of drugs capable of causing the anticholinergic syndrome, including belladonna or other plant alkaloids, phenothiazines, tricyclic antidepressants, and antihistamines. Physostigmine reverses delirium, hallucinations, coma, and some arrhythmias, but is not completely effective in reversing cardiac conduction defects or tachycardia.

Action

- Physostigmine inhibits the breakdown of acetylcholine so that it accumulates and has a prolonged effect. The result is a generalized cholinergic response, including miosis, increased tone of intestinal and skeletal musculature, bronchial and ureteral constriction, bradycardia, increased salivation, lacrimation, sweating, and CNS stimulation.

Time/Action Profile (systemic cholinergic effects)

Onset	Peak	Duration
3–8 min	within 5 min	45–60 min†

†May last up to 5 hr.

Pharmacokinetics

• **Distribution:** Physostigmine is widely distributed and crosses the blood–brain barrier. • **Metabolism and Excretion:** Physostigmine is metabolized by cholinesterases present in many tissues; small amounts are excreted unchanged in the urine. • **Half-life:** The half-life of physostigmine is not known.

Contraindications

• Physostigmine is contraindicated in patients with hypersensitivity to it or to bisulfites. Preparations containing benzyl alcohol should be avoided in newborns. Patients with mechanical obstruction of the GI or GU tracts should not receive physostigmine. Use of physostigmine should be avoided during pregnancy or lactation because 10–20% of newborns will suffer from muscle weakness.

Adverse Reactions and Side Effects*

• **CNS:** dizziness, weakness, <u>restlessness</u>, hallucinations, SEIZURES • **EENT:** miosis, lacrimation • **Resp:** excess respiratory secretions, <u>bronchospasm</u> • **CV:** <u>bradycardia</u>, hypotension • **GI:** <u>abdominal cramps</u>, <u>nausea</u>, <u>vomiting</u>, <u>diarrhea</u>, excess salivation • **Derm:** rash.

---

*<u>Underlines</u> indicate most frequent; CAPITALS indicate life-threatening.

Phytonadione	*Vitamin (fat soluble), Vitamin K₁*
AquaMEPHYTON	**pH 3.7**

 ADMINISTRATION CONSIDERATIONS

Usual Dose

IV use of phytonadione should be reserved for emergencies.

Treatment of Hypoprothrombinemia

ADULTS: 2.5–10 mg; repeat in 6–8 hr (up to 25–50 mg q 4 hr).
CHILDREN: 5–10 mg.
INFANTS: 1–2 mg.

Prevention of Hypoprothrombinemia during Total Parenteral Nutrition

ADULTS: 5–10 mg once weekly.
CHILDREN: 2–5 mg once weekly.

Prevention of Hemorrhagic Disease of Newborn

NEONATES: 0.5–1 mg within 1 hr of birth; may be repeated in 6–8 hr if needed.

Dilution

• **Direct IV:** May be administered **undiluted**. • **Continuous Infusion:** May be **diluted** in D5W, D10W, dextrose and Ringer's or lactated Ringer's combinations, dextrose and saline combinations, 0.9% NaCl, 0.45% NaCl, Ringer's or lactated Ringer's solution, or TPN solutions.

Compatibility

• **Y-site:** ampicillin ♦ epinephrine ♦ famotidine ♦ heparin ♦ hydrocortisone sodium succinate ♦ potassium chloride ♦ tolazoline ♦ vitamin B complex with C.

• **Additive:** amikacin ♦ calcium glucceptate ♦ cephapirin ♦ chloramphenicol ♦ cimetidine ♦ netilmicin ♦ sodium bicarbonate.

Incompatibility

- **Y-site:** dobutamine • phenytoin.
- **Additive:** ranitidine.

Rate of Administration

- **Direct IV:** Administer at a rate not to exceed 1 mg/min.

≋ CLINICAL PRECAUTIONS

- The IM or SC route is preferred for parenteral phytonadione therapy, but because of severe hypersensitivity reactions, IV vitamin K is not generally recommended and should be reserved for emergency situations. If IV administration is required, only the AquaMEPHYTON product should be used.
- Monitor for hypersensitivity reactions. Symptoms may include cramplike pains, convulsive movements, cardiac irregularities, chest pains, cyanosis, dulled consciousness, flushing of the face, a sensation of chest constriction, circulatory collapse, bronchospasm, hyperhidrosis, dyspnea, altered taste, dizziness, weak and rapid pulse, hypotension, shock, and cardiac/respiratory arrest. Reactions can be fatal. Have epinephrine, antihistamines, and resuscitative equipment immediately available.
- Administration of whole blood or plasma may also be required in severe bleeding because of the delayed onset of this medication. Phytonadione is an antidote for warfarin overdose but does not counteract the anticoagulant activity of heparin.
- Monitor for frank and occult bleeding (guaiac test for stools; Hematest for urine and emesis). Monitor pulse and blood pressure frequently; assess for symptoms of internal bleeding or hypovolemic shock. To prevent further trauma, inform all personnel of patient's bleeding tendency. Apply pressure to all venipuncture sites for at least 5 minutes; avoid unnecessary IM injections.
- Use vitamin K cautiously in patients with impaired liver function.
- Large doses of salicylates or broad-spectrum anti-infectives may increase vitamin K requirements. Cholestyramine, colestipol, mineral oil, and sucralfate may decrease vitamin K absorption and increase requirements.

- Safe use in pregnancy or lactation is not established (Pregnancy Category C).

Lab Test Considerations

- Prothrombin time should be monitored prior to and throughout vitamin K therapy to determine response to and need for further therapy.

Patient/Family Teaching

- Caution patient to avoid IM injections and activities leading to injury. Use a soft toothbrush, do not floss, and shave with an electric razor until coagulation defect is corrected. • Advise patient to report any symptoms of unusual bleeding or bruising (bleeding gums; nosebleed; black, tarry stools; hematuria; excessive menstrual flow) to physician. • Foods high in vitamin K include leafy green vegetables, meat, and dairy products. Cooking does not destroy substantial amounts of vitamin K. Patient should not drastically alter diet while taking vitamin K. • Advise patient to always carry identification describing disease process. • Emphasize the importance of frequent lab tests to monitor coagulation factors.

≋ PHARMACOLOGIC PROFILE

Indications

- Phytonadione is used in the prevention and treatment of hypoprothrombinemia, which may be associated with excessive doses of oral anticoagulants, salicylates, or certain anti-infective agents, and with nutritional deficiencies or prolonged total parenteral nutrition. • It is also used to prevent hemorrhagic disease of the newborn.

Action

- Vitamin K is required for hepatic synthesis of blood coagulation factors II (prothrombin), VII, IX, and X.

Time/Action Profile (peak = control of hemorrhage, duration = normal prothrombin time achieved)

Onset	Peak	Duration
1–2 hr	3–6 hr	12 hr

Pharmacokinetics

• **Distribution:** Vitamin K crosses the placenta and enters breast milk. • **Metabolism and Excretion:** Vitamin K is rapidly metabolized by the liver. • **Half-life:** UK.

Contraindications

• Phytonadione is contraindicated in patients with hypersensitivity to it. Preparations containing benzyl alcohol should be avoided in newborns.

Adverse Reactions and Side Effects*

• **GI:** gastric upset, unusual taste • **Derm:** rash, urticaria, flushing • **Hemat:** hemolytic anemia • **Local:** erythema, swelling, pain at injection site • **Misc:** kernicterus, hyperbilirubinemia (large doses in very premature infants), allergic reactions including ANAPHYLAXIS.

Pipecuronium Bromide	Neuromuscular blocking agent (nondepolarizing)
Arduan	pH 6

 ADMINISTRATION CONSIDERATIONS

Usual Dose

Dosage adjustments are required for obesity or renal impairment. In obese patients, dosage should be based on ideal body weight. Dosage reduction is also recommended if using concurrent inhalation anesthetics.

ADULTS: *Intubation*—70–85 mcg (0.07–0.085 mg)/kg. *Following recovery from succinylcholine-assisted intubation*—50 mcg (0.05 mg)/kg. Additional doses of 10–15 mcg (0.01–0.015 mg)/kg may be required as maintenance.

CHILDREN 1–14 yr: 57 mcg (0.057 mg)/kg.

INFANTS 3–12 mo: 40 mcg (0.04 mg)/kg.

---

*Underlines indicate most frequent; CAPITALS indicate life-threatening.

Dilution

- **Direct IV: Reconstitute** with 10 ml of 0.9% NaCl, D5W, D5/0.9% NaCl, lactated Ringer's injection, sterile water for injection, or bacteriostatic water for injection for a concentration of 10 mg/ml. Solutions reconstituted with bacteriostatic water contain benzyl alcohol and should not be used for newborns; use within 5 days. Solutions reconstituted with sterile water or other IV solutions should be refrigerated and used within 24 hours. Do not dilute into or administer from large-volume IV solutions.

Rate of Administration

- **Direct IV:** Administer as a bolus.

≋ CLINICAL PRECAUTIONS

- Assess respiratory status continuously throughout pipecuronium therapy. Pipecuronium should be used only by individuals experienced in endotracheal intubation, and equipment for this procedure should be readily available.
- Neuromuscular response to pipecuronium should be monitored with a peripheral nerve stimulator. Paralysis is initially selective and usually occurs sequentially in the following muscles: levator muscles of eyelids, muscles of mastication, limb muscles, abdominal muscles, muscles of the glottis, intercostal muscles, and the diaphragm. Recovery of muscle function usually occurs in reverse order. Observe the patient for residual muscle weakness and respiratory distress during the recovery period.
- Dose is titrated to patient response. Pipecuronium has no effect on consciousness or the pain threshold. Adequate anesthesia/analgesia should *always* be used when pipecuronium is used as an adjunct to surgical procedures or when painful procedures are performed.
- Doses are listed for nonobese patients with normal renal function.
- Use pipecuronium cautiously in patients with cardiovascular disease or edematous states. Onset time is delayed in elderly patients. Obesity prolongs duration of paralysis; dose should be based on ideal body weight. Use cautiously in patients with electrolyte disturbances or renal impairment.

- Use with *extreme caution* in patients with myasthenia gravis or myasthenic syndromes; duration may be dangerously prolonged. Use cautiously in patients with impaired renal function. Dosage reduction is recommended if creatinine clearance is 60 ml/min or less.
- Intensity and duration of paralysis may be prolonged by pretreatment with aminoglycoside antibiotics, polymyxin B, tetracycline, colistin, clindamycin, lidocaine, quinidine, or procainamide. Additive neuromuscular blockade (prolonged duration and recovery) may occur with inhalation anesthetics (enflurane, isoflurane, halothane).
- Safe use in pregnancy or lactation or in newborns has not been established (Pregnancy Category C). Because of its longer duration of action, pipecuronium is not recommended during cesarean section.

Toxicity and Overdose Alert

- If overdose occurs, use peripheral nerve stimulator to determine the degree of neuromuscular blockade. Maintain airway patency and ventilation until recovery of normal respirations occurs. • Administration of anticholinesterase agents (neostigmine, pyridostigmine) may be used to antagonize the action of pipecuronium once patient has demonstrated some spontaneous recovery from neuromuscular block. Atropine is usually administered prior to or concurrently with anticholinesterase agents. • Administration of fluids and vasopressors may be necessary to treat severe hypotension or shock.

Patient/Family Teaching

- Explain all procedures to patient receiving pipecuronium therapy without anesthesia, as consciousness is not affected by pipecuronium alone. • Reassure patient that communication abilities will return as the medication wears off.

≋ PHARMACOLOGIC PROFILE
Indications

- Pipecuronium is used to produce skeletal muscle paralysis and facilitation of intubation after induction of anesthesia in surgical procedures lasting 90 minutes or more.

Action
• Pipecuronium prevents neuromuscular transmission by blocking the effect of acetylcholine at the myoneural junction. It has no analgesic or anxiolytic effects.

Time/Action Profile (skeletal muscle paralysis)

Onset	Peak	Duration
2.5–3 min	5 min	1–2 hr

Pharmacokinetics
• **Distribution:** UK. • **Metabolism and Excretion:** More than 75% is excreted by the kidneys, mostly as unmetabolized drug. • **Half-life:** 1.7 hours (prolonged in renal impairment).

Contraindications
• Pipecuronium is contraindicated in patients with hypersensitivity to it or to bromides or mannitol. Pipecuronium should not be used in ICU patients requiring prolonged mechanical ventilation. Avoid concurrent use with other nondepolarizing neuromuscular blocking agents. • It is not recommended for use before succinylcholine but may be used following recovery.

Adverse Reactions and Side Effects*
Almost all adverse reactions to pipecuronium are extensions of its pharmacologic effects.
• **Resp:** apnea, respiratory insufficiency • **CV:** hypotension, bradycardia • **MS:** muscle weakness • **Misc:** allergic reactions.

*Underlines indicate most frequent; CAPITALS indicate life-threatening.

Piperacillin Sodium	*Anti-infective*
	(extended-spectrum penicillin)
Pipracil	**pH 5.5–7.5**
	1.85 mEq Na/g

≋ ADMINISTRATION CONSIDERATIONS

Usual Dose

ADULTS: *Meningitis*—4 g q 4 hr or 75 mg/kg q 6 hr; *other serious infections*—3–4 g q 4–6 hr; *complicated urinary tract infections*—3–4 g q 6–8 hr; *uncomplicated urinary tract infections*—1.5–2 g q 6 hr or 3–4 g q 12 hr.

Dilution

• **Direct IV:** The initial **reconstitution** for IV use is made with at least 5 ml of sterile water for injection, 0.9% NaCl, or bacteriostatic water added to each g of piperacillin. Shake well until dissolved. • Reconstituted solution is stable for 24 hours at room temperature and 7 days if refrigerated. • **Intermittent Infusion: Dilute** in at least 50 ml of 0.9% NaCl, D5W, D5/0.9% NaCl, or lactated Ringer's solution.

Compatibility

• **Syringe:** heparin.
• **Y-site:** acyclovir • allopurinol sodium • ciprofloxacin • cyclophosphamide • diltiazem • enalaprilat • esmolol • famotidine • fludarabine • foscarnet • gallium nitrate • hydromorphone • labetalol • magnesium sulfate • melphalan • meperidine • morphine • perphenazine • ranitidine • tacrolimus • verapamil • zidovudine. • Manufacturer recommends temporarily discontinuing primary infusion during piperacillin administration.
• **Additive:** ciprofloxacin • clindamycin • fluconazole • hydrocortisone sodium succinate • ofloxacin • potassium chloride • verapamil.

Incompatibility

• **Y-site:** filgrastim • fluconazole • ondansetron • sargramostim • vinorelbine. • If aminoglycosides and penicillins or cephalosporins must be given concurrently, administer in separate sites at least 1 hour apart.

Rate of Administration

- **Direct IV:** Inject slowly, over 3–5 minutes, to minimize vein irritation. • **Intermittent Infusion:** Administer over 30 minutes via Y-site injection.

☰ CLINICAL PRECAUTIONS

- Change IV sites every 48 hours to prevent phlebitis.
- Assess patient for infection (vital signs; appearance of wound, sputum, urine, and stool; WBC) at beginning and throughout course of therapy.
- Obtain specimens for culture and sensitivity prior to initiating therapy. First dose may be given before receiving results.
- Obtain a history before initiating therapy to determine previous use of and reactions to penicillins or cephalosporins. Persons with a negative history of penicillin sensitivity may still have an allergic response. Observe patient for signs and symptoms of anaphylaxis (rash, pruritus, laryngeal edema, wheezing). Discontinue the drug immediately if these occur. Keep epinephrine, an antihistamine, and resuscitation equipment close by in the event of an anaphylactic reaction.
- In patients with creatinine clearance of 40 ml/min or less, dosing interval should be increased.
- Use cautiously in patients whose sodium intake is restricted.
- Probenecid decreases renal excretion and increases blood levels of piperacillin. Piperacillin may alter excretion of lithium. Concurrent use of diuretics, glucocorticoids, or amphotericin B may increase the risk of hypokalemia. Hypokalemia increases the risk of cardiac glycoside toxicity. The risk of hepatotoxicity is increased by concurrent use of other hepatotoxic agents. Piperacillin may decrease the half-life of aminoglycosides (given by different routes) when used concurrently in patients with renal impairment.
- Safe use in pregnancy or lactation has not been established (Pregnancy Category B).

Lab Test Considerations

- Renal and hepatic function, CBC, serum potassium, and bleeding times should be evaluated prior to and routinely throughout course of therapy. • Piperacillin may cause positive direct Coombs' test results and may cause elevated BUN, creatinine, AST (SGOT), ALT (SGPT), serum bilirubin, and LDH. • In addition, piperacillin may cause elevated serum sodium and decreased serum potassium concentrations.

Patient/Family Teaching

• Advise patient to report the signs of superinfection (black, furry overgrowth on the tongue; vaginal itching or discharge; loose or foul-smelling stools) and allergy.

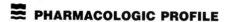 PHARMACOLOGIC PROFILE

Indications

• Piperacillin is used in the treatment of serious infections due to susceptible organisms, including skin and skin structure infections, bone and joint infections, septicemia, respiratory tract infections, intra-abdominal infections, and gynecologic and urinary tract infections. • Combination with an aminoglycoside may be synergistic and is recommended for infection due to *Pseudomonas aeruginosa.* Piperacillin has been combined with other antibiotics in the treatment of infections in immunosuppressed patients. • It has also been used as a perioperative prophylactic anti-infective in abdominal, genitourinary, and head and neck surgery.

Action

• Piperacillin binds to bacterial cell wall membrane, causing cell death. • Its spectrum is extended when compared with other penicillins, with activity against several important Gram-negative aerobic pathogens, notably *P. aeruginosa, Escherichia coli, Proteus mirabilis,* and *Providencia rettgeri.* • It is also active against some anaerobic bacteria, including *Bacteroides.* • It is not active against penicillinase-producing staphylococci or beta-lactamase-producing Enterobacteriaceae.

Time/Action Profile (blood levels)

Onset	Peak
rapid	end of infusion

Pharmacokinetics

• **Distribution:** Piperacillin is widely distributed. It enters CSF in significant amounts only when meninges are inflamed. It crosses the placenta and enters breast milk in low concentrations. • **Metabolism and Excretion:** Piperacillin is mostly (90%) excreted unchanged by the kidneys. Ten percent is excreted in bile. • **Half-life:** 0.7–1.3 hours.

Contraindications

• Piperacillin is contraindicated in patients with hypersensitivity to penicillins.

Adverse Reactions and Side Effects*

• **CNS:** confusion, lethargy, SEIZURES (high doses) • **CV:** congestive heart failure, arrhythmias • **GI:** nausea, diarrhea, hepatotoxicity • **GU:** hematuria (children only), interstitial nephritis • **Derm:** rashes, urticaria • **F and E:** hypokalemia, hypernatremia • **Hemat:** bleeding, blood dyscrasias, increased bleeding time • **Local:** phlebitis at IV site • **Metab:** metabolic alkalosis • **Misc:** superinfection, hypersensitivity reactions including ANAPHYLAXIS and serum sickness.

Piperacillin Sodium/ Tazobactam Sodium	Anti-infective (extended-spectrum penicillin)
{Tazosin}, Zosyn	pH 5.1–5.4 2.35 mEq Na/g

☰ ADMINISTRATION CONSIDERATIONS

Usual Dose

ADULTS: 3.375–4.5 g q 6–8 hr (expressed as 3 g piperacillin sodium with 0.375–0.5 mg tazobactam sodium).

Dilution

• **Intermittent Infusion: Reconstitute** each 1 g of piperacillin with 5 ml of 0.9% NaCl, sterile water for injection,

---

*Underlines indicate most frequent; CAPITALS indicate life-threatening.

{} = Available in Canada only.

D5W, or bacteriostatic saline or water with parabens or benzyl alcohol. Shake well until dissolved. **Further dilute** with at least 50 ml of diluent. • Solution is stable for 24 hours at room temperature and 48 hours to 7 days if refrigerated, depending on the concentration.

Compatibility

• **Y-site:** aminophylline ✦ aztreonam ✦ bleomycin ✦ bumetanide ✦ buprenorphine ✦ butorphanol ✦ calcium gluconate ✦ carboplatin ✦ carmustine ✦ cimetidine ✦ clindamycin ✦ cyclophosphamide ✦ cytarabine ✦ dexamethasone ✦ diphenhydramine ✦ dopamine ✦ enalaprilat ✦ etoposide ✦ floxuridine ✦ fluconazole ✦ fludarabine ✦ fluorouracil ✦ furosemide ✦ gallium nitrate ✦ heparin ✦ hydrocortisone ✦ hydromorphone ✦ ifosfamide ✦ leucovorin ✦ lorazepam ✦ magnesium sulfate ✦ mannitol ✦ meperidine ✦ mesna ✦ methotrexate ✦ methylprednisolone ✦ metoclopramide ✦ metronidazole ✦ morphine ✦ ondansetron ✦ plicamycin ✦ potassium chloride ✦ ranitidine ✦ sargramostim ✦ sodium bicarbonate ✦ thiotepa ✦ trimethoprim/sulfamethoxazole ✦ vinblastine ✦ vincristine ✦ zidovudine.

Incompatibility

• **Y-site:** acyclovir ✦ amphotericin B ✦ chlorpromazine ✦ cisplatin ✦ dacarbazine ✦ daunorubicin ✦ dobutamine ✦ doxorubicin ✦ doxycycline ✦ droperidol ✦ famotidine ✦ ganciclovir ✦ haloperidol ✦ hydroxyzine ✦ idarubicin ✦ miconazole ✦ minocycline ✦ mitomycin ✦ mitoxantrone ✦ nalbuphine ✦ prochlorperazine ✦ promethazine ✦ streptozocin ✦ vancomycin. • If aminoglycosides and penicillins or cephalosporins must be given concurrently, administer in separate sites at least 1 hour apart.

Rate of Administration

• **Intermittent Infusion:** Administer over at least 30 minutes.

≋ CLINICAL PRECAUTIONS

- Monitor for phlebitis. Change IV site every 48 hours to prevent phlebitis.
- Obtain specimens for culture and sensitivity prior to initiating therapy. First dose may be given before results are available.

- Determine history of allergic reactions to penicillins or cephalosporins. Persons with a negative history may still have an allergic response. Observe patient for signs and symptoms of anaphylaxis (rash, pruritus, laryngeal edema, wheezing). Discontinue the drug immediately if these reactions occur. Keep epinephrine, an antihistamine, and resuscitation equipment close by in the event of an anaphylactic reaction.
- Assess patient for infection (vital signs; appearance of wound, sputum, urine, stool; WBC).
- Assess renal function; monitor intake and output, and daily weight. Use cautiously in renal impairment. Piperacillin is excreted primarily by the kidneys. Dosage reduction, increased dosage interval, or both are recommended if creatinine clearance is 40 ml/min or less.
- Safe use in pregnancy, lactation, or children has not been established (Pregnancy Category B).

Lab Test Considerations

 • May cause decreased hemoglobin and hematocrit, thrombocytopenia, and increased platelet count, eosinophilia, leukopenia, neutropenia. Leukopenia and neutropenia are usually associated with prolonged therapy (more than 21 days) and may be reversible. • May cause positive direct Coombs' test results. • May cause elevated AST (SGOT), ALT (SGPT), bilirubin, and alkaline phosphatase levels. • May also cause increases in serum creatinine, BUN, proteinuria, hematuria, and pyuria. • May cause electrolyte abnormalities (sodium, potassium, calcium), hyperglycemia, and decreases in total protein or albumin.

Patient/Family Teaching

 • Advise patient to report the signs of superinfection (black, furry overgrowth on the tongue, vaginal itching or discharge, loose or foul-smelling stools) and allergy.

☰ PHARMACOLOGIC PROFILE

Indications

 • Piperacillin/tazobactam is used in the treatment of the following infections due to piperacillin-resistant, beta-lactamase-producing organisms: appendicitis, skin and skin structure infections, postpartum endometritis or pelvic inflammatory disease, and moderately severe community-acquired pneumonia.

Action

• Piperacillin binds to the bacterial cell wall membrane, causing cell death. Its spectrum is extended when compared with other penicillins. Tazobactam inhibits beta-lactamase, an enzyme that can destroy penicillins. Piperacillin/tazobactam is active against piperacillin-resistant, beta-lactamase-producing *Bacteroides fragilis, Escherichia coli, Staphylococcus aureus,* and *Haemophilus influenzae.*

Time/Action Profile (blood levels)

Onset	Peak
rapid	end of infusion

Pharmacokinetics

• **Distribution:** Piperacillin is widely distributed. It crosses the CSF well only when the meninges are inflamed. It also crosses the placenta and enters breast milk in low concentrations. • **Metabolism and Excretion:** 68% of piperacillin and 80% of tazobactam are excreted unchanged by the kidneys. • **Half-life:** 0.7–1.3 hours.

Contraindications

• Piperacillin/tazobactam is contraindicated in patients with hypersensitivity to penicillins or tazobactam.

Adverse Reactions and Side Effects*

• **CNS:** headache, insomnia, agitation, dizziness, anxiety • **EENT:** rhinitis • **CV:** chest pain, edema, hypertension • **Resp:** dyspnea • **GI:** <u>diarrhea</u>, nausea, constipation, vomiting, abdominal pain, dyspepsia, stool changes • **Derm:** rashes • **Misc:** fever, superinfection.

---

*<u>Underlines</u> indicate most frequent; CAPITALS indicate life-threatening.

Plasma Protein Fraction	*Volume expander*
Plasmanate, Plasma-Plex, Plasmatein, Protenate	pH 6.7–7.3 130–160 mEq Na/L less than 2 mEq K/L

ADMINISTRATION CONSIDERATIONS

Usual Dose

Hypovolemia
ADULTS: 250–500 ml (12.5–25 g protein). Dose should not exceed 250 g in 48 hr.
INFANTS AND YOUNG CHILDREN: 6.6–33 ml/kg (0.33–1.65 g protein/kg). Dose should not exceed 250 g in 48 hr.

Hypoproteinemia
ADULTS: 1000–1500 ml (50–75 g protein).

Dilution
• **Intermittent Infusion:** Administer plasma protein fraction **undiluted** by IV infusion. Infusion must be completed within 4 hours. • Solution may vary from nearly colorless to straw to brownish. Do not use cloudy solutions. Store at room temperature.

Compatibility
• **Additive:** carbohydrate and electrolyte solutions • whole blood • packed RBCs • chloramphenicol.

Incompatibility
• **Additive:** solutions containing protein hydrolysates • amino acids • alcohol • norepinephrine.

Rate of Administration
• **Intermittent Infusion:** Rate of administration is determined by blood volume, indication, and patient response but should not exceed 10 ml/min (5000 ml of 5% solution in 48 hours) to minimize the possibility of hypotension. As the plasma volume approaches normal, the rate of administration should not exceed 5–8 ml/min. The rate for infants and children should not exceed 5–10 ml/min.

≋ CLINICAL PRECAUTIONS

- Administer through a large-gauge (at least 20-g) needle. Use administration set provided by manufacturer. If possible, infusion site should be distal to sites of trauma or infection.
- Monitor vital signs, CVP, pulmonary capillary wedge pressure (PCWP), and intake and output prior to and frequently throughout therapy. Hypotension may result from too-rapid infusion.
- Assess patient for signs of hypervolemia and vascular overload (elevated CVP, elevated PCWP, rales/crackles, dyspnea, hypertension, jugular venous distention) during and following administration. Dehydration should be corrected by additional IV fluids. Underlying causes of hypoproteinemia or hypovolemia should be corrected. Plasma protein fraction serves only as temporary supportive therapy.
- Assess surgical patients for increased bleeding following administration, caused by increased blood pressure and circulating blood volume. Plasma protein fraction does not contain clotting factors.
- Use cautiously in patients with severe hepatic or renal disease.
- Large doses may cause anemia, requiring transfusion.
- There is no danger of serum hepatitis from plasma protein fraction. Crossmatching is not required.
- Safe use in pregnancy or lactation has not been established (Pregnancy Category C).

Lab Test Considerations

- Monitor hemoglobin, hematocrit, serum protein, and electrolytes throughout course of therapy.

Patient/Family Teaching

- Explain the rationale for use of this solution to the patient.

≋ PHARMACOLOGIC PROFILE

Indications

- Plasma protein fraction is used to expand plasma volume and maintain cardiac output in situations associated with deficiencies in circulatory volume, including shock, hemorrhage, and burns. • It is also used as temporary replacement therapy in edema associated with low plasma proteins, such as in the nephrotic syndrome and end-stage liver disease.

Action

• Plasma protein fraction provides colloidal osmotic pressure (in the form of albumin and globulins) within the intravascular space, causing the shift of water from extravascular tissues back into the intravascular space.

Time/Action Profile (intravascular volume expansion)

Onset	Peak	Duration
15–30 min	UK	UK

Pharmacokinetics

• **Distribution:** Plasma protein fraction stays mainly in the intravascular space. • **Metabolism and Excretion:** UK. • **Half-life:** UK.

Contraindications

• Plasma protein fraction is contraindicated in patients with allergic reactions to albumin, severe anemia, or congestive heart failure and those with normal or increased intravascular volume. • It should not be used during cardiopulmonary bypass procedures.

Adverse Reactions and Side Effects*

• **CNS:** headache • **CV:** tachycardia, hypotension, vascular overload • **GI:** nausea, vomiting, excess salivation • **Derm:** erythema, urticaria • **MS:** back pain • **Misc:** fever, chills, flushing.

*Underlines indicate most frequent; CAPITALS indicate life-threatening.

Plicamycin	*Electrolyte modifier (hypocalcemic), Antineoplastic agent (antitumor antibiotic)*
Mithracin, mithramycin	pH 7

≋ ADMINISTRATION CONSIDERATIONS

Usual Dose

Testicular Tumors
ADULTS: 25–30 mcg/kg once daily for 8–10 days or until toxicity occurs (not to exceed 30 mcg/kg/day or more than 10 days); may also be given as 25–50 mcg/kg q other day for 8 doses. Course may be repeated monthly.

Hypercalcemia, Hypercalciuria
ADULTS: 15–25 mcg/kg once daily for 3–4 days; may be repeated q 7 days, may also be given 1–3 times weekly.

Dilution
• **Intermittent Infusion:** To **reconstitute**, add 4.9 ml of sterile water for injection to the 2.5-mg vial of plicamycin to yield a final concentration of 500 mcg/ml. Shake vial to dissolve drug. Use immediately after reconstitution. Discard unused portions. **Add** to 1000 ml of D5W or 0.9% NaCl. • Solution should be prepared in a biologic cabinet. Wear gloves, gown, and mask while handling medication. Discard equipment in designated containers (see Appendix F).

Compatibility
• **Y-site:** allopurinol sodium ◆ filgrastim ◆ melphalan ◆ piperacillin/tazobactam ◆ vinorelbine.

Rate of Administration
• **Direct IV:** Dose may be administered by direct IV push over 20–30 minutes. • **Intermittent Infusion:** Infuse over 4–6 hours. Rapid infusion rate will increase incidence and severity of GI side effects.

≋ CLINICAL PRECAUTIONS
• Ensure patency of the IV. If patient complains of discomfort at the IV site or if extravasation occurs, discontinue IV and restart at another site. Extravasation may cause ir-

ritation and cellulitis. Apply ice to site to prevent pain and swelling. If swelling occurs, application of moderate heat to site may help disperse the medication and decrease the discomfort.

- Monitor for bone marrow suppression. Observe closely for hemorrhagic syndrome (bleeding gums, bruising, petechiae; guaiac test stools, urine, and emesis). This may begin as epistaxis and progress to severe generalized or GI bleeding. May require blood transfusions, fresh frozen plasma, vitamin K, or aminocaproic acid to control bleeding. Avoid giving IM injections and taking rectal temperatures. Apply pressure to venipuncture sites for 10 minutes. Assess for fever, sore throat, and signs of infection.

- Monitor intake and output, appetite, and nutritional intake. Dehydration or volume depletion should be corrected prior to initiating plicamycin therapy. Plicamycin may cause nausea and vomiting, which usually occurs 1–2 hours after therapy is initiated and persists for 12–24 hours and should be treated with prophylactic antiemetics. Adjust diet as tolerated to help maintain fluid and electrolyte balance and nutritional status.

- Monitor symptoms of hypercalcemia (nausea, vomiting, anorexia, thirst, weakness, constipation, paralytic ileus, and bradycardia). Observe patient for evidence of hypocalcemia (paresthesia, muscle twitching, laryngospasm, colic, cardiac arrhythmias, and Chvostek's or Trousseau's sign).

- Use cautiously in patients with other electrolyte abnormalities, especially hypokalemia or hypophosphatemia.

- Additive myelosuppression may occur with other antineoplastic agents or radiation therapy. The risk of bleeding is increased by concurrent use of aspirin, oral anticoagulants, thrombolytic agents, heparin, some cephalosporins, nonsteroidal anti-inflammatory agents, sulfinpyrazone, valproic acid, or dextran. The risk of hepatotoxicity is increased by concurrent use of other hepatotoxic agents. The risk of renal toxicity is increased by concurrent use of other nephrotoxic agents. Use plicamycin cautiously in patients with active infections or other chronic debilitating illnesses. Dosage reduction is required in patients with renal or hepatic impairment.

- Use cautiously in patients with childbearing potential.

Safe use in lactation or children has not been established. Plicamycin is not recommended for use during pregnancy (Pregnancy Category X).

Lab Test Considerations

• Monitor CBC and differential, platelet count, prothrombin time, and bleeding time prior to and periodically throughout therapy. May cause thrombocytopenia, leukopenia, and anemia. • Monitor serum electrolytes prior to and daily during course of therapy. May cause hypocalcemia, hypokalemia, and hypophosphatemia. Correct electrolyte imbalances before beginning therapy. Calcium and phosphate levels may rebound after therapy. • Monitor liver function studies (AST [SGOT], ALT [SGPT], LDH, bilirubin) and renal function studies (BUN, creatinine, urinalysis) prior to and periodically throughout therapy to detect hepatotoxicity and nephrotoxicity.

Patient/Family Teaching

• Advise patient to notify physician promptly in case of fever, chills, sore throat, signs of infection, bleeding gums, bruising, petechiae, or blood in urine, stool, or emesis. Caution patient to avoid crowds and persons with known infections. Instruct patient to use soft toothbrush and electric razor. • Patients should be cautioned not to drink alcoholic beverages or take products containing aspirin, ibuprofen, or naproxen. • Instruct patient to notify physician if weakness, rash, persistent nausea or vomiting, or depression occurs. • Instruct patient to inspect oral mucosa for redness and ulceration. If mouth sores occur, advise patient to use sponge brush and rinse mouth with water after eating and drinking. Consult physician if pain interferes with eating. • Advise patient that although fertility may be decreased with plicamycin, a nonhormonal form of contraception should be used during therapy because of potential teratogenic effects on the fetus. • Patient may also need to avoid products containing calcium or vitamin D. • Instruct patient not to receive any vaccinations without advice of physician. • Emphasize need for periodic lab tests to monitor for side effects.

PHARMACOLOGIC PROFILE

Indications

• Plicamycin is used in the treatment of advanced unresponsive testicular carcinoma. • It is also used in the management of hypercalcemia and hypercalciuria associated with malignancy.

Action

• Plicamycin forms a complex with DNA that subsequently inhibits RNA synthesis, resulting in death of rapidly replicating cells, particularly malignant ones. • It antagonizes the action of vitamin D and inhibits the action of parathyroid hormone on osteoclasts, which results in lowering of serum calcium concentration.

Time/Action Profile

	Onset	Peak	Duration
effects on blood counts	UK	7–10 days	3–4 wk
hypocalcemic effects	24–48 hr	UK	3–15 days

Pharmacokinetics

• **Distribution:** Plicamycin appears to concentrate in the liver, renal tubule, and bone surface. It crosses the blood–brain barrier. • **Metabolism and Excretion:** Plicamycin is excreted primarily by the kidneys. • **Half-life:** UK.

Contraindications

• Plicamycin is contraindicated in patients with hypersensitivity to it or to mannitol. • It should be avoided in patients with bleeding disorders, depressed bone marrow reserve, hypocalcemia, or severe renal or liver disease. • Pregnant patients should not receive plicamycin.

Adverse Reactions and Side Effects*

• **CNS:** drowsiness, weakness, lethargy, malaise, headache, depression, nervousness, irritability, dizziness, fatigue • **EENT:** epistaxis • **GI:** anorexia, nausea, vomiting, stomatitis, diarrhea, hepatitis • **GU:** renal failure, gonadal suppression • **Derm:** facial flushing, rashes • **F and E:** hypocalcemia,

---

*Underlines indicate most frequent; CAPITALS indicate life-threatening.

hypophosphatemia, hypokalemia, rebound hypercalcemia
• **Hemat:** hemorrhagic syndrome, <u>thrombocytopenia</u>, leukopenia, anemia • **Local:** phlebitis at IV site • **Misc:** fever.

Potassium Acetate	*Potassium supplement*
	pH 5.5–8
	10.2 mEq K/g

≋ ADMINISTRATION CONSIDERATIONS

Usual Dose

ADULTS: 10–20 mEq/hour (not to exceed 400 mEq/day or 3 mEq/kg/day). *If serum potassium is >2.5 mEq/liter,* up to 200 mEq/day may be given. *If serum potassium is <2.0 mEq/liter* and is accompanied by ECG changes or paralysis, urgent treatment may consist of up to 400 mEq/day.

INFANTS AND CHILDREN: up to 3 mEq/kg/day or 40 mEq/m²/day.

Dilution

• **Intermittent Infusion:** Do not administer undiluted. Each single dose must be **diluted** and thoroughly mixed.
• **Dilute** to a maximum concentration of 40 mEq/liter in dextrose, saline, Ringer's solution, lactated Ringer's solution, dextrose/saline, dextrose/Ringer's solution, and dextrose/lactated Ringer's solution combinations.

Compatibility

• **Y-site:** ciprofloxacin.
• **Additive:** metoclopramide.

Rate of Administration

• **Intermittent Infusion:** Infuse at a rate not to exceed 20 mEq/hr.

≋ CLINICAL PRECAUTIONS

• Assess patient for signs and symptoms of hypokalemia (weakness, fatigue, U wave on ECG, arrhythmias, polyuria, polydipsia) and hyperkalemia (fatigue, muscle weakness, paresthesia, confusion, dyspnea, peaked T waves, depressed ST segments, prolonged QT segments, widened QRS complexes, loss of P waves, and cardiac arrhythmias).

- Following administration of the initial 40–60 mEq, the need for further potassium should be based on serum potassium determination.
- Concurrent use with potassium-sparing diuretics or angiotensin-converting enzyme inhibitors may lead to hyperkalemia.
- Geriatric patients may require less potassium due to age-related renal impairment.
- Use potassium acetate cautiously in patients with cardiovascular disease or renal impairment. Geriatric patients may require less potassium because of age-related renal impairment.
- Safe use in pregnancy or lactation has not been established. Electrolyte abnormalities should be avoided and, if they occur, treated efficiently.

Toxicity and Overdose Alert

• Symptoms of toxicity are those of hyperkalemia (fatigue, muscle weakness, paresthesia, confusion, dyspnea, peaked T waves, depressed ST segments, prolonged QT segments, widened QRS complexes, loss of P waves, and cardiac arrhythmias). • Treatment includes discontinuation of potassium, administration of sodium bicarbonate to correct acidosis, dextrose and insulin to facilitate passage of potassium into cells, calcium salts to reverse ECG effects (in patients who are not receiving cardiac glycosides), sodium polystyrene used as an exchange resin, and/or dialysis in patients with impaired renal function.

Lab Test Considerations

• Monitor serum potassium levels prior to and periodically throughout therapy. • Monitor renal function, serum bicarbonate, and pH. • Serum magnesium level should be determined in refractory hypokalemia; hypomagnesemia should be corrected to facilitate effectiveness of potassium replacement. • Monitor serum chloride levels; hypochloremia may occur when chloride is not replaced concurrently with potassium.

Patient/Family Teaching

• Advise patient regarding sources of dietary potassium (see Appendix H). Encourage compliance with recommended diet. Instruct patient to avoid salt substitutes unless approved by physician. • Instruct patient to report dark, tarry, or bloody stools; weakness; unusual fatigue; or tingling of extremities promptly. Physician should be notified if nausea, vomiting, diarrhea, or stomach discomfort persists. Dosage may require adjustment. • Emphasize the importance of regular follow-up examinations to monitor serum levels and progress.

PHARMACOLOGIC PROFILE

Indications

• Potassium acetate is used in the treatment or prevention of potassium depletion in patients who are unable to ingest adequate dietary potassium. It is especially useful in patients whose needs are not met by standard fluid and electrolyte preparations.

Action

• Potassium maintains the following cell characteristics: acid-base balance, isotonicity, and electrophysiology. • It serves as an activator in many enzymatic reactions and is essential to many processes, including transmission of nerve impulses; contraction of cardiac, skeletal, and smooth muscle; gastric secretion; renal function; tissue synthesis; and carbohydrate metabolism.

Time/Action Profile (increase in serum potassium levels)

Onset	Peak	Duration
rapid	UK	UK

Pharmacokinetics

• **Distribution:** Potassium enters extracellular fluid and is then actively transported into cells. • **Metabolism and Excretion:** Potassium is excreted by the kidneys. • **Half-life:** UK.

Contraindications

• Potassium acetate is contraindicated in patients with hyperkalemia, severe renal impairment, untreated Addison's disease, severe tissue trauma, acute dehydration, or hyperkalemic familial periodic paralysis.

Adverse Reactions and Side Effects*

• **CNS:** paresthesias, restlessness, confusion, weakness, paralysis • **CV:** <u>arrhythmias</u>, <u>ECG changes</u> (prolonged PR interval, ST-segment depression, tall-tented T waves) • **F and E:** hyperkalemia • **Local:** irritation at IV site.

Potassium Chloride	Potassium supplement
	pH 4–8
	13.4 mEq K/g

≋ ADMINISTRATION CONSIDERATIONS

Usual Dose

ADULTS: 10–20 mEq/hr (not to exceed 400 mEq/day or 3 mEq/kg/day). *If serum potassium is >2.5 mEq/liter,* up to 200 mEq/day may be given. *If serum potassium is <2.0 mEq/liter* and is accompanied by ECG changes or paralysis, urgent treatment may consist of up to 400 mEq/day. In extreme circumstances, higher doses or infusion rates may be needed.

INFANTS AND CHILDREN: 2–3 mEq/kg/day or 40 mEq/m^2.

Dilution

• **Intermittent/Continuous Infusion:** Do not administer undiluted. Each single dose must be **diluted** and thoroughly mixed in 100–1000 ml of dextrose, saline, Ringer's solution, lactated Ringer's solution, dextrose/saline, dextrose/Ringer's solution, or dextrose/lactated Ringer's solution combinations. Vials of concentrated potassium chloride for injection can be identified by black caps and overseals with the words *"Must be diluted"* printed in a contrasting color. Solu-

---

*<u>Underlines</u> indicate most frequent; CAPITALS indicate life-threatening.

tions are also commercially available premixed with many of the above IV solutions. • Concentration is usually limited to 40 mEq/liter of IV solution. In severe hypokalemia, solution may be as concentrated as 80 mEq/liter.

Compatibility

• **Y-site:** acyclovir • allopurinol sodium • aminophylline • ampicillin • amrinone • atropine • betamethasone • calcium gluconate • cephalothin • cephapirin • chlordiazepoxide • chlorpromazine • ciprofloxacin • cyanocobalamin • dexamethasone • digoxin • diltiazem • diphenhydramine • dobutamine • dopamine • droperidol • droperidol/fentanyl • edrophonium • enalaprilat • epinephrine • esmolol • conjugated estrogens • ethacrynate sodium • famotidine • fentanyl • filgrastim • fludarabine • fluorouracil • furosemide • gallium nitrate • hydralazine • idarubicin • indomethacin • insulin • isoproterenol • kanamycin • labetalol • lidocaine • magnesium sulfate • melphalan • menadiol • meperidine • methicillin • methoxamine • methylergonovine • minocycline • morphine • neostigmine • norepinephrine • ondansetron • oxacillin • oxytocin • paclitaxel • penicillin G potassium • pentazocine • phytonadione • piperacillin/tazobactam • prednisolone • procainamide • prochlorperazine • propranolol • pyridostigmine • sargramostim • scopolamine • sodium bicarbonate • succinylcholine • tacrolimus • trimethaphan • trimethobenzamide • vinorelbine • zidovudine.

• **Additive:** aminophylline • atracurium • bretylium • calcium gluconate • cephalothin • cephapirin • chloramphenicol • cimetidine • clindamycin • corticotropin • cytarabine • dimenhydrinate • dopamine • enalaprilat • erythromycin glucepate • erythromycin lactobionate • fluconazole • furosemide • heparin • hydrocortisone sodium succinate • isoproterenol • lidocaine • metaraminol • methicillin • methyldopa • methylprednisolone sodium succinate • metoclopramide • mitoxantrone • nafcillin • netilmicin • oxacillin • penicillin G potassium • phenylephrine • piperacillin • ranitidine • sodium bicarbonate • thiopental • vancomycin • verapamil • vitamin B complex with C.

Incompatibility

• **Y-site:** diazepam • ergotamine tartrate • phenytoin.
• **Additive:** amphotericin B.

Rate of Administration

• **Intermittent Infusion:** Infuse at a rate of 10–20 mEq/hr. As much as 40 mEq/hr has been used in emergency situations. For infants and children, the infusion rate should be 0.5–1 mEq/kg/hr.

≋ CLINICAL PRECAUTIONS

• Assess patient for signs and symptoms of hypokalemia (weakness, fatigue, U wave on ECG, arrhythmias, polyuria, polydipsia) and hyperkalemia (fatigue, muscle weakness, paresthesia, confusion, dyspnea, peaked T waves, depressed ST segments, prolonged QT segments, widened QRS complexes, loss of P waves, and cardiac arrhythmias).

• After administration of the initial 40–60 mg, the need for further potassium should be based on serum potassium determination.

• Concurrent use with potassium-sparing diuretics or angiotensin-converting enzyme inhibitors may lead to hyperkalemia.

• Use potassium chloride cautiously in patients with cardiovascular disease or renal impairment. Geriatric patients may require less potassium due to age-related renal impairment.

• Safe use in pregnancy or lactation has not been established (Pregnancy Category C). Electrolyte abnormalities should be avoided and, if they occur, treated efficiently.

Toxicity and Overdose Alert

• Symptoms of toxicity are those of hyperkalemia (fatigue, muscle weakness, paresthesia, confusion, dyspnea, peaked T waves, depressed ST segments, prolonged QT segments, widened QRS complexes, loss of P waves, and cardiac arrhythmias). • Treatment includes discontinuation of potassium, administration of sodium bicarbonate to correct acidosis, dextrose and insulin to facilitate passage of potassium into cells, calcium salts to reverse ECG effects (in patients who are not receiving cardiac glycosides), sodium polystyrene used as an exchange resin, and/or dialysis in patients with impaired renal function.

Lab Test Considerations

• Monitor serum potassium levels prior to and periodically throughout therapy. • Monitor renal function, serum bicarbonate, and pH. • Serum magnesium level should be determined in refractory hypokalemia; hypomagnesemia should be corrected to facilitate effectiveness of potassium replacement. • Monitor serum chloride levels; hypochloremia may occur when chloride is not replaced concurrently with potassium.

Patient/Family Teaching

• Advise patient regarding sources of dietary potassium (see Appendix H). Encourage compliance with recommended diet. Instruct patient to avoid salt substitutes unless approved by physician. • Instruct patient to promptly report dark, tarry, or bloody stools; weakness; unusual fatigue; or tingling of extremities. Physician should be notified if nausea, vomiting, diarrhea, or stomach discomfort persists. Dosage may require adjustment. • Emphasize the importance of regular follow-up examinations to monitor serum levels and progress.

 PHARMACOLOGIC PROFILE

Indications

• Potassium chloride is used in the treatment or prevention of potassium depletion in patients who are unable to ingest adequate dietary potassium.

Action

• Potassium maintains the following cell characteristics: acid-base balance, isotonicity, and electrophysiology. • It serves as an activator in many enzymatic reactions and is essential to many processes, including transmission of nerve impulses; contraction of cardiac, skeletal, and smooth muscle; gastric secretion; renal function; tissue synthesis; and carbohydrate metabolism.

Time/Action Profile

Onset	Peak	Duration
rapid	UK	UK

Pharmacokinetics

• **Distribution:** Potassium enters extracellular fluid and is then actively transported into cells. • **Metabolism and Excretion:** Potassium is excreted by the kidneys. • **Half-life:** UK.

Contraindications

• Potassium chloride is contraindicated in patients with hyperkalemia, severe renal impairment, untreated Addison's disease, severe tissue trauma, acute dehydration, or hyperkalemic familial periodic paralysis.

Adverse Reactions and Side Effects*

• **CNS:** paresthesias, restlessness, confusion, weakness, paralysis • **CV:** <u>arrhythmias</u>, <u>ECG changes</u> (prolonged PR interval, ST-segment depression, tall-tented T waves) • **F and E:** hyperkalemia • **Local:** irritation at IV site.

Potassium Phosphate(s)	Electrolyte (potassium, phosphate replacement)
	pH 7–7.8 93 mg phosphorus (3 millimoles)/ml 4.4 mEq K/ml

☰ ADMINISTRATION CONSIDERATIONS

Usual Dose

ADULTS: 10–15 mmol phosphorus/day as an infusion.
INFANTS: 1.5–2 mmol/kg phosphorus/day as an infusion.

Dilution

• **Continuous Infusion: Dilute** to a concentration no greater than 160 mEq/liter with 0.45% NaCl, 0.9% NaCl, D5W, D10W, D5/0.45% NaCl, D5/0.9% NaCl, or TPN solutions. • Administer only in dilute concentration. Potassium

---

*<u>Underlines</u> indicate most frequent; CAPITALS indicate life-threatening.

phosphate is a common component of total parenteral nutrition. • Injection is a mixture of dibasic and monobasic potassium phosphate.

Compatibility

• **Y-site:** ciprofloxacin • diltiazem • enalaprilat • esmolol • famotidine • labetalol.

• **Additive:** magnesium sulfate • metoclopramide • verapamil.

Incompatibility

• **Additive:** dobutamine.

• **Solution:** Ringer's or lactated Ringer's solution • D10/0.9% NaCl • D5/LR.

Rate of Administration

• **Continuous Infusion:** Infuse as a continuous infusion at a slow rate.

☰ CLINICAL PRECAUTIONS

- Assess patient for signs and symptoms of hypokalemia (weakness, fatigue, arrhythmias, presence of U waves on ECG, polyuria, polydipsia) and hypophosphatemia (anorexia, weakness, decreased reflexes, bone pain, confusion, blood dyscrasias) throughout course of therapy.
- Monitor pulse, blood pressure, and ECG prior to and periodically throughout IV therapy. Monitor intake and output ratios and daily weights.
- Concurrent use of potassium-sparing diuretics or angiotensin-converting enzyme inhibitors may result in hyperkalemia.
- Use cautiously in patients with hyperparathyroidism, cardiac disease, or renal impairment.
- Safe use in pregnancy or lactation has not been established. Electrolyte abnormalities should be avoided and, if they occur, treated efficiently.

Toxicity and Overdose Alert

• Symptoms of toxicity are those of hyperkalemia (fatigue, muscle weakness, paresthesia, confusion, dyspnea, peaked T waves, depressed ST segments, prolonged QT segments, widened QRS complexes, loss of P waves, and

cardiac arrhythmias) and hyperphosphatemia or hypocalcemia (paresthesia, muscle twitching, laryngospasm, colic, cardiac arrhythmias, or Chvostek's or Trousseau's sign).
• Treatment includes discontinuation of infusion; calcium replacement; and lowering serum potassium (dextrose and insulin to facilitate passage of potassium into cells, sodium polystyrene as an exchange resin, and/or dialysis in patients with impaired renal function).

Lab Test Considerations

• Monitor serum phosphate, potassium, and calcium levels prior to and periodically throughout therapy. Increased phosphate may cause hypocalcemia. • Monitor renal function studies prior to and periodically throughout course of therapy.

Patient/Family Teaching

• Instruct the patient to report diarrhea, weakness, fatigue, muscle cramps, or tremors promptly.

≋ PHARMACOLOGIC PROFILE

Indications

• Potassium phosphates are used in the treatment and prevention of phosphate depletion in patients who are unable to ingest adequate dietary potassium. Phosphate salts of potassium may be used in hypokalemic patients with metabolic acidosis or coexisting phosphorus deficiency.

Action

• Phosphate is present in bone and is involved in energy transfer and carbohydrate metabolism. It serves as a buffer for the excretion of hydrogen ions by the kidney.

Time/Action Profile (effects on serum phosphate level)

Onset	Peak	Duration
rapid	end of infusion	UK (minutes–hours)

Pharmacokinetics

• **Distribution:** Phosphates enter extracellular fluids and are then actively transported to sites of action. • **Metabolism**

and Excretion: More than 90% excretion is renal. • **Half-life:** UK.

Contraindications

• Potassium phosphates are contraindicated in patients with hyperkalemia, hyperphosphatemia, hypocalcemia, severe renal impairment, untreated Addison's disease, severe tissue trauma, or hyperkalemic familial periodic paralysis.

Adverse Reactions and Side Effects*

These are related to hyperphosphatemia, unless indicated.

• **CNS:** listlessness, confusion, weakness • **CV:** ARRHYTHMIAS, ECG changes (absent P waves, widening of the QRS complex with biphasic curve), CARDIAC ARREST, hypotension, hyperkalemia—ARRHYTHMIAS, ECG changes (prolonged PR interval, ST-segment depression, tall-tented T waves) • **F and E:** hypomagnesemia, hyperphosphatemia, hyperkalemia, hypocalcemia • **Local:** phlebitis, irritation at IV site • **MS:** hyperkalemia—muscle cramps; hypercalcemia—tremors • **Neuro:** paresthesias of extremities, flaccid paralysis, heaviness of legs.

Pralidoxime Chloride	*Antidote* (anticholinesterase poisoning)
Protopam	pH 3.5–4.5 (upon reconstitution)

ADMINISTRATION CONSIDERATIONS

Usual Dose

Organophosphate Poisoning

ADULTS: 1–2 g; may be repeated in 1 hr if muscle paralysis is still present, or as a continuous IV infusion at 500 mg/hr. If exposure continues, additional doses may be given q 3–8 hr. Atropine 2–6 mg IV or IM is given concurrently q 5–60 min.

---

*Underlines indicate most frequent; CAPITALS indicate life-threatening.

CHILDREN: 20–40 mg/kg; may be repeated in 1 hr if muscle paralysis is still present or as a continuous infusion at 10–20 mg/kg/hr. If exposure continues, additional doses may be given q 3–8 hr. Atropine 50–100 mcg (0.05–0.1 mg)/kg is given concurrently q 5–10 min.

Anticholinesterase Overdose
ADULTS: 1 g, followed by 250-mg increments q 5 min as needed.

Dilution
• **Reconstitute** vial containing 1 g of powdered pralidoxime with 20 ml of sterile water for injection. • **Direct IV:** May be administered **undiluted** (50 mg/ml) in patients who cannot tolerate IV infusion (for example, pulmonary edema). • **Intermittent Infusion: Further dilute** in 100 ml of 0.9% NaCl.

Rate of Administration
• **Direct IV:** Administer over at least 5 minutes. • **Intermittent Infusion:** Infuse over 15–30 minutes in adults and over 30 minutes in children.

≋ CLINICAL PRECAUTIONS

- Determine insecticide to which patient was exposed and time of exposure. Therapy should begin as soon as possible, within 24 hours of exposure. Contact a poison control center for complete information on the specific insecticide.
- Monitor neuromuscular status prior to and periodically throughout therapy. Document skeletal muscle strength, tidal volume, and vital capacity. Note presence of nicotinic effects of anticholinesterases (twitching, muscle cramps, fasciculations, weakness, pallor, tachycardia, increased blood pressure).
- Closely monitor respirations, pulse, and blood pressure. Rapid IV infusion rate may cause tachycardia, laryngospasm, muscle rigidity, and hypertension. If hypertension occurs, infusion rate may be decreased or infusion discontinued. Phentolamine may be required to control blood pressure.
- Concurrent atropine and supportive measures (suction-

ing, intubation, and ventilation) may be ordered. Atropine 2–6 mg IV in adults (50–100 mcg/kg in children) is given concurrently. If patient is cyanotic, give atropine IM while improving ventilatory status. Atropine is repeated every 5–60 minutes until toxicity is encountered and is then continued for at least 48 hours. Atropine is used to reverse muscarinic effects (bronchoconstriction, dyspnea, cough, increased bronchial secretions, nausea, vomiting, abdominal cramps, diarrhea, increased sweating, salivation, lacrimation, bradycardia, decreased blood pressure, miosis, blurred vision, urinary frequency, incontinence) of anticholinesterases. Pralidoxime is effective only against nicotinic effects. Dosage may need to be repeated every 3–8 hours if the insecticide was ingested; absorption from bowel may continue.

- If dermal exposure to insecticide has occurred, remove clothing and thoroughly wash hair and skin in sodium bicarbonate or alcohol as soon as possible. Health care workers should wear gloves to prevent self-exposure. Carefully dispose of clothing to prevent contamination of others.
- Avoid concurrent use with succinylcholine, morphine, aminophylline, theophylline, reserpine, and respiratory depressants including barbiturates, opioid analgesics, and sedative/hypnotics in patients with anticholinesterase poisoning.
- Use pralidoxime cautiously in patients with myasthenia gravis, as it may precipitate myasthenic crisis. Dosage reduction is required in patients with renal impairment.
- Efficacy in carbamate insecticide poisoning is not known and may increase toxicity.
- Safe use in pregnancy or lactation has not been established (Pregnancy Category C).

Lab Test Considerations

- May cause elevated AST (SGOT), ALT (SGPT), and CPK levels. These usually return to normal in 2 weeks.

Patient/Family Teaching

- Explain purpose of medication to patient.

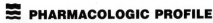

PHARMACOLOGIC PROFILE

Indications
* Pralidoxime is used in the early (first 24–36 hours) treatment of organophosphate anticholinesterase insecticide poisoning, usually with atropine and supportive measures, including mechanical ventilation. It is also used in the management of anticholinesterase (neostigmine, pyridostigmine, ambenonium, or nerve gas) overdosage.

Action
* Pralidoxime reactivates cholinesterase following poisoning with anticholinesterase agents, reversing muscle paralysis following organophosphate poisoning. * It may also directly inactivate organophosphates.

Time/Action Profile (plasma levels)

Onset	Peak	Duration
UK	5–15 min	UK

Pharmacokinetics
* **Distribution:** Pralidoxime is widely distributed throughout extracellular water. It does not appear to enter the CNS. * **Metabolism and Excretion:** 80–90% is excreted unchanged by the kidneys. * **Half-life:** 0.8–2.7 hours.

Contraindications
* Pralidoxime is contraindicated in patients with hypersensitivity to it.

Adverse Reactions and Side Effects*
* **CNS:** dizziness, headache, drowsiness * **EENT:** diplopia, blurred vision, impaired accommodation * **Resp:** hyperventilation, LARYNGOSPASM * **CV:** tachycardia * **GI:** nausea * **Derm:** rash * **MS:** muscle weakness, muscle rigidity, neuromuscular blockade.

---

*Underlines indicate most frequent; CAPITALS indicate life-threatening.

Prednisolone Sodium Phosphate	*Glucocorticoid* *(intermediate acting)*
Hydeltrasol, Key-Pred SP, Predate S, Predicort-RP	pH 7–8

≋ ADMINISTRATION CONSIDERATIONS

Usual Dose

ADULTS: 4–60 mg/day in divided doses q 4–6 hr (up to 400 mg/day).

CHILDREN: *Adrenocortical insufficiency*—140 mcg (0.14 mg)/kg/day or 4 mg/m^2/day in 3 divided doses q third day; or 46–70 mcg (0.046–0.07 mg)/kg/day or 1.33–2 mg/m^2/day as a single dose.

Dilution

• **Direct IV:** Prednisolone sodium phosphate IV may be administered **undiluted** by direct IV push. • Solution is clear and colorless to slightly yellow. • Do not use the acetate or suspension forms of this drug for IV administration. • **Intermittent Infusion:** May be added to 50–1000 ml of D5W or 0.9% NaCl. • Stable for 24 hours.

Compatibility

• **Y-site:** potassium chloride ◆ vitamin B complex with C.

• **Additive:** ascorbic acid ◆ cephalothin ◆ cytarabine ◆ erythromycin lactobionate ◆ fluorouracil ◆ heparin ◆ methicillin ◆ penicillin G potassium ◆ penicillin G sodium ◆ vitamin B complex with C.

Incompatibility

• **Y-site:** calcium gluconate ◆ dimenhydrinate ◆ prochlorperazine edisylate ◆ promazine ◆ promethazine.

• **Additive:** calcium gluceptate ◆ metaraminol ◆ methotrexate ◆ polymyxin B sulfate.

Rate of Administration

• **Direct IV:** Prednisolone sodium phosphate IV may be administered direct IV push at a rate of no more than 10 mg/min. • **Intermittent Infusion:** Administer infusions at prescribed rate.

☰ CLINICAL PRECAUTIONS

- Prednisolone is indicated for many conditions. Assess involved systems prior to and periodically throughout course of therapy.
- Assess patient for signs of adrenal insufficiency (hypotension, weight loss, weakness, nausea, vomiting, anorexia, lethargy, confusion, restlessness) prior to and periodically throughout prolonged courses of therapy.
- Monitor intake and output ratios, and daily weights. Observe patient for the appearance of peripheral edema, steady weight gain, rales/crackles, or dyspnea.
- If dose is ordered daily or every other day, administer in the morning to coincide with the body's normal secretion of cortisol.
- Additive hypokalemia may occur with concurrent use of diuretics, amphotericin B, mezlocillin, piperacillin, or ticarcillin. Hypokalemia may increase the risk of cardiac glycoside toxicity. Prednisolone may increase the requirement for insulin or oral hypoglycemic agents and increase the risk of adverse GI effects with alcohol, aspirin, or nonsteroidal anti-inflammatory agents.
- Chronic treatment should be undertaken with caution, as it will lead to adrenal suppression. Chronic prednisolone therapy should never be abruptly discontinued. Patients receiving chronic therapy require supplemental doses during stress (surgery, infection).
- Prednisolone may mask signs of infections (fever, inflammation). Lowest possible dose for shortest period of time should be used. Geriatric patients may be especially sensitive to the effects of glucocorticoids (osteoporosis, hyperglycemia, and hypertension).
- Safe use in pregnancy or lactation has not been established. Chronic use during pregnancy may result in hypoadrenalism in the newborn.

Lab Test Considerations

- Patients on prolonged courses of therapy should routinely have hematologic values, serum electrolytes, and serum and urine glucose evaluated. Prednisolone may cause decreased WBC counts or hyperglycemia, especially in persons with diabetes. It may cause decreased serum potassium and calcium and increased serum sodium concentrations. • Promptly report presence of guaiac-positive stools. • Prednisolone may increase serum cholesterol and lipid values and may decrease serum protein-bound iodine and thyroxine concentrations. • Reactions to skin tests may be suppressed by prednisolone.

Patient/Family Teaching

• Stopping this medication suddenly after chronic use may result in adrenal insufficiency (anorexia, nausea, fatigue, weakness, hypotension, dyspnea, and hypoglycemia). Advise patient to notify physician immediately if these signs occur. This condition can be life-threatening. • Encourage patients on long-term therapy to eat a diet high in protein, calcium, and potassium and low in sodium and carbohydrates (see Appendix H for foods included). • Prednisolone causes immunosuppression and may mask symptoms of infection. Instruct patient to avoid people with known contagious illnesses and to report possible infections. • Review side effects with patient. Instruct patient to inform physician promptly if severe abdominal pain or tarry stools occur. Patient should also report unusual swelling, weight gain, tiredness, bone pain, bruising, nonhealing sores, visual disturbances, or behavior changes. • Discuss possible effects on body image. Explore coping mechanisms. • Instruct patient to inform physician if symptoms of underlying disease return or worsen. • Advise patient to always carry identification describing disease process and medication regimen in the event of an emergency in which patient cannot relate medical history. • Caution patient to avoid vaccinations without first consulting physician. • Explain need for continued medical follow-up to assess effectiveness and possible side effects of medication. Physician may order periodic lab tests and eye examinations.

☰ PHARMACOLOGIC PROFILE

Indications

• Prednisolone is used systemically in a wide variety of chronic diseases including inflammatory, allergic, hematologic, neoplastic, and autoimmune disorders. • It may be used as replacement therapy in adrenal insufficiency.

Action

- Prednisolone suppresses inflammation and the normal immune response. • It also has numerous intense metabolic effects. Adrenal function is suppressed at chronic doses of 5 mg/day or more. Prednisolone has minimal mineralocorticoid (sodium-retaining) activity.

Time/Action Profile (anti-inflammatory effects)

Onset	Peak	Duration
UK	1 hr	UK

Pharmacokinetics

- **Distribution:** Prednisolone is widely distributed. It crosses the placenta and probably enters breast milk. • **Metabolism and Excretion:** Prednisolone is mostly metabolized by the liver and other tissues. Small amounts are excreted unchanged by the kidneys. • **Half-life:** 115–212 minutes; adrenal suppression lasts 1.25–1.5 days.

Contraindications

- Prednisolone is contraindicated in patients with active untreated infections, except for some forms of meningitis. • Avoid chronic use during lactation. • Prednisolone sodium phosphate contains phenol and bisulfite. Avoid use in patients with known hypersensitivity or intolerance to these additives.

Adverse Reactions and Side Effects*

Adverse reactions occur primarily during chronic therapy.

- **CNS:** headache, restlessness, psychoses, <u>depression</u>, <u>euphoria</u>, personality changes • **EENT:** cataracts, increased intraocular pressure • **CV:** <u>hypertension</u> • **GI:** <u>nausea</u>, vomiting, <u>anorexia</u>, peptic ulceration • **Derm:** <u>decreased wound healing</u>, <u>petechiae</u>, <u>ecchymoses</u>, <u>fragility</u>, <u>hirsutism</u>, <u>acne</u> • **Endo:** <u>adrenal suppression</u>, hyperglycemia • **F and E:** hypokalemia, hypokalemic alkalosis, fluid retention (long-term high doses) • **Hemat:** thromboembolism, thrombophlebitis • **Metab:** weight loss, weight gain • **MS:** <u>muscle wasting</u>, muscle pain, aseptic necrosis of joints, <u>osteoporosis</u> • **Misc:** <u>increased susceptibility to infection</u>, <u>cushingoid appearance (moon face, buffalo hump)</u>.

---

*<u>Underlines</u> indicate most frequent; CAPITALS indicate life-threatening.

Procainamide Hydrochloride	Antiarrhythmic (group IA)
Pronestyl	pH 4–6

 ADMINISTRATION CONSIDERATIONS

Usual Dose

ADULTS: 100-mg bolus over 2 min initially; repeat q 5 min until toxicity response occurs or until a total of 1000 mg is administered, or a loading infusion of 500–600 mg. Either regimen may be followed by an infusion at 2–6 mg/min.

CHILDREN: 3–6 mg/kg (up to 100 mg) over 5 min; repeat as needed (not to exceed 500 mg/30 min). Wait 10 minutes before further dosing. May also be given as a loading infusion of 15 mg/kg over 30 min followed by continuous infusion of 20–80 mcg/kg/min (unlabeled).

INFANTS: 1 mg/kg; may repeat q 5 min (not to exceed 1015 mg/kg total or 100 mg/20 min), may be followed by continuous infusion of 20–50 mcg/kg/min (unlabeled).

Dilution

• **Direct IV:** Dilute each 100 mg with 10 ml of D5W or sterile water for injection. • **Intermittent Infusion:** Prepare IV infusion by adding 200 mg–1 g to 50–500 ml of D5W, for a concentration of 2–4 mg/ml. • Slight yellow color of solution will not alter potency; do not use when darker than light amber or if solution contains a precipitate.

Compatibility

• **Y-site:** famotidine ✦ heparin ✦ hydrocortisone sodium succinate ✦ potassium chloride ✦ ranitidine ✦ vitamin B complex with C.

• **Additive:** atracurium ✦ dobutamine ✦ lidocaine ✦ netilmicin ✦ verapamil.

Incompatibility

• **Y-site:** milrinone.
• **Additive:** esmolol ✦ ethacrynate ✦ milrinone.

Rate of Administration

• **Direct IV:** Administer at a rate not to exceed 25–50 mg/min in adults. Administer at a rate of 3–6 mg/kg over 5 minutes in children and 1 mg/kg over 5 minutes in infants. Rapid administration may cause ventricular fibrillation or asystole. • **Intermittent Infusion:** Administer initial infusion over 25–30 minutes in adults or children. • **Continuous Infusion:** Maintenance infusion should infuse at 2–6 mg/min to maintain control of arrhythmia. Use infusion pump to ensure accurate dosage (see Infusion Rate Table below).

PROCAINAMIDE INFUSION RATE TABLE

Dilution: May be prepared as 1000 mg/500 ml = 2 mg/ml.
Loading dose: 50–100 mg q 5 min until arrhythmia is controlled, adverse reaction occurs, or 1000 mg has been given, *or* 500–600 mg given as a loading infusion over 25–30 min.

Dose (mg/min)	Dose (ml/hr)
PROCAINAMIDE (Pronestyl) INFUSION RATES (ml/hr) *CONCENTRATION = 2 mg/ml*	
1 mg/min	30 ml/hr
2 mg/min	60 ml/hr
3 mg/min	90 ml/hr
4 mg/min	120 ml/hr
5 mg/min	150 ml/hr
6 mg/min	180 ml/hr

≋ CLINICAL PRECAUTIONS

- Monitor ECG, pulse, and blood pressure continuously throughout administration. IV administration is usually discontinued if any of the following occurs: arrhythmia is resolved, QRS complex widens by 50%, PR interval is prolonged, blood pressure drops >15 mm Hg, or toxic side effects develop. Patient should remain supine throughout administration to minimize hypotension. Elderly patients are more prone to hypotensive reactions.
- When converting from IV to oral dose regimen, allow 3–4 hours to elapse between last IV dose and administration of first oral dose.
- Use cautiously in patients with myocardial infarction, cardiac glycoside toxicity, or congestive heart failure. Dosage reduction may be necessary in patients with congestive heart failure and renal or hepatic insufficiency.

- Procainamide may have additive or antagonistic effects with other antiarrhythmics. Additive neurologic toxicity, confusion, or seizures may occur with concurrent use of lidocaine. Antihypertensives and nitrates may potentiate hypotensive effects of procainamide. Procainamide potentiates neuromuscular blocking agents and may partially antagonize the therapeutic effects of anticholinesterase agents in myasthenia gravis. Additive anticholinergic effects may occur with other drugs possessing anticholinergic properties, including antihistamines, antidepressants, atropine, haloperidol, and phenothiazines.
- Safe use in pregnancy, lactation, or children has not been established (Pregnancy Category C).

Toxicity and Overdose Alert

- Serum procainamide and N-acetylprocainamide (NAPA) levels may be monitored periodically during dosage adjustment. Therapeutic blood level of procainamide is 4–10 mg/liter and NAPA is 10–30 mg/liter. Toxicity may occur when the summed concentration of procainamide and NAPA exceeds 25–30 mg/liter. • Signs of toxicity include confusion, dizziness, drowsiness, decreased urination, nausea, vomiting, and tachyarrhythmias.

Lab Test Considerations

- CBC should be monitored every 2 weeks during the first 3 months of therapy. Procainamide rarely causes decreased leukocyte, neutrophil, and platelet counts. Therapy may be discontinued if leukopenia occurs. • Antinuclear antibody (ANA) should be periodically monitored during prolonged therapy or if symptoms of lupuslike reaction occur. Therapy is discontinued if a steady increase in ANA titer occurs. • Procainamide may cause an increase in AST (SGOT), ALT (SGPT), alkaline phosphatase, LDH, and bilirubin, and a positive Coombs' test result.

Patient/Family Teaching

- Procainamide may cause dizziness. Caution patient to avoid activities requiring alertness until response to medication is known. • Advise patient to notify physician immediately if signs of drug-induced lupus syndrome (fever, chills, joint pain or swelling, pain with breathing, skin rash), leukopenia (sore throat, mouth, or gums), or thrombocytopenia (unusual bleeding or bruising) occur. Medication may be discontinued if these occur. • Advise patient to carry identification describing disease process and medication regimen at all times. • Emphasize the importance of routine follow-up examinations to monitor progress.

≋ PHARMACOLOGIC PROFILE

Indications

• Procainamide is used in the treatment of a wide variety of ventricular and atrial arrhythmias, including atrial premature contractions, premature ventricular contractions, ventricular tachycardia, and paroxysmal atrial tachycardia. • It is also used to maintain normal sinus rhythm after conversion from atrial fibrillation or flutter.

Action

• Procainamide decreases myocardial excitability, slows conduction velocity, and may depress myocardial contractility.

Time/Action Profile (anti-arrhythmic effects)

Onset	Peak	Duration
immediate	25–60 min	3–4 hr

Pharmacokinetics

• **Distribution:** Procainamide is rapidly and widely distributed. Procainamide and its active metabolite cross the placenta and enter breast milk. • **Metabolism and Excretion:** Procainamide is converted by the liver to NAPA, an active antiarrhythmic compound. The remainder (40–70%) is excreted unchanged by the kidneys. • **Half-life:** 2.5–4.7 hours (NAPA 5–7 hours), prolonged in renal impairment.

Contraindications

• Procainamide is contraindicated in patients with hypersensitivity to it, and in patients with AV block or myasthenia gravis. • Products containing parabens, benzyl alcohol, or bisulfites should not be given to patients with known intolerance or hypersensitivity.

Adverse Reactions and Side Effects*

• **CNS:** confusion, seizures, dizziness • **CV:** hypotension, ventricular arrhythmias, asystole, heart block • **GI:** nausea, vomiting, bitter taste • **Derm:** rashes • **Hemat:** leukopenia, thrombocytopenia, agranulocytosis, eosinophilia • **Misc:** drug-induced systemic lupus syndrome, fever, chills.

Prochlorperazine Edisylate	*Antiemetic (phenothiazine)*
Cofranzine, Compa-Z, Compazine, Ultrazine-10	pH 4.2–6.2

 ADMINISTRATION CONSIDERATIONS

Usual Dose

ADULTS: 2.5–10 mg, rate not to exceed 5 mg/min; may be repeated in 30 min; single dose not to exceed 10 mg (not to exceed 40 mg/day).

Dilution

• **Direct IV: Dilute** to a concentration of 1 mg/ml. • Slight yellow color will not alter potency. Do not administer solution that is markedly discolored or that contains a precipitate.
• **Intermittent Infusion: Dilute** 20 mg in up to 1 liter dextrose, saline, Ringer's or lactated Ringer's solution, dextrose/saline, dextrose/Ringer's, or lactated Ringer's combinations.

Compatibility

• **Syringe:** Manufacturer does not recommend mixing prochlorperazine with other medications in syringe. • Prochlorperazine has been found to be compatible in syringe for a limited period (15 minutes) with ♦ atropine ♦ butorphanol ♦ cimetidine ♦ diphenhydramine ♦ droperidol ♦ fentanyl ♦ glycopyrrolate ♦ meperidine ♦ metoclopramide ♦ nalbuphine ♦ pentazocine ♦ ranitidine ♦ scopolamine.
• **Y-site:** cisplatin ♦ cyclophosphamide ♦ cytarabine

---

*Underlines indicate most frequent; CAPITALS indicate life-threatening.

✦ doxorubicin ✦ fluconazole ✦ fludarabine ✦ heparin ✦ hydrocortisone sodium succinate ✦ melphalan ✦ methotrexate ✦ paclitaxel ✦ ondansetron ✦ potassium chloride ✦ sargramostim ✦ vinorelbine ✦ vitamin B complex with C.

● **Additive:** amikacin ✦ ascorbic acid ✦ dexamethasone sodium phosphate ✦ dimenhydrinate ✦ erythromycin lactobionate ✦ ethacrynate sodium ✦ lidocaine ✦ nafcillin ✦ sodium bicarbonate ✦ vitamin B complex with C.

Incompatibility

● **Syringe:** dimenhydrinate ✦ ketorolac ✦ midazolam ✦ morphine ✦ pentobarbital ✦ thiopental.

● **Y-site:** allopurinol sodium ✦ aminophylline ✦ chloramphenicol ✦ dexamethasone sodium phosphate ✦ dimenhydrinate ✦ fludarabine ✦ filgrastim ✦ foscarnet ✦ gallium nitrate ✦ heparin ✦ methicillin ✦ penicillin G potassium ✦ phenobarbital ✦ phenytoin ✦ piperacillin/tazobactam ✦ prednisolone sodium phosphate.

● **Additive:** aminophylline ✦ amphotericin B ✦ ampicillin ✦ calcium gluceptate ✦ cephalothin ✦ chloramphenicol ✦ chlorothiazide ✦ furosemide ✦ hydrocortisone sodium succinate ✦ methohexital ✦ penicillin G sodium ✦ phenobarbital ✦ thiopental.

Rate of Administration

● **Direct IV:** Administer no faster than 5 mg/min.

≋ CLINICAL PRECAUTIONS

● To prevent contact dermatitis, avoid getting solution on hands.

● The Canadian product is a different salt form {prochlorperazine mesylate} ({PMS Prochlorperazine}, {Stemetil}).

● Assess patient for nausea and vomiting prior to and 30–60 minutes following administration. Assess fluid, electrolyte, and nutritional status and replace as needed.

● Monitor blood pressure (sitting, standing, lying), pulse, respiratory rate, and level of sedation prior to and frequently during administration. Prochlorperazine may cause Q-wave and T-wave changes in ECG. Additive hypotension may occur with antihypertensive agents, nitrates, or acute ingestion of alcohol.

{} = Available in Canada only.

- Monitor patient for onset of extrapyramidal side effects (akathisia—restlessness; dystonia—muscle spasms and twisting motions; pseudoparkinsonism—mask facies, rigidity, tremors, drooling, shuffling gait, dysphagia). If these symptoms occur, a reduction in dosage or discontinuation of medication may be necessary. Antiparkinsonian agents (trihexyphenidyl, benztropine) or diphenhydramine may be used to control these symptoms.
- Monitor for tardive dyskinesia (rhythmic movement of mouth, face, and extremities). These side effects may be irreversible.
- Monitor for development of neuroleptic malignant syndrome (fever, respiratory distress, tachycardia, convulsions, diaphoresis, hypertension or hypotension, pallor, tiredness).
- Use prochlorperazine cautiously in elderly or debilitated patients. Dosage reduction is recommended in this population. Geriatric patients may be more sensitive to the effects of prochlorperazine.
- Use cautiously in patients with diabetes mellitus, respiratory disease, prostatic hypertrophy, CNS tumors, epilepsy, or intestinal obstruction.
- Phenothiazines should be discontinued 48 hours before metrizamide myelography, and not resumed for 24 hours thereafter, as they lower seizure threshold.
- Additive CNS depression may occur with concurrent use of other CNS depressants, including alcohol, antidepressants, antihistamines, opioid analgesics, sedative/hypnotics, or general anesthetics. Additive anticholinergic effects may occur with other drugs possessing anticholinergic properties, including antihistamines, antidepressants, atropine, haloperidol, and other phenothiazines. Lithium increases the risk of extrapyramidal reactions from prochlorperazine, while early signs of lithium toxicity may be masked. The risk of agranulocytosis is increased by concurrent use of antithyroid agents. Prochlorperazine decreases the beneficial effects of levodopa.
- Safe use in pregnancy or lactation has not been established; prochlorperazine may cause jaundice, hyporeflexia or hyperreflexia, drowsiness, or extrapyramidal reactions in newborns. Children under 2 years should not be given prochlorperazine.

Lab Test Considerations

• CBC and liver function tests should be evaluated periodically throughout course of therapy. • Prochlorperazine may cause false-positive or false-negative pregnancy tests and false-positive urine bilirubin test results. It may also cause increased serum prolactin levels and interfere with gonadorelin test results.

Patient/Family Teaching

• Inform patient of possibility of extrapyramidal symptoms and tardive dyskinesia. Caution patient to report these symptoms immediately to physician. • Advise patient to make position changes slowly to minimize orthostatic hypotension. • Medication may cause drowsiness. Caution patient to avoid driving or other activities requiring alertness until response to medication is known. • Instruct patient to use frequent mouth rinses, good oral hygiene, and sugarless gum or candy to minimize dry mouth. • Caution patient to use sunscreen and protective clothing to prevent photosensitivity. • Inform patient that this medication may turn urine pink to reddish-brown. • Instruct patient to notify physician promptly if sore throat, fever, unusual bleeding or bruising, skin rashes, weakness, tremors, visual disturbances, dark-colored urine, or clay-colored stools are noted.

 PHARMACOLOGIC PROFILE

Indications

• Prochlorperazine is used in the management of severe nausea, vomiting, and anxiety.

Action

• Prochlorperazine alters the effects of dopamine in the CNS. It also possesses significant anticholinergic and alpha-adrenergic blocking activity and depresses the chemoreceptor trigger zone in the CNS.

Time/Action Profile (antiemetic effect)

Onset	Peak	Duration
rapid (minutes)	UK	3–4 hr

Pharmacokinetics

• **Distribution:** Prochlorperazine is widely distributed, achieving high concentrations in the CNS. It crosses the placenta and probably enters breast milk. • **Metabolism and Excretion:** Prochlorperazine is highly metabolized by the liver and GI mucosa. • **Half-life:** UK.

Contraindications

• Prochlorperazine is contraindicated in patients with hypersensitivity to it. Cross-sensitivity with other phenothiazines may exist. • Patients with known hypersensitivity or intolerance to bisulfites or benzyl alcohol should not receive IV prochlorperazine. • Prochlorperazine should not be given to patients with narrow-angle glaucoma, bone marrow depression, or severe liver or cardiovascular disease.

Adverse Reactions and Side Effects*

• **CNS:** sedation, <u>extrapyramidal reactions</u>, tardive dyskinesia, NEUROLEPTIC MALIGNANT SYNDROME • **EENT:** <u>dry eyes</u>, <u>blurred vision</u>, lens opacities • **CV:** hypotension, tachycardia, ECG changes • **GI:** <u>constipation</u>, <u>dry mouth</u>, ileus, anorexia, hepatitis • **GU:** urinary retention, pink or reddish-brown discoloration of urine • **Derm:** rashes, photosensitivity, pigment changes • **Endo:** galactorrhea • **Hemat:** AGRANULOCYTOSIS, leukopenia • **Metab:** hyperthermia • **Misc:** allergic reactions.

Promazine Hydrochloride	Antipsychotic (phenothiazine)
Primazine, Prozine-50, Sparine	pH 4–5.5

 ADMINISTRATION CONSIDERATIONS

Usual Dose

ADULTS: 50–150 mg initially; if required, additional doses may be given after 30 min, up to a total initial dose of 300

---

*<u>Underlines</u> indicate most frequent; CAPITALS indicate life-threatening.

mg. Initial dose in inebriated patients should not exceed 50 mg. Total daily dose should not exceed 1000 mg/day.

Dilution

• **Direct IV:** Use a concentration of 25 mg/ml or less.
• Slight yellow color will not alter potency. Do not administer solution that is markedly discolored or that contains a precipitate.

Compatibility

• **Syringe:** atropine ✦ cimetidine ✦ diphenhydramine ✦ droperidol ✦ fentanyl ✦ glycopyrrolate ✦ hydroxyzine ✦ meperidine ✦ metoclopramide ✦ midazolam ✦ morphine ✦ pentazocine ✦ scopolamine.
• **Additive:** chloramphenicol ✦ erythromycin lactobionate ✦ ethacrynate ✦ heparin ✦ lidocaine ✦ metaraminol ✦ methyldopate.

Incompatibility

• **Syringe:** dimenhydrinate ✦ pentobarbital.
• **Y-site:** aminophylline ✦ chloramphenicol ✦ dimenhydrinate ✦ heparin ✦ hydrocortisone sodium succinate ✦ penicillin G potassium ✦ phenobarbital ✦ phenytoin ✦ prednisolone sodium phosphate.
• **Additive:** aminophylline ✦ chlorothiazide ✦ fibrinogen ✦ fibrinolysin ✦ methohexital ✦ nafcillin ✦ penicillin G potassium ✦ pentobarbital ✦ phenobarbital ✦ thiopental.

Rate of Administration

• **Direct IV:** Administer each 25 mg over at least 1 minute through IV tubing with infusion of dextrose, saline, Ringer's or lactated Ringer's solution, dextrose/saline, dextrose/Ringer's, or lactated Ringer's combinations.

≋ CLINICAL PRECAUTIONS

• To prevent contact dermatitis, avoid getting solution on hands.
• Monitor patient's mental status (orientation to reality and behavior) prior to and periodically throughout therapy. Assess patient for level of sedation following administration. Additive CNS depression may occur with concurrent use of other CNS depressants, includ-

ing alcohol, antihistamines, opioid analgesics, sedative/hypnotics, or general anesthetics.

- Monitor blood pressure (sitting, standing, lying), pulse, and respiratory rate prior to and frequently during the period of dosage adjustment. Keep patient recumbent for at least 30 minutes following injection to minimize hypotensive effects. May cause Q-wave and T-wave changes in ECG. Additive hypotension may occur with concurrent use of antihypertensive agents or nitrates, or with acute ingestion of alcohol.

- Monitor patient for onset of extrapyramidal side effects (akathisia—restlessness; dystonia—muscle spasms and twisting motions; pseudoparkinsonism—mask facies, rigidity, tremors, drooling, shuffling gait, dysphagia). If these symptoms occur, a reduction in dosage or discontinuation of medication may be necessary. Antiparkinsonian agents (trihexyphenidyl or benztropine) or diphenhydramine may be used to control these symptoms.

- Monitor for tardive dyskinesia (rhythmic movements of mouth, face, and extremities). These side effects may be irreversible.

- Monitor for development of neuroleptic malignant syndrome (fever, respiratory distress, tachycardia, convulsions, diaphoresis, hypertension or hypotension, pallor, tiredness).

- Assess fluid intake and bowel function. Increased bulk and fluids in the diet help minimize the constipating effects of this medication.

- Use promazine cautiously in patients with diabetes mellitus, respiratory disease, prostatic hypertrophy, CNS tumors, epilepsy, or intestinal obstruction. Dosage reduction may be necessary in geriatric or debilitated patients. Geriatric patients may be more sensitive to the effects of promazine.

- Phenothiazines should be discontinued 48 hours before metrizamide myelography and not resumed for 24 hours thereafter, as they lower the seizure threshold.

- Additive anticholinergic effects may occur with concurrent use of other drugs possessing anticholinergic properties, including antihistamines, antidepressants, atropine, haloperidol, and other phenothiazines. Lithium increases the risk of extrapyramidal reactions. Promazine

may mask early signs of lithium toxicity. Promazine increases the risk of agranulocytosis with antithyroid agents.
- Safe use in pregnancy or lactation has not been established. Jaundice, hyporeflexia or hyperreflexia, drowsiness, or extrapyramidal reactions may occur in neonates. Safe use in children has not been established.

Lab Test Considerations

- CBC and liver function tests should be evaluated periodically throughout course of therapy. • May cause false-positive or false-negative pregnancy test results and false-positive urine bilirubin test results. • May cause increased serum prolactin levels, thereby interfering with gonadorelin test results.

Patient/Family Teaching

- Inform patient of possibility of extrapyramidal symptoms, tardive dyskinesia, and neuroleptic malignant syndrome. Caution patient to report these symptoms immediately to physician. • Advise patient to make position changes slowly to minimize orthostatic hypotension. • Medication may cause drowsiness. Caution patient to avoid activities requiring alertness until response to medication is known. • Instruct patient to use frequent mouth rinses, good oral hygiene, and sugarless gum or candy to minimize dry mouth. • Instruct patient to notify physician promptly if sore throat, fever, unusual bleeding or bruising, skin rashes, weakness, tremors, visual disturbances, dark-colored urine, or clay-colored stools are noted. • Emphasize the importance of routine follow-up examinations to monitor response to medication and detect side effects. Periodic ocular examinations are indicated. Encourage continued participation in psychotherapy as ordered by physician.

≋ PHARMACOLOGIC PROFILE

Indications

- IV promazine is used in management of severe agitation.

Action

- Promazine alters the effects of dopamine in the CNS. It also possesses significant anticholinergic and alpha-adrenergic blocking activity.

Time/Action Profile (antipsychotic effects)

Onset	Peak	Duration
within 30 min	UK	UK

Pharmacokinetics

- **Distribution:** Promazine is widely distributed, achieving high concentrations in the CNS. It crosses the placenta and probably enters breast milk. • **Metabolism and Excretion:** Promazine is highly metabolized by the liver and GI mucosa. • **Half-life:** UK.

Contraindications

- Promazine is contraindicated in patients with hypersensitivity to it. Cross-sensitivity with other phenothiazines may exist. • Promazine should be avoided in patients with narrow-angle glaucoma, bone marrow depression, or severe liver or cardiovascular disease. • Some products contain bisulfites or formaldehyde and should be avoided in patients with known hypersensitivity or intolerance.

Adverse Reactions and Side Effects*

- **CNS:** sedation, <u>extrapyramidal reactions</u>, tardive dyskinesia, NEUROLEPTIC MALIGNANT SYNDROME • **EENT:** <u>dry eyes</u>, <u>blurred vision</u>, lens opacities • **CV:** hypotension, tachycardia, ECG changes • **GI:** <u>constipation</u>, <u>dry mouth</u>, ileus, anorexia, hepatitis • **GU:** urinary retention, pink or reddish-brown discoloration of urine • **Derm:** rashes, photosensitivity, pigment changes • **Endo:** galactorrhea • **Hemat:** AGRANULOCYTOSIS, leukopenia • **Metab:** hyperthermia • **Misc:** allergic reactions.

---

*<u>Underlines</u> indicate most frequent; CAPITALS indicate life-threatening.

Promethazine Hydrochloride	*Antihistamine, Antiemetic, Sedative/hypnotic (phenothiazine)*
Anergan, Antinaus, Pentazine, Phenazine, Phencen, Phenergan, Phenerzine, Phenoject, Pro-50, Promacot, Pro-Med 50, Promet, Prorex, Prothazine, Shogan, V-Gun	pH 4–5.5

ADMINISTRATION CONSIDERATIONS

Usual Dose

Allergic Conditions
ADULTS: 25 mg; may repeat in 2 hr.

Sedation
ADULTS: 25–50 mg.
CHILDREN: 12.5–25 mg or 0.5–1.1 mg/kg.

Sedation during Labor
ADULTS: 50 mg in early labor; 25–75 mg may be given when labor is established, and additional doses of 25–50 mg may be given 1–2 times at 4-hr intervals (24-hr dose should not exceed 100 mg).

Antiemetic
ADULTS: 12.5–25 mg q 4 hr as needed.
CHILDREN: 0.25–0.5 mg/kg 4–6 times daily.

Dilution
• **Direct IV:** Doses should not exceed a concentration of 25 mg/ml. • Slight yellow color does not alter potency. Do not use if precipitate is present.

Compatibility
• **Syringe:** atropine ◆ butorphanol ◆ cimetidine ◆ diphenhydramine ◆ droperidol ◆ fentanyl ◆ glycopyrrolate ◆ hydromorphone ◆ hydroxyzine ◆ meperidine ◆ metoclopramide ◆ midazolam ◆ pentazocine ◆ ranitidine ◆ scopolamine.

• **Y-site:** ciprofloxacin ◆ cisplatin ◆ cyclophosphamide ◆ cytarabine ◆ doxorubicin ◆ filgrastim ◆ fluconazole ◆ fludarabine ◆ ondansetron ◆ sargramostim ◆ vinorelbine ◆ vitamin B complex with C.

• **Additive:** amikacin ◆ ascorbic acid ◆ netilmicin ◆ vitamin B complex with C.

• **Solution:** dextrose ✦ saline ✦ Ringer's or lactated Ringer's solution ✦ dextrose/saline, dextrose/Ringer's, or lactated Ringer's combinations.

Incompatibility

• **Syringe:** dimenhydrinate ✦ heparin ✦ ketorolac ✦ pentobarbital ✦ thiopental.

• **Y-site:** allopurinol sodium ✦ aminophylline ✦ cefoperazone ✦ chloramphenicol ✦ dimenhydrinate ✦ foscarnet ✦ hydrocortisone sodium succinate ✦ methicillin ✦ penicillin G potassium ✦ phenobarbital ✦ phenytoin ✦ prednisolone.

• **Additive:** aminophylline ✦ chloramphenicol ✦ chlorothiazide ✦ furosemide ✦ heparin ✦ hydrocortisone sodium succinate ✦ methicillin ✦ methohexital ✦ penicillin G ✦ pentobarbital ✦ phenobarbital ✦ thiopental.

Rate of Administration

• **Direct IV:** Administer each 25 mg slowly, over at least 1 minute. Rapid administration may produce a transient fall in blood pressure.

☰ CLINICAL PRECAUTIONS

• Monitor blood pressure, pulse, and respiratory rate frequently in patients receiving IV doses.

• Assess patient for level of sedation following administration. When administering promethazine concurrently with opioid analgesics, supervise ambulation closely to prevent injury due to increased sedation. Additive CNS depression may occur with other CNS depressants, including alcohol, antianxiety agents, other antihistamines, opioid analgesics, and other sedative/hypnotics.

• Monitor patient for onset of extrapyramidal side effects (akathisia—restlessness; dystonia—muscle spasms and twisting motions; pseudoparkinsonism—mask facies, rigidity, tremors, drooling, shuffling gait, dysphagia). If these symptoms occur, antiparkinson agents (trihexyphenidyl, benztropine) or diphenhydramine may be used to treat extrapyramidal symptoms.

• When used as an antiemetic, assess patient for nausea and vomiting prior to and following administration.

- When used for allergies, assess allergic symptoms (rhinitis, conjunctivitis, hives) prior to and periodically throughout course of therapy.
- Use promethazine cautiously in patients with hypertension or sleep apnea.
- Use cautiously in geriatric, debilitated, or emaciated patients; initial dosage reduction may be necessary. Geriatric patients may be more sensitive to the effects of promethazine.
- Additive anticholinergic effects may occur with other drugs possessing anticholinergic properties, including other antihistamines, antidepressants, atropine, haloperidol, other phenothiazines, quinidine, and disopyramide.
- Although promethazine has been used safely during labor, chronic use should be avoided during pregnancy. Safe use in lactation has not been established; drowsiness may occur in the infant. Children under 2 years should not be given promethazine.

Lab Test Considerations

- Promethazine may cause false-positive or false-negative pregnancy tests. • CBC should be evaluated periodically during chronic therapy, as blood dyscrasias may occur. • Promethazine may cause increased serum glucose and may cause false-negative results in skin tests using allergenic extracts. Promethazine should be discontinued 72 hours prior to the test.

Patient/Family Teaching

- Promethazine may cause drowsiness. Caution patient to avoid driving or other activities requiring alertness until response to medication is known. • Advise patient that frequent mouth rinses, good oral hygiene, and sugarless gum or candy may decrease dry mouth. • Advise patient to make position changes slowly to minimize orthostatic hypotension. Elderly patients are at increased risk for this side effect. • Instruct patient to notify physician if sore throat, fever, jaundice, or uncontrolled movements are noted.

≋ PHARMACOLOGIC PROFILE

Indications
- Promethazine is used in the treatment of various allergic conditions, as a preoperative sedative, and in the treatment and prevention of nausea and vomiting.

Action
- Promethazine blocks the effects of histamine. It also has an inhibitory effect on the chemoreceptor trigger zone in the medulla, resulting in antiemetic properties, and alters the effects of dopamine in the CNS. • Promethazine also possesses significant anticholinergic activity. It produces CNS depression by indirectly decreasing stimulation of the CNS reticular system.

Time/Action Profile (antihistaminic effects)

Onset	Peak	Duration
3–5 min	UK	up to 12 hr

Pharmacokinetics
- **Distribution:** Promethazine is widely distributed. It crosses the blood–brain barrier and the placenta. • **Metabolism and Excretion:** Promethazine is metabolized by the liver. • **Half-life:** UK.

Contraindications
- Promethazine is contraindicated in patients with hypersensitivity to it or to bisulfites, edetate, monothioglycerol, or phenol. • Comatose patients and those with prostatic hypertrophy, bladder-neck obstruction, or narrow-angle glaucoma should not receive promethazine. • Children under 2 years old should not be given promethazine.

Adverse Reactions and Side Effects*
- **CNS:** <u>excessive sedation</u>, <u>confusion</u>, <u>disorientation</u>, dizziness, fatigue, extrapyramidal reactions, nervousness, insomnia • **CV:** tachycardia, bradycardia, hypotension, hypertension • **Derm:** rashes, photosensitivity • **EENT:** blurred vision, tinnitus, diplopia • **GI:** dry mouth, hepatitis, constipation • **Hemat:** blood dyscrasias.

---

*<u>Underlines</u> indicate most frequent; CAPITALS indicate life-threatening.

Propiomazine	*Sedative/hypnotic*
Hydrochloride	*(phenothiazine)*
Largon	pH 4.7–5.3

≋ ADMINISTRATION CONSIDERATIONS

Usual Dose

Preoperative
ADULTS: 10–40 mg.
CHILDREN WEIGHING <27 kg: 0.55–1.1 mg/kg.

Dilution
• **Direct IV:** May be administered **undiluted**. Use a concentration of 20 mg/ml or less. • Do not administer solution that contains a precipitate.

Compatibility
• **Syringe:** atropine • glycopyrrolate • pentazocine.

Incompatibility
• **Syringe:** barbiturates.

Rate of Administration
• **Direct IV:** Administer at a rate of 10 mg/ml. Rapid administration may cause a transient fall in blood pressure.

≋ CLINICAL PRECAUTIONS

• Monitor IV site for thrombophlebitis. Propiomazine is irritating to tissues if it extravasates.
• Assess level of anxiety and sedation throughout therapy.
• Monitor blood pressure periodically during administration.
• Monitor for development of neuroleptic malignant syndrome (fever, respiratory distress, tachycardia, convulsions, diaphoresis, hypertension or hypotension, loss of bladder control, pallor, tiredness). Discontinue immediately if these symptoms occur. May be potentially fatal.
• Additive CNS depression may occur with other CNS depressants, including alcohol, antihistamines, opioid analgesics, sedative/hypnotics, or general anesthetics. The risk of hypotension and respiratory depression is in-

creased by concurrent use of ketamine. The risk of hypotension is increased with concurrent use of antihypertensives, nitrates, or with acute ingestion of alcohol. When used concurrently with epinephrine, severe hypotension may occur.
- Propiomazine has been used safely during labor. Problems have not been seen during pregnancy or lactation.

Lab Test Considerations

- May cause false-positive phentolamine test. Propiomazine should be discontinued at least 24 hours, and preferably 47–72 hours, prior to the phentolamine test.

Patient/Family Teaching

- Medication may cause drowsiness and dizziness. Caution patient to avoid driving or other activities requiring alertness until response to medication is known, and for at least 24 hours after administration. • Advise patient to avoid alcohol or other CNS depressants for at least 24 hours following administration. • Instruct patient to use frequent mouth rinses, good oral hygiene, and sugarless gum or candy to minimize dry mouth.

≋ PHARMACOLOGIC PROFILE

Indications
- Propiomazine is used as a preoperative sedative and as an adjunct to analgesia during labor.

Action
- Propiomazine produces CNS depression, probably by altering the effects of dopamine in the CNS. • It also has antihistaminic and antiemetic properties.

Time/Action Profile (sedative effects)

Onset	Peak	Duration
UK	15–30 min	3–6 hr

Pharmacokinetics
- **Distribution:** UK. • **Metabolism and Excretion:** Propiomazine is probably metabolized by the liver. • **Half-life:** UK.

Contraindications

• Propiomazine is contraindicated in patients who have hypersensitivity to it or to formaldehyde. Cross-sensitivity with other phenothiazines may occur.

Adverse Reactions and Side Effects*

• **CNS:** <u>dizziness</u>, <u>prolonged drowsiness</u>, confusion, restlessness • **Resp:** shortness of breath, dyspnea • **CV:** tachycardia • **GI:** <u>dry mouth</u>, nausea, vomiting, diarrhea, abdominal pain • **Derm:** skin rash • **Misc:** NEUROLEPTIC MALIGNANT SYNDROME.

Propofol	*General anesthetic*
disoprofol, Diprivan	pH 7–8.5

≋ ADMINISTRATION CONSIDERATIONS

Usual Dose

General Anesthetic

ADULTS <55 yr: *Induction*—2–2.5 mg/kg given as 40 mg q 10 seconds until induction is achieved. *Maintenance infusion*—100–200 mcg (0.1–0.2 mg)/kg/min. *Maintenance intermittent boluses*—25–50 mg increments as required.

ADULTS ≥55 yr, DEBILITATED OR HYPOVOLEMIC PATIENTS: *Induction*—1–1.5 mg/kg given as 20 mg q 10 seconds until induction is achieved. *Maintenance infusion*—50–100 mcg (0.05–0.1 mg)/kg/min.

NEUROSURGICAL PATIENTS: *Induction*—1–2 mg/kg given as 20 mg q 10 seconds until induction is achieved. *Maintenance*—100–200 mcg (0.1–0.2 mg)/kg/min.

CHILDREN ≥3 yr: *Induction*—2.5–3.5 mg/kg over 20–30 seconds. *Maintenance*—125–300 mcg (0.125–0.3 mg)/kg/min.

Monitored Anesthesia Care (MAC) Patients

ADULTS <55 yr: *Initially*—100–150 mcg (0.1–0.15 mg)/kg/min or slow injection of 500 mcg (0.5 mg)/kg over 3–5

*****<u>Underlines</u> indicate most frequent; CAPITALS indicate lifethreatening.

minutes. *Maintenance*—25–75 mcg (0.025–0.075 mg)/kg/min infusion or incremental boluses of 10–20 mg (infusion method is preferred).

ADULTS ≥55 yr, DEBILITATED OR ASA III, IV PATIENTS: *Initially*—Doses similar to other adults, but slow infusion or slow injection method is recommended over rapid bolus injections. *Maintenance*—20–60 mcg (0.02–0.06 mg)/kg/min infusion (avoid incremental bolus method).

Intensive Care Unit (ICU) Sedation

ADULTS: *Initially*—5 mcg (0.005 mg)/kg/min for at least 5 minutes. Additional increments of 5–10 mcg (0.005–0.01 mg)/kg over 5–10 minutes may be given until appropriate sedation is achieved. *Maintenance*—5–50 mcg (0.005–0.05 mg)/kg/min. Frequent assessment of level of sedation should be carried out.

Dilution

• **Direct IV / Intermittent or Continuous Infusion:** Shake well before use. If diluted prior to administration, use only D5W and **dilute** to a concentration not less than 2 mg/ml. • Solution is opaque, making detection of contaminants difficult. Do not use if separation of the emulsion is evident. Contains no preservatives; maintain sterile technique and administer immediately after preparation. Discard unused portions and IV lines at the end of procedure or every 6 hours.

Compatibility

• **Y-site:** D5W • LR • D5/0.45% NaCl • D5/0.2% NaCl.

Incompatibility

• **Y-site:** blood • plasma.

• **Additive:** Manufacturer does not recommend admixing propofol with other medications.

Rate of Administration

• **Direct IV:** Dose is titrated to patient response.

≋ CLINICAL PRECAUTIONS

• Assess respiratory status, pulse, and blood pressure continuously throughout propofol therapy. Apnea for more than 60 seconds often occurs during induction. Ventilatory support may be required. Propofol should be used only by individuals experienced in endotracheal intubation, and equipment for this procedure should be readily available. The risk of hypotension is increased by the concurrent use of other hypotensive agents. Significant hypotension or bradycardia may be treated with IV fluids, elevation of lower extremities, and the administration of vasopressors or atropine. Higher infusion rates may be required during the initial 10–15 minutes of maintenance, with a decrease of 30–50% following.

- Assess level of sedation and level of consciousness throughout and following administration when used as a general anesthetic. Additive CNS and respiratory depression may occur with alcohol, antihistamines, opioid analgesics, and sedative/hypnotics. Dosage of propofol may need to be reduced when used concurrently with these agents.

- Do not discontinue prior to weaning or for daily wake-up for neurological and respiratory assessments when used for ICU sedation. Rapid awakening may result in anxiety, agitation, and resistance to mechanical ventilation. Light sedation should be maintained through dose titration during these processes.

- Propofol frequently causes pain, burning, and stinging at injection site; use larger veins of the forearm of antecubital fossa or a dedicated IV catheter. Lidocaine 1 ml of a 1% solution IV may be administered prior to injection to minimize pain.

- Propofol has no effect on the pain threshold. Adequate anesthesia/analgesia should *always* be used when propofol is used as an adjunct to surgical procedures. Assess patients receiving propofol for ICU sedation for pain. Signs and symptoms of pain should be treated with opioid analgesics, not an increase in propofol dose.

- Use cautiously in patients with cardiovascular disease, lipid disorders (emulsion may have detrimental effect), increased intracranial pressure, or cerebrovascular disorders and in elderly, debilitated, or hypovolemic patients (dosage reduction recommended).

- Safe use in pregnancy, lactation, or children younger than 3 years has not been established (Pregnancy Category B).

Toxicity and Overdose Alert

• If overdose occurs, monitor pulse, respiration, and blood pressure continuously. Maintain patent airway and assist ventilation as needed. • If hypotension occurs, treatment includes IV fluids, repositioning, and vasopressors.

Patient/Family Teaching

• Inform patient that this medication will decrease mental recall of the procedure. • Propofol causes drowsiness or dizziness. Advise patient to request assistance prior to ambulation and transfer and to avoid driving or other activities requiring alertness for 24 hours following administration. • Advise patient to avoid alcohol or other CNS depressants for 24 hours following administration of propofol.

≋ PHARMACOLOGIC PROFILE

Indications
• Propofol is used in the induction of general anesthesia and in the maintenance of balanced anesthesia when used with other agents. • Propofol is also used to sedate intubated, mechanically ventilated adults in intensive care units (ICU sedation) and during monitored anesthesia care (MAC sedation).

Action
• Propofol is a short-acting hypnotic. Its mechanism of action is unknown. It produces amnesia but has no analgesic properties.

Time/Action Profile (hypnosis)

Onset	Peak	Duration
40 sec	UK	3–5 min†

†Time to recovery is 8 min (up to 19 min if opioid analgesics have been used).

Pharmacokinetics
• **Distribution:** Propofol is rapidly and widely distributed. It crosses the blood–brain barrier well and is rapidly redistributed to other tissues. Propofol crosses the placenta and enters breast milk. • **Metabolism and Excretion:** Propofol

is rapidly metabolized by the liver. • **Half-life:** 3–12 hours (blood–brain equilibration half-life is 2.9 minutes).

Contraindications

• Propofol is contraindicated in patients with hypersensitivity to it or to soybean oil, egg lecithin, or glycerol. • It is not recommended during labor and delivery.

Adverse Reactions and Side Effects*

• **CNS:** dizziness, headache • **Resp:** APNEA, cough • **CV:** bradycardia, hypotension, hypertension • **GI:** nausea, vomiting, abdominal cramping, hiccups • **Derm:** flushing • **Local:** pain, burning, stinging, tingling, numbness, coldness at IV site • **MS:** perioperative myoclonia, involuntary muscle movements • **Misc:** fever.

Propranolol Hydrochloride	*Antiarrhythmic (group II), Beta-adrenergic blocker (nonselective)*
Inderal	pH 2.8–3.5

≋ ADMINISTRATION CONSIDERATIONS

Usual Dose

ADULTS: 1–3 mg; may repeat in 2 min if needed. Subsequent doses may be repeated q 4 hr.

CHILDREN: 10–100 mcg/kg (not to exceed 1 mg/dose in infants or 3 mg in children). May be repeated in 6–8 hr (unlabeled).

Dilution

• **Direct IV:** Administer **undiluted, or dilute** each 1 mg in 10 ml of D5W for injection. • **Intermittent Infusion:** May also be diluted for infusion in 50 ml of 0.9% NaCl, D5W, D5/0.45% NaCl, D5/0.9% NaCl, or lactated Ringer's injection.

---

*Underlines indicate most frequent; CAPITALS indicate life-threatening.

Compatibility

- **Syringe:** amrinone ◆ benzquinamide ◆ milrinone.
- **Y-site:** alteplase ◆ amrinone ◆ heparin ◆ hydrocortisone sodium succinate ◆ meperidine ◆ milrinone ◆ morphine ◆ potassium chloride ◆ tacrolimus ◆ vitamin B complex with C.
- **Additive:** dobutamine ◆ verapamil.

Incompatibility

- **Y-site:** diazoxide.

Rate of Administration

- **Direct IV:** Administer at a rate not to exceed 1 mg/min.
- **Intermittent Infusion:** Infuse at a rate of 1 mg over 10–15 minutes. Infuse slowly at a rate of 10–20 mcg over 10 minutes in children.

≋ CLINICAL PRECAUTIONS

- Monitor blood pressure and pulse frequently when adjusting dose and periodically throughout therapy. If bradycardia (less than 50 bpm) occurs, dosage alteration or discontinuation may be required. Patients receiving propranolol IV must have continuous ECG monitoring and may have pulmonary capillary wedge pressure or central venous pressure monitoring during and for several hours after administration. Assess for orthostatic hypotension when assisting patient up from supine position.
- Monitor intake and output ratios, and daily weight. Assess patient routinely for evidence of congestive heart failure (peripheral edema, dyspnea, rales/crackles, fatigue, weight gain, jugular venous distention).
- Oral and parenteral doses are not interchangeable. Check dose carefully. IV dose is roughly 1/10 of oral dose, but must be individualized.
- Use cautiously in patients with thyrotoxicosis or hypoglycemia (may mask symptoms).
- Dosage reduction is recommended in patients with hepatic impairment.
- Geriatric patients may have altered sensitivity (increased or decreased response) to propranolol. Dosage adjustment may be necessary.
- Use cautiously in patients with a history of severe allergic reactions (intensity of reactions may be increased).

- General anesthesia, IV phenytoin, and verapamil may cause additive myocardial depression with propranolol. Additive bradycardia may occur with concurrent use of cardiac glycosides. Additive hypotension may occur with other antihypertensive agents, acute ingestion of alcohol, or nitrates. Concurrent use with amphetamines, cocaine, ephedrine, epinephrine, norepinephrine, phenylephrine, or pseudoephedrine may result in excess alpha-adrenergic stimulation, hypertension, and bradycardia. Propranolol may negate the beneficial beta$_1$-adrenergic cardiac effects of dopamine or dobutamine. Concurrent use with insulin may produce prolonged hypoglycemia. Propranolol may produce hypertension within 14 days of MAO inhibitor therapy. Concurrent thyroid hormone administration may decrease effectiveness. Propranolol may antagonize beta-adrenergic bronchodilators. Cimetidine may decrease metabolism and increase the effects of propranolol.
- Safe use during pregnancy or lactation has not been established. Apnea, low Apgar scores, bradycardia, and hypoglycemia may occur in the newborn (Pregnancy Category C). Safe use in children has not been established.

Lab Test Considerations

- Hepatic and renal function and CBC should be monitored routinely in patients receiving prolonged therapy. Propranolol may cause elevations in serum potassium, uric acid, LDH, glucose, lipoprotein, triglyceride levels, and BUN.

Patient/Family Teaching

- Propranolol may cause drowsiness. Caution patient to avoid activities that require alertness until response to the drug is known. • Diabetic patients should monitor serum glucose closely, especially if weakness, fatigue, or irritability occurs. • Advise patient to notify physician if slow pulse, dizziness, light-headedness, confusion, depression, or skin rash occurs. • Advise patient to always carry identification describing medication regimen.

≋ PHARMACOLOGIC PROFILE

Indications

• Propranolol is used in the management of various tachyarrhythmias, including supraventricular tachyarrhythmias and arrhythmias associated with thyrotoxicosis.

Action

• Propranolol blocks stimulation of $beta_1$- (myocardial) and $beta_2$- (pulmonary, vascular, or uterine) receptor sites, resulting in decreased heart rate, decreased blood pressure, and decreased AV conduction.

Time/Action Profile (antiarrhythmic effect)

Onset	Peak	Duration
immediate	1 min	4–6 hr

Pharmacokinetics

• **Distribution:** Propranolol is widely distributed. It crosses the blood–brain barrier and the placenta and enters breast milk. • **Metabolism and Excretion:** Propranolol is almost completely metabolized by the liver. • **Half-life:** 3.4–6 hours.

Contraindications

• Propranolol is contraindicated in patients with uncompensated congestive heart failure, pulmonary edema, cardiogenic shock, bradycardia, or heart block.

Adverse Reactions and Side Effects*

• **CNS:** <u>fatigue</u>, <u>weakness</u>, <u>depression</u>, memory loss, mental changes, <u>insomnia</u>, drowsiness, confusion, dizziness • **EENT:** dry eyes, blurred vision, nasal stuffiness • **Resp:** bronchospasm, wheezing • **CV:** BRADYCARDIA, CONGESTIVE HEART FAILURE, PULMONARY EDEMA, hypotension, edema • **GI:** constipation, <u>diarrhea</u>, <u>nausea</u>, <u>vomiting</u> • **GU:** impotence, diminished libido • **Derm:** rash • **Endo:** hyperglycemia, hypoglycemia • **Misc:** <u>Raynaud's phenomenon</u>.

---

*<u>Underlines</u> indicate most frequent; CAPITALS indicate life-threatening.

Protamine Sulfate	*Antidote*
	(antiheparin agent)
	pH 6–7

 ADMINISTRATION CONSIDERATIONS

Usual Dose

Heparin Overdose

ADULTS AND CHILDREN: 1 mg protamine for each 100 units of heparin or determine dose based on coagulation tests (not to exceed 50 mg for any 10-min period or 100 mg for any 2-hr period).

Enoxaparin Overdose

ADULTS: 1 mg protamine for each 1 mg of enoxaparin (unlabeled).

Dilution

• **Direct IV: Reconstitute** 50-mg vial with 5 ml of sterile water for injection or bacteriostatic water for injection for a concentration of 10 mg/ml. **Reconstitute** 250-mg vial with 25 ml. Shake vigorously. • Solutions reconstituted with sterile water for injection should be discarded after dose is withdrawn. Preparations of protamine in solution should be stored in the refrigerator. Solutions reconstituted with bacteriostatic water are stable for 24 hours when refrigerated. • **Intermittent Infusion:** May be **diluted** in D5W or 0.9% NaCl.

Compatibility

• **Additive:** cimetidine ✦ ranitidine ✦ verapamil.

Incompatibility

• **Additive:** cephalosporins ✦ penicillins.

Rate of Administration

• **Direct IV:** May be administered slow IV push over 1–3 minutes. • **Intermittent Infusion:** Infuse no faster than 50 mg over 10 minutes. Rapid infusion rate may result in hypotension, bradycardia, flushing, or feeling of warmth. If these symptoms occur, stop infusion. For accurate administration, do not admix.

≋ CLINICAL PRECAUTIONS

- Discontinue heparin infusion. In milder cases, heparin overdose may be treated by heparin withdrawal alone. In severe cases, fresh frozen plasma or whole blood may also be required to control bleeding. Dose varies with type of heparin, route of heparin therapy, and amount of time elapsed since discontinuation of heparin. Do not administer more than 100 mg in 2 hours without re-checking clotting studies, as protamine sulfate has its own anticoagulant properties. See *heparin sodium, heparin calcium* monograph on page 485.
- Assess for bleeding and hemorrhage throughout course of therapy. Hemorrhage may recur 8–9 hours after therapy due to rebound effects of heparin. Rebound may occur as late as 18 hours after therapy in patients heparinized for cardiopulmonary bypass.
- Assess for allergy to fish (salmon), previous reaction to or use of protamine insulin or protamine sulfate. Vasectomized and infertile men also have higher risk of hypersensitivity reaction. Observe patient for signs and symptoms of hypersensitivity reaction (hives, edema, coughing, wheezing). Keep epinephrine, an antihistamine, and resuscitative equipment close by in the event of anaphylaxis.
- Assess for hypovolemia prior to initiation of therapy. Failure to correct hypovolemia may result in cardiovascular collapse from peripheral vasodilating effects of protamine sulfate.
- Safe use in pregnancy, lactation, or children has not been established.

Lab Test Considerations

- Monitor clotting factors, activated clotting time (ACT), activated partial thromboplastin time (aPTT), and thrombin time (TT) 5–15 minutes after therapy and again as necessary.

Patient/Family Teaching

- Explain purpose of the medication to patient. • Instruct patient to report recurrent bleeding immediately.

• Advise patient to avoid activities that may result in bleeding (shaving, brushing teeth, receiving injections, taking rectal temperatures, or ambulation) until risk of hemorrhage has passed.

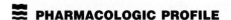 **PHARMACOLOGIC PROFILE**

Indications

• Protamine sulfate is used in the acute management of severe heparin overdosage. It may also be used to neutralize heparin received during dialysis, cardiopulmonary bypass, and other procedures.

Action

• Protamine sulfate is a strong base that forms a complex with heparin (an acid), resulting in inactivation of heparin.

Time/Action Profile (reversal of heparin effect)

Onset	Peak	Duration
30 sec–1 min	UK	2 hr†

†Depends on body temperature.

Pharmacokinetics

• **Distribution:** UK. • **Metabolism and Excretion:** Metabolic fate of protamine is not known. Protamine-heparin complex eventually degrades. • **Half-life:** UK.

Contraindications

• Protamine sulfate is contraindicated in patients with hypersensitivity to protamine or fish. Avoid reconstitution with diluents containing benzyl alcohol if used in neonates.

Adverse Reactions and Side Effects*

• **CV:** hypertension, hypotension, bradycardia, pulmonary hypertension • **Resp:** dyspnea • **GI:** nausea, vomiting • **Derm:** warmth, flushing • **Hemat:** bleeding • **MS:** back pain • **Misc:** hypersensitivity reactions, including angioedema, pulmonary edema, and ANAPHYLAXIS.

---

*Underlines indicate most frequent; CAPITALS indicate life-threatening.

Pyridostigmine Bromide
Cholinergic (anticholinesterase)

Mestinon, Regonol   pH 5

ADMINISTRATION CONSIDERATIONS

Usual Dose

Myasthenia Gravis

ADULTS: 2 mg or ⅟₃₀ of oral dose; may be repeated q 2–3 hr.

NEONATES BORN TO MYASTHENIC MOTHERS: 50–150 mcg (0.05–0.15 mg)/kg q 4–6 hr intramuscularly (IV use in neonates is unlabeled).

INTRAPARTUM ADULTS: 1 mg 1 hr before completion of second stage of labor.

Antidote for Nondepolarizing Neuromuscular Blockers

ADULTS: 10–20 mg; pretreat with 600 mcg (0.6 mg)–1.2 mg atropine IV.

Dilution

- **Direct IV:** Administer **undiluted**. Do not add to IV solutions. May be given through Y-site or 3-way stopcock of solutions of D5W, 0.9% NaCl, lactated Ringer's solution, D5/Ringer's solution, or D5/LR.

Compatibility

- **Syringe:** glycopyrrolate.
- **Y-site:** heparin • hydrocortisone sodium succinate • potassium chloride • vitamin B complex with C.

Rate of Administration

- **Direct IV:** Administer injection very slowly. • For myasthenia gravis, administer each 0.5 mg over 1 minute. • For reversal of nondepolarizing neuromuscular blocking agents, administer each 5 mg over 1 minute.

≋ CLINICAL PRECAUTIONS

- Assess pulse, respiratory rate, and blood pressure prior to administration for significant changes in heart rate.
- *Myasthenia Gravis:* Assess neuromuscular status, includ-

ing vital capacity, ptosis, diplopia, chewing, swallowing, hand grasp, and gait prior to administering and at peak effect. Patients with myasthenia gravis may be advised to keep a daily record of their condition and the effects of this medication.

- Assess patient for overdosage and underdosage/resistance. Both have similar symptoms (muscle weakness, dyspnea, dysphagia), but symptoms of overdosage usually occur within 1 hour of administration, while symptoms of underdosage occur 3 or more hours after administration. Overdosage (cholinergic crisis) symptoms may also include increased respiratory secretions and saliva, bradycardia, nausea, vomiting, cramping, diarrhea, and diaphoresis. Differentiation is important in neonates. A Tensilon test (edrophonium chloride) may be used to differentiate between overdosage and underdosage (see *edrophonium chloride* monograph on page 372). For patients who have difficulty chewing, pyridostigmine may be administered 30 minutes before meals.

- Pyridostigmine should be discontinued or dosage decreased during concurrent glucocorticoid therapy or use of a ventilator.

- In myasthenic mothers, intrapartum use provides strength during labor and protects infant for a short period of time after birth.

- *Antidote to Nondepolarizing Neuromuscular Blocking Agents:* Monitor reversal of effect of neuromuscular blocking agents with a peripheral nerve stimulator. Recovery usually occurs consecutively in the following muscles: diaphragm, intercostal muscles, muscles of the glottis, abdominal muscles, limb muscles, muscles of mastication, and levator muscles of eyelids. Closely observe patient for residual muscle weakness and respiratory distress throughout the recovery period. Maintain airway patency and ventilation until recovery of normal respirations occurs.

- When used as an antidote to nondepolarizing neuromuscular blocking agents, atropine may be ordered prior to or currently with large doses of pyridostigmine to prevent or to treat bradycardia and other side effects.

- Oral dose is not interchangeable with IV dose. Parenteral form is 30 times more potent.

- Cholinergic effects may be antagonized by other drugs

possessing anticholinergic properties, including antihistamines, antidepressants, atropine, haloperidol, phenothiazines, procainamide, quinidine, or disopyramide. Pyridostigmine prolongs the action of depolarizing muscle-relaxing agents including demecarium, echothiophate, and isoflurophate. Antimyasthenic effects may be decreased by concurrent use of guanadrel, guanethidine, or trimethaphan.

- Use cautiously in patients with a history of asthma, ulcer disease, cardiovascular disease, epilepsy, or hyperthyroidism.
- Use cautiously in pregnancy or lactation. Pyridostigmine may cause uterine irritability following administration near term; 20% of newborns may display transient muscle weakness.

Lab Test Considerations

- Atropine is the antidote.

Patient/Family Teaching

- Advise patient to carry identification describing disease and medication regimen at all times. • Instruct patient to space activities to avoid fatigue.

PHARMACOLOGIC PROFILE

Indications

- Pyridostigmine is used to increase muscle strength in the symptomatic treatment of myasthenia gravis. • It is also used to reverse nondepolarizing neuromuscular blocking agents.

Action

- Pyridostigmine inhibits the breakdown of acetylcholine so that it has a prolonged effect. Effects include miosis, increased skeletal and intestinal muscle tone, bronchial and ureteral construction, bradycardia, increased salivation, lacrimation, and sweating.

Time/Action Profile (cholinergic effects)

Onset	Peak	Duration
UK	UK	UK

Pharmacokinetics

• **Distribution:** Pyridostigmine appears to cross the placenta. • **Metabolism and Excretion:** It is metabolized by plasma cholinesterases and the liver. • **Half-life:** 1.9 hours.

Contraindications

• Pyridostigmine is contraindicated in patients with hypersensitivity to it. • Its use should be avoided in patients with mechanical obstruction of the GI or GU tract. • Products containing benzyl alcohol should not be used in newborns.

Adverse Reactions and Side Effects*

• **CNS:** SEIZURE, dizziness, weakness • **EENT:** miosis, lacrimation • **Resp:** excessive secretions, bronchospasm • **CV:** bradycardia, hypotension • **GI:** abdominal cramps, nausea, vomiting, diarrhea, excessive salivation • **Derm:** sweating, rashes.

Pyridoxine Hydrochloride	Vitamin (water soluble)
Beesix, PyriRodex, Vitabee 6, vitamin B₆	pH 2–3.8

 ADMINISTRATION CONSIDERATIONS

Usual Dose

Pyridoxine Deficiency
ADULTS: 10–20 mg/day for 3 wk, followed by 2–5 mg/day PO as a multiple vitamin preparation.

Dietary Supplementation
ADULTS AND CHILDREN: 2 mg (2.5–10 mg/day during pregnancy).

Drug-Induced Deficiency (Isoniazid, Hydralazine, Penicillamine)—Treatment
ADULTS: 50–200 mg/day for 3 wk, then 25–100 mg/day.

---

*Underlines indicate most frequent; CAPITALS indicate life-threatening.

Pyridoxine-Dependency Syndrome

ADULTS: Up to 600 mg/day (initial treatment), followed by 30 mg/day for life.

INFANTS: 10–100 mg initially, followed by oral therapy of 2–100 mg/day, followed by 2–10 mg/day orally for life.

Isoniazid Overdosage (>10 g)

ADULTS: Amount equivalent to isoniazid ingested given as 4 g pyridoxine IV, followed by 1 g IM q 30 min.

Dilution

• **Direct IV:** May be administered **undiluted**. • **Continuous Infusion:** May be administered as an infusion in standard IV solutions. • Protect parenteral solution from light, as decomposition will occur.

Incompatibility

• **Additive:** alkaline solutions • erythromycin • iron salts • kanamycin • riboflavin • streptomycin.

Rate of Administration

• **Direct IV:** May be administered as a bolus. • **Continuous Infusion:** Administer at prescribed rate.

≋ CLINICAL PRECAUTIONS

- Administration of parenteral vitamin B_6 is limited to patients who are NPO, have nausea and vomiting, or have malabsorption syndromes. Because of infrequency of single B-vitamin deficiencies, combinations are commonly administered.

- Assess patient for signs of vitamin B_6 deficiency (anemia, dermatitis, cheilosis, irritability, seizures, nausea, and vomiting) prior to and periodically throughout therapy. Institute seizure precautions in pyridoxine-dependent infants. B_6-dependent seizures should cease within 2–3 minutes of IV administration of pyridoxine.

- Pyridoxine interferes with the therapeutic response to levodopa. Requirements for pyridoxine are increased by isoniazid, hydralazine, chloramphenicol, penicillamine, estrogens, and immunosuppressants. Large doses of pyridoxine may decrease serum levels of phenobarbital or phenytoin.

- Pyridoxine may be used safely during pregnancy (Pregnancy Category A). Doses greater than RDA may suppress lactation. Chronic ingestion of large doses during pregnancy may produce pyridoxine-dependency syndrome in newborn.

Lab Test Considerations

May cause false elevations in urobilinogen concentrations.

Patient/Family Teaching

• Encourage patient to comply with physician's diet recommendations. Explain that the best source of vitamins is a well-balanced diet with foods from the four basic food groups. Foods high in vitamin B_6 include bananas, wholegrain cereals, potatoes, lima beans, and meats. Patients self-medicating with vitamin supplements should be cautioned not to exceed RDA (see Appendix H). • Emphasize the importance of follow-up examinations to evaluate progress.

 PHARMACOLOGIC PROFILE

Indications

• Pyridoxine is used in the treatment and prevention of pyridoxine deficiency, which may be associated with poor nutritional status or chronic debilitating illnesses, and in the treatment and prevention of neuropathy, which may develop from isoniazid, penicillamine, or hydralazine therapy.

Action

• Pyridoxine is required for amino acid, carbohydrate, and lipid metabolism. It is used in the transport of amino acids, formation of neurotransmitters, and synthesis of heme.

Time/Action Profile

Onset	Peak	Duration
UK	UK	UK

Pharmacokinetics

• **Distribution:** Pyridoxine is stored in liver, muscle, and brain. It crosses the placenta and enters breast milk. • **Metabolism and Excretion:** Amounts of pyridoxine in excess of requirements are excreted unchanged by the kidneys. • **Half-life:** 15–20 days.

Contraindications
• There are no known contraindications; however, preparations containing benzyl alcohol should be avoided in newborns.

Adverse Reactions and Side Effects*
Adverse reactions listed are seen with excessive doses only.
• **Neuro:** sensory neuropathy • **Misc:** pyridoxine-dependency syndrome.

Quinidine Gluconate	Antiarrhythmic (group IA)
	pH 5.5–7

ADMINISTRATION CONSIDERATIONS
Usual Dose
ADULTS: Infuse at 16 mg/min (not to exceed 5 g/day).

Dilution
• **Intermittent Infusion:** Dilute 800 mg of quinidine gluconate (10 ml) in at least 40 ml of D5W for injection for a maximum concentration of 16 mg/ml. • Use only clear, colorless solution. Solution is stable for 24 hours at room temperature.

Compatibility
• **Y-site:** diazepam • milrinone.
• **Additive:** bretylium • cimetidine • milrinone • ranitidine • verapamil.

Incompatibility
• **Y-site:** furosemide.
• **Additive:** atracurium.

---

*Underlines indicate most frequent; CAPITALS indicate life-threatening.

Rate of Administration

- **Intermittent Infusion:** Administer at a rate not to exceed 1 ml (16 mg)/min. Administer via infusion pump to ensure accurate dose. Rapid administration may cause hypotension.

≋ CLINICAL PRECAUTIONS

- Monitor ECG, pulse, and blood pressure continuously throughout IV administration. IV administration is usually discontinued if any of the following occurs: arrhythmia is resolved, QRS complex widens by 50%, PR or QT intervals are prolonged, frequent ventricular ectopic beats or tachycardia develops. Patient should remain supine to minimize hypotension.
- Quinidine increases serum digoxin levels and may cause toxicity (dosage reduction of digoxin recommended). Phenytoin, phenobarbital, or rifampin may increase metabolism and decrease effectiveness of quinidine. Cimetidine decreases metabolism and may increase blood levels of quinidine. Quinidine potentiates neuromuscular blocking agents and oral anticoagulants. Additive hypotension may occur with antihypertensives, nitrates, and acute ingestion of alcohol. Quinidine may antgonize anticholinesterase therapy in patients with myasthenia gravis. Drugs that alkalinize the urine, including high-dose antacid therapy or sodium bicarbonate, increase blood levels and the risk of toxicity. Foods that alkalinize the urine (see Appendix H) may increase serum quinidine levels and the risk of toxicity.
- Patients with congestive heart failure or severe liver disease require reduced doses of quinidine.
- Higher doses of quinidine may be required to correct atrial arrhythmias than those required for ventricular arrhythmias.
- Safety in pregnancy, lactation, or children has not been established (Pregnancy Category C).

Toxicity and Overdose Alert

- Serum quinidine levels should be monitored periodically during dosage adjustment. Therapeutic serum concentrations are 3–6 mcg/ml. Toxic effects usually occur at concentrations greater than 8 mcg/ml. • Signs and symptoms of toxicity or cinchonism include tinnitus, visual disturbances, headache, and dizziness. Cardiac signs of toxicity include QRS complex widening, cardiac asystole, ventricular ectopic beats, idioventricular rhythms (ventricular tachycardia, ventricular fibrillation), paradoxical tachycardia, and arterial embolization.

Lab Test Considerations

• Hepatic and renal function, CBC, and serum potassium levels should be periodically monitored during prolonged therapy.

Patient/Family Teaching

• Quinidine may cause dizziness or blurred vision. Caution patient to avoid activities requiring alertness until response to medication is known. • Inform patient that quinidine may cause increased sensitivity to light. Dark glasses may minimize this effect. • Advise patient to consult physician if diarrhea is severe or persistent. • Advise patient to always carry identification describing disease process and medication regimen.

 PHARMACOLOGIC PROFILE

Indications

• Quinidine is used in the management of a wide variety of atrial and ventricular arrhythmias, including atrial premature contractions, premature ventricular contractions, ventricular tachycardia, and paroxysmal atrial tachycardia. • It is also used to maintain normal sinus rhythm after conversion from atrial fibrillation or flutter.

Action

• Quinidine decreases myocardial excitability and slows conduction velocity.

Time/Action Profile

Onset	Peak	Duration
1–5 min	rapid	6–8 hr

Pharmacokinetics

• **Distribution:** Quinidine is widely distributed. It crosses the placenta and enters breast milk. • **Metabolism and Excretion:** Quinidine is metabolized by the liver; 10–30% is excreted unchanged by the kidneys. • **Half-life:** 6–8 hours (increased in congestive heart failure or severe liver impairment).

Contraindications

• Quinidine is contraindicated in patients with hypersensitivity to it or to phenol or edetate. Patients with conduction defects or cardiac glycoside toxicity should not receive quinidine.

Adverse Reactions and Side Effects*

• **CNS:** vertigo, headache, dizziness • **EENT:** tinnitus, blurred vision, photophobia, mydriasis, diplopia • **CV:** hypotension, tachycardia, arrhythmias • **GI:** <u>diarrhea</u>, <u>nausea</u>, <u>cramping</u>, <u>anorexia</u>, bitter taste, hepatitis • **Derm:** rashes • **Hemat:** thrombocytopenia, hemolytic anemia • **Misc:** fever.

Ranitidine Hydrochloride	_Histamine H_2 antagonist, Gastrointestinal (antiulcer)_
Zantac	pH 6.7–7.3

 ADMINISTRATION CONSIDERATIONS

Usual Dose

Short-Term Treatment of Active Ulcers

ADULTS: 50 mg q 6–8 hr or 6.25-mg/hr infusion (not to exceed 400 mg/day).
CHILDREN: 2–4 mg/kg/day.

---

*<u>Underlines</u> indicate most frequent; CAPITALS indicate life-threatening.

Gastric Hypersecretory Conditions (Zollinger-Ellison syndrome)

ADULTS: 1 mg/kg/hr initially by continuous infusion. Based on gastric acid output after 4 hr, may increase by 0.5 mg/kg/hr up to 2.5 mg/kg/hr.

Prevention of Aspiration Pneumonia

ADULTS: 50 mg 45–60 min prior to anesthesia induction (unlabeled).

Adjunctive Therapy of Acute Hypersensitivity Reactions

ADULTS: 50 mg (unlabeled).

Dilution

• **Direct IV: Dilute** each 50 mg in 20 ml of 0.9% NaCl or D5W for injection. • **Intermittent Infusion: Dilute** each 50 mg in 100 ml of 0.9% NaCl or D5W. • Diluted solution is stable for 48 hours at room temperature. Do not use solution that is discolored or that contains precipitate. • **Continuous Infusion: Add** ranitidine to D5W for a concentration of 150 mg/250 ml (no greater than 2.5 mg/ml for Zollinger-Ellison patients).

Compatibility

• **Syringe:** atropine • cyclizine • dexamethasone • dimenhydrinate • diphenhydramine • fentanyl • glycopyrrolate • hydromorphone • isoproterenol • meperidine • metoclopramide • morphine • nalbuphine • oxymorphone • pentazocine • perphenazine • prochlorperazine edisylate • promethazine • scopolamine • thiethylperazone.

• **Y-site:** acyclovir • allopurinol sodium • aminophylline • atracurium • aztreonam • bretylium • ciprofloxacin • cisplatin • cyclophosphamide • cytarabine • diltiazem • dobutamine • dopamine • doxorubicin • enalaprilat • esmolol • filgrastim • fludarabine • foscarnet • gallium nitrate • heparin • idarubicin • labetalol • melphalan • meperidine • methotrexate • morphine • nitroglycerin • ondansetron • paclitaxel • pancuronium • piperacillin • piperacillin/tazobactam • procainamide • sargramostim • tacrolimus • vecuronium • vinorelbine • zidovudine.

• **Additive:** acetazolamide • amikacin • aminophylline • chloramphenicol • dexamethasone • dobutamine • dopamine • doxycycline • erythromycin lactobionate • furosemide • gentamicin • heparin • lidocaine • nitroprusside

* norepinephrine * penicillin G * potassium chloride
* protamine * quinidine gluconate * ticarcillin * tobramycin
* vancomycin.

Incompatibility

* **Syringe:** hydroxyzine * methotrimeprazine * midazolam * pentobarbital * phenobarbital.
* **Additive:** amphotericin B * atracurium * cefamandole
* cefoxitin * ceftazidime * cephalothin * clindamycin.

Rate of Administration

* **Direct IV:** Administer over at least 5 minutes. Rapid administration may cause hypotension and arrhythmias. * **Intermittent Infusion:** Administer over 15–20 minutes.
* **Continuous Infusion:** Administer at a rate of 6.25 mg/hr
for ulcer patients. In patients with Zollinger-Ellison syndrome, start infusion at 1 mg/kg/hr. If gastric acid output is
greater than 10 mEq/hr or patient becomes symptomatic after
4 hours, adjust the dose by 0.5-mg/kg/hr increments and re-
measure gastric output.

≋ CLINICAL PRECAUTIONS

* Assess patient routinely for epigastric or abdominal pain
  and frank or occult blood in the stool, emesis, or gastric
  aspirate.
* Assess elderly and severely ill patients routinely for confusion. Use ranitidine cautiously in elderly patients and
  patients with renal or hepatic impairment due to increased risk of confusion. Increased dosing interval is
  recommended if creatinine clearance is less than 50 ml/
  min. Further dosage alteration may be required if hepatic function is impaired or confusion occurs.
* Ranitidine reduces absorption of ketoconazole.
* Safe use in pregnancy or lactation has not been established (Pregnancy Category B).

Lab Test Considerations

* CBC with differential should be monitored periodically throughout therapy. May cause transient increase in
serum transaminase and serum creatinine. * Antagonizes
the effects of pentagastrin and histamine during gastric

acid secretion test. Avoid administration for 24 hours preceding the test. • May cause false-positive results for urine protein; test with sulfosalicylic acid. May cause false-negative results in skin tests using allergen extracts. Ranitidine should be discontinued 24 hours prior to the test.

Patient/Family Teaching

• Inform patient that smoking interferes with the action of ranitidine. Encourage patient to quit smoking or at least not to smoke after last dose of the day. • Ranitidine may cause drowsiness or dizziness. Caution patient to avoid activities requiring alertness until response to the drug is known. • Advise patient to avoid alcohol, products containing aspirin, ibuprofen, or naproxen, and foods that may cause an increase in GI irritation. • Advise patient to report onset of black, tarry stools; diarrhea; dizziness; rash; or confusion to physician or nurse promptly.

 PHARMACOLOGIC PROFILE

Indications

• IV ranitidine is used in the treatment (short-term) and prevention (long-term) of active duodenal ulcers, short-term treatment of benign gastric ulcers, and management of gastroesophageal reflux disease (GERD) and erosive gastritis. • It is also used in the treatment of gastric hypersecretory states (Zollinger-Ellison syndrome). • Ranitidine may be used to prevent aspiration pneumonia during surgery and as adjunctive therapy in acute hypersensitivity reactions (*unlabeled uses*).

Action

• Ranitidine inhibits the action of histamine at the H_2 receptor site located primarily in gastric parietal cells. This results in inhibition of gastric acid secretion.

Time/Action Profile (inhibition of gastric acid secretion)

Onset	Peak	Duration
UK	15 min	8–12 hr

Pharmacokinetics

• **Distribution:** Ranitidine is widely distributed. It enters breast milk and probably crosses the placenta, crossing the blood–brain barrier only in small amounts. • **Metabolism and Excretion:** Ranitidine is metabolized by the liver, mostly on first pass. Up to 70–80% may be eliminated unchanged by the kidneys following parenteral dosing. • **Half-life:** 1.7–3 hours (increased in renal impairment).

Contraindications

• Ranitidine is contraindicated in patients with hypersensitivity to it or to phenol.

Adverse Reactions and Side Effects*

• **CNS:** confusion, dizziness, <u>headache</u>, <u>malaise</u>, drowsiness • **CV:** bradycardia, tachycardia, premature ventricular contractions • **Derm:** rashes • **EENT:** ocular pain, blurred vision • **Endo:** gynecomastia • **GI:** nausea, constipation, hepatitis, abdominal pain, diarrhea • **GU:** impotence.

Rifampin	Antitubercular
Rifadin IV	pH 7.8–8.8

ADMINISTRATION CONSIDERATIONS

Usual Dose

Tuberculosis

ADULTS: 10 mg/kg/day (up to 600 mg/day) as a single dose; may also be given twice weekly.

GERIATRIC PATIENTS: 10 mg/kg/day as a single dose.

INFANTS AND CHILDREN: 10–20 mg/kg/day (not to exceed 600 mg/day) as a single dose or 2–3 times weekly.

Asymptomatic Carriers of Meningococcus

ADULTS: 600 mg b.i.d. for 2 days.

INFANTS AND CHILDREN ≥1 mo: 10 mg/kg q 12 hr for 2 days.

INFANTS <1 mo: 5 mg/kg q 12 hr for 2 days.

---

*<u>Underlines</u> indicate most frequent; CAPITALS indicate life-threatening.

Dilution

• **Intermittent Infusion: Reconstitute** 600-mg vial with 10 ml of sterile water for injection and swirl gently to completely dissolve. • Manufacturer recommends that preparation and administration time not exceed 4 hours. However, sources suggest that the solution is stable for as long as 24 hours at room temperature. **Dilute further** in 500 ml of D5W or 0.9% NaCl. • May also be added to 100 ml of diluent.

Incompatibility

• **Additive:** Do not admix with other solutions or medications.

Rate of Administration

• **Intermittent Infusion:** Administer solutions diluted in 500 ml over 3 hours. • Administer solutions diluted in 100 ml over 30 minutes.

≋ CLINICAL PRECAUTIONS

- Mycobacterial studies and susceptibility tests should be performed prior to and periodically throughout therapy to detect possible resistance.
- Assess lung sounds and character and amount of sputum periodically throughout therapy.
- Rifampin stimulates liver enzymes, which may increase metabolism and decrease the effectiveness of other drugs, including glucocorticoids, disopyramide, quinidine, opioid analgesics, oral hypoglycemic agents, oral anticoagulants, estrogens, and oral contraceptive agents. The risk of hepatotoxicity is increased by concurrent use of other hepatotoxic agents, including alcohol, isoniazid, ketoconazole, and miconazole.
- Use rifampin cautiously in patients with a history of liver disease or during concurrent use of other hepatotoxic agents.
- Rifampin has been used safely during pregnancy (Pregnancy Category C). Bleeding problems may occur in the mother and baby at term. Vitamin K may be required. Safe use during lactation has not been established, although adverse effects have not been noted.

Lab Test Considerations

• Hepatic function tests should be monitored prior to and monthly, and renal function, CBC, and urinalysis should be evaluated periodically throughout course of therapy. Rifampin may cause increased BUN, AST (SGOT), ALT (SGPT), and serum alkaline phosphatase, bilirubin, and uric acid concentrations and may cause false-positive direct Coombs' test results. • In addition, rifampin may interfere with folic acid and vitamin-B_{12} assays.

Patient/Family Teaching

• Emphasize the importance of continuing therapy even after symptoms have subsided. Course of therapy commonly lasts for 1–2 years. • Advise patient to notify physician promptly if signs and symptoms of hepatitis (yellow eyes and skin, nausea, vomiting, anorexia, unusual tiredness, weakness) or thrombocytopenia (unusual bleeding or bruising) occur. • Caution patient to avoid the use of alcohol during this therapy, as this may increase the risk of hepatotoxicity. • Instruct patient to report the occurrence of flu-like symptoms (fever, chills, myalgia, headache) promptly. • Rifampin may occasionally cause drowsiness. Caution patient to avoid driving or other activities requiring alertness until response to medication is known. • Inform patient that saliva, sputum, sweat, tears, urine, and feces may become red-orange to red-brown, and that soft contact lenses may become permanently discolored. • Advise patient that this medication has teratogenic properties. Counsel patient to use a nonhormonal form of contraception throughout therapy. • Emphasize the importance of regular follow-up examinations to monitor progress and to check for side effects.

≋ PHARMACOLOGIC PROFILE

Indications

• Rifampin is used in combination with other agents in the management of active tuberculosis. It is also used to eliminate carriers of meningococcal disease.

Action

• Rifampin inhibits RNA synthesis by blocking RNA transcription in susceptible organisms, resulting in bactericidal action. Rifampin is active against mycobacteria, *Staphylococcus aureus, Haemophilus influenzae, Legionella pneumophila,* and *Neisseria meningitidis.*

Time/Action Profile (blood levels)

Onset	Peak	Duration
rapid	end of infusion	UK

Pharmacokinetics
• **Distribution:** Rifampin is widely distributed into many body tissues and fluids, including CSF. It crosses the placenta and enters breast milk. • **Metabolism and Excretion:** Rifampin is mostly metabolized by the liver. Sixty percent is eliminated in the feces via biliary elimination. • **Half-life:** 3 hours.

Contraindications
• Rifampin is contraindicated in patients with hypersensitivity to it.

Adverse Reactions and Side Effects*
• **CNS:** headache, drowsiness, confusion, fatigue, ataxia, weakness • **GI:** nausea, vomiting, heartburn, abdominal pain, flatulence, diarrhea, hepatitis • **Hemat:** hemolytic anemia, thrombocytopenia • **MS:** myalgia, arthralgia • **Misc:** flu-like syndrome, red discoloration of all body fluids.

Ritodrine Hydrochloride	Tocolytic (beta-adrenergic agonist)
Yutopar	pH 4.8–5.5

≋ ADMINISTRATION CONSIDERATIONS
Usual Dose
ADULTS: 50–100 mcg (0.05–0.1 mg)/min; increase by 50 mcg (0.05 mg)/min q 10 min until desired response, followed by infusion at 150–350 mcg (0.15–0.35 mg)/min.

---

*Underlines indicate most frequent; CAPITALS indicate life-threatening.

Dilution

• **Continuous Infusion:** Prepare infusion by **diluting** 150 mg (three 50-mg ampules) in 500 ml of D5W for a concentration of 300 mcg/ml. Do not use solutions containing saline, as this increases the risk of fluid overload. • Solution is stable for 48 hours following dilution. Do not use solutions that are cloudy or contain a precipitate.

Incompatibility

• Information unavailable. Do not mix with other drugs or solutions.

Rate of Administration

• **Continuous Infusion:** Rate is titrated according to patient's response and side effects. Usual rate ranges 150–350 mcg/min (0.50–1.17 ml/min). • An infusion pump should be used to ensure accurate dosage. Monitor infusion carefully to prevent circulatory overload.

≋ CLINICAL PRECAUTIONS

- Uterine activity should be assessed frequently throughout therapy.
- Monitor maternal blood pressure and pulse and fetal heart rate frequently throughout administration. Patient should be placed in left lateral position to reduce blood pressure changes. Monitor for tachycardia or arrhythmias. IV ritodrine causes increased maternal heart rate, increased maternal systolic blood pressure, and decreased maternal diastolic blood measure in 80–100% of patients. Use baseline ECG to rule out maternal cardiac disease, and monitor immediately in patients complaining of chest pain or tightness during ritodrine therapy.
- Monitor intake and output ratios for significant discrepancies in totals.
- Assess patient frequently during IV infusion for signs and symptoms of pulmonary edema (dyspnea, rales/crackles, frothy pink-tinged sputum). The risk of pulmonary edema is increased when used concurrently with glucocorticoids. Cardiovascular effects may be additive with other sympathomimetic agents, including epinephrine, terbutaline, metaproterenol, albuterol, or isoproterenol. Therapeutic effects may be antagonized by con-

current use of beta-adrenergic blocking agents. The risk of hypotension is increased when used with general anesthetics.

- Infusion should be continued for 12–24 hours after contractions have stopped, then followed by oral administration. Patients may usually resume ambulation gradually after 36–48 hours if contractions do not recur.
- Use with caution in patients who have had premature rupture of membranes or who have hypotension, diabetes mellitus, or mild to moderate pre-eclampsia.
- Although ritodrine is used during pregnancy, it may cause neonatal hypoglycemia, tachycardia, ileus, and fatal ketoacidosis (Pregnancy Category B).

Toxicity and Overdose Alert

- Symptoms of overdose include tachycardia, arrhythmias, severe nausea and vomiting, anxiety, severe tremor, and shortness of breath. • Treatment includes administration of beta-adrenergic blockers.

Lab Test Considerations

- Blood glucose and electrolytes should be monitored carefully during prolonged therapy, especially for diabetic patients or those receiving glucocorticoids, potassium-depleting diuretics, or digitalis glycosides. May cause transient increases in serum glucose, insulin, and free fatty acid concentrations, but these usually return to pretreatment levels within 24–72 hours, even with continued infusion. Serum potassium levels may be decreased during IV infusion, with a maximum effect 2 hours after initiation of infusion and a return to normal within 30 minutes–24 hours after infusion is discontinued. • May cause elevated AST (SGOT) and ALT (SGPT) concentrations.

Patient/Family Teaching

- Instruct patient to notify nurse or physician immediately if contractions begin again or if water breaks.

≋ PHARMACOLOGIC PROFILE

Indications

- Ritodrine is used to stop preterm labor (Pregnancy Category B).

Action

• Ritodrine stimulates beta-adrenergic receptors, particularly those in uterine, bronchial, and vascular smooth muscle. Stimulation of beta receptors in uterine muscles results in inhibition of uterine contractions.

Time/Action Profile (suppression of contractions)

Onset	Peak†	Duration‡
rapid	5 min	30 min

†After stabilizing dose has been determined.
‡After discontinuation.

Pharmacokinetics

• **Distribution:** Ritodrine crosses the placenta and probably crosses the blood–brain barrier. • **Metabolism and Excretion:** Ritodrine is metabolized by the liver. • **Half-life:** 10 hours.

Contraindications

• Ritodrine is contraindicated in patients with hypersensitivity to bisulfites or in situations where continuation of pregnancy is hazardous, such as antepartum hemorrhage, eclampsia, intrauterine death, abruptio placentae, placenta previa, chorioamnionitis, or fetal malformation incompatible with life. • Ritodrine should be avoided in patients with hypovolemia, cardiac disease, arrhythmias, pulmonary hypertension, uncontrolled hypertension, pheochromocytoma, hyperthyroidism, uncontrolled diabetes mellitus, severe asthma, or pregnancy of <20 weeks duration.

Adverse Reactions and Side Effects*

• **CNS:** tremor, nervousness, restlessness, malaise, weakness • **Resp:** dyspnea, hyperventilation • **CV:** tachycardia (maternal and fetal), increased systolic pressure, decreased diastolic pressure, palpitations, chest pain, arrhythmias, murmurs, PULMONARY EDEMA • **GI:** nausea, vomiting, ileus, bloating, diarrhea, constipation • **Derm:** erythema, rash, sweating • **Endo:** hyperglycemia • **F and E:** KETOACIDOSIS, hypokalemia, lactic acidosis • **Misc:** ANAPHYLACTIC SHOCK.

---

*Underlines indicate most frequent; CAPITALS indicate life-threatening.

Rocuronium Bromide	*Neuromuscular blocking agent (nondepolarizing)*
Zemuron	pH 4

≋ ADMINISTRATION CONSIDERATIONS

Usual Dose

ADULTS: *Rapid sequence intubation*—600 mcg (0.6 mg)–1.2 mg/kg; *Tracheal intubation*—600 mcg (0.6 mg)/kg (smaller doses of 450 mcg [0.45 mg]/kg and larger boluses of 900 mcg [0.9 mg]–1.2 mg/kg have been used); *Maintenance dosing*—100–200 mcg (0.1–0.2 mg)/kg; *Continuous infusion*—10–12 mcg (0.01–0.012 mg)/kg/min [range 4–16 mcg (0.004–0.016 mg)/kg/min].

CHILDREN: *Intubation dose*—600 mcg (0.6 mg)/kg; *Maintenance dose*—75–125 mcg (0.075–0.125 mg)/kg; *Continuous Infusion*—12 mcg (0.012 mg)/kg/min.

Dilution

• **Direct IV:** Administer **undiluted**. • **Continuous Infusion:** May be **diluted** in solution with 0.9% NaCl, sterile water for injection, D5W, lactated Ringer's solution, or D5/0.9% NaCl for infusion. • Solution is stable for 24 hours at room temperature.

Incompatibility

• **Syringe/Y-site:** alkaline solutions • barbiturates.

Rate of Administration

• **Direct IV:** Titrate according to patient response. • **Continuous Infusion:** Infusion rates of 4–16 mcg (0.004–0.016 mg)/kg/min have been used. Rate of infusion should be titrated according to the patient's twitch response as monitored with the use of a peripheral nerve stimulator.

≋ CLINICAL PRECAUTIONS

• Rocuronium should be used only by individuals experienced in endotracheal intubation, and equipment for this procedure should be immediately available.
• Rocuronium has no effect on consciousness or the pain

threshold. Adequate anesthesia and analgesia should *always* be used when rocuronium is used as an adjunct to surgical procedures or when painful procedures are performed. If eyes remain open throughout prolonged administration, protect corneas with artificial tears.

- Assess respiratory status continuously throughout use of rocuronium. Neuromuscular response to rocuronium should be monitored intraoperatively with a peripheral nerve stimulator. Paralysis is initially selective and usually occurs consecutively in the following muscles: levator muscles of eyelids, muscles of mastication, limb muscles, abdominal muscles, muscles of the glottis, intercostal muscles, and the diaphragm. Recovery of muscle function usually occurs in reverse order. Monitor ECG, heart rate, and blood pressure throughout use of rocuronium. Observe patient for residual muscle weakness and respiratory distress during the recovery period.

- Monitor infusion site frequently. If signs of local irritation or extravasation occur, discontinue IV and restart in another site.

- When used following succinylcholine, rocuronium should not be given until recovery from succinylcholine has occurred.

- In obese patients, the initial dose of rocuronium should be based on actual body weight. Larger initial doses for rapid sequence induction may be required in patients with ascites. Duration of action may be prolonged in these patients.

- Neuromuscular blockade from rocuronium is enhanced by concurrent use of inhalation anesthetics, especially enflurane or isoflurane. Infusion rate of rocuronium should be decreased by 30–50% at 45–60 minutes following the intubating dose.

- Use cautiously in patients with any history of pulmonary or cardiovascular disease or renal or liver impairment, elderly or debilitated patients, patients with electrolyte disturbances, myasthenia gravis or myasthenic syndromes (use extreme caution). Rocuronium may increase pulmonary vascular resistance and should be used with caution in patients with pulmonary hypertension or valvular heart disease.

- Intensity and duration of paralysis may be prolonged by pretreatment with succinylcholine, general anesthesia, aminoglycoside antibiotics, polymyxin B, colistin, clindamycin, lidocaine, quinidine, procainamide, beta-adrenergic blocking agents, potassium-losing diuretics, and magnesium.

- Patients receiving anticonvulsants concurrently may require higher infusion rates.
- Safe use in pregnancy or lactation has not been established (Pregnancy Category B). Rocuronium is not recommended for rapid sequence induction in patients undergoing cesarean section.

Toxicity and Overdose Alert

- If overdose occurs use peripheral nerve stimulator to determine the degree of neuromuscular blockade. Maintain airway patency and ventilation until recovery of normal respiration occurs. Administer anticholinesterase agents (edrophonium, neostigmine, pyridostigmine) to antagonize the action of rocuronium. Atropine is usually administered prior to or concurrently with anticholinesterase agents to counteract the muscarinic effects. Administration of fluids and vasopressors may be necessary to treat severe hypotension or shock.

Patient/Family Teaching

- Explain all procedures to patients receiving rocuronium therapy without anesthesia, as consciousness is not affected by rocuronium alone. Provide emotional support.
- Reassure patient that communication abilities will return as the medication wears off.

≋ PHARMACOLOGIC PROFILE

Indications

- Rocuronium is used to produce skeletal muscle paralysis and facilitation of intubation after induction of anesthesia in surgical procedures and during mechanical ventilation.

Action

- Rocuronium prevents neuromuscular transmission by blocking the effect of acetylcholine at the myoneural junction.
- Rocuronium has no analgesic or anxiolytic effects.

Time/Action Profile (skeletal muscle paralysis)†

Time to ≥80% Block	Time to Maximal Block	Duration
1 min	1.8 min	31 min

†Following 0.6 mg/kg dose in adult patients.

Pharmacokinetics

• **Distribution:** The distribution of rocuronium is not known. • **Metabolism and Excretion:** Rocuronium is mostly metabolized by the liver. • **Half-life:** 1.4 hours (increased in patients with hepatic impairment).

Contraindications

• Rocuronium is contraindicated in patients with known hypersensitivity to it or to bromides.

Adverse Reactions and Side Effects*

• **CV:** transient hypotension/hypertension.

Sargramostim	*Colony-stimulating factor*
Leukine, Prokine, rhuGM-CSF	pH 7.1–7.7

ADMINISTRATION CONSIDERATIONS

Usual Dose

Dose may be rounded to nearest vial size.

Myeloid Reconstitution Following Autologous Bone Marrow Transplantation

ADULTS: 250 mcg/m²/day for 21 days as a 2-hr infusion.

Bone Marrow Transplant Failure or Engraftment Delay

ADULTS: 250 mcg/m²/day for 14 days as a 2-hr infusion; may be repeated after 7 days if engraftment has not occurred. A third course of 500 mcg/m²/day for 14 days should be given after 7 days if engraftment has still not happened.

---

*Underlines indicate most frequent; CAPITALS indicate life-threatening.

Dilution

• **Intermittent Infusion: Reconstitute** with 1 ml of sterile water without preservatives injected toward the side of the vial. Swirl gently to avoid foaming. Solution should be clear and colorless. • **Dilute** in 0.9% NaCl. If the final concentration is less than 10 mcg/ml, add a final concentration of 0.1% human albumin to 0.9% NaCl prior to addition of sargramostim to prevent absorption of the components of the drug delivery system. • Administer within 6 hours of reconstitution and dilution. Refrigerate, but do not freeze powder, reconstituted solution, or diluted solution. Do not shake. Discard if left at room temperature for more than 6 hours. Vial is for one-time use only.

Compatibility

• **Y-site:** amikacin • aminophylline • aztreonam • bleomycin • butorphanol • calcium gluconate • carboplatin • carmustine • cefazolin • cefotaxime • cefotetan • ceftizoxime • ceftriaxone • cefuroxime • cimetidine • cisplatin • clindamycin • cyclophosphamide • cyclosporine • cytarabine • dacarbazine • dactinomycin • dexamethasone • diphenhydramine • dopamine • doxorubicin • doxycycline • droperidol • etoposide • famotidine • fentanyl • floxuridine • fluconazole • fluorouracil • furosemide • gentamicin • heparin • idarubicin • ifosfamide • immune globulin IV • magnesium sulfate • mannitol • mechlorethamine • meperidine • mesna • methotrexate • metoclopramide • metronidazole • mezlocillin • miconazole • minocycline • mitoxantrone • netilmicin • pentostatin • piperacillin/tazobactam • potassium chloride • prochlorperazine • promethazine • ranitidine • teniposide • ticarcillin • ticarcillin/clavulanate • trimethoprim/sulfamethoxazole • vinblastine • vincristine • zidovudine.

Incompatibility

• **Y-site:** acyclovir • ampicillin • ampicillin/sulbactam • cefonicid • cefoperazone • chlorpromazine • ganciclovir • haloperidol • hydrocortisone sodium phosphate • hydrocortisone sodium succinate • hydromorphone • hydroxyzine • imipenem/cilastatin • lorazepam • methylprednisolone • mitomycin • morphine • nalbuphine • ondansetron • piperacillin • sodium bicarbonate • tobramycin.

• **Additive:** Do not admix with other medications.

Rate of Administration
- **Intermittent Infusion:** Infuse over 2 hours without an in-line filter.

≋ CLINICAL PRECAUTIONS

- Monitor heart rate, blood pressure, and respiratory status during and immediately following infusion. If dyspnea develops, slow infusion rate by half; reassess; medication may need to be discontinued. Assess for peripheral edema daily throughout therapy.
- *Myeloid reconstitution following autologous bone marrow transplantation:* Administer sargramostim 2–4 hours after bone marrow transplant and no earlier than 24 hours following cytotoxic chemotherapy or 12 hours after last dose of radiotherapy.
- *Bone marrow transplant failure or engraftment delay:* If engraftment does not happen, treatment may be repeated after a 7-day rest period. If there is no response, a third course may be given at twice the dose following a 7-day rest period.
- Monitor for first-dose reaction (flushing, hypotension, syncope, weakness). Does not recur with first dose of each course but may occur with first dose of more than one course.
- Fever, unrelated to leukopenia, occurs in 50% of patients receiving sargramostim. Fever resolves with discontinuation of sargramostim or administration of antipyretics.
- May cause arthralgias or myalgias, usually in lower extremities, which tend to occur when granulocyte counts are returning to normal. May also cause mild to moderate bone pain, possibly due to bone marrow expansion. Usually occurs over 1–3-day period before myeloid recovery and occurs in the sternum, spine, pelvis, and long bones. Treat with analgesics.
- Lithium or glucocorticoids may potentiate myeloproliferative effects of sargramostim.
- Use sargramostim cautiously in patients with pre-existing fluid retention, congestive heart failure, pulmonary infiltrates, or pre-existing cardiac disease. Patients with myeloid malignancies, previous extensive radiation, or

chemotherapy may have a limited response to sargramostim.

- Safe use in pregnancy, lactation, or children is not established (Pregnancy Category C).

Lab Test Considerations

- Obtain a CBC and platelet count prior to chemotherapy and twice weekly during therapy to avoid leukocytosis. Monitor absolute neutrophil count (ANC); may increase rapidly. If ANC is more than 20,000/mm^3 or 10,000/mm^3 after the nadir has occurred, or platelet count is more than 500,000/mm^3, interrupt administration and reduce dose by half or discontinue. Excessive blood levels usually return to baseline 3–7 days following discontinuation of therapy. If blast cells appear, sargramostim should be discontinued. • Monitor renal and hepatic function prior to and biweekly throughout therapy in patients with renal or hepatic dysfunction.

Patient/Family Teaching

- Advise patient to notify nurse or physician if dyspnea or palpitations occur.

≋ PHARMACOLOGIC PROFILE

Indications

- Sargramostim is used to accelerate bone marrow recovery (myeloid reconstruction) following autologous bone marrow transplantation in patients with non-Hodgkin's lymphoma, acute lymphoblastic leukemia, or Hodgkin's disease. It is used in the management of bone marrow transplant failure or delayed engraftment. • Chemotherapy-induced neutropenia has also been managed with sargramostim (unlabeled use).

Action

- Sargramostim consists of a glycoprotein produced by recombinant DNA technique that is capable of binding to and stimulating the production, division, differentiation, and activation of granulocytes and macrophages. Administration of sargramostim results in accelerated recovery of bone marrow function with a decreased risk of infection and other complications.

Time/Action Profile (noted as effects on blood counts)

Onset	Peak	Duration
rapid	UK	3–7 days

Pharmacokinetics

• **Distribution**: UK. • **Metabolism and Excretion:** UK.
• **Half-life:** UK.

Contraindications

• Sargramostim is contraindicated in the presence of 10% or more leukemic myeloid blast cells in bone marrow or peripheral blood. • Patients who have hypersensitivity to granulocyte-macrophage colony-stimulating factors (GM-CSF), yeast products, or additives (mannitol, tromethamine, or sucrose) should not receive sargramostim.

Adverse Reactions and Side Effects*

• **CNS:** weakness, malaise • **Resp:** dyspnea • **CV:** transient supraventricular tachycardia, peripheral edema, pericardial effusion, diarrhea • **Derm:** rash • **MS:** arthralgia, myalgia, bone pain • **Misc:** fever, chills.

Scopolamine Hydrochloride	*Anticholinergic (antimuscarinic)*
	pH 3.5–6.5

≋ ADMINISTRATION CONSIDERATIONS

Usual Dose

ADULTS: *Anticholinergic, antiemetic*—300–600 mcg (0.3–0.6 mg); *sedation/hypnosis* (anesthesia adjunct)—600 mcg (0.6 mg) 3–4 times daily; *amnestic* (anesthesia adjunct)—320–650 mcg (0.32–0.65 mg).
CHILDREN: 6 mcg (0.006 mg)/kg or 200 mcg (0.2 mg)/m^2.

---

*Underlines indicate most frequent; CAPITALS indicate life-threatening.

Dilution

- **Direct IV:** Scopolamine should be **diluted** with sterile water for injection prior to IV administration.

Compatibility

- **Syringe:** atropine ✦ benzquinamide ✦ butorphanol ✦ chlorpromazine ✦ cimetidine ✦ dimenhydrinate ✦ diphenhydramine ✦ droperidol ✦ fentanyl ✦ glycopyrrolate ✦ hydromorphone ✦ hydroxyzine ✦ meperidine ✦ metoclopramide ✦ midazolam ✦ morphine ✦ nalbuphine ✦ pentazocine ✦ pentobarbital ✦ perphenazine ✦ prochlorperazine edisylate ✦ promazine ✦ promethazine ✦ ranitidine ✦ thiopental.
- **Y-site:** heparin ✦ hydrocortisone sodium succinate ✦ potassium chloride ✦ vitamin B complex with C.
- **Additive:** furosemide ✦ meperidine ✦ succinylcholine.

Rate of Administration

- **Direct IV:** Inject slowly.

≋ CLINICAL PRECAUTIONS

- Assess patient for signs of urinary retention periodically throughout course of therapy.
- Monitor heart rate periodically throughout parenteral therapy.
- Assess patient for pain prior to administration. Scopolamine may act as a stimulant in the presence of pain, producing delirium if used without opioid analgesics.
- The risk of adverse reactions is increased in elderly patients, infants, and children. Geriatric patients are more sensitive to the effects of scopolamine. Use cautiously in patients with possible intestinal obstruction; prostatic hypertrophy; or chronic renal, hepatic, pulmonary, or cardiac disease.
- Additive anticholinergic effects may occur with concurrent use of antihistamines, antidepressants, quinidine, or disopyramide. Additive CNS depression may occur with alcohol, antidepressants, antihistamines, opioid analgesics, or other sedative/hypnotics.
- Safe use in pregnancy or lactation has not been established (Pregnancy Category C).

Patient/Family Teaching

• Scopolamine may cause drowsiness or blurred vision. Caution patient to avoid driving or other activities requiring alertness until response to medication is known. • Inform patient that frequent mouth rinses, good oral hygiene, and sugarless gum or candy may minimize dry mouth.

PHARMACOLOGIC PROFILE

Indications

• Scopolamine is used preoperatively to produce sedation and amnesia. It also decreases salivation and excessive respiratory secretions and has antiemetic properties.

Action

• Scopolamine inhibits the muscarinic activity of acetylcholine. Effects include sedation, preoperative amnesia, and decreased secretions.

Time/Action Profile (antisecretory effects)

Onset	Peak	Duration
30 min	UK	4 hr

Pharmacokinetics

• **Distribution:** Scopolamine crosses the placenta and blood–brain barrier. • **Metabolism and Excretion:** Scopolamine is mostly metabolized by the liver. • **Half-life:** 8 hours.

Contraindications

• Scopolamine is contraindicated in patients with hypersensitivity to it, and in patients with narrow-angle glaucoma, acute hemorrhage, or tachycardia secondary to cardiac insufficiency or thyrotoxicosis.

Adverse Reactions and Side Effects*

• **CNS:** <u>drowsiness</u>, confusion • **EENT:** <u>blurred vision</u>, mydriasis, photophobia • **CV:** palpitations, <u>tachycardia</u> • **GI:** <u>dry mouth</u>, constipation • **GU:** <u>urinary hesitancy</u>, urinary retention • **Derm:** decreased sweating.

---

*<u>Underlines</u> indicate most frequent; CAPITALS indicate life-threatening.

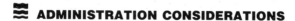

Secobarbital	*Sedative/hypnotic (barbiturate)*
	pH 9.5–10.5

Schedule II

≋ ADMINISTRATION CONSIDERATIONS

Usual Dose

Hypnotic
ADULTS: 50–250 mg.

Anticonvulsant (tetanus)
ADULTS: 5.5 mg/kg; may be repeated q 3–4 hr.
CHILDREN: 3–5 mg/kg (125 mg/m^2)/dose.

Dilution
• **Direct IV:** May be administered **undiluted** or **diluted** with sterile water for injection, 0.9% NaCl, or Ringer's solution. Do not dilute with lactated Ringer's solution. • Do not use solution that is discolored or that contains particulate matter.

Compatibility
• **Additive:** amikacin • aminophylline.

Incompatibility
• **Syringe:** benzquinamide • cimetidine • glycopyrrolate • pentazocine.
• **Additive:** atracurium • chlorpromazine • clindamycin • codeine • droperidol • ephedrine • erythromycin gluceptate • hydrocortisone sodium succinate • insulin • levorphanol • methadone • norepinephrine • pancuronium • pentazocine • phenytoin • procaine • propiomazine • sodium bicarbonate • streptomycin • succinylcholine • vancomycin.

Rate of Administration
• **Direct IV:** Administer each 50 mg over at least 1 minute. Titrate slowly for desired response. Rapid administration may result in respiratory depression, apnea, laryngospasm, bronchospasm, or hypertension.

≋ CLINICAL PRECAUTIONS

- Monitor respiratory status, pulse, and blood pressure frequently in patients receiving secobarbital IV. Equipment for resuscitation and artificial ventilation should be readily available.
- Secobarbital sodium is highly alkaline; avoid extravasation, which may cause tissue damage and necrosis. If extravasation occurs, infiltration with 5% procaine solution into affected area and application of moist heat may be ordered.
- Supervise ambulation and transfer of patients following administration. Remove cigarettes. Side rails should be raised and call bell within reach at all times.
- Assess sleep patterns prior to and periodically throughout course of therapy. Hypnotic doses of secobarbital suppress REM sleep. Patient may experience an increase in dreaming upon discontinuation of medication. Prolonged therapy may lead to psychological or physical dependence.
- Assess postoperative patients for pain. Secobarbital may increase responsiveness to painful stimuli.
- Additive CNS depression may occur with concurrent use of other CNS depressants including alcohol, antihistamines, antidepressants, opioid analgesics, and other sedative/hypnotics. Valproates may decrease metabolism and increase CNS depression.
- Use cautiously in patients with chronic obstructive pulmonary disease or hepatic or renal impairment. Geriatric or debilitated patients may experience excitement, confusion, or excessive CNS depression; dosage reduction may be necessary.
- Secobarbital should be used cautiously in patients with childbearing potential. Chronic use may result in physical dependence, coagulation defects, or respiratory depression in the newborn (Pregnancy Category C).

Patient/Family Teaching

- Discuss the importance of preparing environment for sleep (dark room, quiet, avoidance of nicotine and caffeine). Medication may cause daytime drowsiness. • Caution patient to avoid activities requiring alertness until response to medication is known. • Instruct patient to contact physician immediately if pregnancy is planned or suspected.

 PHARMACOLOGIC PROFILE

Indications
• Secobarbital is used as an adjunct to regional or spinal anesthesia, as a sedative/hypnotic, and as an anticonvulsant (tetanus).

Action
• Secobarbital produces all levels of CNS depression, resulting in induction of sleep and sedation.

Time/Action Profile (hypnotic effect)

Onset	Peak	Duration
rapid	1–3 min	15 min

Pharmacokinetics
• **Distribution:** Secobarbital is widely distributed, highest concentrations occurring in brain and liver. It crosses the placenta; small amounts enter breast milk. • **Metabolism and Excretion:** Secobarbital is metabolized by the liver. • **Half-life:** 30 hours.

Contraindications
• Secobarbital is contraindicated in patients with hypersensitivity to it or to propylene glycol or phenol. • Secobarbital should not be administered to patients with pre-existing CNS depression or uncontrolled severe pain. It should not be used during pregnancy or lactation.

Adverse Reactions and Side Effects*
• **CNS:** <u>drowsiness</u>, <u>lethargy</u>, vertigo, depression, <u>hangover</u>, excitation, delirium • **Resp:** respiratory depression, LARYNGOSPASM, bronchospasm • **CV:** hypotension • **GI:** nausea, vomiting, diarrhea, constipation • **Derm:** rashes, urticaria,

---

*<u>Underlines</u> indicate most frequent; CAPITALS indicate life-threatening.

photosensitivity • **Local:** phlebitis at IV site • **MS:** arthralgia, myalgia • **Neuro:** neuralgia • **Misc:** hypersensitivity reactions, including ANGIOEDEMA and serum sickness; psychological dependence, physical dependence.

Sodium Bicarbonate	*Electrolyte modifier (alkalinizing agent)*
	pH 7–8.5
	contains 12 mEq of Na/g

 ## ADMINISTRATION CONSIDERATIONS

Usual Dose

Dose should be determined on the basis of frequent lab assessment.

Metabolic Acidosis

ADULTS AND CHILDREN >12 yr: 2–5 mEq/kg as a 4–8-hr infusion.

Cardiopulmonary Resuscitation

ADULTS AND CHILDREN: 1 mEq/kg; may repeat 0.5 mEq/kg q 10 min.

Dilution

• **Direct IV:** Administer direct IV push in arrest situation. Use premeasured ampules or prefilled syringes to assure accurate dosage. Available in various concentrations as follows: *4.2% sodium bicarbonate solution*—5 mEq/10 ml (0.5 mEq/ml); *5% sodium bicarbonate solution*—297.5 mEq/500 ml (0.6 mEq/ml); *7.5% sodium bicarbonate solution*—44.6 mEq/50 ml (0.9 mEq/ml); *8.4% sodium bicarbonate solution*—50 mEq/50 ml or 10 mEq/10 ml (1 mEq/ml). Doses should be based on arterial blood gas (ABG) test results. Dose may be repeated every 10 minutes. For children, 4.2% or more dilute solution is preferred. • Flush IV line before and after administration to prevent incompatible medications used in arrest management from precipitating. • **Intermittent/Continuous Infusion:** May be **diluted** in dextrose, saline, and dextrose/saline combinations.

Compatibility

- **Syringe:** milrinone • pentobarbital.
- **Y-site:** acyclovir • famotidine • fludarabine • filgrastim • fludarabine • gallium nitrate • indomethacin • insulin • melphalan • morphine • paclitaxel • piperacillin/tazobactam • potassium chloride • tacrolimus • tolazoline • vitamin B complex with C.
- **Additive:** amikacin • aminophylline • amobarbital • amphotericin B • atropine • bretylium • calcium chloride • calcium gluceptate • cefoxitin • ceftazidime • cephalothin • cephapirin • chloramphenicol • chlorothiazide • cimetidine • clindamycin • cytarabine • droperidol/fentanyl • ergonovine maleate • erythromycin • furosemide • heparin • hyaluronidase • hydrocortisone sodium phosphate • hydrocortisone sodium succinate • kanamycin • lidocaine • metaraminol • methotrexate • methyldopate • multivitamins • nafcillin • netilmicin • oxacillin • oxytocin • phenobarbital • phenylephrine • phenytoin • phytonadione • potassium chloride • prochlorperazine • thiopental • verapamil.

Incompatibility

- **Syringe:** glycopyrrolate • metoclopramide • thiopental.
- **Y-site:** allopurinol sodium • amrinone • calcium chloride • idarubicin • ondansetron • sargramostim • verapamil • vinorelbine.
- **Additive:** ascorbic acid • carboplatin • carmustine • cefotaxime • cisplatin • codeine • corticotropin • dobutamine • epinephrine • hydromorphone • imipenem/cilastatin • insulin • isoproterenol • labetalol • levorphanol • magnesium sulfate • methadone • morphine • norepinephrine • pentazocine • pentobarbital • procaine • secobarbital • streptomycin • succinylcholine.
- **Solution:** Do not add to Ringer's solution, lactated Ringer's solution, or Ionosol products, as compatibility varies with concentration.

Rate of Administration

- **Direct IV:** Administer as a bolus. Rapid injection (10 ml/min) of hypertonic sodium bicarbonate may cause hypernatremia, a decrease in CSF pressure, and possible intracranial hemorrhage, especially in neonates and children under 2 years. Inject at a rate no faster than 1–2 mEq/kg/min in children. Do not administer more than 8 mEq/kg/day of a

4.2% solution. Injecting sodium bicarbonate too rapidly may produce severe alkalosis, resulting in hyperirritability and tetany. • **Intermittent Infusion:** Infuse over 4–8 hours.

≋ CLINICAL PRECAUTIONS

- Assess fluid balance (intake and output, daily weights, edema, lung sounds) throughout therapy. Monitor for symptoms of fluid overload (hypertension, edema, dyspnea, rales/crackles, frothy sputum).
- Assess patient throughout therapy for signs of acidosis (disorientation, headache, weakness, dyspnea, hyperventilation), alkalosis (confusion, irritability, paresthesia, tetany, altered breathing pattern), hypernatremia (edema, weight gain, hypertension, tachycardia, fever, flushed skin, mental irritability), or hypokalemia (weakness, fatigue, U wave on ECG, arrhythmias, polyuria, polydipsia).
- Flush IV line before and after administration to prevent incompatible medications used in arrest management from precipitating.
- Observe IV site closely. Avoid extravasation of hypertonic solution (8.4%), as tissue irritation or cellulitis may occur. If infiltration occurs, may be treated with elevation of extremity, application of warm compresses, and infiltration of the site with lidocaine or hyaluronidase.
- Use cautiously in patients with congestive heart failure, renal insufficiency, or concurrent glucocorticoid therapy.
- If urinary alkalinization occurs, this may result in decreased salicylate or barbiturate blood levels or increased blood levels of quinidine, mexiletine, flecainide, or amphetamines.
- Although sodium bicarbonate has been used without adverse effects, safe use in pregnancy or lactation has not been established (Pregnancy Category C).

Lab Test Considerations

• Monitor serum sodium, potassium, calcium, bicarbonate concentrations, serum osmolarity, acid/base balance, and renal function prior to and periodically throughout course of therapy. • ABGs should be obtained frequently in emergency situations. • Monitor urine pH frequently when used for urinary alkalinization. • Sodium bicarbonate antagonizes effects of pentagastrin and histamine during gastric acid secretion test. Avoid administration during the 24 hours preceding the test.

Patient/Family Teaching

• Review symptoms of electrolyte imbalance with patients receiving chronic therapy; instruct patient to notify physician if these symptoms occur. • Emphasize the importance of regular follow-up examinations to monitor serum electrolyte levels and acid-base balance and to monitor progress.

≋ PHARMACOLOGIC PROFILE

Indications

• Sodium bicarbonate is used in the management of metabolic acidosis. • It is also used to alkalinize urine and promote the excretion of certain drugs in overdose situations (phenobarbital, aspirin).

Action

• Sodium bicarbonate acts as an alkalinizing agent by releasing bicarbonate ions.

Time/Action Profile (alkalinization)

Onset	Peak	Duration
immediate	rapid	UK

Pharmacokinetics

• **Distribution:** Sodium bicarbonate is widely distributed into extracellular fluid. • **Metabolism and Excretion:** Sodium and bicarbonate are excreted by the kidneys. • **Half-life:** UK.

Contraindications

• Sodium bicarbonate is contraindicated in metabolic or respiratory alkalosis, hypocalcemia, or excessive chloride loss.

Adverse Reactions and Side Effects*

• **CV:** edema • **F and E:** sodium and water retention, <u>metabolic alkalosis</u>, hypocalcemia • **Local:** irritation at IV site • **Neuro:** tetany.

---

*<u>Underlines</u> indicate most frequent; CAPITALS indicate life-threatening.

Sodium Chloride *Electrolyte modifier*
(replacement solution)

pH 5–5.8

ADMINISTRATION CONSIDERATIONS

Usual Dose

0.9% Sodium Chloride (isotonic)
ADULTS: 1 liter (contains 150 mEq sodium per liter).

0.45% Sodium Chloride (hypotonic)
ADULTS: 1–2 liters (contains 75 mEq sodium per liter).

3%, 5% Sodium Chloride (hypertonic)
ADULTS: Not more than 100 ml over 1 hr (3% contains 50 mEq sodium per 100 ml; 5% contains 83.3 mEq sodium per 100 ml).

Dilution
• **Intermittent Infusion:** Hypertonic solutions may be administered **undiluted**. • **Continuous Infusion:** Administer 0.45% and 0.9% sodium chloride **undiluted**.

Compatibility
• **Additive:** D5W ◆ D10W ◆ Ringer's and lactated Ringer's injection ◆ dextrose/Ringer's solution combinations ◆ dextrose/lactated Ringer's solution combinations ◆ dextrose/saline combinations ◆ ⅙ M sodium lactate.

Incompatibility
• **Additive:** amphotericin B ◆ mannitol ◆ streptomycin.

Rate of Administration
• **Intermittent Infusion:** Rate of hypertonic sodium chloride solutions should not exceed 100 ml/hr.

≋ CLINICAL PRECAUTIONS

- Assess fluid balance (intake and output, daily weights, edema, lung sounds) throughout course of therapy.
- Assess patient for symptoms of hyponatremia (headache, tachycardia, lassitude, dry mucous membranes, nausea, vomiting, muscle cramps) or hypernatremia (edema, weight gain, hypertension, tachycardia, fever, flushed

skin, mental irritability) throughout therapy. Sodium is measured in relation to its concentration to fluid in the body, and symptoms may change based on patient's hydration status.

- Dosage of sodium chloride depends on patient's age, weight, condition, fluid and electrolyte balance, and acid/base balance.

- Do not administer bacteriostatic sodium chloride containing benzyl alcohol as a preservative to neonates or use to reconstitute or dilute solutions or to flush intravascular catheters in neonates. Benzyl alcohol has been associated with a fatal "gasping" syndrome in neonates.

- Administer 3% or 5% NaCl via a large vein and prevent infiltration.

- Excessive amounts of sodium chloride may partially antagonize the effects of antihypertensive medications. Use of sodium chloride with glucocorticoids may result in excess sodium retention.

- Use cautiously in patients prone to metabolic, acid/base, or fluid and electrolyte abnormalities, including geriatric patients, or those with nasogastric suctioning, vomiting, diarrhea, diuretic therapy, glucocorticoid therapy, fistulas, congestive heart failure, severe renal failure, or severe liver diseases, as additional electrolytes may be required.

Lab Test Considerations

- After the first 100 ml of hypertonic saline, sodium, chloride, and bicarbonate concentrations should be reevaluated to determine the need for further administration.
- Monitor serum sodium, potassium, bicarbonate, and chloride concentrations and acid/base balance periodically for patients receiving prolonged therapy with sodium chloride. • Monitor serum osmolarity in patients receiving hypertonic saline solutions.

Patient/Family Teaching

- Explain to patient the purpose of the infusion.

≋ PHARMACOLOGIC PROFILE

Indications

- Sodium chloride is used for hydration and provision of sodium chloride in deficiency states and for maintenance of fluid and electrolyte status in situations when losses may be excessive (excess diuresis or severe salt restriction). • 0.45% ("half-normal saline") solution is most commonly used for hydration and in the treatment of hyperosmolar diabetes. • 0.9% ("normal saline") solution is used for replacement, to treat metabolic alkalosis, as a priming fluid for hemodialysis, and to begin and end blood transfusions. Small volumes of 0.9% sodium chloride (preservative-free or bacteriostatic) are used to reconstitute or dilute other medications. • Hypertonic saline solutions (3%, 5%) may be required in situations in which rapid replacement of sodium is necessary, such as hyponatremia, hypochloremia, renal failure, or heart failure.

Action

• Sodium is a major cation in extracellular fluid and helps maintain water distribution, fluid and electrolyte balance, acid/base equilibrium, and osmotic pressure. Chloride is the major anion in extracellular fluid and is involved in maintaining acid-base balance. Solutions of sodium chloride resemble extracellular fluid.

Time/Action Profile (electrolyte effects)

Onset	Peak	Duration
rapid	end of infusion	UK

Pharmacokinetics

• **Distribution:** Sodium chloride is rapidly and widely distributed. • **Metabolism and Excretion:** Sodium chloride is excreted primarily by the kidneys. • **Half-life:** UK.

Contraindications

• There are no known contraindications to IV sodium chloride.

Adverse Reactions and Side Effects*

• **CV:** edema, congestive heart failure, pulmonary edema
• **F and E:** hypokalemia, hypervolemia, hypernatremia
• **Local:** extravasation, irritation at IV site.

---

*Underlines indicate most frequent; CAPITALS indicate life-threatening.

Sodium Nitrite

Antidote
(cyanide)

pH 7–9

≋ ADMINISTRATION CONSIDERATIONS

Usual Dose
ADULTS: 300 mg (4–6 mg/kg); may repeat with 50% of initial dose in 2 hr if toxicity persists.

CHILDREN: 180–240 mg/m^2 (4–6 mg/kg, not to exceed 300 mg); 50% of initial dose may be repeated in 2 hr if toxicity persists.

Dilution
• **Direct IV:** For adults, administer 300 mg as 10 ml of 3% solution.

Rate of Administration
• **Direct IV:** Administer over 2–4 minutes.

≋ CLINICAL PRECAUTIONS

• Assess patient for sources of cyanide and signs of cyanide poisoning (absence of reflexes, coma, distant heart sounds, hypotension, imperceptible pulse, metabolic acidosis, pink color, very shallow breathing, widely dilated pupils). Begin treatment at the first sign of toxicity if cyanide poisoning is known or strongly suspected. Amyl nitrite should be inhaled (crush a 0.3-ml ampule every minute and have patient inhale vapors) for 15–30 seconds while sodium nitrite IV is started. In adults, follow amyl nitrite with sodium nitrite. This is followed by sodium thiosulfate 12.5 g. If symptoms recur after 2 hours, treatment may be repeated at half the dose. Oxygen therapy may also be used.

• Monitor pulse and blood pressure continuously. Sodium nitrite may cause transient vasodilation and hypotension.

• Sodium nitrite converts as much hemoglobin to methemoglobin as the patient can safely tolerate, usually about 10%. Methylene blue should not be used to reduce methemoglobin levels as this level of methemoglobinemia is not dangerous.

- Use cautiously in children; adjust dose based on methemoglobin levels.
- Safe use in pregnancy has not been established (Pregnancy Category C).

Patient/Family Teaching

- Explain purpose and procedure of therapy to patient.
- Caution patient to make position changes slowly to minimize orthostatic hypotension.

≋ PHARMACOLOGIC PROFILE

Indications

- Sodium nitrite, with amyl nitrite and sodium thiosulfate, is used in the management of cyanide poisoning.

Action

- During cyanide poisoning, recommended doses of nitrites (amyl nitrite, sodium nitrite) act as a buffer, combining with 10% of hemoglobin to form methemoglobin. Methemoglobin combines with cyanogen to form cyanmethemoglobin, a nontoxic complex. Cyanogen is then slowly released from this complex. Subsequent administration of sodium thiosulfate results in the formation of sodium thiocyanate, which is readily excreted by the kidneys.

Time/Action Profile

Onset	Peak	Duration
rapid	UK	UK

Pharmacokinetics

- **Distribution:** Sodium nitrite is widely distributed.
- **Metabolism and Excretion:** UK. • **Half-life:** UK.

Contraindications

- None.

Adverse Reactions and Side Effects*

- **CV:** transient vasodilation and hypotension.

---

*Underlines indicate most frequent; CAPITALS indicate lifethreatening.

Sodium Phosphate   *Electrolyte*
(potassium replacement,
phosphate replacement)

pH 5–6
contains 3 mmol phosphate/ml
contains 4 mEq Na/ml

≋ ADMINISTRATION CONSIDERATIONS

Usual Dose
ADULTS: 10–15 mmol phosphorus/liter of TPN.
INFANTS: 1.5–2 mmol phosphorus/kg/day, added to TPN.

Dilution
• **Continuous Infusion:** Administer IV only in dilute concentrations. • May be administered as a component of TPN.

Compatibility
• **Y-site:** ciprofloxacin.

Incompatibility
• **Additive:** calcium ◆ magnesium.

Rate of Administration
• **Continuous Infusion:** Infuse slowly; dose and rate of administration are based on patient's condition.

≋ CLINICAL PRECAUTIONS

- Assess patient for signs and symptoms of hypophosphatemia (anorexia, weakness, decreased reflexes, bone pain, confusion, blood dyscrasias) throughout therapy.
- Monitor pulse, blood pressure, and ECG prior to and periodically throughout IV therapy.
- Monitor intake and output ratios, and daily weights.
- Use cautiously in patients with hyperparathyroidism, cardiac disease, or renal impairment.
- Safe use during pregnancy or lactation has not been established (Pregnancy Category C). Adverse effects have not been noted. However, if electrolyte abnormalities occur, prompt treatment is indicated.

Toxicity and Overdose Alert

• Symptoms of toxicity are those of hyperphosphatemia or hypocalcemia (paresthesia, muscle twitching, laryngospasm, colic, cardiac arrhythmias, or Chvostek's or Trousseau's sign) or hypernatremia (thirst, dry flushed skin, fever, tachycardia, hypotension, irritability, decreased urine output). Treatment includes discontinuation of infusion and calcium replacement.

Lab Test Considerations

• Monitor serum phosphate and calcium levels prior to and periodically throughout therapy. Increased phosphate may cause hypocalcemia. • Monitor renal function studies prior to and periodically throughout course of therapy.

Patient/Family Teaching

• Instruct the patient to report diarrhea, weakness, fatigue, muscle cramps, or tremors promptly.

≋ PHARMACOLOGIC PROFILE

Indications

• Sodium phosphate is used in the treatment and prevention of phosphate depletion in patients who are unable to ingest adequate dietary phosphorus.

Action

• Phosphate is present in bone and is involved in energy transfer and carbohydrate metabolism. It serves as a buffer for the excretion of hydrogen ions by the kidney.

Time/Action Profile (effects on serum phosphate levels)

Onset	Peak	Duration
rapid	end of infusion	UK (min–hr)

Pharmacokinetics

• **Distribution:** Phosphates enter extracellular fluids and are then actively transported to sites of action. • **Metabolism and Excretion:** Excretion occurs >90% by the kidneys. • **Half-life:** UK.

Contraindications

• Sodium phosphate is contraindicated in patients with hyperphosphatemia, hypocalcemia, severe renal impairment, untreated Addison's disease, or severe tissue trauma.

Adverse Reactions and Side Effects*

These are related to hyperphosphatemia, unless indicated.

• **CNS:** listlessness, confusion, weakness • **CV:** ARRHYTHMIAS, ECG changes (absent P waves, widening of the QRS complex with biphasic curve), CARDIAC ARREST, hypotension • **F and E:** hypomagnesemia, hyperphosphatemia, hypocalcemia • **Local:** phlebitis, irritation at IV site • **MS:** tremors (hypercalcemia) • **Neuro:** paresthesias of extremities, flaccid paralysis, heaviness of legs.

Sodium Thiosulfate	*Antidote* *(arsenic, cyanide)*
	pH 6–9.5

 ADMINISTRATION CONSIDERATIONS

Usual Dose

Cyanide Poisoning

ADULTS AND CHILDREN: 150–200 mg/kg immediately following sodium nitrite. Entire regimen may be repeated at 50% of initial dose in 2 hr if toxicity persists.

Dilution

• **Direct IV:** May be administered **undiluted**.

Rate of Administration

• **Direct IV:** Administer 12.5 g (50 ml of 25% solution) over 10 minutes.

---

*Underlines indicate most frequent; CAPITALS indicate life-threatening.

≋ CLINICAL PRECAUTIONS

- *Cyanide Poisoning:* Assess patient for sources of cyanide and signs of cyanide poisoning (absence of reflexes, coma, distant heart sounds, hypotension, imperceptible pulse, metabolic acidosis, pink color, very shallow breathing, widely dilated pupils). Begin treatment at the first sign of toxicity if cyanide poisoning is known or strongly suspected. Amyl nitrite should be inhaled (crush a 0.3-ml ampule every minute and have patient inhale vapors) for 15–30 seconds while sodium nitrite IV is started. In adults, follow amyl nitrite with 300 mg (10 ml of 3% solution) of sodium nitrite at a rate of 2–2.5 ml/min. This is followed by sodium thiosulfate. Oxygen therapy may also be used. If symptoms recur, treatment may be repeated at half the dose.
- Sodium nitrite converts as much hemoglobin to methemoglobin as the patient can safely tolerate, usually about 10%. Methylene blue should not be used to reduce methemoglobin levels as this level of methemoglobinemia is not dangerous.
- Safe use in pregnancy has not been established (Pregnancy Category C). Use cautiously in children with cyanide poisoning; adjust dose based on methemoglobin levels.

Patient/Family Teaching

- Explain purpose and procedure of therapy to patient.
- Caution patient to make position changes slowly to minimize orthostatic hypotension.

≋ PHARMACOLOGIC PROFILE

Indications

- Sodium thiosulfate, with amyl nitrite and sodium nitrite, is used in the management of cyanide poisoning.

Action

- In acute cyanide poisoning, nitrites (amyl nitrite and sodium nitrite) are given to form methemoglobin, which combines with cyanide, forming a nontoxic compound (cyanmethemoglobin). Cyanide is then liberated as cyanogen, which is taken up by thiosulfate (from sodium thiosulfate) in the form of thiocyanate. Thiocyanate is readily excreted by the kidneys.

Time/Action Profile

Onset	Peak	Duration
rapid	UK	UK

Pharmacokinetics

• **Distribution:** Thiosulfate is widely distributed. • **Metabolism and Excretion:** Thiosulfate combines with cyanide to form thiocyanate, which is excreted by the kidneys. • **Half-life:** 0.65 hours.

Contraindications

• None.

Adverse Reactions and Side Effects*

• None.

Streptokinase	*Thrombolytic*
Kabikinase, Streptase	pH depends on diluent

 ADMINISTRATION CONSIDERATIONS

Usual Dose

Myocardial Infarction
ADULTS: 1,500,000 IU. *Intracoronary*—20,000-IU bolus, followed by 2000-IU/min infusion.

Deep Vein Thrombosis, Pulmonary Emboli, Arterial Embolism, or Thromboses
ADULTS: 250,000-IU loading dose, followed by 100,000 IU/hr for 24 hours for pulmonary emboli, 72 hours for recurrent

---

*<u>Underlines</u> indicate most frequent; CAPITALS indicate life-threatening.

pulmonary emboli or deep vein thrombosis, 24–72 hours for arterial thrombosis or embolism.

Arteriovenous Cannula Occlusion

ADULTS: 100,000–250,000 IU into each occluded limb of cannula; clamp for 2 hr; then aspirate, flush, and reconnect.

Dilution

• **Direct IV:** For arteriovenous cannula occlusion, **dilute** 250,000 IU in 2 ml of 0.9% NaCl or D5W. • **Dilute** intracoronary doses in 20 ml of 0.9% NaCl or D5W. • **Intermittent Infusion: Reconstitute** the 250,000-IU, 600,000-IU, and 750,000-IU vials with 5 ml and the 1,500,000-IU vial with 10 ml of 0.9% NaCl or D5W (direct slowly to sides of vial) and swirl gently; do not shake. **Dilute further** with 0.9% NaCl for a total volume of 45–500 ml. • Administer through 0.8-micron pore size filter. • Use reconstituted solution within 24 hours of preparation.

Compatibility

• **Y-site:** dobutamine • dopamine • heparin • lidocaine • nitroglycerin. • However, manufacturer recommends that streptokinase not be admixed or administered via Y-site with any other medication.

Rate of Administration

• **Direct IV:** Administer intracoronary bolus over 15 seconds–2 minutes. • Administer dose for arteriovenous cannula occlusion over 25–30 minutes. • **Intermittent Infusion:** Intracoronary bolus should be followed by an intracoronary maintenance infusion of 2000 IU/min for 60 minutes. • Loading dose for deep vein thrombosis or pulmonary embolism may be infused over 30 minutes, followed by an infusion of 100,000 IU/hr. Infuse via infusion pump to ensure accurate dosage.

≋ CLINICAL PRECAUTIONS

- Streptokinase should be used only in settings where hematologic function and clinical response can be adequately monitored.
- Invasive procedures such as IM injections or arterial punctures should be avoided during streptokinase ther-

apy. If such procedures must be performed, apply pressure to IV puncture sites for at least 15 minutes and to arterial puncture sites for at least 30 minutes. Systemic anticoagulation with heparin is usually begun several hours after the completion of thrombolytic therapy.

- Monitor vital signs, including temperature, at least every 4 hours during course of therapy. Do not use lower extremities for blood pressure determinations. Acetaminophen may be ordered to control fever.

- Assess patient carefully for bleeding every 15 minutes during the first hour of therapy, every 15–30 minutes during the next 8 hours, and at least every 4 hours for the duration of therapy. Frank bleeding may occur from invasive sites or body orifices. Internal bleeding may also occur (decreased neurologic status, abdominal pain with coffee-ground emesis or black tarry stools, joint pain). If bleeding not controllable by local pressure occurs, stop medication immediately. Concurrent use with anticoagulants, cefamandole, cefotetan, plicamycin, or agents affecting platelet function (including aspirin, nonsteroidal anti-inflammatory agents, valproates, and dipyridamole) increases the risk of bleeding.

- Inquire about previous reaction to streptokinase therapy. Assess patient for hypersensitivity reaction (rash, dyspnea, fever). Keep epinephrine, an antihistamine, and resuscitation equipment close by in the event of an anaphylactic reaction. Use cautiously in patients with a history of severe hypersensitivity reaction to previous streptokinase or anistreplase therapy.

- Inquire about recent streptococcal infection. Streptokinase may not be effective if administered between 5 days and 6 months of a streptococcal infection, or within 12 months of previous streptokinase/anistreplase therapy.

- Monitor ECG continuously for significant arrhythmias in patients with coronary thrombosis. IV lidocaine or procainamide (Pronestyl) may be ordered prophylactically. Cardiac enzymes should be monitored. Coronary angiography and/or radionuclide myocardial scanning may be used to monitor effectiveness of therapy.

- Monitor pulse, blood pressure, hemodynamics, and respiratory status (rate, degree of dyspnea, ABGs) in patients with pulmonary embolism.

- Observe extremities for circulatory impairment and palpate pulses of affected extremities every hour in patients with deep vein thrombosis or acute arterial occlusion. Computerized tomography, impedance plethysmography, quantitative Doppler effect determination, and/or angiography or venography may be used to determine restoration of blood flow and duration of therapy; however, repeated venograms are not recommended.

- Monitor ability to aspirate blood as indicator of patency in patients with a cannula or catheter occlusion. To prevent air embolism, ensure that patient exhales and holds breath when connecting and disconnecting IV syringe.

- Assess neurological status throughout therapy. Altered sensorium or neurological changes may be indicative of intracranial bleeding. Due to increased risk of cerebral emboli, use cautiously in patients with recent minor trauma or surgery (within 2 months), cerebrovascular disease, diabetic hemorrhagic retinopathy, recent streptococcal infection, recent streptokinase therapy, in patients 75 years or older (increased risk of CNS bleeding), or patients with arterial emboli originating in the left side of the heart.

- Use with *extreme caution* in patients who have been receiving oral anticoagulants or who are 10 days or less postpartum. Safe use in pregnancy, lactation, or children has not been established (Pregnancy Category C).

Toxicity and Overdose Alert

- If local bleeding occurs, apply pressure to site. If severe or internal bleeding occurs, discontinue infusion. Clotting factors and/or blood volume may be restored through infusions of whole blood, packed red blood cells, fresh frozen plasma, or cryoprecipitate. Do not administer dextran, which has antiplatelet activity. Aminocaproic acid (Amicar) may be used as an antidote.

Lab Test Considerations

- Hematocrit, hemoglobin, platelet count, fibrin/fibrinogen degradation product (FDP/fdp) titer, fibrinogen concentration, prothrombin time, thrombin time, and activated partial thromboplastin time should be evaluated prior to and frequently throughout course of therapy.
- Bleeding time may be assessed prior to therapy if patient

has received platelet aggregation inhibitors. • Obtain type and crossmatch and have blood available at all times in case of hemorrhage.

Patient/Family Teaching

• Explain the purpose of the medication to the patient. • Instruct patient to report hypersensitivity reactions (rash, dyspnea) and bleeding or bruising. • Explain need for bed rest and minimal handling during therapy to avoid injury.

 PHARMACOLOGIC PROFILE

Indications

• Streptokinase is used in the treatment of coronary thrombosis associated with acute transmural myocardial infarction. It is also used in the treatment of recent, severe, or massive deep vein thrombosis, pulmonary emboli, arterial embolism, or thrombosis and has been used in the management of occluded arteriovenous cannulas.

Action

• Streptokinase directly activates plasminogen, which subsequently dissolves fibrin deposits, including those required for normal hemostasis.

Time/Action Profile (fibrinolysis)

Onset	Peak	Duration
immediate	rapid	4 hr (up to 12 hr)

Pharmacokinetics

• **Distribution:** Streptokinase does not cross the placenta.
• **Metabolism and Excretion:** Streptokinase is rapidly cleared from circulation following IV administration by antibodies and the reticuloendothelial system. • **Half-life:** 23 minutes (streptokinase/plasmin complex).

Contraindications

• Streptokinase is contraindicated in patients with hypersensitivity to it. • It should be avoided in patients with active internal bleeding, recent (within 2 months) cerebrovascular accident, intracranial or intraspinal surgery, intracranial neoplasms, thoracic surgery, or severe uncontrolled hypertension.

Adverse Reactions and Side Effects*

• **CV:** reperfusion arrhythmias • **EENT:** periorbital edema • **Derm:** <u>urticaria</u>, flushing • **Hemat:** <u>bleeding</u> • **Local:** phlebitis at IV site • **Misc:** <u>fever</u>, hypersensitivity reactions including ANAPHYLAXIS, bronchospasm.

Streptomycin Sulfate	*Anti-infective (aminoglycoside), Antitubercular*
	pH 4.5–7

 ADMINISTRATION CONSIDERATIONS

Streptomycin is not approved for IV use. All IV doses are unlabeled.

Usual Dose

Tuberculosis

ADULTS: 15 mg/kg daily (not to exceed 1 g/dose) or 25–30 mg/kg 2–3 times weekly (not to exceed 1.5 g/dose).

CHILDREN: 20–40 mg/kg/day (not to exceed 1 g/dose) or 25–35 mg/kg 2–3 times weekly (not to exceed 1.5 g/dose).

Other Infections

ADULTS: 250 mg–1 g q 6 hr or 500 mg–2 g q 12 hr.

CHILDREN: 5–10 mg/kg q 6 hr or 10–20 mg/kg q 12 hr.

Dilution

• **Intermittent Infusion: Reconstitute** with 4.5 or 3.5 ml of sterile water or 0.9% NaCl for injection for a concentration of 200 or 250 mg/ml. Solution is stable for 48 hours at room temperature and 14 days if refrigerated. Also available in 1 g/2.5 ml ampules for a concentration of 400 mg/ml. • **Dilute further** in 100 ml of 0.9% NaCl or D5W.

---

*<u>Underlines</u> indicate most frequent; CAPITALS indicate life-threatening.

Compatibility

- **Y-site:** esmolol. • If aminoglycosides and penicillins or cephalosporins must be given concurrently, administer in separate sites, at least 1 hour apart.
- **Additive:** bleomycin.

Incompatibility

- **Syringe:** heparin.
- **Additive:** amobarbital ✦ amphotericin B ✦ chlorothiazide ✦ erythromycin glucoptate ✦ heparin ✦ methohexital ✦ norepinephrine ✦ pentobarbital ✦ phenobarbital ✦ phenytoin ✦ secobarbital ✦ sodium bicarbonate.

≋ CLINICAL PRECAUTIONS

- Assess patient for infection (vital signs; appearance of wound, sputum, urine, and stool; WBC) at beginning and throughout course of therapy.
- Obtain specimens for culture and sensitivity prior to initiating therapy. First dose may be given before receiving results.
- Evaluate eighth cranial nerve function by audiometry prior to and throughout course of therapy. Hearing loss is usually in the high-frequency range. Prompt recognition and intervention are essential in preventing permanent damage. Also monitor for vestibular dysfunction (vertigo, ataxia, nausea, vomiting). Eighth cranial nerve dysfunction is associated with persistently elevated peak streptomycin levels. Caloric stimulation tests may also be used to assess ototoxicity.
- Use cautiously in obese patients; dosage should be based on ideal body weight.
- Monitor intake and output and weight to assess hydration status and renal function. Decreased dose and/or increased dosing interval is recommended if creatinine clearance is >80 ml/min.
- Assess patient for signs of superinfection (fever, upper respiratory infection, vaginal itching or discharge, increasing malaise, diarrhea).
- Safe use during pregnancy or lactation has not been established. Use of streptomycin during pregnancy may cause deafness in the newborn. Risks and benefits

should be carefully assessed prior to use in the pregnant patient (Pregnancy Category D).

Lab Test Considerations

• Monitor renal function (urinalysis, specific gravity, BUN, creatinine, and creatinine clearance) prior to and during therapy. • Blood levels should be monitored periodically during therapy. Draw peak blood levels 15–30 minutes following infusion; peak streptomycin levels should not exceed 20–25 mcg/ml in patients with renal impairment. Trough levels (prior to a dose) should not be >5 mcg/ml. • Streptomycin may cause increased AST (SGOT), ALT (SGPT), LDH, bilirubin, and serum alkaline phosphatase levels. • Serum calcium, magnesium, sodium, and potassium levels may be decreased.

Patient/Family Teaching

• Instruct patients receiving streptomycin to report signs of hypersensitivity, tinnitus, vertigo, or hearing loss.

≋ PHARMACOLOGIC PROFILE

Indications

• Streptomycin is used in combination therapy of active tuberculosis. It has also been used in combination with a penicillin in the treatment of streptococcal or enterococcal endocarditis. Plague and tularemia may be treated with streptomycin. The use of streptomycin should be reserved for infections due to organisms not sensitive to less toxic anti-infectives or when contraindications to their use exist.

Action

• Streptomycin inhibits protein synthesis in bacteria at the level of the 30S ribosome, resulting in bactericidal action against susceptible organisms. Despite a broad spectrum of activity against many Gram-negative pathogens, toxicity precludes its use in many clinical situations. Streptomycin is most notable for its activity against *Mycobacterium tuberculosis, Brucella, Nocardia, Erysipelothrix, Pasteurella multocida,* and *Yersinia pestis.* In the treatment of enterococcal infections, synergy with a penicillin is required.

Time/Action Profile (blood levels)

Onset	Peak
rapid	end of infusion

Pharmacokinetics

• **Distribution:** Streptomycin crosses the placenta; small amounts enter breast milk. Penetration of streptomycin into CSF is poor. • **Metabolism and Excretion:** Excretion of streptomycin is >90% renal. • **Half-life:** 2–3 hours (increased in renal impairment).

Contraindications

• Streptomycin should not be used in patients with hypersensitivity to it. Cross-sensitivity with other aminoglycosides may occur.

Adverse Reactions and Side Effects*

• **EENT:** <u>ototoxicity</u> (vestibular and cochlear) • **GU:** <u>nephrotoxicity</u> • **Neuro:** enhanced neuromuscular blockade • **Misc:** hypersensitivity reactions.

Streptozocin	*Antineoplastic agent (antitumor antibiotic)*
Zanosar	pH 3.5–4.5

≋ ADMINISTRATION CONSIDERATIONS

Usual Dose

ADULTS: 500 mg/m^2/day for 5 days q 4–6 wk or 1 g/m^2/wk for 2 wk. Dose may be increased as tolerated (not to exceed 1.5 g per dose).

Dilution

• **Intermittent Infusion: Reconstitute** vial with 9.5 ml of D5W or 0.9% NaCl, for a concentration of 100 mg/ml. May be **further diluted** in 10–200 ml of D5W or 0.9% NaCl.

---

*<u>Underlines</u> indicate most frequent; CAPITALS indicate life-threatening.

• Solution is pale gold. Do not use if dark brown. Stable for 12 hours at room temperature, 96 hours at 2–8°C. • Solution should be prepared in a biologic cabinet. Wear gloves, gown, and mask while handling medication. Discard equipment in designated containers (see Appendix F).

Compatibility

• **Y-site:** filgrastim ✦ melphalan ✦ ondansetron ✦ vinorelbine.

Incompatibility

• **Y-site:** allopurinol sodium ✦ piperacillin/tazobactam.
• **Additive:** Do not admix.

Rate of Administration

• **Direct IV:** May be administered via rapid IV injection.
• **Intermittent Infusion:** Infuse over 10–15 minutes to decrease venous irritation. May also be infused over 6 hours.

≋ CLINICAL PRECAUTIONS

• Monitor vital signs prior to and periodically during therapy.
• Monitor intake and output, and daily weights. If significant discrepancies or dependent edema occurs, may indicate nephrotoxicity. Encourage fluids to 3000 ml/day to reduce risk of renal damage. The risk of nephrotoxicity is increased with concurrent use of other nephrotoxic agents (aminoglycoside antibiotics).
• IV dextrose should be immediately available, as hypoglycemia may occur in response to initial dose.
• Monitor IV site carefully and ensure patency. Discontinue infusion immediately if severe discomfort, erythema along vein, or infiltration occurs. Streptozocin is a vesicant. Tissue ulceration and necrosis may result from infiltration.
• Monitor for bone marrow depression. Assess for fever and chills, sore throat, and signs of infection. Monitor platelet count throughout therapy. Assess for bleeding (bleeding gums, bruising, petechiae; guaiac test stools, urine, and emesis). If thrombocytopenia occurs, avoid IM injections and rectal temperatures and apply pressure to venipuncture sites for 10 minutes. Anemia may occur. Monitor for increased fatigue, dyspnea, and or-

thostatic hypotension. Additive myelosuppression may occur with other antineoplastic agents.

• Monitor hydration status, appetite, and nutritional intake. Severe, protracted nausea and vomiting usually occur 2–4 hours after beginning infusion. Nausea and vomiting may worsen with subsequent doses. Administration of an antiemetic and adjusting diet as tolerated may help maintain fluid and electrolyte balance and nutritional status.

• Use cautiously in patients with renal disease. Dosage reduction is recommended in this population. Use cautiously in patients with liver disease, active infections, or decreased bone marrow reserve or other chronic debilitating illnesses.

• Concurrent use with phenytoin may decrease therapeutic effects of streptozocin. Streptozocin may increase the toxicity of doxorubicin.

• Use cautiously in patients with childbearing potential. Safe use in pregnancy, lactation, or children has not been established (Pregnancy Category C). Avoid using during pregnancy or lactation.

Lab Test Considerations

• Monitor renal status prior to and frequently throughout therapy and for 4 weeks after course of therapy. Nephrotoxicity is common and may be manifested by elevated BUN and creatinine, decreased creatinine clearance, and presence of protein in urine. Reduction or discontinuation of streptozocin may allow reversal of renal damage. • Monitor for hepatotoxicity, evidenced by increased AST (SGOT), ALT (SGPT), LDH, serum bilirubin, and alkaline phosphatase or decreased serum albumin. • Monitor serum glucose prior to and after initial dose and periodically during therapy. • Monitor serum uric acid level prior to and periodically throughout therapy. • Monitor CBC, differential, and platelet count prior to and throughout therapy. • Serial fasting insulin concentrations may be used to determine response to therapy.

Patient/Family Teaching

• Instruct patient to notify nurse immediately if pain or redness develops at IV site. • Instruct patient to notify nurse immediately if symptoms of hypoglycemia occur (anxiety, chills, cold sweats, confusion, cool pale skin, difficulty in concentration, drowsiness, excessive hunger, headache, irritability, nausea, nervousness, shakiness, unusual tiredness, or weakness). • Instruct patient to notify physician if decreased urine output, swelling of lower extremities, yellowing of skin, fever, chills, sore throat, signs of infection, bleeding gums, bruising, petechiae, or blood in urine, stool, or emesis occurs. • Caution patient to avoid crowds and persons with known infections. Instruct patient to use soft toothbrush and electric razor. Patient should be cautioned not to drink alcoholic beverages or take products containing aspirin, ibuprofen, or naproxen. • This drug may cause gonadal suppression; however, patient should continue to use a nonhormonal method of birth control. Advise patient to inform physician immediately if pregnancy is suspected. • Instruct patient not to receive any vaccinations without advice of physician. Streptozocin may decrease antibody response to live virus vaccines and increase the risk of adverse reactions. • Advise patient of need for medical follow-up and frequent lab tests.

 PHARMACOLOGIC PROFILE

Indications

• Streptozocin is used in the management of metastatic islet cell carcinoma of the pancreas. • It is also used in the management of metastatic carcinoid tumor, Hodgkin's disease, pancreatic adenocarcinoma, and colorectal cancer (*unlabeled uses*).

Action

• Streptozocin inhibits DNA synthesis by cross-linking DNA strands (cell cycle–phase nonspecific) resulting in death of rapidly replicating cells, particularly malignant ones.

Time/Action Profile

	Onset	Peak	Duration
effects on blood counts	UK	1–2 wk	UK
tumor response	17 days	35 days	UK

Pharmacokinetics

• **Distribution:** Streptozocin is rapidly distributed. High concentrations are achieved in the liver, pancreas, kidneys, and intestine. It probably crosses the placenta. An active metabolite enters the CSF. • **Metabolism and Excretion:** Streptozocin is highly metabolized in liver and kidneys; 10–20% is excreted unchanged by the kidneys. Small amounts are excreted in expired air (5%) and feces (1%). • **Half-life:** 35–40 minutes.

Contraindications

• Streptozocin is contraindicated in patients with hypersensitivity to it. • Pregnant or lactating patients should not receive streptozocin.

Adverse Reactions and Side Effects*

• **CNS:** confusion, lethargy, depression • **F and E:** hypophosphatemia • **GI:** <u>nausea</u>, <u>vomiting</u>, hepatitis, diarrhea, duodenal ulcer • **GU:** proteinuria, <u>nephrotoxicity</u>, gonadal suppression • **Hemat:** leukopenia, thrombocytopenia, anemia • **Metab:** HYPOGLYCEMIA (first dose), hyperglycemia, diabetes • **Local:** <u>phlebitis</u> at IV site • **Misc:** fever.

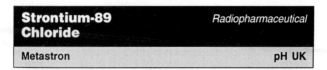

Strontium-89 Chloride	*Radiopharmaceutical*
Metastron	**pH UK**

≋ ADMINISTRATION CONSIDERATIONS

Usual Dose

ADULTS: 148 Mbq (4 mcCi) or 1.5–2.2 Mbq/kg (40–60 mcCi/kg). The dose should not be repeated for at least 90 days.

Dilution

• **Direct IV:** Administer undiluted.

---

*<u>Underlines</u> indicate most frequent; CAPITALS indicate life-threatening.

Incompatibility

• Information unavailable. Do not admix or administer with any other solution or medication.

Rate of Administration

• Administer slowly over 1–2 minutes. If injected more rapidly (over less than 30 seconds), a flushing sensation may occur.

≋ CLINICAL PRECAUTIONS

• Strontium should only be used in facilities with personnel experienced in the safe use and handling of radiopharmaceuticals.

• Assess pain (intensity, location) periodically throughout therapy. Patient may experience a transient increase in bone pain for 2–3 days beginning 2–3 days after administration. Increased analgesic dosage may be required during this time. Pain should begin to diminish after 1–2 weeks or longer and may allow for reduction or discontinuation of analgesics. Effects may continue for several months.

• Incontinent patients should have indwelling catheters placed prior to administration of strontium-89 chloride to decrease the risk of radioactive contamination of clothing, linens, and the environment.

• The risk of bone marrow depression is increased by concurrent use of antineoplastic agents or radiation therapy. Calcium supplements decrease binding of strontium-89 to metastatic sites and may decrease the effectiveness of therapy.

• Use cautiously in patients with childbearing potential. Avoid use during pregnancy or lactation (Pregnancy Category D). Safe use of strontium-89 chloride in children has not been established.

Lab Test Considerations

• Monitor hematologic parameters (WBCs, platelets) at least once every other week during therapy. Platelets are usually decreased by 30% from preadministration levels. The nadir of thrombocytopenia is at 12–16 weeks. Leukopenia may also occur. Recovery to preadministration levels usually occurs within 6 months. • A pregnancy test should be performed before administration.

Patient/Family Teaching

• Instruct patient to continue taking pain medication until strontium-89 chloride becomes effective. Analgesic doses may be decreased once strontium's effects are known. • Inform patient that no changes in eating or drinking requirements are necessary. Alcohol and caffeine should not necessarily be avoided. • Calcium supplements should not be taken for 2 weeks before and 2 weeks after strontium-89 therapy. • Strontium-89 chloride remains in blood and urine for 1 week following administration. During the first week, the patient should be instructed to use a toilet (not a urinal) and to flush twice after use. Spilled urine or blood from a cut should be wiped up with a tissue and flushed. Good handwashing should be observed, and any linen or clothing contaminated with blood or urine should be immediately washed separately from other items and thoroughly rinsed. Similar practices should be followed if urine-collecting devices are used. • Instruct patient to notify other care providers of strontium-89 chloride treatment. • Instruct patient to report any increase in pain that may occur as the effects of strontium-89 chloride decrease. • Advise the patient to notify a physician if pregnancy is planned or suspected. • Emphasize the importance of periodic blood tests during treatment.

 PHARMACOLOGIC PROFILE

Indications

• Management of bone pain in patients with painful skeletal metastases.

Action

• Strontium-89 chloride is preferentially taken up by bone tumors and metastatic bone lesions, where selective irradiation takes place.

Time/Action Profile (decreased pain)

Onset	Peak	Duration
7–20 days	variable	variable

Pharmacokinetics

• **Distribution:** Strontium-89 chloride is selectively taken up and retained by metastatic bone lesions. • **Metabolism and Excretion:** 67% of strontium-89 chloride is excreted in urine, 33% in feces. • **Half-life:** 55 days (physical half-life).

Contraindications

• Strontium-89 chloride should not be used in pregnant or lactating patients.

Adverse Reactions and Side Effects*

• **Hemat:** <u>neutropenia</u>, <u>thrombocytopenia</u>, <u>anemia</u> • **MS:** transient increase in bone pain.

Succinylcholine Chloride	*Neuromuscular blocking agent* *(depolarizing)*
Anectine, Quelicin, Scoline, Sucostrin	pH 4

ADMINISTRATION CONSIDERATIONS

Usual Dose

Test Dose

ADULTS: A test dose of 10 mg or 0.1 mg/kg may be administered to determine patient's sensitivity and recovery time.

Short Procedures

ADULTS: 600 mcg (0.6 mg)/kg (range 300 mcg–1.1 mg/kg); additional doses depend on response.
CHILDREN: 1–2 mg/kg; additional doses depend on response.

Prolonged Procedures

ADULTS: 2.5 mg/min infusion (range 500 mcg–10 mg/min); or 600 mcg (0.6 mg)/kg (range 300 mcg–1.1 mg/kg) initially, then 40–70 mcg (0.04–0.07 mg)/kg as necessary.

---

*<u>Underlines</u> indicate most frequent; CAPITALS indicate life-threatening.

Dilution

• **Direct IV:** May be administered **undiluted**. • **Continuous Infusion: Dilute** to a 0.1–0.2% solution (1–2 mg/ml) in dextrose/Ringer's or lactated Ringer's combinations, dextrose/saline combinations, 0.45% NaCl, 0.9% NaCl, D5W, D10W, Ringer's or lactated Ringer's injection. • Solution is stable for 24 hours at room temperature. Administer only clear solutions. Discard any unused solution.

Compatibility

• **Syringe:** heparin.
• **Y-site:** potassium chloride • vitamin B complex with C.
• **Additive:** amikacin • cephapirin • isoproterenol • meperidine • methyldopa • morphine • norepinephrine • scopolamine.

Incompatibility

• **Additive:** barbiturates • nafcillin • sodium bicarbonate.

Rate of Administration

• **Direct IV:** Usual adult dose is administered over 10–30 seconds. Dose is titrated to patient response. • **Continuous Infusion:** Administer at a rate of 0.5–10 mg/min; usual rate is 2.5–4.3 mg/min. Titrate dose to patient response and degree of paralysis required.

≋ CLINICAL PRECAUTIONS

• Assess respiratory status continuously throughout use of succinylcholine. Succinylcholine should be used only by individuals experienced in endotracheal intubation, and equipment for this procedure should be immediately available.

• Monitor neuromuscular response to succinylcholine with a peripheral nerve stimulator intraoperatively. Paralysis is initially selective and usually occurs consecutively in the following muscles: levator muscles of eyelids, muscles of mastication, limb muscles, abdominal muscles, muscles of the glottis, intercostal muscles, and the diaphragm.

• Monitor ECG, heart rate, and blood pressure throughout use of succinylcholine. Assess patient for history of malignant hyperthermia prior to administration. Monitor for signs of malignant hyperthermia (tachycardia, tachypnea, hypercarbia, jaw muscle spasm, lack of laryngeal relaxation, hyperthermia) throughout administration.

- Observe patient for residual muscle weakness and respiratory distress during the recovery period.

- Succinylcholine has no effect on consciousness or pain threshold. Adequate anesthesia/analgesia should *always* be used when succinylcholine is used as an adjunct to surgical procedures or when painful procedures are performed. Benzodiazepines and/or analgesics should be administered concurrently when prolonged succinylcholine therapy is used for ventilator patients, as patient is awake and able to feel all sensations.

- If eyes remain open throughout prolonged administration, protect corneas with artificial tears.

- To prevent excessive salivation or bradycardia, patients may be premedicated with atropine or scopolamine.

- A small dose of a nondepolarizing agent may be used prior to succinylcholine to decrease the severity of muscle fasciculations.

- Use cautiously in patients with a history of malignant hyperthermia, pulmonary disease, or renal or liver impairment; elderly or debilitated patients; patients with glaucoma or electrolyte disturbances or those receiving cardiac glycosides; and patients with fractures or muscular spasm, myasthenia gravis, or myasthenic syndromes.

- Concurrent administration of cholinesterase inhibitors (echothiophate, isoflurophate, and demecarium eyedrops) reduces pseudocholinesterase activity and intensifies paralysis. The intensity and duration of paralysis may be prolonged by pretreatment with general anesthesia, aminoglycoside antibiotics, polymyxin B, colistin, clindamycin, lidocaine, quinidine, procainamide, beta-adrenergic blocking agents, potassium-losing diuretics, and magnesium.

- Succinylcholine has been used in pregnant women undergoing cesarean section. Use cautiously in neonates and children due to increased risk of malignant hyperthermia, rhabdomyolysis, and adverse cardiovascular reactions (infusion method not recommended).

Toxicity and Overdose Alert

• If overdose occurs, use peripheral nerve stimulator to determine degree of neuromuscular blockade. Maintain airway patency and ventilation until recovery of normal respirations occurs.

Lab Test Considerations

• Succinylcholine may cause hyperkalemia, especially in patients with severe trauma, burns, or neurologic disorders.

Patient/Family Teaching

• Explain all procedures to patient receiving succinylcholine therapy without anesthesia, as consciousness is not affected by succinylcholine alone. Provide emotional support. • Reassure patient that communication abilities will return as the medication wears off.

PHARMACOLOGIC PROFILE

Indications

• Succinylcholine is used to produce skeletal muscle paralysis after induction of anesthesia in surgical procedures.

Action

• Succinylcholine prevents neuromuscular transmission by blocking the effect of acetylcholine at the myoneural junction. • It has agonist activity initially, producing fasciculation. • It also causes the release of histamine. • Succinylcholine has no analgesic or anxiolytic effects.

Time/Action Profile (skeletal muscle paralysis)

Onset	Peak	Duration
0.5–1 min	1–2 min	4–10 min

Pharmacokinetics

• **Distribution:** Succinylcholine is widely distributed into extracellular fluid and crosses the placenta in small amounts. • **Metabolism and Excretion:** 90% of succinylcholine is metabolized by pseudocholinesterase in plasma; 10% is excreted unchanged by the kidneys. • **Half-life:** UK.

Contraindications

• Succinylcholine is contraindicated in patients with hypersensitivity to it and should not be given to patients with plasma pseudocholinesterase deficiency.

Adverse Reactions and Side Effects*

Most adverse reactions to succinylcholine are extensions of pharmacologic effects.

• **EENT:** excess salivation • **CV:** hypotension, arrhythmias • **Resp:** bronchospasm, apnea • **F and E:** hyperkalemia • **MS:** muscle fasciculation, rhabdomyolysis • **Misc:** MALIGNANT HYPERTHERMIA.

Sufentanil Citrate	Opioid analgesic (agonist)
Sufenta	pH 3.5–6

Schedule II

 ADMINISTRATION CONSIDERATIONS

Usual Dose

Low-Dose Anesthesia Adjunct

ADULTS: 0.5–1 mcg/kg initially; additional doses of 10–25 mcg may be given if needed (not to exceed 1 mcg/kg/hr when administered with nitrous oxide and oxygen).

Moderate-Dose Anesthesia Adjunct

ADULTS: 2–8 mcg/kg initially; additional doses of 10–50 mcg may be given if needed (not to exceed 1 mcg/kg/hr when administered with nitrous oxide and oxygen for procedures lasting up to 8 hr).

Primary Anesthesia (with 100% oxygen)

ADULTS: 8–30 mcg/kg initially; additional doses of 25–50 mcg may be given if needed.

CHILDREN: *Cardiovascular surgery*—10–25 mcg/kg initially; additional doses of up to 25–50 mcg may be given.

---

*Underlines indicate most frequent; CAPITALS indicate life-threatening.

Dilution

- **Direct IV:** May be administered **undiluted**.

Rate of Administration

- **Direct IV:** Administer slowly, over at least 1–2 minutes. Slow IV administration may reduce the incidence or severity of muscle rigidity, bradycardia, or hypotension. • **Continuous Infusion:** When used as a primary anesthetic agent, a continuous infusion of sufentanil may be administered with or following the initial loading dose to provide immediate and sustained effects throughout a prolonged surgical procedure.

≋ CLINICAL PRECAUTIONS

- Monitor respiratory rate and blood pressure frequently throughout course of therapy. The respiratory depressant effects of sufentanil last longer than the analgesic effects. Subsequent opioid doses should be reduced by ¼ to ⅓ of the usually recommended dose. Monitor closely.

- Use cautiously in obese patients (>20% over ideal body weight). Dosage should be based on ideal body weight in these patients.

- Benzodiazepines may be administered prior to administration of sufentanil to reduce the induction dose requirements and to decrease the time until loss of consciousness. This combination may increase the risk of hypotension. Opioid antagonist, oxygen, and resuscitative equipment should be readily available during the administration of sufentanil.

- Concurrent use of alcohol, antihistamines, antidepressants, or sedative/hypnotics results in additive CNS and respiratory depression. MAO inhibitors should be avoided for 14 days prior to use. Cimetidine or erythromycin may prolong duration of recovery. Nalbuphine or pentazocine may decrease response to sufentanil. Concurrent use with succinylcholine may increase the risk and severity of cardiovascular adverse reactions.

- Use cautiously in elderly patients, debilitated or severely ill patients, diabetic patients, and those with severe pulmonary disease, hepatic disease, CNS tumors, increased intracranial pressure, head trauma, adrenal insufficiency, undiagnosed abdominal pain, hypothyroidism, alcoholism, or cardiac disease (arrhythmias).

- Sufentanil has been used in women undergoing cesarean section and may cause drowsiness in the infant (Pregnancy Category C). Safe use in lactation has not been established.

Toxicity and Overdose Alert

- Atropine may be used to treat bradycardia; or use of a neuromuscular blocking agent with vagolytic activity, such as pancuronium or gallamine, may prevent bradycardia caused by sufentanil. • If respiratory depression persists following surgery, prolonged mechanical ventilation may be necessary. If an opioid antagonist is required to reverse respiratory depression or coma, naloxone (Narcan) is the antidote. Dilute the 0.4-mg ampule of naloxone in 10 ml of 0.9% NaCl and administer 0.5 ml (0.02 mg) by direct IV push every 2 minutes. For children and patients weighing <40 kg, dilute 0.1 mg of naloxone in 10 ml of 0.9% NaCl for a concentration of 10 mcg/ml and administer 0.5 mcg every 1–2 minutes. Titrate the dose to avoid withdrawal, seizures, and severe pain. Administration of naloxone in these circumstances, especially in cardiac patients, has resulted in hypertension and tachycardia, occasionally causing left ventricular failure and pulmonary edema. Monitor respiratory status continuously; the duration of respiratory depression may exceed the duration of a dose of naloxone. Continuous infusion of naloxone may be required (see *naloxone hydrochloride* monograph on page 690). • If hypotension occurs, administer parenteral fluids, position patient to improve venous return to the heart when surgical conditions permit, and administer a vasopressor as necessary. • If muscle rigidity occurs during surgery, a neuromuscular blocking agent and mechanical ventilation should be used. Muscle rigidity occurring upon emergence may be treated with naloxone.

Lab Test Considerations

- May cause elevated serum amylase and lipase concentrations.

Patient/Family Teaching

- Caution patient to make position changes slowly to minimize orthostatic hypotension. • Medication causes dizziness and drowsiness. Advise patient to call for assistance during ambulation and transfer, and to avoid driving or other activities requiring alertness for at least 24 hours after administration of sufentanil following outpatient surgery and until response to medication is known. • Instruct patient to avoid alcohol and other CNS depressants for 24 hours after administration when sufentanil is used during outpatient surgery.

PHARMACOLOGIC PROFILE

Indications

• Sufentanil is used as an analgesic adjunct when given in the maintenance of balanced anesthesia with barbiturate/nitrous oxide/oxygen. • It is also used as an analgesic administered by continuous IV infusion with nitrous oxide/oxygen while maintaining general anesthesia. • It may also be used in primary induction of anesthesia in major surgical procedures with 100% oxygen.

Action

• Sufentanil binds to opiate receptors in the CNS, altering the response to and perception of pain and causing generalized CNS depression.

Time/Action Profile (analgesia)†

Onset	Peak	Duration
within 1 min	UK	5 min

†At anesthesia adjunct dose.

Pharmacokinetics

• **Distribution:** Sufentanil does not readily penetrate adipose tissue. It crosses the placenta and enters breast milk. • **Metabolism and Excretion:** Sufentanil is mostly metabolized by the liver, with some metabolism in the small intestine. • **Half-life:** 2.7 hours (increased during cardiopulmonary bypass).

Contraindications

• Sufentanil is contraindicated in patients with hypersensitivity or known intolerance.

Adverse Reactions and Side Effects*

• **CNS:** dizziness, sleepiness, drowsiness • **EENT:** blurred vision • **Resp:** apnea, postoperative respiratory depression • **CV:** bradycardia, tachycardia, <u>hypotension</u>, hypertension, arrhythmias • **GI:** nausea, vomiting • **Derm:** itching, erythema • **MS:** thoracic muscle rigidity, intraoperative muscle movement • **Misc:** chills.

Tacrolimus	*Immunosuppressant*
Prograf	**pH UK**

≋ ADMINISTRATION CONSIDERATIONS

Usual Dose
ADULTS: 0.05–0.1 mg/kg/day continuous infusion.
CHILDREN: 0.1 mg/kg/day continuous infusion.

Dilution
• **Continuous Infusion: Dilute** in 0.9% NaCl or D5W for a concentration between 0.004–0.02 mg/ml prior to use.
• May be stored in polyethylene or glass containers for 24 hours following dilution. Do not store in PVC containers.

Rate of Administration
• **Continuous Infusion:** Administer daily dose as a continuous infusion over 24 hours.

≋ CLINICAL PRECAUTIONS

• Therapy with tacrolimus should be started no sooner than 6 hours post-transplant. Concurrent therapy with glucocorticoids is recommended in the early postoperative period. Oral therapy is preferred due to the risk of anaphylactic reactions with IV tacrolimus and should be initiated as soon as possible. Epinephrine and resuscita-

---

*<u>Underlines</u> indicate most frequent; CAPITALS indicate life-threatening.

tive equipment should be readily available. Observe for the development of anaphylaxis (rash, pruritus, laryngeal edema, wheezing) for at least 30 minutes following the first dose and frequently after. If signs develop, stop infusion and initiate treatment.

- IV therapy should be replaced with oral therapy as soon as possible. Initial oral dosage in adults is 0.15 mg/kg/day given in two divided doses every 12 hours and in children 0.3 mg/kg/day in two divided doses every 12 hours. The first oral dose may be given 8–12 hours after stopping IV infusion of tacrolimus.

- Monitor blood pressure closely during therapy. Hypertension is a common complication of tacrolimus therapy and should be treated. Hyperkalemia occurs frequently. Avoid using potassium-sparing diuretics or angiotensin-converting enzyme (ACE) inhibitors.

- Hyperglycemia occurs frequently and may require treatment.

- Concurrent use of tacrolimus with aminoglycoside anti-infectives, amphotericin B, cisplatin, or cyclosporine increases the risk of nephrotoxicity. Tacrolimus and cyclosporine should not be used at the same time. Allow 24 hours to lapse after stopping cyclosporine before beginning tacrolimus.

- The following drugs may increase blood levels of tacrolimus: antifungals, bromocriptine, calcium channel blockers, cimetidine, clarithromycin, cyclosporine, danazol, erythromycin, methylprednisolone, metoclopramide, nicardipine, and verapamil. Tacrolimus blood levels may be decreased by concurrent use of carbamazepine, phenobarbital, phenytoin, or rifamycins.

- The occurrence of hepatic or renal impairment may require dosage adjustment of tacrolimus. Use lower end of dosage range. If oliguria occurs, wait 48 hours before initiating tacrolimus.

- Vaccinations may be less effective if given concurrently with tacrolimus. Avoid use of live vaccinations.

- Children under the age of 12 years generally require higher doses (higher end of dosing range) than adults to maintain adequate blood levels of tacrolimus.

- Hyperkalemia and renal impairment have occurred in the newborn following use of tacrolimus during pregnancy (Pregnancy Category C). Use of tacrolimus in pregnancy is recommended only if benefit to mother justifies the risk to the fetus. Breast-feeding should be avoided.

Lab Test Considerations

• Tacrolimus blood level monitoring may be helpful in the evaluation of rejection and toxicity, dose adjustments, and assessment of compliance. Tacrolimus whole blood concentrations measured with ELISA are variable during the first week post-transplantation. After the first week, median trough blood concentrations range from 9.8–19.4 ng/ml. • Monitor serum creatinine, potassium, and glucose closely. Elevated serum creatinine and decreased urine output may indicate nephrotoxicity. May cause hyperkalemia. Do not use potassium-sparing diuretics. Frequently causes hyperglycemia; may require insulin therapy. • May also cause hyperuricemia, hypokalemia, hypomagnesemia, acidosis, alkalosis, hyperlipidemia, hyperphosphatemia, hypophosphatemia, hypocalcemia, hyponatremia. • Monitor CBC and platelet count. May cause anemia, leukocytosis, and thrombocytopenia.

Patient/Family Teaching

• Emphasize the importance of repeated lab tests during tacrolimus therapy. • Advise patient of the risk of taking tacrolimus during pregnancy. • Inform paient of the increased risk of lymphoma with tacrolimus therapy.

PHARMACOLOGIC PROFILE

Indications

• Tacrolimus is used to prevent organ rejection in patients who have undergone allogeneic liver transplantation.

Action

• Tacrolimus inhibits T-lymphocyte activation.

Time/Action Profile (immunosuppression)

Onset	Peak	Duration
UK	UK	UK

Pharmacokinetics

• **Distribution:** Tacrolimus crosses the placenta and enters breast milk. The remainder of distribution of tacrolimus is not known. • **Metabolism and Excretion:** Tacrolimus is mostly (99%) metabolized by the liver. • **Half-life:** 11.7 hours (liver transplant patients), 21.2 hours (healthy volunteers).

Contraindications

• Tacrolimus should not be used in patients who have hypersensitivity to it or to HCO-60 polyoxyl 60 hydrogenated castor oil (a component of the injection). Concurrent use with cyclosporine should be avoided. • Pregnant or lactating patients should not be given tacrolimus.

Adverse Reactions and Side Effects*

• **CNS:** <u>tremor</u>, <u>headache</u>, SEIZURES, <u>insomnia</u>, abnormal dreams, anxiety, agitation, confusion, depression, dizziness, emotional lability, hallucinations, psychoses, somnolence • **EENT:** abnormal vision, amblyopia, tinnitus, rhinitis, sinusitis, voice change • **Resp:** asthma, bronchitis, cough, pulmonary edema, pharyngitis, pneumonia • **CV:** <u>hypertension</u>, <u>ascites</u>, <u>peripheral edema</u> • **GI:** <u>nausea</u>, <u>vomiting</u>, <u>anorexia</u>, <u>diarrhea</u>, <u>abdominal pain</u>, cholangitis, cholestatic jaundice, dyspepsia, dysphagia, flatulence, GI PERFORATION, GI HEMORRHAGE, increased appetite, jaundice, increased liver function studies, oral thrush, peritonitis • **GU:** <u>nephrotoxicity</u>, <u>urinary tract infection</u> • **Derm:** <u>pruritus</u>, <u>rash</u>, alopecia, herpes simplex, hirsutism, photosensitivity • **F and E:** <u>hyperkalemia</u>, hypokalemia, <u>hyperglycemia</u>, <u>hypomagnesemia</u>, acidosis, alkalosis, hyperlipidemia, hyperphosphatemia, hyperuricemia, hypophosphatemia, hypocalcemia, hyponatremia • **Hemat:** <u>anemia</u>, <u>lymphocytosis</u>, <u>thrombocytopenia</u>, leukopenia, coagulation defects • **MS:** hypertonia, arthralgia, muscle spasm, leg cramps, myalgia, myasthenia, osteoporosis • **Neuro:** <u>paresthesia</u>, neuropathy • **Misc:** allergic reactions including ANAPHYLAXIS, <u>generalized pain</u>, fever, abnormal healing, chills, sweating, increased risk of lymphoma.

---

*<u>Underlines</u> indicate most frequent; CAPITALS indicate life-threatening.

Teniposide	*Antineoplastic agent*
	(podophyllotoxin derivative)
VM-26, Vumon	**pH 5.1**

≋ ADMINISTRATION CONSIDERATIONS

Usual Dose

Several regimens have been used. These are examples.

CHILDREN: Teniposide 165 mg/m^2 in combination with cytarabine 300 mg/m^2 IV twice weekly for 8–9 doses (see *cytarabine* monograph on page 262). Another regimen used teniposide 250 mg/m^2 in combination with vincristine 1.5 mg/m^2 IV weekly for 4–8 wk and with prednisone 40 mg/m^2/day PO for 28 days (see *vincristine sulfate* monograph on page 1030).

Dilution

• **Intermittent Infusion:** Dilute with D5W or 0.9% NaCl for a final concentration of 0.1, 0.2, 0.4, or 1 mg/ml.
• Concentrated teniposide is clear but may develop a slight opalescence when diluted in solution. Do not shake or agitate unnecessarily. Precipitation may occur at recommended concentrations. Solution must be prepared and administered in nonplastic equipment to prevent cracking of plastic and possible drug leakage. Glass or polyolefin plastic bags or containers should be used; PVC containers are not recommended.
• Solutions should be prepared in a biologic cabinet. Wear gloves, gown, and mask while handling medication. Discard equipment in specially designated containers (see Appendix F). • Concentrations of 1 mg/ml should be administered within 4 hours of dilution. Diluted solutions are stable for 24 hours at room temperature. Do not refrigerate.

Compatibility

• **Y-site:** ondansetron ♦ sargramostim.
• **Solution:** D5W ♦ 0.9% NaCl ♦ lactated Ringer's injection.

Incompatibility

• **Y-site/Additive:** heparin. Flush IV line with D5W or 0.9% NaCl only. Do not admix or administer via Y-site with other medications or solutions.

Rate of Administration

- **Intermittent Infusion:** Administer over 30–60 minutes or longer. Do not give by rapid infusion; may result in hypotension.

≋ CLINICAL PRECAUTIONS

- Ensure patency of IV prior to administration. Teniposide is an irritant. Observe IV frequently for redness or irritation. Extravasation may lead to local tissue necrosis, or thrombophlebitis may occur. If extravasation occurs, mix 150 units of hyaluronidase with 1 ml of 0.9% NaCl for a concentration of 150 units/ml and inject 1–4 ml, 1 ml for each ml extravasated, through existing IV cannula or inject SC if the needle has been removed. This enhances absorption and dispersion of extravasated teniposide. Apply warm compresses to increase the systemic absorption of the drug.
- Observe infusion frequently as occlusion of central venous access devices may occur.
- Monitor blood pressure frequently during infusion.
- Monitor for hypersensitivity reaction (fever, chills, pruritus, urticaria, bronchospasm, tachycardia, hypotension). If these occur, stop the infusion. Keep epinephrine, an antihistamine, and resuscitative equipment close by in the event of an anaphylactic reaction.
- Monitor for bone marrow depression. Assess for fever, chills, sore throat, and signs of infection. Assess for bleeding (bleeding gums, bruising, petechiae; guaiac test stools, urine, and emesis). Avoid giving IM injections and taking rectal temperatures. Apply pressure to venipuncture sites for 10 minutes. Additive bone marrow depression may occur with other antineoplastic agents or radiation therapy.
- Monitor intake and output, appetite, and nutritional intake. Teniposide causes nausea and vomiting in 30% of patients. Antiemetics may be used prophylactically. Adjust diet as tolerated to help maintain fluid and electrolyte balance and nutritional status.
- Use cautiously in patients with Down's syndrome as these patients are more susceptible to the myelosuppressive effects of teniposide. Initial dose of first course of therapy should be reduced by 50%.

- Use with caution in patients with hepatic impairment, active infections, decreased bone marrow reserve, or other chronic debilitating illnesses.
- Use cautiously in patients with childbearing potential. Avoid using teniposide during pregnancy or lactation (Pregnancy Category D).

Lab Test Considerations

- Monitor CBC and differential prior to and periodically throughout therapy. Nadirs for leukopenia and thrombocytopenia occur on days 16–18 of therapy. Recovery occurs in approximately 15 days. Anemia occurs infrequently. Therapy may be discontinued if platelet count is less than 50,000/mm^3 or absolute neutrophil count is less than 500/mm^3. • Monitor liver function studies (AST [SGOT], ALT [SGPT], LDH, bilirubin) and renal function studies (BUN, creatinine) prior to and periodically throughout therapy to detect hepatotoxicity and nephrotoxicity. • May cause increased uric acid. Monitor levels periodically during therapy.

Patient/Family Teaching

- Advise patient to notify physician if fever, chills, sore throat, signs of infection, bleeding gums, bruising, petechiae, or blood in urine, stool, or emesis occurs. Caution patient to avoid crowds and persons with known infections. Instruct patient to use soft toothbrush and electric razor. • Patient should be cautioned not to drink alcoholic beverages or take products containing aspirin, ibuprofen, or naproxen. • Instruct patient to notify physician if abdominal pain, yellow skin, weakness, paresthesia, or gait disturbances occur. • Instruct patient to inspect oral mucosa for redness and ulceration. If mouth sores occur, advise patient to use sponge brush and rinse mouth with water after eating and drinking. • Discuss with patient the possibility of hair loss. Explore coping strategies. • Advise patient to use a nonhormonal method of contraception. • Instruct patient not to receive any vaccinations without advice of physician. • Emphasize the need for periodic lab tests to monitor for side effects.

PHARMACOLOGIC PROFILE

Indications
• Teniposide is used in combination with other agents for induction therapy for refractory acute lymphoblastic leukemia in children.

Action
• Teniposide damages DNA prior to mitosis (cycle-dependent and phase specific), resulting in death of rapidly replicating cells, particularly malignant ones.

Time/Action Profile (effects on blood counts)

Onset	Peak	Duration
UK	UK	UK

Pharmacokinetics
• **Distribution:** Teniposide has limited distribution into the CSF. • **Metabolism and Excretion:** 44% of teniposide is excreted by the kidneys; 10% or less is eliminated in feces. • **Half-life:** 5 hours.

Contraindications
• Teniposide is contraindicated in patients with hypersensitivity to it and should be avoided in patients with known intolerance to castor oil, ethyl alcohol, or benzyl alcohol. • Pregnant or lactating patients should not receive teniposide. • Preparations containing benzyl alcohol should be avoided in newborns.

Adverse Reactions and Side Effects*
• **CNS:** acute CNS depression, transient cortical blindness • **CV:** hypotension • **GI:** <u>nausea</u>, <u>vomiting</u>, <u>mucositis</u>, <u>diarrhea</u> • **Derm:** alopecia, rashes • **Endo:** gonadal suppression • **Hemat:** <u>leukopenia</u>, <u>thrombocytopenia</u>, <u>anemia</u> • **Local:** phlebitis at IV site • **Neuro:** peripheral neurotoxicity • **Misc:** allergic reactions including ANAPHYLAXIS, fever.

---

*<u>Underlines</u> indicate most frequent; CAPITALS indicate life-threatening.

Terbutaline Sulfate
Tocolytic
(beta-adrenergic agonist)

Brethine, Bricanyl   pH 3–5

 ADMINISTRATION CONSIDERATIONS

Terbutaline is not approved for IV use. All doses are unlabeled.

Usual Dose

ADULTS: Begin infusion at 10 mcg/min. Increase dosage by 5 mcg q 10 min until contractions cease. Maximal dose is 80 mcg/min. Begin to taper dose in 5-mcg decrements after a 30–60-min contraction-free period is attained. Switch to oral dosage form after patient is contraction-free for 4–8 hr on the lowest effective dose.

Dilution

- **Continuous Infusion:** May be diluted with D5W, 0.45% NaCl, or 0.9% NaCl.

Compatibility

- **Y-site:** insulin.
- **Additive:** aminophylline.

Incompatibility

- **Additive:** bleomycin.

Rate of Administration

- **Continuous Infusion:** Use infusion pump to ensure accurate dosage. See Usual Dose for rate of administration.

 CLINICAL PRECAUTIONS

- Monitor maternal pulse and blood pressure, frequency and duration of contractions, and fetal heart rate. Dose modification or discontinuation may be required if contractions persist or increase in frequency or duration. If symptoms of maternal or fetal distress occur, other interventions may be required. Maternal side effects include tachycardia, palpitations, tremor, anxiety, and headache.
- Assess maternal respiratory status for symptoms of pulmonary edema (increased rate, dyspnea, rales/crackles, frothy sputum).

- Monitor mother and neonate for symptoms of hypoglycemia (anxiety, chills, cold sweats, confusion, cool pale skin, difficulty in concentration, drowsiness, excessive hunger, headache, irritability, nausea, nervousness, rapid pulse, shakiness, unusual tiredness or weakness) and mother for hypokalemia (weakness, fatigue, U wave on ECG, arrhythmias).
- Use cautiously in patients with cardiac disease, hypertension, hyperthyroidism, diabetes mellitus, history of seizures, or glaucoma.
- Terbutaline causes additive adrenergic effects with other adrenergic (sympathomimetic) agents, including decongestants, and vasopressors. Concurrent use with MAO inhibitors may lead to hypertensive crisis. Concurrent use with beta-adrenergic blockers may block therapeutic effect.
- Use cautiously in pregnant patients near term (Pregnancy Category B).

Lab Test Considerations

- Monitor maternal serum glucose and electrolytes. May cause hypokalemia and hypoglycemia. • Monitor neonate's serum glucose, as hypoglycemia may also occur in neonate.

Patient/Family Teaching

- Instruct patient to notify physician or nurse immediately if labor resumes or significant side effects occur.

≋ PHARMACOLOGIC PROFILE

Indications

- Terbutaline is used as a tocolytic to arrest preterm labor (unlabeled).

Action

- Terbutaline is a beta-adrenergic agonist which produces accumulation of cyclic adenosine monophosphate (cAMP). Results of increased levels of cAMP at beta-adrenergic receptors include bronchodilation, CNS and cardiac stimulation, diuresis, gastric acid secretion, and relaxation of uterine smooth muscle. It is relatively selective for beta$_2$ (pulmonary) receptors.

Time/Action Profile

Onset	Peak	Duration
within 15 min	30–60 min	1.5–4 hr

Pharmacokinetics

• **Distribution:** Terbutaline enters breast milk. • **Metabolism and Excretion:** Terbutaline is partially metabolized by the liver. Sixty percent is execreted unchanged by the kidneys and 3% in feces. • **Half-life:** UK.

Contraindications

• Terbutaline is contraindicated in patients with hypersensitivity to adrenergic amines. • Terbutaline should be avoided in situations in which continuation of pregnancy is hazardous (antepartum hemorrhage, eclampsia, intrauterine death, abruptio placentae, placenta previa, chorioamnionitis, fetal malformation incompatible with life).

Adverse Reactions and Side Effects*

• **CNS:** <u>nervousness</u>, <u>restlessness</u>, insomnia, <u>tremor</u>, headache, anxiety, drowsiness • **CV:** hypertension, arrhythmias, angina, tachycardia, palpitations, PULMONARY EDEMA • **GI:** nausea, vomiting, unusual taste • **F and E:** hypokalemia • **MS:** muscle cramps, twitching.

Theophylline	*Bronchodilator (phosphodiesterase inhibitor), Respiratory stimulant*
	pH 4.3

≋ ADMINISTRATION CONSIDERATIONS

Usual Dose

Bronchodilator

ADULTS: 5 mg/kg initially over 20–30 min, then in *otherwise healthy nonsmoking adults*—0.43 mg/kg/hr; *young adult*

---

*<u>Underlines</u> indicate most frequent; CAPITALS indicate life-threatening.

smokers—0.7 mg/kg/hr; *patients >60 yr or patients with cor pulmonale*—0.26 mg/kg/hr; *patients with congestive heart failure or liver disease*—0.2 mg/kg/hr. Maintenance infusion rates may be decreased after 12 hr.

CHILDREN 12–16 yr: 5 mg/kg initially, then in *nonsmokers*—0.5 mg/kg/hr; *smokers*—0.7 mg/kg/hr.

CHILDREN 9–12 yr: 5 mg/kg initially, then 0.7 mg/kg/hr.

CHILDREN 1–9 yr: 5 mg/kg initially, then 0.8 mg/kg/hr.

CHILDREN UP TO 1 yr: 5 mg/kg initially, then dose in mg/kg/hr = (0.008) (age in weeks) + 0.21.

Respiratory Stimulant

NEONATES: 5 mg/kg initially, then 1–1.5 mg/kg q 12 hr.

Dilution

• **Continuous Infusion:** IV theophylline and 5% dextrose is packed in a moisture barrier overwrap. Remove immediately before administration and squeeze bag to check for leaks. Discard if solution is not clear. Available in varying concentrations.

Compatibility

• **Y-site:** acyclovir • diltiazem • famotidine • haloperidol.
• **Additive:** fluconazole • methylprednisolone • verapamil.

Incompatibility

• **Y-site:** hetastarch.
• **Additive:** ascorbic acid • chlorpromazine • corticotropin • dimenhydrinate • erythromycin glucepate • hydralazine • methicillin • papaverine • penicillin G • phenytoin • prochlorperazine • promazine • promethazine • vancomycin.

Rate of Administration

• **Continuous Infusion:** Administer loading dose over 20 minutes. • Do not exceed 20–25 mg/min. Rapid administration may cause hypotension, arrhythmias, syncope, and death. Administer via infusion pump to ensure accurate dosage.

≋ CLINICAL PRECAUTIONS

• Assess blood pressure, pulse, and respiratory status (rate, lung sounds, use of accessory muscles) prior to and throughout therapy. Monitor ECG continuously, as tachyarrhythmias may occur. Ensure that oxygen, fluid, and electrolyte therapy are correctly instituted.

- Monitor intake and output ratios for an increase in diuresis or fluid overload due to volume of medication. Patients with a history of cardiovascular problems should be monitored for ECG changes.

- If patient has had another form of theophylline prior to loading dose, serum theophylline level should be obtained and loading dose proportionately reduced. In emergency situations when serum level is not available, half the usual loading dose may be given if no symptoms of theophylline toxicity are present. Dose should be based on ideal body weight in obese patients.

- Wait at least 4 hours after discontinuing IV therapy to begin immediate-release oral dosage; for extended-release oral dosage form, administer first oral dose at time of IV discontinuation.

- Additive cardiovascular and CNS side effects may occur with concurrent use of adrenergic (sympathomimetic) agents. Theophylline may decrease the therapeutic effect of lithium. Smoking, phenobarbital, rifampin, phenytoin, and ketoconazole increase metabolism and may decrease effectiveness of theophylline. Erythromycin, beta-adrenergic blockers, influenza vaccine, cimetidine, oral contraceptives, glucocorticoids, disulfiram, interferon, mexiletine, fluoroquinolones, thiabendazole, and large doses of allopurinol decrease metabolism and may lead to theophylline toxicity. The risk of arrhythmias is increased by concurrent use of halothane, isoniazid, carbamazepine, or loop diuretics, which may increase or decrease theophylline levels.

- Use theophylline cautiously in patients over 60 years old or those with liver disease as dosage reduction is required. Use with caution in patients with CHF or cor pulmonale. Cigarette smokers may require larger doses.

- Theophylline has been used safely during pregnancy, but may cause tachycardia, jitteriness, irritability, gagging, or vomiting in neonates. Monitor infants born to mothers taking theophylline for potential toxicity (Pregnancy Category C). Since theophylline enters breast milk in significant concentrations, infants of mothers receiving theophylline may experience fretfulness, irritability, or insomnia.

Toxicity and Overdose

• Monitor drug levels routinely. Therapeutic plasma levels range from 10–20 mcg/ml. • Observe patients closely for the appearance of progressive theophylline toxicity (anorexia, nausea, vomiting, restlessness, insomnia, tachycardia, arrhythmias, seizures). Drug levels of more than 20 mcg/ml are associated with progressive toxicity. Caffeine ingestion may falsely elevate drug concentration levels.

Lab Test Considerations

• Monitor ABGs and serum electrolytes prior to and periodically throughout therapy.

Patient/Family Teaching

• Encourage patient to drink adequate liquids (2000 ml/day minimum) to decrease the viscosity of airway secretions. • Advise patient to minimize intake of xanthine-containing foods or beverages (cola, coffee, chocolate) and not to eat charcoal-broiled foods daily. Additive adverse reactions may occur with excessive ingestion of xanthine (caffeine)-containing food or beverages, and excess consumption of charcoal-broiled beef may decrease effectiveness. • Encourage patient not to smoke. Instruct patient to inform physician if smoking pattern changes, as dosage adjustment may be necessary. • Emphasize the importance of having serum levels routinely tested every 6–12 months.

PHARMACOLOGIC PROFILE

Indications

• Theophylline is used as a bronchodilator in reversible airway obstruction due to asthma or COPD. • It is also used as a respiratory and myocardial stimulant in apnea of infancy (unlabeled use).

Action

• Theophylline inhibits phosphodiesterase, producing increased tissue concentrations of cyclic adenosine monophosphate (cAMP). Increased levels of cAMP result in bronchodilation, CNS and cardiac stimulation, diuresis, and gastric acid secretion.

Time/Action Profile (bronchodilation)

Onset	Peak	Duration
rapid	end of infusion	6–8 hr

Pharmacokinetics

• **Distribution:** Theophylline is widely distributed. It crosses the placenta. Breast milk concentrations are 70% of plasma levels. • **Metabolism and Excretion:** Theophylline is mostly metabolized by the liver to caffeine, which may accumulate in neonates. Metabolites are renally excreted. • **Half-life:** 3–13 hours (increased in patients over 60 years of age, neonates, and patients with CHF or liver disease; decreased in cigarette smokers and children).

Contraindications

• Theophylline is contraindicated in patients with uncontrolled arrhythmias or hyperthyroidism.

Adverse Reactions and Side Effects*

• **CNS:** <u>nervousness</u>, <u>anxiety</u>, headache, insomnia, SEIZURES
• **CV:** <u>tachycardia</u>, palpitations, arrhythmias, angina pectoris
• **GI:** <u>nausea</u>, <u>vomiting</u>, anorexia, cramps • **Neuro:** tremor.

Thiamine	*Vitamin* *(water soluble)*
{Betaxin}, Biamine	pH 2.5–4.5

☰ ADMINISTRATION CONSIDERATIONS

Usual Dose

Thiamine Deficiency (Beriberi)

ADULTS: 50–100 mg 3 times daily. *Wet beriberi with heart failure*—10–30 mg 3 times daily.
CHILDREN: 10–25 mg/day.

---

*Underlines indicate most frequent; CAPITALS indicate life-threatening.

{} = Available in Canada only.

Wernicke's Encephalopathy

Adults: 100 mg initially, then 50–100 mg/day until nutritional status improves. Institute therapy prior to high carbohydrate diet or IV dextrose.

Dilution

• **Direct IV:** May be administered **undiluted.** • **Continuous Infusion:** May be **diluted** in dextrose/Ringer's or lactated Ringer's combinations, dextrose/saline combinations, D5W, D10W, Ringer's and lactated Ringer's injection, 0.9% NaCl, or 0.45% NaCl and is usually administered with other vitamins.

Compatibility

• **Y-site:** famotidine.

Incompatibility

• **Additive:** barbiturates • solutions with neutral or alkaline pH, such as carbonates, bicarbonates, citrates, and acetates • erythromycin • kanamycin • streptomycin.

Rate of Administration

• **Direct IV:** Administer each 100 mg over at least 5 minutes.

≋ CLINICAL PRECAUTIONS

• Sensitivity reactions and deaths have occurred from IV administration. An intradermal test dose is recommended in patients with suspected sensitivity. Monitor for erythema and induration. Monitor patients receiving IV thiamine for anaphylaxis (wheezing, urticaria, edema). Parenteral administration is reserved for patients in whom oral administration is not feasible.

• Because of infrequency of single B-vitamin deficiencies, combinations are commonly administered.

• Assess patient for signs and symptoms of thiamine deficiency (anorexia, GI distress, irritability, palpitations, tachycardia, edema, paresthesia, muscle weakness and pain, depression, memory loss, confusion, psychosis, visual disturbances, elevated serum pyruvic acid levels).

• Assess patient's nutritional status (diet, weight) prior to and throughout course of therapy.

- When used in the prevention of Wernicke's encephalopathy, condition may be worsened unless thiamine is administered *before* glucose.
- Thiamine may enhance the effects of neuromuscular blocking agents.
- Thiamine has been used safely during pregnancy (Pregnancy Category A).

Lab Test Considerations

- Thiamine may interfere with certain methods of testing serum theophylline, uric acid, and urobilinogen concentrations.

Patient/Family Teaching

- Encourage patient to comply with physician's dietary recommendations. Explain that the best source of vitamins is a well-balanced diet with foods from the four basic food groups. Teach patient that foods high in thiamine include cereals (whole grain and enriched), meats (especially pork), and fresh vegetables; loss is variable during cooking. Caution patients self-medicating with vitamin supplements not to exceed RDA (see Appendix I).

≋ PHARMACOLOGIC PROFILE

Indications

- Thiamine is used in the treatment of thiamine deficiencies (beriberi), in the prevention of Wernicke's encephalopathy, and as a dietary supplement in patients with GI disease, alcoholism, or cirrhosis.

Action

- Thiamine is required for carbohydrate metabolism.

Time/Action Profile (Time for symptoms of deficiency [edema and heart failure] to resolve; confusion and psychosis take longer to respond.)

Onset	Peak	Duration
hours	days	days–weeks

Pharmacokinetics

• **Distribution:** Thiamine is widely distributed and enters breast milk. • **Metabolism and Excretion:** Thiamine is metabolized by the liver. Excess amounts are excreted unchanged by the kidneys. • **Half-life:** UK.

Contraindications

• Thiamine is contraindicated in patients with hypersensitivity to it or to formaldehyde or chlorobutanol.

Adverse Reactions and Side Effects*

• **CNS:** weakness, restlessness • **EENT:** tightness of the throat • **CV:** hypotension, VASCULAR COLLAPSE, vasodilation • **Resp:** respiratory distress, pulmonary edema • **GI:** nausea, GI bleeding • **Derm:** warmth, tingling, pruritus, urticaria, sweating, cyanosis • **Misc:** angioedema.

Thiopental Sodium	*Anesthetic, Anticonvulsant*
	(barbiturate)
Pentothal	**pH 10–11 (2.5% solution)**

Schedule III

 ADMINISTRATION CONSIDERATIONS

Usual Dose

Dosages must be carefully titrated by patient response.

Test Dose

ADULTS: 25–75 mg.

Anesthesia

ADULTS: 50–100 mg initially, followed by 50–100 mg as needed or 3–5 mg/kg as a single dose.

CHILDREN UP TO 15 yr: 3–5 mg/kg initially, followed by 1 mg/ kg as needed.

---

*Underlines indicate most frequent; CAPITALS indicate life-threatening.

Anticonvulsant

Adults: 50–125 mg (up to 250 mg may be required).

Children: 30 mg/kg loading dose; may be followed by 5–20 mg/kg/hr maintenance dose.

Narcoanalysis

Adults: 100 mg/min until patient becomes confused.

Increased Intracranial Pressure

Adults: 1.5–3.5 mg/kg as needed.

Dilution

• **Direct IV: Dilute** thiopental with sterile water for injection, D5W, or 0.9% NaCl. Solution should be freshly prepared and used within 24 hours of reconstitution. Refrigerate and keep tightly sealed. Do not administer solution containing a precipitate. • **Intermittent Infusion:** 2% or 2.5% concentration (20–25 mg/ml) of thiopental is used for intermittent infusion. • **Continuous Infusion:** Solutions of 0.2–0.4% concentration (2–4 mg/ml) have been administered by continuous infusion to maintain anesthesia when thiopental is the sole agent.

Compatibility

• **Syringe:** aminophylline • hyaluronidase • hydrocortisone sodium succinate • neostigmine • pentobarbital • scopolamine • tubocurarine.

• **Additive:** chloramphenicol • hydrocortisone sodium succinate • oxytocin • potassium chloride • sodium bicarbonate.

• **Solution:** D5/0.45% NaCl, D5W, multiple electrolyte solutions, 0.45% NaCl, 0.9% NaCl, and ⅙ M sodium lactate.

Incompatibility

• **Syringe:** benzquinamide • chlorpromazine • clindamycin • cimetidine • dimenhydrinate • diphenhydramine • doxapram • droperidol • ephedrine • fentanyl • glycopyrrolate • meperidine • morphine • pancuronium • pentazocine • prochlorperazine • promethazine • propiomazine • sodium bicarbonate • trimethaphan.

• **Additive:** amikacin • atracurium • cephapirin • chlorpromazine • cimetidine • clindamycin • codeine • dimenhydrinate • diphenhydramine • droperidol • fentanyl • fibrinolysin • hydromorphone • regular insulin • levorphanol • meperidine • metaraminol • methadone • morphine

• norepinephrine • penicillin G potassium • prochlorperazine • promazine • promethazine • succinylcholine • trimethaphan camsylate.

• **Solution:** dextrose/Ringer's or lactated Ringer's injection combinations • D10/0.9% NaCl • D10W • Ringer's and lactated Ringer's injection.

Rate of Administration

• **Direct IV:** Administer slowly. Rapid administration may cause overdose. • When thiopental is used as the sole anesthetic agent, small repeated doses may be used to maintain desired level of anesthesia.

≋ CLINICAL PRECAUTIONS

• Thiopental should be used only by individuals qualified to administer anesthesia and experienced in endotracheal intubation. Equipment for this procedure should be immediately available.

• A test dose of 25–75 mg (1–3 ml of a 2.5% soution) may be administered to determine tolerance or unusual sensitivity to thiopental. Observe patient for at least 60 seconds.

• Administer premedication with anticholinergics (atropine, glycopyrrolate) to decrease mucous secretions. Opioid analgesics may be administered preoperatively because of the lack of analgesic effects of thiopental. Administer preoperative medications so peak effects are attained shortly before induction of anesthesia.

• Administer muscle relaxants separately. Concurrent use of nitrous oxide 67% decreases the requirements for thiopental by two thirds.

• Assess blood pressure, ECG, heart rate, and respiratory status continuously throughout thiopental therapy. Monitor for apnea immediately after IV injection, especially in the presence of opioid analgesic premedication.

• Monitor IV site carefully. Extravasation may cause pain, swelling, ulceration, and necrosis.

• Assess level of consciousness and intracranial pressure in patients treated for increased intracranial pressure before and throughout therapy.

- Additive CNS depression may occur with other CNS depressants, including alcohol, antihistamines, antidepressants, opioid analgesics, and sedative/hypnotics. The risk of hypotension is increased with antihypertensives, diuretics, or ketamine.
- Use cautiously in patients with severe cardiovascular disease, shock or hypotension, myxedema, Addison's disease, increased intracranial pressure, liver disease, renal disease, or myasthenia gravis.
- Middle-aged, elderly, or debilitated patients may require dosage reduction. Tolerance may develop with repeated doses. Repeated doses, large doses, or prolonged infusion in 24-hour period may result in excessive somnolence or respiratory or circulatory depression. Dosage reduction is required in these situations.
- Safe use in pregnancy or lactation has not been established (Pregnancy Category C). Avoid during pregnancy; CNS depression may occur in newborn.

Toxicity and Overdose Alert

- Monitor for signs of overdose, which may occur from rapid injections (drop in blood pressure, possibly to shock levels) or excessive or repeated injections (respiratory distress, laryngospasm, apnea).

Patient/Family Teaching

- Thiopental may cause psychomotor impairment for 24 hours following administration. Caution patient to avoid driving or other activities requiring alertness for 24 hours. • Advise patient to avoid use of alcohol or other CNS depressants for 24 hours following anesthesia, unless directed by physician or dentist.

≋ PHARMACOLOGIC PROFILE

Indications

- Thiopental is used to provide an unconscious state as part of balanced anesthesia in combination with muscle relaxants and/or analgesics during short surgical procedures. • It is also used in the treatment of seizures, as part of narcoanalysis or narcosynthesis in psychiatric patients, and in the management of increased intracranial pressure.

Action

• Thiopental produces all levels of CNS depression. It depresses the sensory cortex, decreases motor activity, alters cerebellar function, inhibits transmission in the nervous system, and raises the seizure threshold. • Thiopental induces sleep and anesthesia without analgesia (short-acting), decreases seizure activity, and lowers intracranial pressure.

Time/Action Profile (anesthetic effects)

Onset	Peak	Duration
30–60 sec	UK	10–30 min

Pharmacokinetics

• **Distribution:** Thiopental is rapidly distributed to the CNS, then redistributed to viscera (liver, kidneys, heart), then to muscle, and finally to fat. It crosses the placenta readily. Small amounts enter breast milk. • **Metabolism and Excretion:** Thiopental is mostly metabolized by the liver. Small amounts are converted to pentobarbital. • **Half-life:** 12 hours (increased in obese patients and in pregnant patients at term).

Contraindications

• Thiopental is contraindicated in patients with hypersensitivity to it, and in those with porphyria or status asthmaticus.

Adverse Reactions and Side Effects*

• **CNS:** emergence delirium, headache, prolonged somnolence • **EENT:** salivation • **Resp:** respiratory depression, APNEA, laryngospasm, bronchospasm, hiccups, sneezing, coughing • **CV:** hypotension, myocardial depression, arrhythmias • **GI:** nausea, vomiting • **Derm:** erythema, pruritus, urticaria, rashes • **Local:** pain, phlebitis at IV site • **MS:** skeletal muscle hyperactivity • **Misc:** allergic reactions including ANAPHYLAXIS, shivering.

---

*Underlines indicate most frequent; CAPITALS indicate life-threatening.

Thiotepa	*Antineoplastic agent* *(alkylating agent)*
	pH 7.6

☰ ADMINISTRATION CONSIDERATIONS

Usual Dose

Palliative Therapy of Breast, Ovarian Cancer

ADULTS: 300–400 mcg (0.3–0.4 mg)/kg q 1–4 wk *or* 200 mcg (0.2 mg)/kg (6 mg/m^2) daily for 4–5 days q 2–4 wk.

Dilution

• **Direct IV: Reconstitute** 15 mg of powder with 1.5 ml of sterile water for injection for a concentration of 10 mg/ml. • Solution should be prepared in a biologic cabinet. Wear gloves, gown, and mask while handling medication. Discard equipment in designated containers (see Appendix F). • Solution is clear to slightly opaque. Do not use solution that is cloudy or that contains precipitate. Stable for 5 days if refrigerated after reconstitution. • **Intermittent Infusion: Dilute further** in 50–100 ml of 0.9% NaCl, D5W, dextrose/saline combinations, Ringer's or lactated Ringer's solution.

Compatibility

• **Syringe:** procaine hydrochloride 2% ✦ epinephrine 1:1000.

• **Y-site:** allopurinol sodium ✦ melphalan ✦ piperacillin/tazobactam.

Incompatibility

• **Y-site:** filgrastim ✦ vinorelbine.

• **Additive:** cisplatin.

Rate of Administration

• **Direct IV:** Following reconstitution, may be administered undiluted over 1–3 minutes.

☰ CLINICAL PRECAUTIONS

• Monitor vital signs prior to and periodically during therapy.
• Monitor for bone marrow depression. Assess for fever, chills, sore throat, and signs of infection. Assess for

bleeding (bleeding gums, bruising, petechiae; guaiac test stools, urine, and emesis). Avoid IM injections and rectal temperatures. Apply pressure to venipuncture site for 10 minutes. Anemia may occur. Monitor for increased fatigue, dyspnea, and orthostatic hypotension. Additive bone marrow depression may occur with other concurrent use of antineoplastic agents or radiation therapy.

- Monitor intake and output, appetite, and nutritional intake. Assess for nausea, vomiting, and anorexia. Administration of an antiemetic and adjusting diet as tolerated may help maintain fluid and electrolyte balance and nutritional status.

- Monitor for symptoms of gout (increased uric acid, joint pain, edema). Encourage patient to drink at least 2 liters of fluids/day. Allopurinol or alkalinization of urine may be used to decrease uric acid levels.

- Thiotepa may prolong apnea after succinylcholine administration.

- Use cautiously in patients with active infections, decreased bone marrow reserve, chronic debilitating illnesses, or severe hepatic or renal disease.

- Thiotepa should be used cautiously in patients with childbearing potential. Avoid use during pregnancy or lactation. Safe use in children has not been established.

Lab Test Considerations

• Monitor CBC and differential prior to and weekly throughout therapy and for at least 3 weeks after therapy. The nadir of leukopenia occurs after 10–14 days, although it may be delayed up to 1 month. To prevent irreversible bone marrow depression, therapy should be discontinued or dose reduced at the first sign of a sudden large decrease in the leukocyte (especially granulocyte) or platelet count. Resume therapy when leukocyte count is >2000/mm^3 and thrombocyte count is >50,000/mm^3. • Monitor for increased AST (SGOT), ALT (SGPT), LDH, serum bilirubin, uric acid, creatinine, and BUN.

Patient/Family Teaching

• Instruct patient to notify physician in the event of fever, chills, sore throat, signs of infection, bleeding gums, bruising, petechiae, or blood in urine, stool, or emesis.

Caution patient to avoid crowds and persons with known infections. Instruct patient to use soft toothbrush and electric razor. • Caution patient not to drink alcoholic beverages or take products containing aspirin, ibuprofen, or naproxen. • Instruct patient to inspect oral mucosa for redness and ulceration. If ulceration occurs, advise patient to use sponge brush and rinse mouth with water after eating and drinking. Analgesic therapy may be required if pain interferes with eating. • This drug may cause gonadal suppression; however, patient should still use a nonhormonal method of birth control. Advise patient to inform physician immediately if pregnancy is suspected. • Discuss possibility of hair loss with patient. Explore methods of coping. • Instruct patient not to receive any vaccinations without advice of physician. Thiotepa may decrease antibody response to live virus vaccines and increase the risk of adverse reactions. • Advise patient of need for medical follow-up and frequent lab tests.

PHARMACOLOGIC PROFILE

Indications

• IV thiotepa is used in the palliative treatment for breast and ovarian cancer. • It may also be used for intracavitary instillation in the prevention of recurrent malignant effusions in pleura, pericardium, or peritoneum.

Action

• Thiotepa disrupts protein, DNA, and RNA synthesis by cross-linking strands of DNA and RNA (cell cycle–phase nonspecific), resulting in death of rapidly replicating cells, particularly malignant ones. It also has immunosuppressive properties.

Time/Action Profile (noted as effects on blood counts)

Onset	Peak	Duration
10 days	14 days	21 days (up to 30 days)

Pharmacokinetics

• **Distribution:** UK. • **Metabolism and Excretion:** Thiotepa is extensively metabolized. • **Half-life:** UK.

Contraindications

• Thiotepa is contraindicated in patients with hypersensitivity to it. • It should be avoided during pregnancy or lactation.

Adverse Reactions and Side Effects*

• **CNS:** headache, dizziness • **EENT:** tightness of the throat • **GI:** nausea, anorexia, vomiting, stomatitis • **GU:** gonadal suppression • **Derm:** alopecia, rash, pruritus, hives • **Hemat:** <u>thrombocytopenia</u>, <u>leukopenia</u>, <u>anemia</u> • **Local:** pain at IV site • **Metab:** hyperuricemia • **Misc:** fever, allergic reactions.

Ticarcillin Disodium	*Anti-infective*
	(extended-spectrum penicillin)
Ticar	**pH 6–8**
	5.2–6.5 mEq Na/g

≋ ADMINISTRATION CONSIDERATIONS

Usual Dose

ADULTS AND CHILDREN ≥40 kg: *Most serious infections*—3 g q 4 hr or 4 g q 6 hr (up to 24 g/day); *complicated urinary tract infections*—3 g q 6 hr; *uncomplicated urinary tract infections*—1 g q 6 hr.

CHILDREN <40 kg: *Most serious infections*—33.3–50 mg/kg q 4 hr or 50–75 mg/kg q 6 hr; *complicated urinary tract infections*—25–33.3 mg/kg q 4 hr or 37.5–50 mg/kg q 6 hr; *uncomplicated urinary tract infections*—12.5–25 mg/kg q 6 hr or 16.7–33.3 mg/kg q 8 hr.

NEONATES ≥2 kg: 75 mg/kg q 8 hr; increase to 75 mg/kg q 6 hr after 7 days of life.

NEONATES <2 kg: 75 mg/kg q 12 hr; increase to 75 mg/kg q 8 hr after 7 days of life.

---

*<u>Underlines</u> indicate most frequent; CAPITALS indicate life-threatening.

Dilution

• **Direct IV: Constitute with** at least 4 ml of sterile water for injection to each 1-g vial for a concentration of 200 mg/ml. Concentrations of <50 mg/ml are preferred for peripheral administration to avoid vein irritation. Dilution with sterile water for injection for a concentration of 90 mg/ml may be used in patients with fluid restriction. • **Intermittent Infusion: Further dilute** for a concentration of 10–100 mg/ml with 0.9% NaCl, D5W, Ringer's or lactated Ringer's solution. • Solution is stable for 48 hours at room temperature, 14 days if refrigerated.

Compatibility

• **Y-site:** acyclovir • allopurinol sodium • cyclophosphamide • diltiazem • famotidine • filgrastim • fludarabine • hydromorphone • insulin • magnesium sulfate • melphalan • meperidine • morphine • ondansetron • perphenazine • sargramostim • verapamil • vinorelbine.

• **Additive:** ranitidine • verapamil.

Incompatibility

• **Y-site:** fluconazole. • If aminoglycosides and penicillins or cephalosporins must be given concurrently, administer in separate sites, at least 1 hour apart.

Rate of Administration

• **Direct IV:** Administer as slowly as possible to minimize vein irritation. • **Intermittent Infusion:** Administer over 30 minutes–2 hours, 10–20 minutes in neonates.

≋ CLINICAL PRECAUTIONS

• Assess patient for infection (vital signs; appearance of wound, sputum, urine, and stool; WBC) at beginning and throughout course of therapy.

• Obtain specimens for culture and sensitivity prior to initiating therapy. First dose may be given before receiving results.

• Obtain a history before initiating therapy to determine previous use of and reactions to penicillins or cephalosporins. Persons with a negative history of penicillin sensitivity may still have an allergic response. Observe patient for signs and symptoms of anaphylaxis (rash, pruritus, laryngeal edema, wheezing). Discontinue drug immediately if these occur. Keep epinephrine, an antihistamine, and resuscitation equipment close by in the event of an anaphylactic reaction.

- Observe IV site for redness or irritation. Change IV sites every 48 hours to prevent phlebitis.
- Probenecid decreases renal excretion and increases blood levels of ticarcillin. Ticarcillin may alter the excretion of lithium. Diuretics, glucocorticoids, or amphotericin B may increase the risk of hypokalemia. Hypokalemia increases the risk of cardiac glycoside toxicity.
- Use cautiously in patients with renal impairment. Dosage reduction and/or increased dosing interval is required if creatinine clearance is less than 60 ml/min.
- Use with caution in patients with severe liver disease or a history of hypersensitivity reactions to other drugs.
- Safe use in pregnancy and lactation has not been established (Pregnancy Category B).

Lab Test Considerations

- Renal and hepatic function, CBC, serum potassium, and bleeding times should be evaluated prior to and routinely throughout course of therapy. • May cause false-positive urine protein testing and increased BUN, creatinine, AST (SGOT), ALT (SGPT), serum bilirubin, alkaline phosphatase, LDH, and uric acid levels. • May also cause increased bleeding time. • May cause hypernatremia and hypokalemia with high dose.

Patient/Family Teaching

- Advise patient to report the signs of superinfection (black, furry overgrowth on the tongue; vaginal itching or discharge; loose or foul-smelling stools) and allergy.

≋ PHARMACOLOGIC PROFILE

Indications

- Ticarcillin is used in the treatment of the following serious infections due to susceptible organisms: skin and skin structure infections, bone and joint infections, septicemia, respiratory tract infections, intra-abdominal infections, and genitourinary tract infections. • The addition of an amino-glycoside may be synergistic and is recommended against *Pseudomonas.* • Ticarcillin has been combined with other anti-infectives in the treatment of infections in immunosuppressed patients.

Action

• Ticarcillin binds to bacterial cell wall membrane, causing cell death. • Its spectrum is similar to penicillin but greatly extended to include several important Gram-negative aerobic pathogens, notably *Pseudomonas aeruginosa, Escherichia coli, Proteus mirabilis,* and *Providencia rettgeri.* • It is also active against some anaerobic bacteria, including *Bacteroides,* but is not active against penicillinase-producing staphylococci or beta-lactamase-producing Enterobacteriaceae.

Time/Action Profile (blood levels)

Onset	Peak
rapid	end of infusion

Pharmacokinetics

• **Distribution:** Ticarcillin is widely distributed. It enters CSF well only when meninges are inflamed. It also crosses the placenta and enters breast milk in low concentrations. • **Metabolism and Excretion:** 10% is metabolized by the liver; 90% is excreted unchanged by the kidneys. • **Half-life:** 0.9–1.3 hours (increased in renal impairment).

Contraindications

• Ticarcillin is contraindicated in patients with hypersensitivity to penicillins.

Adverse Reactions and Side Effects*

• **CNS:** confusion, lethargy, SEIZURES (high doses) • **CV:** congestive heart failure, arrhythmias • **GI:** nausea, diarrhea • **GU:** hematuria (children only) • **Derm:** rashes, urticaria • **F and E:** hypokalemia, hypernatremia • **Hemat:** bleeding, blood dyscrasias, increased bleeding time • **Local:** phlebitis • **Metab:** metabolic alkalosis • **Misc:** superinfection, hypersensitivity reactions including ANAPHYLAXIS and serum sickness.

---

*Underlines indicate most frequent; CAPITALS indicate life-threatening.

Ticarcillin Disodium/ Clavulanate Potassium

Anti-infective (extended-spectrum penicillin)

Timentin	pH 5.5–7.5
	4.75 mEq Na/g ticarcillin
	0.15 mEq K/100 mg clavulanate

 ADMINISTRATION CONSIDERATIONS

Usual Dose

Systemic/Urinary Tract Infections

ADULTS ≥60 kg: *Systemic/urinary tract infections*—3.1 g q 4 hr (3.1 g = 3 g ticarcillin plus 100 mg clavulanate). *Gynecologic infections*—50 mg/kg q 4–6 hr (based on ticarcillin content).

ADULTS <60 kg: 33.5–50 mg/kg q 4 hr *or* 50–75 mg/kg q 6 hr (based on ticarcillin content).

CHILDREN 1 mo–12 yr: 50 mg/kg q 4–6 hr (based on ticarcillin content).

Dilution

• **Intermittent Infusion: Add** 13 ml of sterile water or 0.9% NaCl for injection to each 3.1-g vial, to provide a concentration of ticarcillin 200 mg/ml and clavulanic acid 6.7 mg/ml. Shake well. Solution should be colorless to pale yellow. **Further dilute** in 0.9% NaCl, D5W, Ringer's or lactated Ringer's solution. • Stable for 6 hours at room temperature, 72 hours if refrigerated.

Compatibility

• **Y-site:** allopurinol sodium • cyclophosphamide • diltiazem • famotidine • filgrastim • fluconazole • fludarabine • foscarnet • gallium nitrate • insulin • melphalan • meperidine • morphine • ondansetron • perphenazine • sargramostim • vinorelbine.

Incompatibility

• **Y-site:** If aminoglycosides and penicillins or cephalosporins must be given concurrently, administer in separate sites, at least 1 hour apart.

• **Additive:** sodium bicarbonate.

Rate of Administration

• **Intermittent Infusion:** Administer over 30 minutes via Y-site or direct IV.

☰ CLINICAL PRECAUTIONS

• Assess patient for infection (vital signs; appearance of wound, sputum, urine, and stool; WBC) at beginning and throughout course of therapy.

• Obtain specimens for culture and sensitivity prior to initiating therapy. First dose may be given before receiving results.

• Obtain a history before initiating therapy to determine previous use of and reactions to penicillins or cephalosporins. Persons with a negative history of penicillin sensitivity may still have an allergic response. Observe patient for signs and symptoms of anaphylaxis (rash, pruritus, laryngeal edema, wheezing). Discontinue drug immediately if these occur. Keep epinephrine, an antihistamine, and resuscitation equipment close by in the event of an anaphylactic reaction.

• Assess IV site frequently for redness or irritation. Change IV sites every 48 hours to prevent phlebitis.

• Use cautiously in patients with renal impairment. Dosage reduction and/or increased dosing interval is required if creatinine clearance is less than 60 ml/min.

• Use cautiously in patients with a history of hypersensitivity reactions to other drugs or severe liver disease.

• Probenecid decreases renal excretion and increases blood levels of ticarcillin/clavulanate. Ticarcillin/clavulanate may alter excretion of lithium. Diuretics, glucocorticoids, or amphotericin B may increase the risk of hypokalemia. Hypokalemia increases the risk of cardiac glycoside toxicity.

• Safe use in pregnancy or lactation has not been established (Pregnancy Category B).

Lab Test Considerations

• Renal and hepatic function, CBC, serum potassium, and bleeding times should be evaluated prior to and routinely throughout course of therapy. • Ticarcillin/clavulanate may cause false-positive urine protein testing and in-

creased BUN, creatinine, AST (SGOT), ALT (SGPT), serum
bilirubin, alkaline phosphatase, LDH, and uric acid levels.
• It may also cause increased bleeding time, hypernatremia,
and hypokalemia with high doses.

Patient/Family Teaching

• Advise patient to report the signs of superinfection
(black, furry overgrowth on the tongue; vaginal itching or
discharge; loose or foul-smelling stools) and allergy.

≋ PHARMACOLOGIC PROFILE

Indications

• Ticarcillin/clavulanate is used in the treatment of the following serious infections due to susceptible organisms: skin
and skin structure infections, bone and joint infections, septicemia, respiratory tract infections, intra-abdominal infections,
and genitourinary tract infections. • Addition of an aminoglycoside may be synergistic and is recommended against
Pseudomonas. • It has also been combined with other anti-
infectives in the treatment of infections in immunosuppressed
patients.

Action

• Ticarcillin binds to bacterial cell wall membrane, causing
cell death. • Addition of clavulanate enhances resistance to
beta-lactamase, an enzyme produced by bacteria capable of
inactivating some penicillins. • The spectrum of ticarcillin/
clavulanate is similar to that of penicillin but greatly extended
to include several important Gram-negative aerobic pathogens, notably *Pseudomonas aeruginosa, Escherichia coli, Proteus
mirabilis,* and *Providencia rettgeri.* • It is also active against
some anaerobic bacteria, including *Bacteroides,* but is not
active against penicillinase-producing staphylococci or beta-
lactamase-producing Enterobacteriaceae.

Time/Action Profile (blood levels)

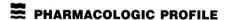

Onset	Peak
rapid	end of infusion

Pharmacokinetics

• **Distribution:** Ticarcillin/clavulanate is widely distributed. It enters CSF well only when meninges are inflamed. It also crosses the placenta and enters breast milk in low concentrations. • **Metabolism and Excretion:** 10% of ticarcillin is metabolized by the liver; 90% is excreted unchanged by the kidneys. Clavulanate is metabolized by the liver. • **Half-life:** ticarcillin—0.9–1.3 hours (increased in renal impairment); clavulanate—1.1–1.5 hours.

Contraindications

• Ticarcillin/clavulanate is contraindicated in patients with hypersensitivity to penicillins or cephalosporins.

Adverse Reactions and Side Effects*

• **CNS:** confusion, lethargy, SEIZURES (high doses) • **CV:** congestive heart failure, arrhythmias • **GI:** nausea, <u>diarrhea</u> • **GU:** hematuria (children only) • **Derm:** <u>rashes</u>, urticaria • **F and E:** <u>hypokalemia</u>, hypernatremia • **Hemat:** bleeding, blood dyscrasias, increased bleeding time • **Local:** <u>phlebitis</u> • **Metab:** metabolic alkalosis • **Misc:** superinfection, <u>hypersensitivity reactions</u> including ANAPHYLAXIS and serum sickness.

Tobramycin Sulfate	Anti-infective (aminoglycoside)
Nebcin	pH 3–6.5

≋ ADMINISTRATION CONSIDERATIONS

Usual Dose

All doses after initial loading dose should be determined by renal function/blood levels.

ADULTS: 0.75–1.25 mg/kg q 6 hr *or* 1–1.7 mg/kg q 8 hr.

CHILDREN: 2.5 mg/kg q 8–16 hr or 1.5–1.9 mg/kg q 6 hr (interval may vary from q 4–q 24 hr).

NEONATES <1 wk: up to 2 mg/kg q 12–24 hr.

---

*<u>Underlines</u> indicate most frequent; CAPITALS indicate life-threatening.

Dilution

• **Intermittent Infusion: Dilute** each dose of tobramycin in 50–100 ml of D5W, D10W, D5/0.9% NaCl, 0.9% NaCl, Ringer's or lactated Ringer's injection. Pediatric doses may be diluted in proportionately smaller amounts for a concentration no greater than 40 mg/ml. • Stable for 24 hours at room temperature, 96 hours if refrigerated. Also available in commercially mixed piggyback injections.

Compatibility

• **Y-site:** acyclovir • ciprofloxacin • cyclophosphamide • diltiazem • enalaprilat • esmolol • filgrastim • fluconazole • fludarabine • foscarnet • furosemide • hydromorphone • insulin • labetalol • magnesium sulfate • melphalan • meperidine • morphine • perphenazine • tacrolimus • tolazoline • vinorelbine • zidovudine.

• **Additive:** aztreonam • bleomycin • calcium gluconate • cefoxitin • ciprofloxacin • clindamycin • furosemide • metronidazole • ofloxacin • ranitidine • verapamil.

Incompatibility

• **Syringe:** cefamandole • clindamycin • heparin.
• **Y-site:** allopurinol sodium • heparin • hetastarch • indomethacin • sargramostim. • If aminoglycosides and penicillins or cephalosporins must be given concurrently, administer in separate sites, at least 1 hour apart.

Rate of Administration

• **Intermittent Infusion:** Infuse slowly, over 20–60 minutes in both adult and pediatric patients. Flush IV line with D5W or 0.9% NaCl following administration.

☰ CLINICAL PRECAUTIONS

• Assess patient for infection (vital signs; appearance of wound, sputum, urine, and stool; WBC) at beginning and throughout course of therapy.
• Obtain specimens for culture and sensitivity prior to initiating therapy. First dose may be given before receiving results.
• Evaluate eighth cranial nerve function by audiometry prior to and throughout course of therapy. Hearing loss

is usually in the high-frequency range. Prompt recognition and intervention is essential in preventing permanent damage. Also monitor for vestibular dysfunction (vertigo, ataxia, nausea, vomiting). Eighth cranial nerve dysfunction is usually associated with persistently elevated peak tobramycin levels. These parameters may be difficult to evaluate in very young or geriatric patients.

- Monitor intake and output and daily weights to assess hydration status and renal function. Keep patient well hydrated (1500–2000 ml/day) during therapy.
- Dosage adjustments (decreased dose and/or increased dosing interval) are required for any degree of renal impairment, especially if creatinine clearance is less than 70 ml/min.
- Use cautiously in obese patients. Dose should be based on ideal body weight.
- Use cautiously in patients with neuromuscular diseases such as myasthenia gravis.
- Use cautiously in geriatric patients due to age-related decrease in renal function. Geriatric patients are more likely to develop ototoxicity and nephrotoxicity.
- Tobramycin is inactivated by penicillins when coadministered to patients with renal insufficiency. Possible respiratory paralysis may occur after inhalation anesthetics (ether, cyclopropane, halothane, or nitrous oxide) or neuromuscular blockers (tubocurarine, succinylcholine, decamethonium). The risk of ototoxicity is increased by concurrent use of loop diuretics (bumetanide, furosemide). The risk of nephrotoxicity is increased by concurrent use of other nephrotoxic drugs (cisplatin).
- Tobramycin may cause congenital deafness or fetal nephrotoxicity if used during pregnancy (Pregnancy Category D). Safe use during lactation has not been established.

Toxicity and Overdose Alert

• Blood levels should be monitored periodically during therapy. Timing of blood levels is important in interpreting results. Draw blood for peak levels 15–30 minutes after IV infusion is completed. Trough levels should be drawn just prior to next dose. Acceptable peak level is 4–10 mcg/ml; trough level should not be more than 2 mcg/ml.

Lab Test Considerations

• Monitor renal function by urinalysis, specific gravity, BUN, creatinine, and creatinine clearance prior to and throughout therapy. • Tobramycin may cause increased AST (SGOT), ALT (SGPT), LDH, bilirubin, and serum alkaline phosphatase levels. • Tobramycin may also cause decreased serum calcium, magnesium, sodium, and potassium levels.

Patient/Family Teaching

• Instruct patient to report signs of hypersensitivity, tinnitus, vertigo, or hearing loss.

≋ PHARMACOLOGIC PROFILE

Indications

• Tobramycin is used in the treatment of serious Gram-negative bacillary infections and infections due to staphylococci when penicillins or other less toxic drugs are contraindicated or resistance to gentamicin has occurred. • It is used in the treatment of the following infections due to susceptible organisms: bone infections, CNS infections (intrathecal administration required in addition to IV), respiratory tract infections, skin and soft tissue infections, abdominal infections, complicated urinary tract infections, endocarditis, and septicemia.

Action

• Tobramycin inhibits protein synthesis in bacteria at the level of the 30S bacterial ribosome, resulting in bactericidal action against susceptible bacteria. • It is active against important Gram-negative pathogens where resistance to gentamicin has occurred, including *Pseudomonas aeruginosa, Klebsiella pneumoniae, Escherichia coli, Proteus, Serratia,* and *Acinetobacter.* • It is also active against *Staphylococcus aureus.* • Treatment of enterococcal infections requires synergy with a penicillin.

Time/Action Profile (blood levels)

Onset	Peak
rapid	end of infusion

Pharmacokinetics

• **Distribution:** Tobramycin crosses the placenta but has poor penetration into CSF. • **Metabolism and Excretion:** Excretion of tobramycin is mainly renal (more than 90%). Minimal amounts are metabolized by the liver. • **Half-life:** 2–3 hours (increased in renal impairment).

Contraindications

• Tobramycin is contraindicated in patients with hypersensitivity to it or to bisulfites. Cross-sensitivity with other aminoglycosides may occur.

Adverse Reactions and Side Effects*

• **EENT:** <u>ototoxicity</u> (vestibular and cochlear) • **GU:** <u>nephrotoxicity</u> • **Neuro:** enhanced neuromuscular blockade • **Misc:** hypersensitivity reactions.

Tolazoline Hydrochloride	Antihypertensive (alpha-adrenergic blocker)
Priscoline	pH 3–4

≋ ADMINISTRATION CONSIDERATIONS

Usual Dose

NEWBORNS: 1–2 mg/kg over 5–10 min through scalp vein initially, then 1–2 mg/kg/hr IV infusion. Initial dose may be repeated if necessary.

Dilution

• **Direct IV:** Administer initial dose **undiluted**. Follow with maintenance infusion. Initial bolus may be repeated during infusion if needed. • **Continuous Infusion:** May be **diluted** in D5W, D10W, 0.45% NaCl, 0.9% NaCl, Ringer's or lactated Ringer's solution, dextrose/saline combinations, dextrose/Ringer's or lactated Ringer's combinations. • Do not use diluents containing benzyl alcohol for neonates; *fatal reaction may occur.*

---

*<u>Underlines</u> indicate most frequent; CAPITALS indicate life-threatening.

Compatibility

- **Y-site:** aminophylline • ampicillin • calcium gluconate • cefotaxime • cimetidine • dobutamine • dopamine • furosemide • gentamicin • phytonadione • sodium bicarbonate • tobramycin • vancomycin.
- **Additive:** verapamil.

Incompatibility

- **Y-site:** indomethacin.
- **Additive:** ethacrynate.

Rate of Administration

- **Direct IV:** Administer initial dose over 10 minutes via scalp vein or directly into pulmonary artery. • **Continuous Infusion:** Administer at a rate of 1–2 mg/kg/hr via infusion pump for accurate dosage. Response should be evident within 30 minutes of initial dose.

≋ CLINICAL PRECAUTIONS

- Administer only in a neonatal intensive care area equipped to provide trained personnel and respiratory support.
- If scalp vein site is not available for initial dose, tolazoline may be given into any right upper extremity vein with drainage into the superior vena cava, ensuring maximal delivery to the pulmonary artery. Tolazoline may also be administered via pulmonary artery catheter.
- Antacids may be ordered prior to therapy to minimize GI bleeding.
- Monitor arterial blood pressure, ECG, and heart rate routinely throughout administration. Tolazoline should be discontinued if systolic blood pressure cannot be maintained at more than 40–50 mm Hg.
- Monitor pulmonary artery pressure (PAP) and pulmonary capillary wedge pressure (PCWP) frequently throughout administration. Volume expanders should be available before treatment is begun.
- Monitor intake and output and daily weights throughout therapy. Patients with renal impairment require smaller doses. Decreased infusion rate is recommended if urine output is less than 0.9 ml/kg/hr.
- Assess patient for bleeding, bruising, petechiae, or blood in stools, urine, or emesis throughout therapy.

- Concurrent use with epinephrine or norepinephrine may result in initial hypotension, followed by rebound hypertension. Tolazoline may antagonize the vasopressor effects of dopamine, ephedrine, metaraminol, methoxamine, or phenylephrine.
- Use cautiously in patients with acidosis (effect may be decreased), mitral stenosis (paradoxical response may occur), gastritis, or history of GI bleeding.

Toxicity and Overdose Alert

- If profound hypotension occurs, keep patient's head low and administer IV fluids. Do not administer epinephrine or norepinephrine, as further hypotension followed by rebound hypertension may occur. Dopamine may be infused simultaneously with tolazoline if IV fluids fail to maintain blood pressure.

Lab Test Considerations

- Monitor arterial blood gases, CBC, and serum electrolytes, especially potassium and chloride, routinely throughout therapy. If hypochloremic metabolic acidosis occurs, wean patient from tolazoline and administer potassium and chloride. • Hematest gastric aspirate periodically to assess for GI bleeding.

Patient/Family Teaching

- Explain purpose of medication to parents. Provide emotional support.

 PHARMACOLOGIC PROFILE

Indications

- Tolazoline is used in the treatment of pulmonary hypertension in newborns when oxygenation cannot be provided by other methods (oxygen therapy, mechanical ventilation).

Action

- Tolazoline is a direct-acting vasodilator. It also causes vasodilation by alpha-adrenergic blockade, resulting in decreased pulmonary arterial pressure and decreased vascular resistance.

Time/Action Profile (vascular response)

Onset	Peak	Duration
30 min	UK	UK

Pharmacokinetics

• **Distribution:** UK. • **Metabolism and Excretion:** Tolazoline is excreted mostly unchanged by the kidneys. • **Half-life:** 3–10 hours (neonates).

Contraindications

• Tolazoline should not be used in hypotensive patients. • Patients with known intolerance to chlorobutanol should not receive tolazoline.

Adverse Reactions and Side Effects*

• **EENT:** mydriasis • **CV:** <u>hypotension</u>, tachycardia, SHOCK • **GI:** <u>GI bleeding</u>, diarrhea, nausea, vomiting • **GU:** <u>acute oliguric renal failure</u> • **Derm:** flushing, piloerection • **F and E:** <u>hypochloremic alkalosis</u> • **Hemat:** <u>thrombocytopenia</u>.

Tolbutamide Sodium	Hypoglycemic agent, Diagnostic agent (sulfonylurea)
Orinase Diagnostic	pH 8.5–9.8

 ADMINISTRATION CONSIDERATIONS

Usual Dose

ADULTS: 1 g.

Dilution

• **Direct IV:** Reconstitute 1 g of tolbutamide sodium with 20 ml of diluent provided.

Rate of Administration

• **Direct IV:** Administer at a constant rate over 2–3 minutes.

---

*<u>Underlines</u> indicate most frequent; CAPITALS indicate life-threatening.

≋ CLINICAL PRECAUTIONS

- For 3 days prior to Fajans test, patient should eat a diet that includes at least 150–300 g of carbohydrate/day.
- Observe patient for signs and symptoms of hypoglycemia (sweating, hunger, weakness, dizziness, tremor, tachycardia, anxiety). When hypoglycemia occurs, it is not usually severe. Some nondiabetic patients may experience moderate to severe symptoms. Use cautiously in patients with atherosclerosis. In these patients, test should be stopped after 30 minutes and followed by administration of a carbohydrate.
- Assess for the development of acute hypersensitivity reactions (shortness of breath, wheezing, rash). Have epinephrine, antihistamines, and resuscitation equipment available in case a reaction occurs.
- Use cautiously in patients with impaired hepatic or renal function. These patients may experience prolonged hypoglycemia.
- Salicylates, sulfonamides, oxyphenbutazone, beta blockers, chloramphenicol, phenylbutazone, MAO inhibitors, and probenecid may interfere with test results by producing more severe and prolonged hypoglycemia. Beta blockers may also diminish the response to tolbutamide.
- Safe use in pregnancy has not been established (Pregnancy Category C); prolonged hypoglycemia may occur in the newborn. Avoid using during pregnancy or lactation.

Toxicity and Overdose Alert

- If hypoglycemia occurs, discontinue test and administer 12.5–25 g of glucose (in a 25–50% solution) IV immediately.

Lab Test Considerations

- Blood specimens may be drawn at 20, 30, 45, 60, 90, 120, 150, and 180 minutes after the midpoint of the injection of tolbutamide. • In normal patients, there is a rapid decrease in blood sugar occurring 30–45 minutes following the injection. This returns to baseline in the following 90–100 minutes. Serum insulin levels peak 20 minutes following the injection. • Patients with insulinoma have a greater decrease in blood sugar with a more dramatic rise in insulin levels. • Patients with adenomas have markedly prolonged hypoglycemia.

Patient/Family Teaching

• Review signs of hypoglycemia and hyperglycemia with patient. Advise patient to notify physician if hypoglycemia occurs. • Encourage patient to follow prescribed diet during the 3 days prior to the test. • Caution patient to avoid other medications, especially those containing aspirin, and alcohol while taking this test without first consulting physician or pharmacist. Concurrent use of alcohol and tolbutamide may cause a disulfiram-like reaction (abdominal cramps, nausea, vomiting, flushing, headache, hypoglycemia).

 PHARMACOLOGIC PROFILE

Indications

• IV tolbutamide is used in the diagnosis of pancreatic islet cell adenomas.

Action

• Tolbutamide lowers blood sugar by stimulating the release of insulin from the pancreas.

Time/Action Profile

	Onset	Peak	Duration
fall in blood sugar in normal subjects	rapid	30–45 min	120–210 min
increase in serum insulin levels	rapid	20 min	UK

Pharmacokinetics

• **Distribution:** UK. • **Metabolism and Excretion:** Tolbutamide is mostly metabolized by the liver. • **Half-life:** 7 hours (range 4–25 hours).

Contraindications

• IV tolbutamide should not be used in children or in patients with hypersensitivity to tolbutamide. Cross-sensitivity to other sulfonylurea hypoglycemics may occur. • Avoid using during pregnancy or lactation.

Adverse Reactions and Side Effects*

• **Endo:** hypoglycemia • **Local:** burning along vein, thrombophlebitis with thrombosis • **MS:** shoulder pain • **Misc:** allergic reactions, including ANAPHYLAXIS.

Torsemide	Loop diuretic
Demadex	pH 8.3–9.5

ADMINISTRATION CONSIDERATIONS

Usual Dose

ADULTS: *Congestive heart failure*—10–20 mg once daily; *Chronic renal failure*—20 mg; *Hepatic cirrhosis*—5–10 mg. Dose may be doubled until response is obtained, up to 200 mg for congestive heart failure or renal failure or up to 40 mg for cirrhosis.

Dilution

• **Direct IV:** Administer **undiluted**. • Do not administer if solution is discolored or contains particulate matter.

Rate of Administration

• **Direct IV:** Administer slowly over 2 minutes.

CLINICAL PRECAUTIONS

• Assess fluid status throughout therapy. Monitor daily weight, intake and output ratios, amount and location of edema, lung sounds, skin turgor, and mucous membranes. Assess patient for thirst, dry mouth, lethargy, weakness, hypotension, or oliguria. Monitor blood pressure and pulse before and during administration. Additive hypotension occurs with concurrent administration of antihypertensives or nitrates.

• Assess patient receiving cardiac glycosides for anorexia, nausea, vomiting, muscle cramps, paresthesia, confu-

---

*Underlines indicate most frequent; CAPITALS indicate life-threatening.

sion. Hypokalemia increases the risk of cardiac glycoside toxicity. Notify physician if these symptoms occur. Additive hypokalemia occurs with other diuretics, mezlocillin, piperacillin, amphotericin B, and glucocorticoids.

- Doses for the IV and oral routes are the same.
- Use torsemide cautiously in patients with severe hepatic disease accompanied by ascites or cirrhosis. Sudden changes in fluid and electrolyte balance may precipitate hepatic coma. Concurrent use with aldosterone antagonists or potassium-sparing diuretics is recommended for patients with cirrhosis.
- Assess patient for tinnitus and hearing loss. Audiometry is recommended for patients receiving prolonged therapy. Hearing loss is most common following rapid or high-dose IV administration in patients with decreased renal function or those taking other ototoxic drugs (aminoglycosides or cisplatin). This parameter may be difficult to assess in geriatric patients.
- Assess for allergy to sulfonamides. Cross-sensitivity may occur.
- Use torsemide cautiously in patients with electrolyte depletion, diabetes mellitus, or increasing azotemia.
- Salicylate toxicity may occur in patients receiving high-dose salicylate therapy and concurrent torsemide. Concurrent use with nonsteroidal anti-inflammatory agents may increase the risk of renal dysfunction. Concurrent use with indomethacin in patients whose sodium intake is restricted may decrease the effectiveness of torsemide. The diuretic activity of torsemide is decreased by concurrent use of probenecid. Torsemide may decrease lithium excretion and increase the risk of toxicity.
- Safe use in pregnancy, lactation, or children has not been established (Pregnancy Category B).

Lab Test Considerations

- Monitor electrolytes, renal and hepatic function, serum glucose, and uric acid levels prior to and periodically throughout therapy. Torsemide may cause abnormalities of serum potassium, sodium, chloride, or acid/base balance. May also cause increased BUN, serum creatinine, glucose, and uric acid levels. • Torsemide may cause increases in total plasma cholesterol and lipids during initial therapy. These elevations usually return to normal with chronic therapy.

Patient/Family Teaching

• Caution patient to make position changes slowly to minimize orthostatic hypotension. • Advise patient to contact physician immediately if muscle weakness, cramps, nausea, dizziness, numbness, or tingling of extremities occurs. • Instruct patient to consult physician regarding a diet high in potassium (see Appendix H). • Advise patients on antihypertensive regimen to continue taking medication and monitoring blood pressure routinely, even if feeling better. Torsemide controls but does not cure hypertension. Reinforce the need to continue additional therapies for hypertension (weight loss, restricted sodium intake, stress reduction, regular exercise, moderation of alcohol consumption, cessation of smoking). • Emphasize the importance of routine follow-up examinations.

☰ PHARMACOLOGIC PROFILE

Indications

• IV torsemide is indicated when a rapid onset of diuresis is desired or oral administration is impractical in the management of edema associated with CHF, renal, or hepatic disease. Torsemide is also used alone or with other agents in the management of hypertension.

Action

• Torsemide exerts its action in the lumen of the thick ascending limb of the loop of Henle, where it increases the renal excretion of sodium, chloride, and water. Torsemide induces diuresis with subsequent mobilization of excess fluid (edema, ascites, pleural effusions). It also possesses vasodilatory activity that reduces cardiac preload and afterload. Its antihypertensive effect occurs at doses less than those required for diuresis.

Time/Action Profile (diuretic effect)

Onset	Peak	Duration
within 10 min	within 60 min	6–8 hr

Pharmacokinetics

• **Distribution:** Distribution of torsemide is not known.
• **Metabolism and Excretion:** 80% of torsemide is metabolized by the liver, 20% is excreted in urine. • **Half-life:** 210 minutes.

Contraindications

• Torsemide is contraindicated in patients with known hypersensitivity. Cross-sensitivity with sulfonamides may occur. Use of torsemide should be avoided in patients with pre-existing uncorrected electrolyte imbalance, hepatic coma, or anuria.

Adverse Reactions and Side Effects*

• **CNS:** headache, dizziness, weakness, nervousness, insomnia • **Resp:** increased cough, rhinitis, sore throat • **CV:** hypotension, ECG abnormalities, chest pain • **GI:** nausea, constipation, dyspepsia • **GU:** excessive urination • **MS:** arthralgia, myalgia • **F and E:** hypomagnesemia, hypokalemia.

Trace Metal Combination Additive	Nutritional supplement

ConTE-PAK-4, M.T.E.-4, M.T.E.-5, M.T.E.-5 Concentrated, M.T.E.-6, M.T.E.-6 Concentrated, M.T.E.-7, MulTE-PAK-4, MulTE-PAK-5, Multiple Trace Element, Multiple Trace Element Concentrated, Multiple Trace Element Neonatal, Multiple Trace Element Pediatric, Multiple Trace Element with Selenium, Multiple Trace Element with Selenium Concentrated, Neotrace-4, PedTE-PAK-4, Pedtrace-4, PTE-5, Trace Metals Additive in 0.9% NaCl

---

≋ ADMINISTRATION CONSIDERATIONS

Contains chromium, copper, manganese, and zinc. Some products also contain iodine, molybdenum, and selenium.

---

*Underlines indicate most frequent; CAPITALS indicate life-threatening.

Usual Dose

ADULTS AND CHILDREN: Amount necessary to maintain normal trace element levels.

Chromium

ADULTS: 10–15 mcg (0.01–0.015 mg)/day (20 mcg [0.02 mg]/day if stable but with intestinal fluid loss).
CHILDREN: 0.14–0.2 mcg (0.00014–0.0002 mg)/kg/day.

Copper

ADULTS: 500 mcg (0.5 mg)–1.5 mg/day.
CHILDREN: 20 mcg (0.02 mg)/kg/day.

Iodine

ADULTS: 1–2 mcg/kg/day (75–150 mcg/day).
PREGNANT OR LACTATING WOMEN, CHILDREN: 2–3 mcg/kg/day.

Manganese

ADULTS: 150–800 mcg (0.15–0.8 mg)/day.
CHILDREN: 2–10 mcg (0.002–0.01 mg)/kg/day.

Molybdenum

ADULTS: 20–120 mcg (0.02–0.120 mg)/day (163 mcg [0.163 mg]/day for 21 days in deficiency secondary to prolonged TPN).

Selenium

ADULTS: 20–40 mcg (0.02–0.04 mg)/day (100 mcg [0.01 mg]/day for 24 or 31 days in deficiency secondary to prolonged TPN).
CHILDREN: 3 mcg (0.003 mg)/kg/day.

Zinc

ADULTS: 2.5–4 mg/day with additional 2 mg/day in catabolic states (12.2 mg additional zinc/1000 ml TPN fluid or 17.7 mg/kg of stool or ileostomy output).
CHILDREN <5 yr AND FULL-TERM INFANTS: 100 mcg (0.1 mg)/kg/day.
PREMATURE INFANTS: 300 mcg (0.3 mg)/kg/day.

Dilution

• **Continuous Infusion:** Must be diluted prior to administration. **Dilute** each dose in at least 1 liter of IV solution.
• Solution usually does not contain preservatives; discard unused portion.

Compatibility
• **Additive:** Usually compatible with electrolytes and dextrose/amino acid combinations used for TPN.

Rate of Administration
• **Continuous Infusion:** Administer at prescribed rate for TPN infusion.

☰ CLINICAL PRECAUTIONS

• Monitor patient for signs and symptoms of trace metal deficiencies prior to and throughout therapy, as follows: *Chromium*—glucose intolerance, ataxia, peripheral neuropathy, confusion. *Copper*—leukopenia, neutropenia, anemia, iron deficiency, skeletal abnormalities, defective tissue formation. *Iodine*—impaired thyroid function, goiter, cretinism. *Manganese*—nausea, vomiting, weight loss, dermatitis, changes in hair. *Molybdenum*—tachycardia, tachypnea, headache, night blindness, nausea, vomiting, edema, lethargy, disorientation, coma, hypouricemia, hypouricosuria. *Selenium*—cardiomyopathy, muscle pain, kwashiorkor, Keshan disease. *Zinc*—diarrhea, apathy, depression, anorexia, hypogonadism, growth retardation, anemia, hepatosplenomegaly, impaired wound healing.
• Use cautiously in patients with nasogastric suction, fistula drainage, prolonged vomiting, or diarrhea. These patients may have increased requirements. Patients with renal impairment or biliary obstruction may have increased risk of toxicities.
• Use cautiously in patients with isolated trace element deficiency (other additives may be excessive; use only those required).
• Use cautiously during pregnancy or lactation (Pregnancy Category C).

Lab Test Considerations
• Serum trace metal concentrations should be monitored periodically throughout TPN therapy.

Patient/Family Teaching
• Explain purpose of infusion of TPN and components to patient.

PHARMACOLOGIC PROFILE

Indications

• Trace metal additive is administered as a component in total parenteral nutrition (TPN, parenteral hyperalimentation). • It may contain any or all of the following: chromium ♦ copper ♦ iodine ♦ manganese ♦ molybdenum ♦ selenium ♦ zinc.

Action

• Trace metals serve as cofactors or catalysts for numerous diverse homeostatic processes. Administration serves as replacement in deficiency states when oral ingestion is not feasible.

Time/Action Profile (replacement)

Onset	Peak	Duration
rapid	UK	UK

Pharmacokinetics

• **Distribution:** Trace elements are widely distributed.
• **Metabolism and Excretion:** *Copper*—80% in bile, 16% in intestinal wall, 4% in urine; *chromium*—kidneys and bile; *iodine*—kidneys and bile; *manganese*—bile, unless obstruction is present, when it is returned to intestinal lumen or lost in pancreatic juice; *molybdenum*—mostly renal, some bile; *selenium*—urine, feces, lung, skin; *zinc*—90% in feces, the rest in urine and perspiration. • **Half-life:** UK.

Contraindications

• Trace metal additive is contraindicated in patients with hypersensitivity to iodine (iodine-containing products only). • In neonates, avoid using products that contain benzyl alcohol.

Adverse Reactions and Side Effects*

Listed for individual trace metals and usually associated with toxicity.

• **Chromium:** nausea, vomiting, GI ulceration, renal damage, hepatic damage, SEIZURES, coma • **Copper:** behavioral changes, weakness, diarrhea, photophobia, peripheral edema, progressive marasmus • **Iodine:** metallic taste, sore mouth,

---

*<u>Underlines</u> indicate most frequent; CAPITALS indicate life-threatening.

increased salivation, runny nose, sneezing, headache, swelling of eyelids, parotitis, acneform skin lesions • **Manganese:** irritability, speech difficulties, gait disturbances, headache, anorexia, impotence, apathy • **Molybdenum:** goutlike syndrome • **Selenium:** hair loss, weak nails, mental depression, nervousness, vomiting, garlic-like breath, garlic-like sweat, metallic taste, GI discomfort • **Zinc:** toxicity poorly defined but may include hypothermia, blurred vision, loss of consciousness, tachycardia, pulmonary edema, jaundice, oliguria, hypotension, vomiting.

Tranexamic Acid	*Hemostatic (plasminogen inactivator), Antifibrinolytic agent*
Cyklokapron	**pH 6.5–7.5**

 ADMINISTRATION CONSIDERATIONS

Usual Dose

Dental Extraction in Patients with Hemophilia

ADULTS AND CHILDREN: 10 mg/kg before surgery, then 3 to 4 times daily for 2–8 days.

Dilution

• **Intermittent Infusion:** May be diluted with most solutions, such as electrolyte, carbohydrate, amino acid, and dextran solutions. • Prepare mixture on the day of infusion.

Compatibility

• **Additive:** heparin.

Incompatibility

• **Additive:** blood • penicillin.

Rate of Administration

• **Intermittent Infusion:** Infuse at a rate not to exceed 100 mg (1 ml)/min. More rapid administration has resulted in hypotension.

≋ CLINICAL PRECAUTIONS

- Observe site of surgery for excessive bleeding.
- Because of visual abnormalities, patients on therapy for more than several days should have ophthalmological examinations before therapy and at regular intervals thereafter.
- Concurrent use of clotting factor complexes may increase the risk of thrombotic complications. To avoid problems, tranexamic acid may be given 8 hours following clotting factor replacement therapy. The risk of thrombosis may be increased by concurrent estrogen therapy.
- Tranexamic acid will antagonize the effects of thrombolytic agents.
- Use cautiously in patients with renal impairment. Increased dosing interval is recommended if serum creatinine is more than 1.36 mg/dl.
- Oral bioavailability is diminished, necessitating larger oral than IV doses.
- Safe use in pregnancy or lactation has not been established (Pregnancy Category B).

Patient/Family Teaching

• Patients should inform physician of any changes in vision. Inform patients on prolonged therapy of the need for regular ophthalmological follow-up. • Signs and symptoms of thrombosis (severe, sudden headache; pains in chest, groin, or legs, especially calves; sudden loss of coordination; sudden and unexplained shortness of breath; slurred speech; visual changes; weakness or numbness in arm or leg) should be reported to physician. • Patient should avoid products containing aspirin, ibuprofen, or naproxen.

≋ PHARMACOLOGIC PROFILE

Indications

• Tranexamic acid is used to prevent hemorrhage following dental surgery in hemophiliacs.

Action

• Tranexamic acid inhibits activation of plasminogen, thereby preventing the conversion of plasminogen to plasmin.

Time/Action Profile (blood levels)

Onset	Peak	Duration
UK	3 hr	7–8 hr†

†Antifibrinolytic concentration in plasma. Tissue levels persist for 17 hr.

Pharmacokinetics

• **Distribution:** Tranexamic acid penetrates readily into joint fluid and synovial membranes. • **Metabolism and Excretion:** 95% is excreted unchanged in urine. • **Half-life:** 2 hours (increased in renal impairment); 3 hours in joint fluid.

Contraindications

• Tranexamic acid is contraindicated in patients with hypersensitivity to it or in patients with acquired defective color vision or subarachnoid hemorrhage.

Adverse Reactions and Side Effects*

• **CNS:** dizziness • **CV:** hypotension, thrombosis, thromboembolism • **GI:** nausea, vomiting, diarrhea • **EENT:** visual abnormalities.

Trimethaphan Camsylate	*Antihypertensive (ganglionic blocker)*
Arfonad	pH 5

≋ ADMINISTRATION CONSIDERATIONS

Usual Dose

Severe Hypertension, Hypertensive Emergencies

ADULTS: 500 mcg (0.5 mg)–1 mg/min initially; may be increased gradually to achieve desired response (range 1–5 mg/min).

Aortic Dissection

ADULTS: 1–4 mg/min initially, increased as needed to maintain systolic blood pressure of 100–200 mm Hg.

---

*Underlines indicate most frequent; CAPITALS indicate life-threatening.

Controlled Hypotension during Anesthesia

ADULTS: 3–4 mg/min initially, followed by 300 mcg (0.3 mg)–6 mg/min infusion.

Pediatric Dose

CHILDREN: 50–150 mcg (0.05–0.15 mg)/kg/min.

Dilution

• **Continuous Infusion: Dilute** 500-mg (10-ml) vial in 500 ml of D5W, 0.9% NaCl, or Ringer's solution, for a final concentration of 1 mg/ml. • Vial should be stored under refrigeration. Prepare solution immediately prior to use. Solution is stable for 24 hours after reconstitution.

Compatibility

• **Y-site:** heparin ◆ hydrocortisone ◆ potassium chloride ◆ vitamin B complex with C.

Incompatibility

• **Additive:** alkaline solutions ◆ bromides ◆ gallamine triethiodide ◆ thiopental sodium ◆ tubocurarine. • Admixture is not recommended with any medication.

Rate of Administration

• **Continuous Infusion:** Infusion rate must be regulated by IV pump or controller and titrated to patient's blood pressure.

≋ CLINICAL PRECAUTIONS

• Monitor blood pressure, pulse, and respirations at least every 5 minutes during initial adjustment of dosage and at least every 15 minutes throughout course of therapy. Titrate infusion rate according to predetermined parameters. Elevating the head of the bed will enhance the hypotensive effects. Position the patient to avoid cerebral anoxia. Patients with cardiac history should be monitored with continuous ECG.

• Monitor intake and output ratios and weights and assess for edema, jugular vein distention, dyspnea, and rales/crackles, especially in patients with pulmonary edema.

• Patients with any allergy are more prone to development of tachyphylaxis, because of the drug's effect on histamine release.

- Use cautiously in geriatric patients due to increased sensitivity to hypotensive effects of trimethaphan.
- Pupil examination will be inaccurate because of mydriatic (dilating) effect.
- Monitor for nausea and vomiting; protect airway in patients with diminished level of consciousness. Monitor abdominal status (distention, bowel sounds); risk of paralytic ileus is increased in patients on therapy more than 48 hours. Use cautiously in patients with allergies, cardiovascular disease, degenerative CNS disease, diabetes mellitus, hepatic or renal impairment, or Addison's disease. Use with *extreme caution* in children, elderly, or debilitated patients.
- Additive hypotension may occur with concurrent use of other antihypertensives, nitrates, diuretics, anesthetics (especially spinal anesthesia), or procainamide. Trimethaphan may prolong neuromuscular blockade from succinylcholine or tubocurarine.
- Trimethaphan may cause meconium ileus or neonatal paralytic ileus when used in pregnant patients. Excessive hypotension may also have adverse effects on the fetus (Pregnancy Category D).

Toxicity and Overdose Alert

- Toxicity is manifested by severe hypotension. Stop infusion and administer vasopressors.

Lab Test Considerations

- May cause slightly decreased serum potassium and may prevent surgically induced elevation in serum glucose.

Patient/Family Teaching

- Explain purpose of medication to patient. • Instruct alert patients to remain supine throughout course of therapy to prevent orthostatic hypotension.

≋ PHARMACOLOGIC PROFILE

Indications

- Trimethaphan is used for rapid reduction of blood pressure in the management of hypertensive emergencies. It is particularly useful in lowering blood pressure in patients with acute aortic dissection. • It is also used to produce controlled hypotension in patients undergoing head and neck surgery.

Action

• Trimethaphan blocks nerve transmission at sympathetic and autonomic ganglia. It produces vasodilation and histamine release, increases peripheral blood flow, and decreases blood pressure.

Time/Action Profile (antihypertensive effect)

Onset	Peak	Duration
immediate	UK	10–15 min

Pharmacokinetics

• **Distribution:** Trimethaphan crosses the placenta. • **Metabolism and Excretion:** It is mainly excreted unchanged by the kidneys. Small amounts may be metabolized by pseudocholinesterase. • **Half-life:** UK.

Contraindications

• Trimethaphan is contraindicated in patients with hypersensitivity to it or to phenol, parabens, or edetate. • It should be avoided in patients with anemia, hypovolemia, shock, asphyxia, glaucoma, or respiratory insufficiency. • Trimethaphan should not be used during pregnancy or lactation.

Adverse Reactions and Side Effects*

• **CNS:** weakness, restlessness • **EENT:** cycloplegia, mydriasis • **Resp:** APNEA, RESPIRATORY ARREST (large doses only) • **CV:** <u>hypotension</u>, tachycardia, angina • **GI:** anorexia, nausea, vomiting, dry mouth, ileus (if therapy is longer than 48 hours) • **GU:** urinary retention • **Derm:** urticaria, itching • **Misc:** tachyphylaxis.

---

*<u>Underlines</u> indicate most frequent; CAPITALS indicate life-threatening.

Trimethoprim/ Sulfamethoxazole	*Anti-infective* *(sulfonamide)*
Bactrim, co-trimoxazole, Septra, SMX/ TMP, Sulfamethoprim, TMP/SMX	pH 10

ADMINISTRATION CONSIDERATIONS

Usual Dose

TMP = trimethoprim, SMX = sulfamethoxazole.

Anti-infective Dosing (bacterial infections)

ADULTS AND CHILDREN >2 mo: 2–2.5 mg/kg TMP/10–12.5 mg/kg SMX q 6 hr *or* 2.7–3.3 mg/kg TMP/13.3–16.7 mg/kg SMX q 8 hr *or* 4–5 mg/kg TMP/20–25 mg/kg SMX q 12 hr.

Antiprotozoal Dosing (*Pneumocystis carinii* pneumonia)

ADULTS AND CHILDREN: 3.75–5 mg/kg TMP/18.7–25 mg/kg SMX q 6 hr *or* 5–6.7 mg/kg TMP/25–33.3 mg/kg SMX q 8 hr.

Dilution

• **Intermittent Infusion:** Dilute each 5-ml ampule with 100–125 ml of D5W. May reduce diluent to 75 ml if fluid restriction required. • Do not use if solution is cloudy or contains a precipitate. Solution is stable for 6 hours in standard dilution and 2 hours in fluid-restricted dilution at room temperature. Do not refrigerate.

Compatibility

• **Syringe:** heparin.
• **Y-site:** acyclovir • atracurium • cyclophosphamide • diltiazem • enalaprilat • esmolol • filgrastim • fludarabine • gallium nitrate • hydromorphone • labetalol • magnesium sulfate • melphalan • meperidine • morphine • pancuronium • perphenazine • piperacillin/tazobactam • sargramostim • tacrolimus • vecuronium • zidovudine.
• **Additive/Solution:** D5/0.45% NaCl • 0.45% NaCl. However, manufacturer recommends not mixing with other medications or solutions.

Incompatibility
- **Y-site:** fluconazole ✦ vinorelbine.
- **Additive:** fluconazole ✦ verapamil.

Rate of Administration
- **Intermittent Infusion:** Infuse over 60–90 minutes. Do not administer rapidly or by bolus injection.

☰ CLINICAL PRECAUTIONS

- Assess patient for infection (vital signs; appearance of wound, sputum, urine, and stool; WBC) at beginning and throughout therapy.
- Obtain specimens for culture and sensitivity prior to initiating therapy. First dose may be given before results are available.
- Inspect IV site frequently. Phlebitis is common.
- Assess patient for allergy to sulfonamides.
- Monitor intake and output ratios. Fluid intake should be sufficient to maintain a urine output of at least 1200–1500 ml daily to prevent crystalluria and stone formation.
- Patients with impaired hepatic or renal function may require dosage reduction. Dosage reduction is recommended if creatinine clearance is less than 30 ml/min. Patients receiving prolonged therapy should have liver function studies performed. Hepatic necrosis is an unusual but potentially fatal complication of therapy.
- Observe skin frequently; a variety of rashes may occur. Some rashes are indications of serious systemic reactions. HIV-positive patients have an increased incidence of adverse reactions, especially rashes.
- Trimethoprim/sulfamethoxazole may increase half-life, decrease clearance, and exaggerate folic acid deficiency caused by phenytoin. It may also enhance the effects of oral hypoglycemic agents and oral anticoagulants. Observe for hypoglycemia or bleeding in patients receiving these agents concurrently.
- The toxicity of methotrexate is increased by concurrent use of trimethoprim/sulfamethoxazole.
- Elderly patients receiving thiazide diuretics have an increased risk of thrombocytopenia while receiving trimethoprim/sulfamethoxazole.

- Concurrent use with cyclosporine increases efficacy of cyclosporine and increases risk of nephrotoxicity.
- Trimethoprim/sulfamethoxazole should not be used at term, as it may cause jaundice, hemolytic anemia, or kernicterus in the newborn. Use in pregnant or lactating patients only if benefits outweigh risks (Pregnancy Category C).

Lab Test Considerations

- Monitor CBC and urinalysis periodically throughout therapy. May produce elevated serum bilirubin, creatinine, and alkaline phosphatase.

Patient/Family Teaching

- Caution patient to use sunscreen and protective clothing to prevent photosensitivity reactions. • Advise patient to notify physician if skin rash, sore throat, fever, mouth sores, or unusual bleeding or bruising occurs. • Instruct patient to notify physician if symptoms do not improve within a few days.
- **Home Care Issues:** Instruct family or care-giver on dilution, rate, and administration of drug and proper care of IV equipment.

≋ PHARMACOLOGIC PROFILE

Indications

- IV use of trimethoprim/sulfamethoxazole is reserved for treatment of the following infections due to susceptible organisms: severe urinary tract infections, *Shigella* enteritis, acute exacerbations of chronic bronchitis, and *Pneumocystis carinii* pneumonia. • The unlabeled uses of trimethoprim/sulfamethoxazole include: biliary tract infections, osteomyelitis, burn and wound infections, endocarditis, intra-abdominal infections, nocardiosis, and sinusitis.

Action

- The combination of trimethoprim and sulfamethoxazole inhibits the metabolism of folic acid in bacteria at two different points. This combination is active against many strains of Gram-positive aerobic pathogens, including *Streptococcus pneumoniae, Staphylococcus aureus,* group A beta-hemolytic streptococci, *Nocardia,* and *Enterococcus.* • It also has activity against many aerobic Gram-negative pathogens, such as: *Acinetobacter, Enterobacter, Klebsiella pneumoniae, Escherichia coli, Proteus mirabilis, Shigella,* and *Haemophilus influenzae* (including ampicillin-resistant strains). • In addition, it is active against a pathogenic protozoa, *Pneumocystis carinii.* • It is not active against *Pseudomonas aeruginosa.*

Time/Action Profile (blood levels)

Onset	Peak
rapid	end of infusion

Pharmacokinetics

• **Distribution:** Trimethoprim/sulfamethoxazole is widely distributed, crosses the placenta, and enters breast milk. • **Metabolism and Excretion:** Some metabolism occurs in the liver (20%); remainder excreted unchanged by the kidneys. • **Half-life:** trimethoprim, 8–11 hours; sulfamethoxazole, 7–12 hours.

Contraindications

• Trimethoprim/sulfamethoxazole must not be used in patients with hypersensitivity to sulfonamides, trimethoprim, or bisulfites. • Patients who have megaloblastic anemia secondary to folate deficiency should not be treated with trimethoprim/sulfamethoxazole. • Trimethoprim/sulfamethoxazole is contraindicated in pregnancy near term or in neonates under 2 months. IV trimethoprim/sulfamethoxazole contains ethyl alcohol and benzyl alcohol and should be avoided in patients with known intolerance. • Severe renal impairment is an additional situation where trimethoprim/sulfamethoxazole should be avoided.

Adverse Reactions and Side Effects*

• **CNS:** headache, insomnia, fatigue, depression, hallucinations • **GI:** <u>nausea</u>, <u>vomiting</u>, stomatitis, diarrhea, HEPATIC NECROSIS • **GU:** crystalluria • **Derm:** <u>rashes</u>, TOXIC EPIDERMAL NECROLYSIS, photosensitivity • **Hemat:** APLASTIC ANEMIA, AGRANULOCYTOSIS, leukopenia, thrombocytopenia, megaloblastic anemia,

---

*<u>Underlines</u> indicate most frequent; CAPITALS indicate life-threatening.

hemolytic anemia • **Local:** <u>phlebitis at IV site</u> • **Misc:** allergic reactions including STEVENS-JOHNSON SYNDROME, ERYTHEMA MULTI-FORME, fever.

<table>
<tr><td>Trimetrexate
Glucuronate</td><td>Antiprotozoal</td></tr>
<tr><td>NeuTrexin</td><td>pH 4.8</td></tr>
</table>

ADMINISTRATION CONSIDERATIONS

Usual Dose

ADULTS: 45 mg/m^2 (1.2 mg/kg) once daily for 21 days. Concurrent leucovorin dose is 20 mg/m^2 PO or IV q 6 hr for 24 days.

Dilution

• **Intermittent Infusion: Reconstitute** each vial of trimetrexate with 2 ml of D5W or sterile water for injection for a concentration of 12.5 mg/ml. Complete dissolution should occur within 30 seconds. Reconstituted solution is greenish-yellow. Do not administer if solution is cloudy or contains particulate matter. • Filter the solution with a 0.22-micron filter prior to further dilution. • **Further dilute** solution with D5W for a final concentration of 0.25–2 mg/ml. • Solution should be prepared in a biologic cabinet. Wear gloves, gown, and mask while handling medication. Discard IV equipment in specially designated containers (see Appendix F). • Solution is stable for 24 hours at room temperature. Discard unused solution.

Incompatibility

• **Y-site/Additive:** 0.9% NaCl • leucovorin • sodium chloride. Administer trimetrexate and leucovorin separately. Flush IV lines with at least 10 ml of D5W between infusions.

Rate of Administration

• **Intermittent Infusion:** Administer over 60–90 minutes.

≋ CLINICAL PRECAUTIONS

- Concurrent leucovorin (leucovorin protection) must be administered during and for 72 hours after the last dose of trimetrexate to prevent life-threatening toxicity. The initial dose of leucovorin is given IV prior to the first dose of trimetrexate (see *leucovorin calcium* monograph on page 554).
- Monitor IV site frequently for signs of infection and extravasation. Should extravasation occur, apply warm compresses to the site and restart infusion at a new site. Trimetrexate is not a vesicant.
- Monitor temperature daily. If patient becomes febrile an antipyretic may be administered. Assess for fever, chills, sore throat, and signs of infection. Assess for bleeding (bleeding gums, bruising, petechiae; guaiac test stools, urine, and emesis). Avoid giving IM injections and taking rectal temperatures. Apply pressure to venipuncture sites for 10 minutes. Initiate bleeding precautions for platelet counts $\leq 50,000/mm^3$ and infection control measures for absolute neutrophil counts (ANC) $\leq 1000/mm^3$ (see Patient/Family Teaching). Other myelosuppressive or nephrotoxic agents may be stopped during trimetrexate therapy.
- The concurrent use of the following medications may alter blood levels and effectiveness of trimetrexate: acetaminophen, erythromycin, rifampin, rifabutin, ketoconazole, and fluconazole. Toxicity of trimetrexate may be increased by concurrent cimetidine, clotrimazole, ketoconazole, or miconazole.
- Concurrent leucovorin may decrease the effectiveness of phenobarbital, phenytoin, or primidone as anticonvulsants.
- Use trimetrexate cautiously in patients with childbearing potential (Pregnancy Category D). Avoid use during pregnancy or lactation. Safe use of trimetrexate in children under 18 years of age has not been established.

Lab Test Considerations

- Monitor hematologic, renal, and hepatic functions twice weekly during therapy. May cause decreased ANC and platelet counts. Dose adjustment is required for concurrent hematologic toxicity (neutrophils less than 1000/mm³ or platelets less than 75,000/mm³). May cause increased serum creatinine, BUN, AST (SGOT), ALT (SGPT), and alkaline phosphatase levels.

Patient/Family Teaching

• Instruct the patient about the purpose of trimetrexate and leucovorin and the importance of complying with the full course of therapy. • Instruct the patient to take his or her temperature at least once daily, and more frequently if fever is suspected. • Advise the patient with ANC ≤1000/mm³ to practice infection control measures (rigorous hand-washing, coverage of IV site during showers or when bathing, thorough washing of fresh fruit, avoidance of raw or undercooked meat and vegetables, elimination of fresh flowers and live house plants, and avoidance of crowds and persons with known infections). • Instruct patients with a platelet count of ≤50,000/mm³ to practice bleeding precautions (use soft toothbrush; use electric razor; be especially careful to avoid falls; avoid alcoholic beverages and medications containing aspirin, ibuprofen, or naproxen, as these may precipitate gastric bleeding). • Advise the patient to use a nonhormonal form of contraception throughout therapy. • Instruct the patient to report fever ≥101°F, rash, flu-like symptoms, numbness or tingling in the extremities, nausea or vomiting, abdominal pain, mouth sores, increased bruising or bleeding, or black tarry stools to the physician promptly. • Emphasize the importance of frequent lab tests to monitor side effects.

≋ PHARMACOLOGIC PROFILE

Indications

• Trimetrexate is used for the treatment of moderate to severe *Pneumocystis carinii* pneumonia (PCP) in immunocompromised patients who are unable to tolerate therapy with trimethoprim/sulfamethoxazole (co-trimoxazole, TMP/SMX).

Action

• Trimetrexate inhibits dihydrofolate reductase, thereby acting as a folic acid antagonist. Concurrent administration of leucovorin prevents bone marrow depression from trimetrexate while allowing its antiprotozoal action on *P. carinii* to continue.

Time/Action Profile (blood levels)

Onset	Peak
rapid	end of infusion

Pharmacokinetics

• **Distribution:** Distribution of trimetrexate is not known. • **Metabolism and Excretion:** Trimetrexate is metabolized by the liver; some metabolites may have folate antagonist activity. About 10–30% is excreted unchanged by the kidneys. • **Half-life:** 11 hours.

Contraindications

• Trimetrexate is contraindicated in patients with hypersensitivity to trimetrexate, methotrexate, or leucovorin. ◆ Pregnant or lactating patients should not receive trimetrexate.

Adverse Reactions and Side Effects*

• **CNS:** confusion, fatigue • **GI:** nausea, vomiting, <u>increased AST/ALT</u>, increased alkaline phosphatase, increased bilirubin • **GU:** increased serum creatinine • **Derm:** rash, pruritus • **F and E:** hyponatremia, hypocalcemia • **Hemat:** <u>neutropenia</u>, <u>thrombocytopenia</u>, anemia • **Misc:** fever.

Tromethamine	*Electrolyte modifier (alkalinizing-agent)*
Tham, tris buffer	pH 8.6

≋ ADMINISTRATION CONSIDERATIONS

Usual Dose

Can be calculated by the following formula: tromethamine solution (ml of 0.3 M) = body weight (kg) × base deficit (mEq/liter) × 1.1.

---

*<u>Underlines</u> indicate most frequent; CAPITALS indicate life-threatening.

ADULTS: *Acidosis during cardiac bypass surgery*—9 ml/kg. Total dose of 500 ml (150 mEq or 18 g) is sufficient in most adult patients, up to 1000 ml (not to exceed 500 mg/kg in 1 hr); *acidosis in cardiac arrest*—3.6–10.8 g (111–333 ml), additional doses may be required.

CHILDREN: 3–6 ml/kg (1–2 mEq/kg) single dose *or* 3–16 ml/kg/hr as an infusion, up to 33–40 ml/kg/day.

Dilution

• **Direct IV:** Administer undiluted in a concentration of 36 mg/ml. • **Intermittent/Continuous Infusion:** Available as a commercially prepared 0.3-*M* solution or may be prepared by adding 36 g of tromethamine to 1 liter of sterile water for injection. • Tromethamine solution should be discarded 24 hours after reconstitution. • Available in combination with sodium, potassium, and chloride (Tham-E). Tham and Tham-E are not interchangeable.

Rate of Administration

• **Direct IV:** Administer at a rate of 3–5 mg/kg over 3–5 minutes. • **Intermittent Infusion:** Administer by slow infusion. • **Continuous Infusion:** May be administered continuously at a rate of 3–16 mg/kg/hr.

≋ CLINICAL PRECAUTIONS

- Administer via large needle or, preferably, catheter into largest antecubital vein for peripheral vein infusion. Elevate limb. Observe IV site frequently for redness or irritation. Solution is highly alkaline. Extravasation may lead to thrombosis, phlebitis, necrosis, and sloughing. If extravasation occurs, discontinue infusion. Extravasated area may be infiltrated with procaine hydrochloride 1% and hyaluronidase or phentolamine.
- Assess patient for signs of acidosis (disorientation, headache, weakness, dyspnea, hyperventilation) and alkalosis (confusion, irritability, paresthesia, tetany, altered breathing pattern) throughout therapy.
- Assess respiratory status throughout therapy. Use with caution in patients with respiratory depression. Additive respiratory depression may occur with concurrent use of sedative/hypnotics or opioid analgesics.
- Monitor intake and output throughout therapy.

- Use cautiously in neonates due to increased risk of hypoglycemia and hemorrhagic hepatic necrosis. Use cautiously in patients with renal impairment due to increased risk of acid/base and electrolyte abnormalities.
- Tromethamine should not be used for more than 1 day.
- May also be administered directly into ventricular cavity or into acid citrate dextrose blood during cardiac bypass surgery.
- Safe use in pregnancy has not been established (Pregnancy Category C).

Lab Test Considerations

- Monitor pH, pCO_2, bicarbonate, glucose, and electrolytes before, frequently during, and after administration. • May cause transient decreases in serum glucose. • Arterial blood gases should be obtained frequently in emergency situations.

Patient/Family Teaching

- Explain the reason for administration of tromethamine to the patient.

≋ PHARMACOLOGIC PROFILE

Indications

- Tromethamine is used in the management of metabolic acidosis associated with cardiac bypass surgery or cardiac arrest.

Action

- Tromethamine acts as a proton acceptor in the treatment of acidosis. It is capable of combining with hydrogen ions to form bicarbonate and a buffer. • It also acts as an osmotic diuretic.

Time/Action Profile

Onset	Peak	Duration
rapid (minutes)	UK	UK

Pharmacokinetics

- **Distribution:** 30% reaches equilibrium in body water at normal pH (7.4). • **Metabolism and Excretion:** Excreted mainly by the kidneys. • **Half-life:** UK.

Contraindications

• Tromethamine is contraindicated in patients with anuria or uremia.

Adverse Reactions and Side Effects*

• **Resp:** respiratory depression • **GI:** hemorrhagic hepatic necrosis (neonates) • **Endo:** hypoglycemia (neonates) • **F and E:** alkalosis • **Local:** phlebitis, thrombosis at injection site.

Tubocurarine Chloride	*Neuromuscular blocking agent (nondepolarizing)*
{Tubarine}	pH 2.5–5

 ADMINISTRATION CONSIDERATIONS

Usual Dose

Adjunct to General Anesthesia

ADULTS: 6–9 mg initially, followed by 3–4.5 mg in 3–5 min if needed. Additional doses of 3 mg (0.165 mg/kg) may be given as need is determined.

INFANTS AND CHILDREN: 500 mcg (0.5 mg)/kg.

NEONATES−4 wk: 250–500 mcg (0.25–0.5 mg)/kg initially, then in increments of ⅓–⅙ of initial dose.

Adjunct to Electroconvulsive Therapy

ADULTS: 165 mcg (0.165 mg)/kg (initial doses should be 3 mg less than calculated dose).

Aid to Mechanical Ventilation

ADULTS: 1 mg or 16.5 mcg (0.0165 mg)/kg; subsequent doses may be given as necessary.

Diagnosis of Myasthenia Gravis

ADULTS: 4–33 mcg (0.004–0.033 mg)/kg. Profound myasthenic symptoms may occur and may be reversed with

---

*Underlines indicate most frequent; CAPITALS indicate life-threatening.

{} = Available in Canada only.

neostigmine (see *neostigmine methylsulfate* monograph on page 695).

Dilution

• **Direct IV:** Administer **undiluted** in a concentration not greater than 3 mg/ml.

Compatibility

• **Syringe:** pentobarbital ✦ thiopental.

• **Solution:** dextrose in Ringer's or lactated Ringer's combinations ✦ dextrose in saline combinations ✦ D5W ✦ D10W ✦ 0.45% NaCl ✦ 0.9% NaCl ✦ Ringer's and lactated Ringer's injection.

Incompatibility

• **Additive:** most barbiturates ✦ sodium bicarbonate ✦ trimethaphan.

Rate of Administration

• **Direct IV:** Administer dose over 60–90 seconds. Rapid injection or large doses cause histamine release, resulting in hypotension and bronchospasm. Titrate dose to patient response.

≋ CLINICAL PRECAUTIONS

• Tubocurarine should be used only by individuals experienced in endotracheal intubation, and equipment for this procedure should be immediately available.

• Assess respiratory status continuously throughout use of tubocurarine. Neuromuscular response to tubocurarine should be monitored intraoperatively with a peripheral nerve stimulator. Paralysis is initially selective and usually occurs consecutively in the following muscles: levator muscles of eyelids, muscles of mastication, limb muscles, abdominal muscles, muscles of the glottis, intercostal muscles, and the diaphragm. Recovery of muscle function usually occurs in reverse order.

• Monitor ECG, heart rate, and blood pressure throughout use of tubocurarine.

• Observe patient for residual weakness and respiratory distress during the recovery period.

• Tubocurarine has no effect on consciousness or the pain threshold. Adequate anesthesia/analgesia should *always* be used when tubocurarine is used as an adjunct to surgical procedures or when painful procedures are performed. Benzodiazepines and/or analgesics should be administered concurrently when prolonged tubocurarine therapy is used for ventilator patients, as patient is awake and able to feel all sensations.

- If eyes remain open throughout prolonged administration, protect corneas with artificial tears.
- Use cautiously in patients with a history of pulmonary disease or renal or liver impairment, in elderly or debilitated patients, and in patients with electrolyte disturbances, myasthenia gravis, or myasthenic syndromes.
- Intensity and duration of paralysis may be prolonged by pretreatment with succinylcholine, general anesthesia, aminoglycoside antibiotics, polymyxin B, colistin, clindamycin, lidocaine, quinidine, procainamide, beta-adrenergic blocking agents, potassium-losing diuretics, and magnesium. Dosage should be reduced by ⅔ if concurrent ether is used, ⅓ if methoxyflurane is used, and ⅕ if halothane or cyclopropane is used. Doxapram masks residual effects.
- Safe use in pregnancy or lactation has not been established (Pregnancy Category C).

Toxicity and Overdose Alert

- If overdose occurs, use peripheral nerve stimulator to determine the degree of neuromuscular blockade. Maintain airway patency and ventilation until recovery of normal respiration occurs. Administer anticholinesterase agents (edrophonium, neostigmine, pyridostigmine) to antagonize the action of tubocurarine. Atropine is usually administered prior to or concurrently with anticholinesterase agents to counteract the muscarinic effects. Administration of fluids and vasopressors may be necessary to treat severe hypotension or shock.

Patient/Family Teaching

- Explain all procedures to patient receiving tubocurarine therapy without anesthesia, as consciousness is not affected by tubocurarine alone. Provide emotional support.
- Reassure patient that communication abilities will return as the medication wears off.

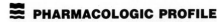

PHARMACOLOGIC PROFILE

Indications

- Tubocurarine is used to produce skeletal muscle paralysis after induction of anesthesia in surgical procedures. • It is also used during mechanical ventilation to improve pulmonary compliance, as an adjunct to electroconvulsive therapy, and as a diagnostic agent in myasthenia gravis.

Action

- Tubocurarine prevents neuromuscular transmission by blocking the effect of acetylcholine at the myoneural junction. • It has no anxiolytic or analgesic effects.

Time/Action Profile (skeletal muscle paralysis)

Onset	Peak	Duration
1 min	2–5 min	20–90 min†

†Duration increases with repeated dosing.

Pharmacokinetics

- **Distribution:** Tubocurarine is extensively distributed and subsequently redistributed to various tissue compartments. Saturation of compartments occurs, explaining prolonged duration of action following repeated doses. It crosses the placenta. • **Metabolism and Excretion:** 30–75% is excreted unchanged by the kidneys; 11% excreted in bile. Small amounts are metabolized by the liver. • **Half-life:** 2 hours.

Contraindications

- Tubocurarine is contraindicated in patients with hypersensitivity to it. Some products contain benzyl alcohol or bisulfites and should be avoided in patients with hypersensitivity or intolerance to these ingredients.

Adverse Reactions and Side Effects*

- **CV:** hypotension, arrhythmias • **EENT:** excess salivation • **Resp:** bronchospasm, APNEA • **GI:** decreased GI tone, decreased GI motility • **MS:** muscle weakness • **Misc:** allergic reactions.

---

*Underlines indicate most frequent; CAPITALS indicate life-threatening.

Urokinase	Thrombolytic
Abbokinase,	
Abbokinase Open-Cath	pH 6–7.5

ADMINISTRATION CONSIDERATIONS

Usual Dose

Pulmonary Emboli, Deep Vein Thrombosis
ADULTS: 4400 IU/kg loading dose over 10 min followed by 4400 IU/kg/hr for 12 hr.

Occluded IV Catheters
ADULTS: 1–1.8 ml of 5000 IU/ml solution injected into catheter, then aspirated; may repeat q 5 min for 30 min; if no result, may cap and leave in catheter for 30–60 min, then aspirate. After clearance, flush catheter.

Lysis of Coronary Thrombi, Myocardial Infarction
ADULTS: *Intracoronary* (preceded by 2500–10,000 units of heparin IV) 6000 IU/min for up to 2 hr (see *heparin sodium, heparin calcium* monograph on page 485).

Dilution
• **Intermittent Infusion:** **Reconstitute** each 250,000-IU vial with 5 ml of sterile water for injection without preservatives (direct to sides of vial) and swirl gently; do not shake. • Solution is light straw-colored. Do not administer solutions that are discolored or contain a precipitate. Use reconstituted solution immediately after preparation. • **Dilute further** with 190 ml of 0.9% NaCl or D5W for treatment of *pulmonary emboli.* • For intracoronary infusion, **add** the contents of three reconstituted 250,000-IU vials to 500 ml of D5W or 0.9% NaCl for a solution containing 1500 IU/ml. • **Cannula/ Catheter Clearance:** **Add** 1 ml of the previously reconstituted drug to 9 ml of sterile water for injection without preservatives. • Available in a dual-chamber vial, which reconstitutes to 5000 IU/ml concentration for clearance of occluded cannulae and catheters.

Incompatibility
• **Additive:** Manufacturer recommends not admixing with any medications.

Rate of Administration

- **Intermittent Infusion:** Infuse through a 0.45-micron filter. Administer via infusion pump to ensure accurate dosage. For *pulmonary emboli,* administer loading dose over 10 minutes and follow with infusion of 4400 IU/kg/hr for 12 hours. For *intracoronary* infusion, administer at a rate of 6000 IU (4 ml)/min until the artery is maximally opened, up to 2 hours. • **Cannula/Catheter Clearance:** Inject 1 ml slowly and gently into occluded cannula, and then clamp for 5 minutes. Aspirate contents carefully to remove clot. If unsuccessful, reclamp for 5 minutes. Repeat aspiration every 5 minutes until clot clears, up to 30 minutes. If still unsuccessful, clamp for 30–60 minutes and attempt to aspirate again. A second dose of urokinase may be needed. Once catheter is patent, aspirate 4–5 ml of blood, then irrigate the catheter with 10 ml of 0.9% NaCl in a separate syringe.

≋ CLINICAL PRECAUTIONS

- Urokinase should be used only in settings where hematologic function and clinical response can be adequately monitored. Invasive procedures, such as IM injections or arterial punctures, should be avoided with this therapy. If such procedures must be performed, apply pressure to IV puncture site for at least 15 minutes and to arterial puncture sites for at least 30 minutes.
- Assess patient for bleeding every 15 minutes during the first hour of therapy, every 15–30 minutes during the next 8 hours, and at least every 4 hours for the duration of therapy. Frank bleeding may occur from invasive sites or body orifices. Internal bleeding may also occur (decreased neurologic status, abdominal pain with coffee-ground emesis or black tarry stools, joint pain). If uncontrollable bleeding occurs, stop medication immediately.
- Monitor vital signs, including temperature, every 4 hours during course of therapy. Do not use lower extremities to measure blood pressure.
- Inquire about previous reaction to urokinase therapy. Assess patient for hypersensitivity (rash, dyspnea) or fever. Keep epinephrine, an antihistamine, and resuscitation equipment close by in the event of an anaphylactic reaction.

- Systemic anticoagulation with heparin is usually begun several hours after the completion of thrombolytic therapy.
- Monitor pulse, blood pressure, hemodynamics, and respiratory status (rate, degree of dyspnea, ABGs) in patients with pulmonary embolism.
- Observe extremities and palpate pulses of affected extremities every hour in patients with deep vein thrombosis or acute arterial occlusion for circulatory impairment. Computerized tomography, impedance plethysmography, quantitative Doppler effect determination, and/or angiography or venography may be used to determine effects and duration of therapy.
- Assess ability to aspirate blood as an indicator of patency. When connecting and disconnecting IV syringe, ensure that patient exhales and holds breath to prevent air embolism in patients with cannula or catheter occlusion.
- Monitor ECG continuously in patients with coronary thrombosis for significant arrhythmias. IV lidocaine or procainamide (Pronestyl) may be ordered prophylactically. Cardiac enzymes should be monitored. Coronary angiography or radionuclide myocardial scanning may be used to assess effectiveness of therapy.
- Concurrent use with other anticoagulants, cefamandole, cefotetan, plicamycin, or agents affecting platelet function, including aspirin, nonsteroidal anti-inflammatory agents, valproates, or dipyridamole, increases the risk of bleeding.
- Assess neurological status throughout therapy. Altered sensorium or mental changes may be indicative of intracranial bleeding.
- Urokinase should be used cautiously in patients with recent (<12 months) minor trauma or surgery, patients who are at risk of left heart thrombus, and in patients with cerebrovascular disease or diabetic hemorrhagic retinopathy. Elderly patients are at increased risk of intracranial bleeding.
- Safe use in pregnancy, lactation, or children has not been established (Pregnancy Category B). Use with *extreme caution* in the early (10 days) postpartum period.

Toxicity and Overdose Alert

• If local bleeding occurs, apply pressure to site. If severe or internal bleeding occurs, discontinue infusion. Clotting factors and/or blood volume may be restored through infusions of whole blood, packed RBCs, fresh frozen plasma, or cryoprecipitate. Do not administer dextran, as it has antiplatelet activity. Aminocaproic acid (Amicar) may be used as an antidote.

Lab Test Considerations

• Hematocrit, hemoglobin, platelet count, prothrombin time, thrombin time, activated partial thromboplastin time, and fibrinolytic activity should be evaluated prior to and frequently throughout course of therapy. Bleeding time may be assessed prior to therapy if patient has received platelet aggregation inhibitors. • Obtain type and crossmatch and have blood available at all times in case of hemorrhage. • Stools should be tested for occult blood loss and urine tested for hematuria periodically during therapy.

Patient/Family Teaching

• Explain purpose of medication to patient. • Instruct patient to report hypersensitivity reactions (rash, dyspnea), bleeding, or bruising. • Explain need for rest and minimal handling during therapy to avoid injury.

≋ PHARMACOLOGIC PROFILE

Indications

• Urokinase is used in the treatment of acute, massive pulmonary emboli and in the management of occluded IV catheters. It is also used to lyse coronary thrombi when given by the intracoronary route.

Action

• Urokinase directly activates plasminogen.

Time/Action Profile (thrombolysis)

Onset	Peak	Duration
immediate	rapid	up to 12 hr

Pharmacokinetics

• **Distribution:** UK. • **Metabolism and Excretion:** Urokinase is metabolized by the liver. • **Half-life:** 10–20 minutes.

Contraindications

• Urokinase is contraindicated in patients with hypersensitivity to it, and in patients with active internal bleeding, recent (<12 months) cerebrovascular accident, intracranial or intraspinal surgery, or intracranial neoplasm.

Adverse Reactions and Side Effects*

• **Resp:** bronchospasm • **Derm:** rash • **Hemat:** <u>BLEEDING</u> • **Misc:** fever, hypersensitivity reactions including ANAPHYLAXIS.

Vancomycin Hydrochloride	*Anti-infective (miscellaneous)*
Lyphocin, Vancocin, Vancoled	pH 2.5–4.5

≋ ADMINISTRATION CONSIDERATIONS

Usual Dose

Serious Systemic Infections

ADULTS: 500 mg (7.5 mg/kg) q 6 hr or 1 g (15 mg/kg) q 12 hr (up to 4 g/day).

CHILDREN: 10 mg/kg q 6 hr or 20 mg/kg q 12 hr (up to 60 mg/kg/day).

INFANTS: 10 mg/kg q 6 hr.

NEONATES 1 wk–1 mo: 15 mg/kg initially, then 10 mg/kg q 8 hr.

NEONATES <1 wk: 15 mg/kg initially, then 10 mg/kg q 8–12 hr.

Endocarditis Prophylaxis in Penicillin-Allergic Patients

ADULTS AND CHILDREN >27 kg: 1-g single dose 1 hr before procedure; may be repeated 8 hr later (see Appendix K).

---

*<u>Underlines</u> indicate most frequent; CAPITALS indicate life-threatening.

CHILDREN <**27 kg:** 20-mg/kg single dose 1 hr before procedure; may be repeated 8 hr later (see Appendix K).

Dilution

• **Intermittent Infusion: Dilute** each 500-mg vial with 10 ml of sterile water for injection. **Dilute further** with 100–200 ml of 0.9% NaCl, D5W, D10W, or lactated Ringer's solution. • Solution is stable for 14 days after initial reconstitution if refrigerated. After further dilution, solution is stable for 96 hours if refrigerated. • **Continuous Infusion:** May also be prepared as a continuous infusion with 1–2 g in sufficient volume to infuse over 24 hours. Thrombophlebitis can be minimized by diluting to 2.5–5 mg/ml and rotating injection sites. • Should be used only if intermittent infusion is not feasible.

Compatibility

• **Y-site:** acyclovir ◆ allopurinol sodium ◆ atracurium ◆ cyclophosphamide ◆ diltiazem ◆ enalaprilat ◆ esmolol ◆ filgrastim ◆ fluconazole ◆ fludarabine ◆ gallium nitrate ◆ hydromorphone ◆ insulin ◆ labetalol ◆ magnesium sulfate ◆ melphalan ◆ meperidine ◆ methotrexate ◆ morphine ◆ ondansetron ◆ paclitaxel ◆ pancuronium ◆ perphenazine ◆ tacrolimus ◆ tolazoline ◆ vecuronium ◆ vinorelbine ◆ zidovudine.

• **Additive:** amikacin ◆ atracurium ◆ calcium gluconate ◆ cimetidine ◆ corticotropin ◆ dimenhydrinate ◆ hydrocortisone sodium succinate ◆ potassium chloride ◆ ranitidine ◆ verapamil ◆ vitamin B complex with C.

Incompatibility

• **Syringe:** heparin.
• **Y-site:** albumin ◆ aztreonam ◆ idarubicin ◆ piperacillin/tazobactam.
• **Additive:** amobarbital ◆ chloramphenicol ◆ chlorothiazide ◆ dexamethasone ◆ methicillin ◆ pentobarbital ◆ phenobarbital ◆ secobarbital.

Rate of Administration

• **Intermittent Infusion:** Administer over at least 20–30 minutes. Do not administer rapidly or as a bolus. Administration over more than 60 minutes may minimize risk of thrombophlebitis, hypotension, and "red-man" or "red-neck syndrome" (sudden severe hypotension, flushing, and/or maculopapular rash of face, neck, chest, upper extremities). If reaction is severe, antihistamines, glucocorticoids, and IV fluids may be required. • **Continuous Infusion:** Administer slowly over 24 hours.

≋ CLINICAL PRECAUTIONS

- Assess patient for infection (vital signs; appearance of wound, sputum, urine, and stool; WBC) at beginning and throughout course of therapy.
- Obtain specimens for culture and sensitivity prior to initiating therapy. First dose may be given before receiving results.
- Monitor IV site closely. Vancomycin is irritating to tissues and causes necrosis and severe pain with extravasation. Rotate infusion site.
- Monitor blood pressure throughout IV infusion.
- Evaluate eighth cranial nerve function by audiometry and serum vancomycin levels prior to and throughout course of therapy in patients with borderline renal function or those over 60 years of age. Geriatric patients are more prone to ototoxicity and nephrotoxicity because of age-related renal impairment and difficulty in assessing hearing. Prompt recognition and intervention is essential in preventing permanent damage. Monitor intake and output ratios and daily weights. Cloudy or pink urine may be a sign of nephrotoxicity. May cause additive ototoxicity and nephrotoxicity when used concurrently with other ototoxic and nephrotoxic drugs (aspirin, aminoglycosides, cyclosporine, cisplatin, loop diuretics). When used with anesthetics in children, vancomycin causes erythema and histamine-like flushing. Use vancomycin cautiously in patients with renal impairment; increased dosing interval is recommended if creatinine clearance is 80 ml/min or less. Use cautiously in patients with hearing impairment. Vancomycin may potentiate neuromuscular blocking.
- Assess patient for signs of superinfection (black, furry overgrowth on tongue; vaginal itching or discharge; loose or foul-smelling stools).
- Safe use in pregnancy and lactation has not been established (Pregnancy Category C). Vancomycin has been

used during the second and third trimesters without adverse effects.

Toxicity and Overdose Alert

• Peak serum vancomycin levels should not exceed 25–40 mcg/ml. Trough concentrations should not exceed 5–10 mcg/ml.

Lab Test Considerations

• Monitor for casts, albumin, or cells in the urine or decreased urine specific gravity, CBC, and renal function periodically throughout course of therapy. Vancomycin may cause increased BUN levels.

Patient/Family Teaching

• Instruct patient to report signs of hypersensitivity, tinnitus, vertigo, or hearing loss. • Patients with a history of rheumatic heart disease or valve replacement need to be taught the importance of using antimicrobial prophylaxis prior to invasive dental or medical procedures.

≋ PHARMACOLOGIC PROFILE

Indications

• Vancomycin is used in the treatment of potentially life-threatening infections when less toxic anti-infectives are contraindicated. • It is particularly useful in staphylococcal infections such as endocarditis, osteomyelitis, pneumonia, septicemia, and soft tissue infections in patients who have allergies to penicillin or its derivatives or where sensitivity testing demonstrates resistance to methicillin. • It is also used as part of endocarditis prophylaxis in high-risk patients who are allergic to penicillin.

Action

• Vancomycin binds to bacterial cell wall, resulting in bactericidal action against susceptible organisms. • It is active against Gram-positive pathogens, including staphylococci (including methicillin-resistant strains of *Staphylococcus aureus*), Group A beta-hemolytic streptococci, *Streptococcus pneumoniae, Corynebacterium,* and *Clostridium.*

Time/Action Profile (blood levels)

Onset	Peak
rapid	end of infusion

Pharmacokinetics

• **Distribution:** Vancomycin is widely distributed. There is some penetration (20–30%) of CSF. It crosses the placenta.
• **Metabolism and Excretion:** IV vancomycin is eliminated almost entirely by the kidneys. • **Half-life:** 6 hours (increased in renal impairment).

Contraindications

• Vancomycin is contraindicated in patients with hypersensitivity to it.

Adverse Reactions and Side Effects*

• **EENT:** <u>ototoxicity</u> • **CV:** hypotension • **GI:** nausea • **GU:** <u>nephrotoxicity</u> • **Derm:** rashes • **Hemat:** leukopenia, eosinophilia • **Local:** <u>phlebitis</u> • **MS:** back and neck pain • **Misc:** hypersensitivity reactions including ANAPHYLAXIS, fever, chills, "red-man" syndrome, superinfection.

Vecuronium Bromide

Neuromuscular blocking agent (nondepolarizing)

Norcuron   pH 4

≋ ADMINISTRATION CONSIDERATIONS

Usual Dose

ADULTS AND CHILDREN ≥**10 yr:** *For intubation*—80–100 mcg/ kg after steady-state anesthesia is achieved; *after anesthesia with enflurane or isoflurane*—60–85 mg/kg; *after succinylcholine-assisted intubation and inhalation anesthesia*—40– 60 mcg/kg (wait for disappearance of succinylcholine effects); *after succinylcholine-assisted intubation and balanced*

---

*Underlines indicate most frequent; CAPITALS indicate life-threatening.

anesthesia—50–60 mcg/kg (wait for disappearance of succinylcholine effects). Up to 150–280 mcg/kg has been used in some patients during halothane anesthesia. *Maintenance*—10–15 mcg/kg 25–40 min after initial dose; then q 12–15 min as needed or as a continuous infusion at 1 mcg/kg/min (range 0.8–1.2 mcg/kg/min).

CHILDREN **1–10 yr:** Individualize dose. Slightly greater initial doses and more frequent supplemental doses may be necessary.

Dilution

• **Reconstitute** vecuronium with bacteriostatic water (may be provided by manufacturer), D5W, 0.9% NaCl, D5/0.9% NaCl, or lactated Ringer's injection. Solution reconstituted with bacteriostatic water is stable if refrigerated for 5 days. If other diluents are used, solution is stable for 24 hours if refrigerated. Discard all unused solutions. • **Direct IV: Reconstitute** each dose in 5–10 ml. • **Continuous Infusion:** Dilute 10–20 mg of vecuronium in 100 ml for a concentration of 0.1–0.2 mg/ml.

Compatibility

• **Y-site:** aminophylline ♦ cefazolin ♦ cefuroxime ♦ cimetidine ♦ dobutamine ♦ dopamine ♦ epinephrine ♦ esmolol ♦ fentanyl ♦ gentamicin ♦ heparin ♦ hydrocortisone sodium succinate ♦ isoproterenol ♦ lorazepam ♦ midazolam ♦ morphine ♦ nitroglycerin ♦ nitroprusside ♦ ranitidine ♦ trimethoprim/sulfamethoxazole ♦ vancomycin.

Incompatibility

• **Y-site:** diazepam ♦ most barbiturates.

Rate of Administration

• **Direct IV:** Administer via rapid injection. • **Continuous Infusion:** Titrate rate of infusion according to patient response.

≋ CLINICAL PRECAUTIONS

• Vecuronium should be used only by individuals experienced in endotracheal intubation, and equipment for this procedure should be immediately available.
• Assess respiratory status continuously throughout use of vecuronium. Neuromuscular response to vecuronium

should be monitored intraoperatively with a peripheral nerve stimulator. Paralysis is initially selective and usually occurs consecutively in the following muscles: levator muscles of eyelids, muscles of mastication, limb muscles, abdominal muscles, muscles of the glottis, intercostal muscles, and the diaphragm. Recovery of muscle function usually occurs in reverse order.

- Monitor ECG, heart rate, and blood pressure throughout use of vecuronium.
- Observe patient for residual muscle weakness and respiratory distress during the recovery period.
- Vecuronium has no effect on consciousness or the pain threshold. Adequate anesthesia/analgesia should *always* be used when vecuronium is used as an adjunct to surgical procedures or when painful procedures are performed. Benzodiazepines and/or analgesics should be administered concurrently when prolonged vecuronium therapy is used for ventilator patients, as patient is awake and able to feel all sensations.
- If eyes remain open throughout prolonged administration, protect corneas with artificial tears.
- Use cautiously in patients with any history of pulmonary or cardiovascular disease or renal or liver impairment, in elderly or debilitated patients, and in patients with electrolyte disturbances, myasthenia gravis, or myasthenic syndromes (*extreme caution*).
- Intensity and duration of paralysis may be prolonged by pretreatment with succinylcholine, general anesthesia, aminoglycoside antibiotics, polymyxin B, colistin, clindamycin, lidocaine, quinidine, procainamide, beta-adrenergic blocking agents, potassium-losing diuretics, and magnesium. Additive neuromuscular blockade may occur with inhalation anesthetic—decrease vecuronium dose by 15% when used with enflurane or isoflurane, and decrease dose of anesthetic by 30–50%.
- Safe use in pregnancy, lactation, or infants younger than 7 weeks has not been established (Pregnancy Category C). Children 7 weeks–1 year display increased sensitivity, resulting in prolonged recovery time.

Toxicity and Overdose Alert

- If overdose occurs, use peripheral nerve stimulator to determine the degree of neuromuscular blockade. Maintain airway patency and ventilation until recovery of normal respiration occurs. Administer anticholinesterase agents (edrophonium, neostigmine, pyridostigmine) to antagonize the action of vecuronium. Atropine is usually administered prior to or concurrently with anticholinesterase agents to counteract the muscarinic effects. Administration of fluids and vasopressors may be necessary to treat severe hypotension or shock.

Patient/Family Teaching

• Explain all procedures to patient receiving vecuronium therapy without anesthesia, as consciousness is not affected by vecuronium alone. Provide emotional support.
• Reassure patient that communication abilities will return as the medication wears off.

≋ PHARMACOLOGIC PROFILE

Indications

• Vecuronium is used to produce skeletal muscle paralysis and facilitation of intubation after induction of anesthesia in surgical procedures. It is also used during mechanical ventilation to increase pulmonary compliance.

Action

• Vecuronium prevents neuromuscular transmission by blocking the effect of acetylcholine at the myoneural junction.
• It has no analgesic or anxiolytic effects.

Time/Action Profile (skeletal muscle paralysis)

Onset	Peak	Duration
1 min	3–5 min	15–25 min

Pharmacokinetics

• **Distribution:** Vecuronium is rapidly distributed in extracellular fluid. Minimal penetration occurs into the CNS.
• **Metabolism and Excretion:** Some metabolism occurs in the liver (20%), with conversion to at least one active metabolite. Thirty-four percent is excreted unchanged by the kidneys. • **Half-life:** 31–80 minutes (decreased near term in pregnant patients, increased in patients with hepatic impairment).

Contraindications

• Vecuronium is contraindicated in patients with hypersensitivity to it or to bromides.

Adverse Reactions and Side Effects*

Most adverse reactions to vecuronium are extensions of pharmacologic effects.

• **Resp:** APNEA, respiratory insufficiency • **MS:** muscle weakness • **Misc:** allergic reactions.

Verapamil Hydrochloride	Antiarrhythmic (group IV), Calcium channel blocker
Isoptin	pH 4.1–6

 ADMINISTRATION CONSIDERATIONS

Usual Dose

ADULTS: 5–10 mg (75–150 mcg/kg); may repeat in 30 min.

CHILDREN 1–15 yr: 0.1–0.3 mg/kg over 2 min; may repeat in 30 min. Initial dose not to exceed 5 mg; repeat dose not to exceed 10 mg.

CHILDREN <1 yr: 0.1–0.2 mg/kg (usual range 0.75–2 mg per dose) over 2 min; may repeat in 30 min (not to exceed 5 mg/dose).

Dilution

• **Direct IV:** May be administered **undiluted**.

Compatibility

• **Syringe:** amrinone • heparin • milrinone.

• **Y-site:** amrinone • ciprofloxacin • dobutamine • dopamine • famotidine • hydralazine • meperidine • methicillin • milrinone • penicillin G potassium • piperacillin • ticarcillin.

---

*Underlines indicate most frequent; CAPITALS indicate life-threatening.

- **Solution:** D5W ✦ 0.9% NaCl ✦ 0.45% NaCl ✦ Ringer's injection ✦ lactated Ringer's injection ✦ D5/LR ✦ D5/0.9% NaCl ✦ D5/0.45% NaCl.

Incompatibility

- **Y-site:** albumin ✦ ampicillin ✦ mezlocillin ✦ nafcillin ✦ oxacillin ✦ sodium bicarbonate.

Rate of Administration

- **Direct IV:** Administer through Y-site or 3-way stopcock over 2 minutes for each single dose in adults and children. Administer over 3 minutes in geriatric patients.

≋ CLINICAL PRECAUTIONS

- Monitor blood pressure and pulse before and frequently during parenteral administration. Patients should remain recumbent for at least 1 hour following IV administration to minimize hypotensive effects.
- ECG should be monitored continuously during IV administration for symptomatic bradycardia or prolonged hypotension. Emergency equipment and medication should be available.
- Monitor intake and output ratios and daily weights. Assess patient for signs of congestive heart failure (peripheral edema, rales/crackles, dyspnea, weight gain, jugular venous distention).
- Patients receiving cardiac glycosides concurrently with verapamil should have serum digitalis levels routinely monitored and be monitored for signs and symptoms of cardiac glycoside toxicity.
- Use cautiously in patients with liver disease; dosage reduction is recommended. Use cautiously in patients with hypertrophic cardiomyopathy (when accompanied by paroxysmal nocturnal dyspnea, orthopnea, left ventricular obstruction, SA node dysfunction, heart block, or elevated pulmonary wedge pressure), congestive heart failure, sick sinus syndrome, or Duchenne's muscular dystrophy (may precipitate respiratory muscle failure).
- Geriatric patients may be more sensitive to the hypotensive and constipating effects of verapamil.
- The risk of bradycardia, congestive heart failure, and arrhythmias is increased by concurrent use of beta-adren-

ergic blocking agents or disopyramide. Additive hypotension may occur with acute ingestion of alcohol, or with concurrent use of antihypertensive agents, nitrates, or quinidine. Verapamil decreases the effectiveness of oral rifampin and increases the muscle relaxant effects of nondepolarizing neuromuscular blockers. Concurrent administration with calcium and vitamin D may result in decreased effectiveness of verapamil. Verapamil may decrease metabolism of and increase risk of toxicity from carbamazepine, cyclosporine, prazosin, or quinidine. The anesthetic effect of etomidate may be increased by verapamil. Severe hypotension may occur with concurrent use of fentanyl. Verapamil may increase risk of toxicity from theophylline.

- Safe use in pregnancy, lactation, or children has not been established (Pregnancy Category C). Maternal hypotension may result in fetal distress. Newborns may experience adverse hemodynamic reactions.

Lab Test Considerations

- May cause elevated alkaline phosphatase, CPK, LDH, AST (SGOT), and ALT (SGPT) levels.

Patient/Family Teaching

- Caution patient to make position changes slowly to minimize orthostatic hypotension. • Verapamil may cause dizziness. Advise patient to avoid activities requiring alertness until response to the medication is known.

≋ PHARMACOLOGIC PROFILE

Indications

- IV verapamil is used to control supraventricular tachyarrhythmias and rapid ventricular rates in atrial flutter or fibrillation.

Action

- Verapamil inhibits calcium transport into myocardial and vascular smooth muscle cells, resulting in inhibition of excitation-contraction coupling and subsequent contraction. It decreases SA and AV conduction and prolongs the AV node refractory periods in cardiac conduction tissue.

Time/Action Profile

	Onset	Peak	Duration
antiarrhythmic effects	1–5 min	3–5 min	2 hr
hemodynamic effects	3–5 min	UK	10–20 min

Pharmacokinetics

• **Distribution:** UK. Small amounts enter breast milk.
• **Metabolism and Excretion:** Verapamil is mostly metabolized by the liver, much of it on first-pass through the liver.
• **Half-life:** 4.5–12 hours.

Contraindications

• Verapamil is contraindicated in patients with hypersensitivity to it, and in patients with sinus bradycardia, advanced heart block, or severe congestive heart failure.

Adverse Reactions and Side Effects*

• **CNS:** <u>dizziness</u>, headache, fatigue • **CV:** <u>bradycardia</u>, <u>hypotension</u>, <u>edema</u>, heart block, congestive heart failure, SINUS ARREST, ASYSTOLE • **GI:** <u>constipation</u>, nausea, abdominal discomfort • **Resp:** pulmonary edema.

Vinblastine Sulfate
*Antineoplastic agent
(vinca alkaloid)*

Velban, {Velbe}, Velsar   pH 3.5–5

 ADMINISTRATION CONSIDERATIONS

Usual Dose

Doses may vary greatly depending on tumor, schedule, condition of patient, and blood counts.

ADULTS: 3.7 mg/m^2 (100 mcg/kg) single dose; increase at weekly intervals as tolerated by 1.8–1.9 mg/m^2 (50 mcg/kg) to a maximum of 18.5 mg/m^2 (150–200 mcg/kg) (usual dose is 5.5–7.4 mg/m^2). Maintenance dose is one

---

*<u>Underlines</u> indicate most frequent; CAPITALS indicate life-threatening.

{} = Available in Canada only.

decrement smaller than initial tolerated dose given q 7–14 days or 10 mg once or twice monthly.

Children: 2.5 mg/m^2 single dose; increase as tolerated at weekly intervals by 1.25 mg/m^2 to a maximum of 7.5 mg/m^2. Maintenance dose is one decrement smaller than initial tolerated dose given q 7–14 days.

Dilution

• **Direct IV: Dilute** each 10 mg with 10 ml of 0.9% NaCl for injection with phenol or benzyl alcohol. • Solution should be prepared in a biologic cabinet. Wear gloves, gown, and mask while handling medication. Discard IV equipment in specially designated containers (see Appendix F). • Reconstituted medication is stable for 30 days if refrigerated. • **Intermittent Infusion:** May be **further diluted** with 50–100 ml of 0.9% NaCl.

Compatibility

• **Syringe:** bleomycin • cisplatin • cyclophosphamide • droperidol • fluorouracil • leucovorin • methotrexate • metoclopramide • mitomycin • vincristine.

• **Y-site:** allopurinol sodium • bleomycin • cisplatin • cyclophosphamide • doxorubicin • droperidol • filgrastim • fludarabine • fluorouracil • heparin • leucovorin • melphalan • methotrexate • metoclopramide • mitomycin • ondansetron • paclitaxel • piperacillin/tazobactam • sargramostim • vincristine • vinorelbine.

Incompatibility

• **Syringe:** furosemide.
• **Y-site:** furosemide.

Rate of Administration

• **Direct IV:** Administer each single dose over 1 minute through Y-site injection or 3-way stopcock of a free-flowing infusion of 0.9% NaCl or D5W. • **Intermittent Infusion:** Administer over 15–30 minutes. Administering medication over a longer period or with more diluent may increase irritation of vein.

☰ CLINICAL PRECAUTIONS

• Monitor blood pressure, pulse, and respiratory rate during course of therapy. Assess patient for respiratory distress throughout therapy. Bronchospasm can be life-threatening and may occur at time of infusion or several hours later.

- Monitor for bone marrow depression. Assess for fever, sore throat, and signs of infection. Assess for bleeding (bleeding gums, bruising, petechiae; guaiac test stools, urine, and emesis). Avoid IM injections and rectal temperatures. Apply pressure to venipuncture sites for 10 minutes. Anemia may occur. Monitor for increased fatigue and dyspnea. Additive bone marrow depression may occur with other antineoplastic agents or radiation therapy.

- Vinblastine may cause nausea and vomiting. Monitor fluid intake and output, appetite, and nutritional intake. Prophylactic antiemetics may be used. Adjust diet as tolerated.

- Assess injection site frequently for redness, irritation, or inflammation. Vinblastine is a vesicant. If extravasation occurs, infusion must be stopped and restarted elsewhere to avoid damage to SC tissue. Inject 1–4 ml of a solution of hyaluronidase and 0.9% NaCl (150 units/ml), 1 ml for each ml extravasated, through existing IV cannula, or SC if needle has been removed, to enhance the absorption and dispersion of the extravasated drug. Apply warm compresses to increase the systemic absorption of the drug.

- Do not administer SC, IM, or IT. *Intrathecal administration* is fatal.

- Use cautiously in patients with impaired liver function. Decrease dose by 50% if serum bilirubin is greater than 3 mg/100 ml.

- Monitor for symptoms of gout (increased uric acid, joint pain, edema). Encourage patient to drink at least 2 liters of fluid per day. Allopurinol or alkalinization of urine may be used to decrease uric acid levels.

- Bronchospasm may occur in patients who have been previously treated with mitomycin.

- Do not confuse with vincristine (see *vincristine sulfate* monograph on page 1030).

- Use cautiously in patients with untreated active infections, decreased bone marrow reserve, or other chronic debilitating illnesses.

- Use cautiously in patients with childbearing potential.

Avoid using during pregnancy or lactation (Pregnancy Category D).

Lab Test Considerations

• Monitor CBC prior to and routinely throughout course of therapy. If WBC <2000, subsequent doses are usually withheld until WBC is at least 4000. The nadir of leukopenia occurs in 5–10 days, and recovery usually occurs 7–14 days later. Thrombocytopenia may also occur in patients who have received radiation or other chemotherapy agents. • Monitor liver function studies (AST [SGOT], ALT [SGPT], LDH, bilirubin) and renal function studies (BUN, creatinine) prior to and periodically throughout therapy. • Vinblastine may cause increased serum and urine uric acid. Monitor periodically during therapy.

Patient/Family Teaching

• Instruct patient to notify nurse immediately if redness, swelling, or pain at the injection site occurs. • Advise patient to notify physician in case of fever, chills, sore throat, signs of infection, bleeding gums, bruising, petechiae, or blood in urine, stool, or emesis. Caution patient to avoid crowds and persons with known infections. Instruct patient to use soft toothbrush and electric razor. • Caution patient not to drink alcoholic beverages or take products containing aspirin, ibuprofen, or naproxen, as these may precipitate gastric bleeding. • Instruct patient to inspect oral mucosa for redness and ulceration. If ulceration occurs, advise patient to avoid spicy foods, use sponge brush, and rinse mouth with water after eating and drinking. Treatment with analgesics may be required if pain interferes with eating. • Instruct patient to report symptoms of neurotoxicity (paresthesia, pain, difficulty walking, persistent constipation). • Advise patient that this medication may have teratogenic effects. A nonhormonal method of contraception should be used during therapy and for at least 2 months after therapy is concluded. • Discuss the possibility of hair loss with patient. Explore coping strategies. • Instruct patient not to receive any vaccinations without advice of physician. Vinblastine may decrease antibody response to live virus vaccines and increase the risk of adverse reactions. • Emphasize need for periodic lab tests to monitor for side effects.

≋ PHARMACOLOGIC PROFILE

Indications

• Vinblastine is used in combination chemotherapy as part of the treatment of lymphomas, nonseminomatous testicular carcinoma, advanced breast cancer, and other tumors.

Action

• Vinblastine binds to proteins of mitotic spindle, causing metaphase arrest. Cell replication is stopped as a result (cell cycle–specific for M phase). These effects result in death of rapidly replicating cells, particularly malignant ones. • It also has immunosuppressive properties.

Time/Action Profile (effects on WBC counts)

Onset	Peak	Duration
5–7 days	10 days	7–14 days

Pharmacokinetics

• **Distribution:** Vinblastine does not cross the blood–brain barrier well. • **Metabolism and Excretion:** Vinblastine is converted by the liver to an active antineoplastic compound. It is excreted in the feces via biliary excretion, with some renal elimination. • **Half-life:** 24 hours.

Contraindications

• Vinblastine is contraindicated in patients with hypersensitivity to it; and in pregnancy or lactation.

Adverse Reactions and Side Effects*

• **CNS:** neurotoxicity, depression, weakness, SEIZURES • **Resp:** BRONCHOSPASM • **GI:** nausea, vomiting, anorexia, diarrhea, stomatitis, constipation • **GU:** gonadal suppression • **Derm:** dermatitis, vesiculation, alopecia • **Hemat:** anemia, leukopenia, thrombocytopenia • **Local:** phlebitis at IV site • **Metab:** hyperuricemia • **Neuro:** peripheral neuropathy, paresthesia, neuritis.

---

*Underlines indicate most frequent; CAPITALS indicate life-threatening.

Vincristine Sulfate

*Antineoplastic agent
(vinca alkaloid)*

Oncovin, Vincasar PFS, Vincrex   pH 3.5–5.5

☰ ADMINISTRATION CONSIDERATIONS

Usual Dose

Many other protocols are used.

ADULTS: 10–30 mcg/kg or 0.4–1.4 mg/m^2; may repeat weekly.

CHILDREN >10 kg: 1.5–2-mg/m^2 single dose; may repeat weekly.

CHILDREN <10 kg: 50-mcg/kg (0.05 mg/kg) single dose; may repeat weekly.

Dilution

• **Direct IV: Reconstitute** by adding 5 ml of sterile water for injection to each vial for a concentration of 1 mg/ml. • Administer **undiluted**. • Solution should be prepared in a biologic cabinet. Wear gloves, gown, and mask while handling medication. Discard IV equipment in specially designated containers (see Appendix F).

Compatibility

• **Syringe:** bleomycin ◆ cisplatin ◆ cyclophosphamide ◆ doxapram ◆ doxorubicin ◆ droperidol ◆ fluorouracil ◆ heparin ◆ leucovorin calcium ◆ methotrexate ◆ metoclopramide ◆ mitomycin ◆ vinblastine.

• **Y-site:** allopurinol sodium ◆ bleomycin ◆ cisplatin ◆ cyclophosphamide ◆ doxorubicin ◆ droperidol ◆ filgrastim ◆ fludarabine ◆ fluorouracil ◆ heparin ◆ leucovorin calcium ◆ melphalan ◆ methotrexate ◆ metoclopramide ◆ mitomycin ◆ ondansetron ◆ paclitaxel ◆ piperacillin/tazobactam ◆ sargramostim ◆ vinblastine ◆ vinorelbine.

Incompatibility

• **Syringe:** furosemide.
• **Y-site:** furosemide.

Rate of Administration

• **Direct IV:** Administer each single dose direct IV push over 1 minute through Y-site injection or 3-way stopcock of a free-flowing infusion of 0.9% NaCl or D5W.

≋ CLINICAL PRECAUTIONS

- Monitor blood pressure, pulse, and respiratory rate for significant changes during course of therapy.
- Monitor neurologic status. Assess for paresthesia (numbness, tingling, pain), loss of deep tendon reflexes (Achilles reflex is usually first involved), weakness (wrist or foot drop, gait disturbances), cranial nerve palsies (jaw pain, hoarseness, ptosis, visual changes), autonomic dysfunction (ileus, difficulty voiding, orthostatic hypotension, impaired sweating), and CNS dysfunction (decreased level of consciousness, agitation, hallucinations). If these symptoms develop, they may persist for months.
- Monitor intake and output ratios and daily weights. Decreased urine output with concurrent hyponatremia may indicate syndrome of inappropriate secretion of antidiuretic hormone (SIADH), which usually responds to fluid restriction.
- Assess infusion site frequently for redness, irritation, or inflammation. Vincristine is a vesicant. If extravasation occurs, infusion must be stopped and restarted elsewhere to avoid damage to SC tissue. Cellulitis and discomfort may be minimized by infiltration with 1–4 ml of hyaluronidase mixed with 0.9% NaCl, 1 ml for each ml extravasated, through existing IV cannula, or SC if needle has been removed, to enhance the absorption and dispersion of the extravasated drug. Apply warm compresses to increase the systemic absorption of the drug.
- Do not administer SC, IM, or IT. *Intrathecal administration is fatal.*
- Assess nutritional status. An antiemetic may be used to minimize nausea and vomiting.
- Use cautiously in patients with impaired liver function. Decrease dose by 50% if serum bilirubin is greater than 3 mg/100 ml.
- Monitor for symptoms of gout (increased uric acid, joint pain, edema). Encourage patient to drink at least 2 liters of fluid per day. Allopurinol or alkalinization of urine may be used to decrease uric acid levels.
- Bronchospasm may occur in patients who have been

previously treated with mitomycin. L-asparaginase may decrease hepatic metabolism of vincristine (give vincristine 12–24 hours prior to asparaginase).

- Assess patient for constipation periodically during therapy. Prophylactic administration of a laxative or enema may be used to prevent upper colon impaction. Lactulose may also be effective.
- Do not confuse with vinblastine (see *vinblastine sulfate* monograph on page 1025).
- Use vincristine cautiously in patients with active untreated infections, decreased bone marrow reserve, or other chronic debilitating illnesses. Dosage reduction is recommended in patients with hepatic impairment.
- Use cautiously in patients with childbearing potential. Avoid use during pregnancy or lactation (Pregnancy Category D).

Lab Test Considerations

• Monitor CBC prior to and periodically throughout course of therapy. May cause slight leukopenia 4 days after therapy, which resolves within 7 days. Platelet count may increase or decrease. • Monitor liver function studies (AST [SGOT], ALT [SGPT], LDH, bilirubin) and renal function studies (BUN, creatinine) prior to and periodically throughout therapy. • May cause increased serum and urine uric acid concentrations. Monitor periodically during therapy.

Patient/Family Teaching

• Instruct patient to notify nurse immediately if redness, swelling, or pain at the injection site occurs. • Instruct patient to report symptoms of neurotoxicity (paresthesia, pain, difficulty walking, persistent constipation). Inform patient that increased fluid intake, dietary fiber, and exercise may minimize constipation. Stool softeners or laxatives may be required. Patient should inform physician if severe constipation or abdominal discomfort occur, as this may be a sign of neuropathy. • Advise patient to notify physician if fever; chills; sore throat; signs of infection; bleeding gums; bruising; petechiae; blood in urine, stool, or emesis; or mouth sores occur. Caution patient to avoid crowds and persons with known infections. • Advise patient that this medication may have teratogenic effects. A nonhormonal method of contraception should be used during therapy and for at least 2 months after therapy is concluded. • Discuss the possibility of hair loss with patient. Explore coping strategies. • Instruct patient not to receive any vaccinations without advice of physician. Vincristine may decrease antibody response to live virus vaccines and increase the risk of adverse reactions. • Emphasize need for periodic lab tests to monitor for side effects.

PHARMACOLOGIC PROFILE

Indications

• Vincristine is used alone and in combination with other treatment modalities (antineoplastic agents, surgery, or radiation therapy) in the treatment of Hodgkin's disease, leukemias, neuroblastoma, malignant lymphomas, rhabdomyosarcoma, Wilms' tumor, and other tumors.

Action

• Vincristine binds to proteins of mitotic spindle, causing metaphase arrest. Cell replication is stopped as a result (cell cycle–specific for M phase). This results in death of rapidly replicating cells, particularly malignant ones. It has little or no effect on bone marrow. • In addition, vincristine has immunosuppressive properties.

Time/Action Profile (effects on blood counts, which are usually mild)

Onset	Peak	Duration
UK	UK	7 days

Pharmacokinetics

• **Distribution:** Vincristine is rapidly and widely distributed. • **Metabolism and Excretion:** Vincristine is extensively metabolized by the liver and eliminated in the feces via biliary elimination. • **Half-life:** 10.5–37.5 hours.

Contraindications

• Vincristine is contraindicated in patients with hypersensitivity to it or to mannitol. • It should not be used in pregnancy or lactation.

Adverse Reactions and Side Effects*

• **CNS:** mental status changes, depression, agitation, insomnia • **Resp:** bronchospasm • **GI:** <u>nausea</u>, <u>vomiting</u>, anorexia, stomatitis, constipation, ileus, abdominal cramps • **GU:** urinary retention, nocturia, oliguria, gonadal suppression • **Derm:** alopecia • **Endo:** SIADH • **Hemat:** anemia, leukopenia, thrombocytopenia (mild and brief) • **Local:** <u>phlebitis</u> at IV site • **Metab:** hyperuricemia • **Neuro:** <u>neurotoxicity</u> (ascending peripheral neuropathy).

Vinorelbine Tartrate	*Antineoplastic agent*
	(vinca alkaloid)
Navelbine	**pH 3.5**

≋ ADMINISTRATION CONSIDERATIONS

Usual Dose

ADULTS: 30 mg/m^2 once weekly.

Dilution

• **Direct IV: Dilute** vinorelbine to a concentration of 1.5–3 mg/ml with 0.9% NaCl or D5W. • **Intermittent Infusion: Dilute** vinorelbine to a concentration of 0.5–2 mg/ml with 0.9% NaCl, D5W, 0.45% NaCl, D5/0.45% NaCl, Ringer's or lactated Ringer's injection. • Solution should be colorless to pale yellow. Do not administer solutions that are discolored or contain particulate matter. • Solution should be prepared in a biologic cabinet. Wear gloves, gown, and mask while handling medication. Discard IV equipment in specially designated containers (see Appendix F). • Diluted solution is stable for 24 hours at room temperature.

Compatibility

• **Y-site:** amikacin ✦ aztreonam ✦ bleomycin ✦ bumetanide ✦ buprenorphine ✦ butorphanol ✦ calcium gluconate ✦ car-

---

*<u>Underlines</u> indicate most frequent; CAPITALS indicate life-threatening.

boplatin ✦ carmustine ✦ cefotaxime ✦ ceftazidime ✦ ceftizoxime ✦ chlorpromazine ✦ cimetidine ✦ cisplatin ✦ clindamycin
✦ cyclophosphamide ✦ cytarabine ✦ dacarbazine ✦ dactinomycin ✦ daunorubicin ✦ dexamethasone sodium phosphate
✦ diphenhydramine ✦ doxorubicin ✦ doxycycline ✦ droperidol
✦ enalaprilat ✦ etoposide ✦ famotidine ✦ floxuridine ✦ fluconazole ✦ fludarabine ✦ gallium nitrate ✦ gentamicin ✦ haloperidol ✦ heparin ✦ hydrocortisone ✦ hydromorphone ✦ hydroxyzine ✦ idarubicin ✦ ifosfamide ✦ imipenem/cilastatin
✦ lorazepam ✦ mannitol ✦ mechlorethamine ✦ melphalan
✦ meperidine ✦ mesna ✦ methotrexate ✦ metoclopramide
✦ metronidazole ✦ miconazole ✦ minocycline ✦ mitoxantrone ✦ morphine ✦ nalbuphine ✦ netilmicin ✦ ondansetron
✦ plicamycin ✦ potassium chloride ✦ prochlorperazine ✦ promethazine ✦ ranitidine ✦ streptozocin ✦ ticarcillin ✦ ticarcillin/
clavulanate ✦ tobramycin ✦ vancomycin ✦ vinblastine ✦ vincristine ✦ zidovudine.

Incompatibility

- **Y-site:** acyclovir ✦ aminophylline ✦ amphotericin B
✦ ampicillin ✦ cefazolin ✦ cefoperazone ✦ ceforanide ✦ cefotetan ✦ ceftriaxone ✦ cefuroxime ✦ fluorouracil ✦ furosemide
✦ ganciclovir ✦ methylprednisolone ✦ mitomycin ✦ piperacillin ✦ sodium bicarbonate ✦ thiotepa ✦ trimethoprim/
sulfamethoxazole.

Rate of Administration

- **Direct IV:** Administer via slow IV push, over at least 1
minute. • **Intermittent Infusion:** Infuse over 6–10 minutes
into the Y-site closest to the bag of a free-flowing IV or into a
central line. • Flush the vein with at least 75–125 ml of 0.9%
NaCl or D5W administered over 10 minutes or more following administration.

≋ CLINICAL PRECAUTIONS

- Assess infusion site frequently for redness, irritation, or
inflammation. If extravasation occurs, infusion must be
stopped and restarted elsewhere to avoid damage to SC
tissue. Treatment of extravasation includes application
of warm compresses over the area immediately for 30–
60 minutes, then alternating on/off every 15 minutes
for 1 day. Hyaluronidase 150 units diluted in 1–2 ml of

0.9% NaCl should be injected through the existing cannula into the site of extravasation or SC if the needle has been removed, to enhance absorption and dispersion of the extravasated drug.

- Monitor blood pressure, pulse, and respiratory rate during course of therapy. Note significant changes. Acute shortness of breath and severe bronchospasm may occur infrequently shortly after administration. The risk of this adverse reaction may be increased by concurrent use of mitomycin or chest radiation therapy. Treatment with corticosteroids, bronchodilators, and supplemental oxygen may be required, especially in patients with a history of pulmonary disease.
- Assess frequently for signs of infection (sore throat, fever, cough, mental status changes), especially when a nadir of granulocytopenia is expected.
- Monitor neurologic status. Assess for paresthesia (numbness, tingling, pain); loss of deep tendon reflexes (Achilles reflex is usually first involved); weakness (wrist or foot drop, gait disturbances); cranial nerve palsies (jaw pain, hoarseness, ptosis, visual changes); autonomic dysfunction (constipation, ileus, difficulty voiding, orthostatic hypotension, impaired sweating); and CNS dysfunction (decreased level of consciousness, agitation, hallucinations). These symptoms may persist for months. The incidence of neurotoxicity associated with vinorelbine is less than that of other vinca alkaloids.
- Monitor intake and output ratios and weight for significant discrepancies.
- Assess nutritional status. Mild to moderate nausea is common. An antiemetic may be used to minimize nausea and vomiting.
- Monitor for symptoms of gout (increased uric acid, joint pain, edema). Encourage patient to drink at least 2 liters of fluid per day. Allopurinol or alkalinization of urine may decrease uric acid levels.
- Use cautiously in patients with impaired hepatic function. Dosage reduction is recommended if total bilirubin >2 mg/dl.
- Concurrent use with cisplatin increases the risk and severity of bone marrow depression.
- Vinorelbine should be used cautiously in patients with active infections, decreased bone marrow reserve, or

other chronic debilitating illnesses. Safe use in children has not been established.

- Use cautiously in patients with childbearing potential. Avoid use during pregnancy or lactation (Pregnancy Category D). Safe use in children has not been established.

Lab Test Considerations

- Monitor CBC prior to each dose and routinely throughout course of therapy. The nadir of granulocytopenia usually occurs 7–10 days after vinorelbine administration, and recovery usually follows within 7–14 days. If granulocyte count is <1500/mm^3, dosage reduction or temporary interruption of vinorelbine may be warranted. If repeated episodes of fever and/or sepsis occur during granulocytopenia, future dosage of vinorelbine should be modified. May also cause mild to moderate anemia. Thrombocytopenia rarely occurs. • Monitor liver function studies (AST [SGOT], ALT [SGPT], LDH, bilirubin) and renal function studies (BUN, creatinine) prior to and periodically throughout therapy. May cause increased uric acid. Monitor periodically during therapy.

Patient/Family Teaching

- Instruct patient to report symptoms of neurotoxicity (paresthesia, pain, difficulty walking, persistent constipation). • Inform patient that increased fluid intake, dietary fiber, and exercise may minimize constipation. Stool softeners or laxatives may be necessary. Patient should be advised to report severe constipation or abdominal discomfort as this may be a sign of ileus, which may occur as a consequence of neuropathy. • Advise patient to notify physician if fever, chills, sore throat, signs of infection, bleeding gums, bruising, petechiae, mouth sores, or blood in urine, stool, or emesis occurs. • Caution patient to avoid crowds and persons with known infections. • Advise patient that this medication may have teratogenic effects. Contraception should be used during and for at least 2 months after therapy is concluded. • Discuss with patient the possibility of hair loss and explore coping strategies. • Instruct patient not to receive any vaccinations without advice of physician. • Emphasize need for periodic lab tests to monitor for side effects.

≋ PHARMACOLOGIC PROFILE

Indications
- Vinorelbine is used alone or in combination with cis-platin in the treatment of ambulatory patients with advanced inoperable non–small cell cancer of the lung.

Action
- Vinorelbine binds to a protein (tubulin) of cellular microtubules, where it interferes with microtubule assembly. Cell replication is stopped as a result (cell cycle–specific for M phase), causing death of rapidly replicating cells, particularly malignant ones.

Time/Action Profile (effect on WBC counts)

Onset	Peak	Duration
UK	7–10 days	7–14 days

Pharmacokinetics
- **Distribution:** Vinorelbine has a high degree of binding to platelets and lymphocytes. The remainder of its distribution is not known. • **Metabolism and Excretion:** Vinorelbine is metabolized by the liver. At least one metabolite has antineoplastic activity. Large amounts are eliminated in feces; 11% is excreted unchanged in urine. • **Half-life:** 28–44 hours.

Contraindications
- Vinorelbine is contraindicated in patients with hypersensitivity to it. Its use should be avoided during pregnancy or lactation. Patients with pretreatment granulocyte counts <1000/mm^3 should not receive vinorelbine.

Adverse Reactions and Side Effects*
- **CNS:** <u>fatigue</u> • **Resp:** shortness of breath • **CV:** chest pain • **GI:** <u>constipation</u>, <u>nausea</u>, vomiting, diarrhea, anorexia, transient elevation of liver enzymes • **Hemat:** <u>neutropenia</u>, <u>anemia</u>, thrombocytopenia • **Derm:** <u>alopecia</u> • **Local:** <u>irritation at IV site</u>, <u>skin reactions</u>, phlebitis, rashes • **MS:** jaw pain, myalgia, arthralgia • **Neuro:** <u>neurotoxicity</u>.

---

*<u>Underlines</u> indicate most frequent; CAPITALS indicate life-threatening.

Zidovudine *Antiviral*

azidothymidine, AZT, Retrovir pH 5.5

≋ ADMINISTRATION CONSIDERATIONS

Usual Dose

ADULTS AND CHILDREN: 1–2 mg/kg infused over 60 min q 4 hr. Change to oral therapy as soon as possible.

INTRAPARTUM ADULTS: 2 mg/kg initially, then 1 mg/kg/hr while in labor and until the umbilical cord is clamped.

Dilution

• **Intermittent Infusion:** Remove the calculated dose from the vial and **dilute** with D5W or 0.9% NaCl for a concentration of no greater than 4 mg/ml. • Do not use solutions that are discolored. Stable for 8 hours at room temperature or 24 hours if refrigerated.

Compatibility

• **Y-site:** acyclovir • allopurinol sodium • amikacin • amphotericin B • aztreonam • ceftazidime • ceftriaxone • cimetidine • clindamycin • dexamethasone • dobutamine • dopamine • erythromycin lactobionate • filgrastim • fluconazole • fludarabine • gentamicin • heparin • imipenem/cilastatin • lorazepam • melphalan • metoclopramide • morphine • nafcillin • ondansetron • oxacillin • paclitaxel • pentamidine • phenylephrine • piperacillin • piperacillin/tazobactam • potassium chloride • ranitidine • sargramostim • tobramycin • trimethoprim/sulfamethoxazole • trimetrexate • vancomycin • vinorelbine.

Incompatibility

• **Additive:** blood products • protein solutions.

Rate of Administration

• **Intermittent Infusion:** Infuse at a constant rate over 1 hour. Avoid rapid infusion or bolus injection.

≋ CLINICAL PRECAUTIONS

• Patients should receive the IV infusion only until oral therapy can be administered.

- Assess patient for change in severity of symptoms of acquired immunodeficiency syndrome (AIDS) and for symptoms of opportunistic infections throughout therapy.
- Use zidovudine cautiously in patients with decreased bone marrow reserve; dosage reduction is required for granulocytopenia or anemia. Dosage modification may be required for impaired renal or hepatic function.
- Additive bone marrow depression may occur with other agents having bone marrow–depressing properties (antineoplastic agents or radiation therapy). Additive neurotoxicity may occur with acyclovir. Toxicity may be increased by concurrent administration of acetaminophen, amphotericin B, aspirin, benzodiazepines, cimetidine, indomethacin, interferon, pentamidine, sulfonamides, or probenecid.
- Although AZT is a common name for this drug, avoid using this abbreviation as it may be confused with other drugs (azathioprine, aztreonam) and lead to medication errors.
- Zidovudine has been used safely during pregnancy and in children, although safety is not established (Pregnancy Category C). Breast feeding should be avoided because the HIV virus may be transmitted to the infant in breast milk.

Lab Test Considerations

• Monitor CBC every 2 weeks for the first 8 weeks and then monthly if the first 2 months are well tolerated in symptomatic patients. Patients who are asymptomatic or have early symptoms should have CBC monitored monthly for the first 3 months and every 3 months thereafter, unless indicated for other reasons. Zidovudine commonly causes granulocytopenia and anemia. Anemia may occur 2–4 weeks after initiation of therapy. Granulocytopenia usually occurs after 6–8 weeks of therapy. Dosage reduction, discontinuation of therapy, or blood transfusions should be considered if hemoglobin is <7.5 g/dl and/or granulocyte count is <750/mm^3. Treatment with epoetin (see *epoetin alfa* monograph on page 385) or sargramostim (see *sargramostim* monograph on page 895) may be necessary. Therapy may be gradually resumed when bone marrow recovery is evident.

Patient/Family Teaching

- Zidovudine may cause dizziness or fainting. Caution patient to avoid driving or other activities requiring alertness until response to medication is known. • Inform patient that zidovudine does not cure AIDS and does not reduce the risk of transmission of HIV to others through sexual contact or blood contamination. Caution patient to avoid sexual contact, use a condom, and avoid sharing needles or donating blood, to prevent spreading the AIDS virus to others. • Instruct patient to notify physician promptly if fever, sore throat, or signs of infection occur. Caution patient to avoid crowds and persons with known infections. Instruct patient to use soft toothbrush, to use caution when using toothpicks or dental floss, and to have dental work done prior to therapy or deferred until blood counts return to normal. • Advise patient to avoid taking any over-the-counter medications without consulting physician or pharmacist. • Emphasize the importance of regular follow-up examinations and blood counts to determine progress and monitor for side effects.

 PHARMACOLOGIC PROFILE

Indications

- Zidovudine is used in the management of symptomatic human immunodeficiency virus (HIV, AIDS) and selected patients with ARC.

Action

- Following intracellular conversion to its active form, zidovudine inhibits viral RNA synthesis by inhibiting the enzyme DNA polymerase (reverse transcriptase). This effect prevents viral replication. Although not curative, zidovudine may slow the progression or decrease the severity of the disease and its associated sequelae.

Time/Action Profile (blood levels)

Onset	Peak
rapid	end of infusion

Pharmacokinetics

• **Distribution:** Zidovudine is widely distributed and enters the CSF. It probably crosses the placenta. • **Metabolism and Excretion:** Zidovudine is mostly metabolized by the liver; 15–20% is excreted unchanged by the kidneys. • **Half-life:** 1 hour.

Contraindications

• Zidovudine is contraindicated in patients with hypersensitivity to it. • It should not be used during lactation.

Adverse Reactions and Side Effects*

• **CNS:** <u>headache</u>, <u>weakness</u>, malaise, somnolence, restlessness, insomnia, anxiety, confusion, depression, decreased mental acuity, dizziness, fainting • **GI:** <u>nausea</u>, <u>abdominal pain</u>, <u>diarrhea</u>, dyspepsia, anorexia, vomiting, hepatitis • **Derm:** nail pigmentation • **Hemat:** <u>anemia</u>, <u>granulocytopenia</u>, thrombocytosis • **MS:** back pain, myalgia • **Neuro:** tremor.

---

*<u>Underlines</u> indicate most frequent; CAPITALS indicate life-threatening.

APPENDIX A
Schedules of Controlled Substances

Classes or schedules are determined by the Drug Enforcement Agency (DEA) of the United States Department of Justice and are selected based on the potential for abuse and the dependence liability (physical and psychological) of the medication.

Schedule I (C-I)
Potential for abuse is unacceptably high. May be used for research with appropriate limitations (e.g., LSD and heroin).

Schedule II (C-II)
High potential for abuse and extreme liability for dependence (e.g., amphetamines, opioid analgesics, cannabinoids, certain barbiturates). Outpatient prescriptions must be in writing. In emergencies telephone orders may be acceptable, if a written prescription is provided within 72 hours; no refills are allowed.

Schedule II Drugs Included in *Davis's Guide to IV Medications*:

alfentanil	meperidine
amobarbital	morphine
droperidol/fentanyl	oxymorphone
fentanyl	pentobarbital
hydromorphone	secobarbital
levorphanol	sufentanil

Schedule III (C-III)
Intermediate potential for abuse (less than C-II) and intermediate liability for dependence (e.g., certain nonbarbiturate sedatives, certain nonamphetamine central nervous system stimulants, limited dosages of certain opioid analgesics). Outpatient prescriptions can be refilled five times within 6 months from date of issue, if authorized by prescriber; telephone orders are acceptable.

Schedule III Drugs Included in *Davis's Guide to IV Medications*:

thiopental

(Continued)

APPENDIX A
Schedules of Controlled Substances
(Continued)

<u>Schedule IV (C-IV)</u>
Less abuse potential than Schedule III with minimal liability for dependence (e.g., certain sedative/hypnotics, certain antianxiety agents, some barbiturates, benzodiazepines, pentazocine). Outpatient prescriptions can be refilled five times within 6 months from date of issue if authorized by prescriber; telephone orders are acceptable.

<u>Schedule IV Drugs Included in *Davis's Guide to IV Medications*</u>:

chlordiazepoxide	midazolam
diazepam	pentazocine
lorazepam	phenobarbital

<u>Schedule V (C-V)</u>
Minimal abuse potential. Number of outpatient refills determined by prescriber.

<u>Schedule V Drugs Included in *Davis's Guide to IV Medications*</u>:

buprenorphine

Individual states may have stricter prescription regulations.

APPENDIX B
Equianalgesic Tables

DOSING DATA FOR OPIOID ANALGESICS*

Drug	Approximate Equianalgesic Dose		Recommended Starting Dose (adults more than 50 kg body weight)		Recommended Starting Dose (children and adults less than 50 kg body weight)[1]	
	Oral	Parenteral	Oral	Parenteral	Oral	Parenteral
Opioid Agonist						
Morphine[2]	30 mg q 3–4 hr (around-the-clock dosing) 60 mg q 3–4 hr (single dose or intermittent dosing)	10 mg q 3–4 hr	30 mg q 3–4 hr	10 mg q 3–4 hr	0.3 mg/kg q 3–4 hr	0.1 mg/kg q 3–4 hr
Codeine[3]	180–200 mg q 3–4 hr	130 mg q 3–4 hr	60 mg q 3–4 hr	60 mg q 2 hr (intramuscular/subcutaneous)	1 mg/kg q 3–4 hr[4]	Not recommended
Hydromorphone[2] (Dilaudid)	7.5 mg q 3–4 hr	1.5 mg q 3–4 hr	6 mg q 3–4 hr	1.5 mg q 3–4 hr	0.06 mg/kg q 3–4 hr	0.015 mg/kg q 3–4 hr

(Continued)

APPENDIX B
Equianalgesic Tables (*Continued*)

DOSING DATA FOR OPIOID ANALGESICS*

Drug	Approximate Equianalgesic Dose		Recommended Starting Dose (adults more than 50 kg body weight)		Recommended Starting Dose (children and adults less than 50 kg body weight)[1]	
	Oral	Parenteral	Oral	Parenteral	Oral	Parenteral
Hydrocodone (in Lorcet, Lortab, Vicodin, others)	30 mg q 3–4 hr	Not available	10 mg q 3–4 hr	Not available	0.2 mg/kg q 3–4 hr[4]	Not available
Levorphanol (Levo-Dromoran)	4 mg q 6–8 hr	2 mg q 6–8 hr	4 mg q 6–8 hr	2 mg q 6–8 hr	0.04 mg/kg q 6–8 hr	0.02 mg/kg q 6–8 hr
Meperidine (Demerol)	300 mg q 2–3 hr	100 mg q 3 hr	Not recommended	100 mg q 3 hr	Not recommended	0.75 mg/kg q 2–3 hr
Methadone (Dolophine, others)	20 mg q 6–8 hr	10 mg q 6–8 hr	20 mg q 6–8 hr	10 mg q 6–8 hr	0.2 mg/kg q 6–8 hr	0.1 mg/kg q 6–8 hr

Drug						
Oxycodone (Roxicodone, also in Percocet, Percodan, Tylox, others)	30 mg q 3–4 hr	Not available	10 mg q 3–4 hr	Not available	0.2 mg/kg q 3–4 hr[4]	Not available
Oxymorphone[2] (Numorphan)	Not available	1 mg q 3–4 hr	Not available	1 mg q 3–4 hr	Not recommended	Not recommended
Opioid Agonist-Antagonist and Partial Agonist						
Buprenorphine (Buprenex)	Not available	0.3–0.4 mg q 6–8 hr	Not available	0.4 mg q 6–8 hr	Not available	0.004 mg/kg q 6–8 hr
Butorphanol (Stadol)	Not available	2 mg q 3–4 hr	Not available	2 mg q 3–4 hr	Not available	Not recommended
Dezocine (Dalgan)	Not available	10 mg q 3–4 hr	Not available	10 mg q 3–4 hr	Not available	Not recommended
Nalbuphine (Nubain)	Not available	10 mg q 3–4 hr	Not available	10 mg q 3–4 hr	Not available	0.1 mg/kg q 3–4 hr
Pentazocine (Talwin, others)	150 mg q 3–4 hr	60 mg q 3–4 hr	50 mg q 4–6 hr	Not recommended	Not recommended	Not recommended

Note: Published tables vary in the suggested doses that are equianalgesic to morphine. Clinical response is the criterion that must be applied for each patient; titration to clinical response is necessary. Because there is not complete cross tolerance among these drugs, it is usually necessary to use a lower than equianalgesic dose when changing drugs and to retitrate to response.

(Continued)

APPENDIX B
Equianalgesic Tables
(Continued)

Caution: Recommended doses do not apply to patients with renal or hepatic insufficiency or other conditions affecting drug metabolism and kinetics.

[1] **Caution:** Doses listed for patients with body weight less than 50 kg cannot be used as initial starting doses in babies less than 6 months of age. Consult the *Clinical Practice Guideline for Acute Pain Management: Operative or Medical Procedures and Trauma* section on management of pain in neonates for recommendations.

[2] For morphine, hydromorphone, and oxymorphone, rectal administration is an alternate route for patients unable to take oral medications, but equianalgesic doses may differ from oral and parenteral doses because of pharmacokinetic differences.

[3] **Caution:** Codeine doses above 65 mg often are not appropriate due to diminishing incremental analgesia with increasing doses but continually increasing constipation and other side effects. Oral doses refer to combination with aspirin or acetaminophen.

[4] **Caution:** Doses of aspirin and acetaminophen in combination opioid/NSAID preparations must also be adjusted to the patient's body weight.

*Adapted from Acute Pain Management Guideline Panel: *Acute Pain Management in Adults: Operative Procedures. Quick Reference Guide for Clinicians.* Agency for Health Care Policy and Research, Public Health Service, U.S. Department of Health and Human Services, Rockville, MD. AHCPR Publication No. 92-0019.

(Continued)

FENTANYL TRANSDERMAL DOSE BASED ON DAILY MORPHINE EQUIVALENCE DOSE*

Oral 24-hr Morphine (mg/day)	IM 24-hr Morphine (mg/day)	Fentanyl Transdermal (mcg/hr)
45–134	8–22	25
135–224	23–37	50
225–314	38–52	75
315–404	53–67	100
405–494	68–82	125
495–584	83–97	150
585–674	98–112	175
675–764	113–127	200
765–854	128–142	225
855–944	143–157	250
945–1034	158–172	275
1035–1124	173–187	300

*A 10-mg IM or 60-mg oral dose of morphine every 4 hr for 24 hr (total of 60 mg/day IM or 360 mg/day oral) was considered approximately equivalent to fentanyl transdermal 100 mcg/hr.

APPENDIX B
Equianalgesic Tables
(*Continued*)

OPIOID ANALGESICS COMMONLY USED FOR MILD TO MODERATE PAIN

Name	Starting Dose* Adults (mg)	Starting Dose* Children (mg/kg)	Comments	Precautions and Contraindications
Morphine-like Agonists				
Codeine	30–60	0.5–1	Many preparations include combination with nonopioid analgesics.†	Caution in patients with impaired ventilation, bronchial asthma, increased intracranial pressure, liver failure.
Hydrocodone (in Lorcet, Lortab, Vicodin, Zydone, others)	5–10	0.2 mg/kg	Preparations include acetaminophen, which limits daily dose.	Same as codeine.
Oxycodone	5–10	0.1	Shorter acting; many preparations include acetaminophen, which limits dose to 12 tabs/day.†	Same as for codeine.

Meperidine (Demerol)	NR‡	Shorter acting; biotransformed to normeperidine, a toxic metabolite.	Normeperidine accumulates with repetitive dosing, causing CNS excitation; avoid in patients with impaired renal function or who are receiving monoamine oxidase inhibitors; avoid any chronic use.
Propoxyphene (Darvon)	65–130	Weak analgesic; many preparations include nonopioid analgesics; biotransformed to potentially toxic metabolite (norpropoxyphene).	Propoxyphene and metabolite accumulate with repetitive dosing; overdose complicated by convulsions.
Mixed Agonist-Antagonist			
Pentazocine (Talwin)	50	Some preparations include naloxone to discourage parenteral abuse.	May cause psychotomimetic effects; may precipitate withdrawal in opioid-dependent patients.

*Starting doses are approximately equianalgesic to aspirin 650 mg (adults) or 10–15 mg/kg (children). The optimal dose for each patient is determined by titration.

†In children, opioid-acetaminophen formulations must not exceed the maximum safe dose of acetaminophen, 90 mg/kg/day.

‡NR = not recommended.

Adapted from American Pain Society: *Principles of Analgesic Use in the Treatment of Acute Pain and Cancer Pain*, ed 3, 1992.

APPENDIX C
Infusion Control Devices

Because of the accuracy of drug delivery required by the IV route, in terms of drug dosage and volume infused, a variety of systems to precisely control rates have evolved over the years.

In many commonly encountered clinical situations, gravity-driven flow control devices will suffice. These devices are usually in-line and alter rate of flow by pinching the tubing, changing its diameter and flow rate (roller clamps, screw clamps), or having the tubing either open or closed (slide clamps, pinch clamps). More accurate flow regulators were developed, which were also in-line systems. However, these systems were often not responsive to changes in the position of the patient and were limited in terms of rates and volumes reproducibly achieved.

Mechanical infusion control devices (ICDs) are becoming more commonly used in a variety of patient care settings. Since the 1960s, modern technology has greatly advanced the degree of sophistication of these instruments, making them safe, accurate, and convenient. The advances in technology were fueled by the increasing use of more toxic drugs (antineoplastic agents) and use of drugs requiring close titration (cardiovascular agents, thrombolytics). Many patient populations require specific doses or volumes using systems that allow close titration as well as transportability (neonates, home care patients). The availability of accurate microelectric circuitry has enhanced the development of ICDs.

ICDs can be divided into two basic categories: *controllers,* which are gravity dependent, and *positive pressure pumps:*

Controllers maintain a constant rate of fluid administration in a gravity flow system by electronically measuring and adjusting for changes in flow rate. Controllers are more accurate than gravity flow clamp-controlled systems. They do not generate pressure, but control the delivery rate by monitoring drop rate or a similar parameter and thus determining flow through tubing. Viscous fluids such as blood, fat emulsion, or hypertonic dextrose cannot be delivered with these systems.

Positive pressure pumps are able to deliver a variety of fluids at varying rates and can overcome back pressure. Positive pressure pumps can be of several types, depending on the mechanism of operation. *Peristaltic pumps* use a massaging action on tubing to produce small pulses of fluid per unit of time and can employ either linear peristaltic motion (finger-like projections move the fluid along) or rotary peristaltic motion (uses rollers to propel fluid). *Cassette pumps* consist of a plastic chamber and tubing that use sequential filling and emptying to deliver fluid, using either a syringe mechanism, a piston, or a dual-piston-activated mechanism. *Syringe pumps* use a motor-driven lead screw or gear mechanism to move the syringe or plunger. *Nonelectric pumps* may work by either elastomeric or vacuum pressure and do not require an external power source. The advantages and disadvantages of various pumps are compared in the following table.

Several pumps combine the advantages of controllers with positive-pressure devices to offer units adaptable to a variety of clinical situations.

ICDs may also be grouped by use. *Patient-controlled analgesia (PCA) pumps* allow programming of a chosen constant infusion rate and a limited number of intermittent bolus doses separated by a specific lockout time during which no further boluses may be selected. These instruments allow rapid and flexible alteration of dosing to produce rapid control of pain. *Ambulatory infusion pumps* refer to the size and weight of the ICD and its ability to run without an external power source. The Verifuse (from Block Medical) is an example. *Implantable pumps,* ICDs with very small reservoirs, are implanted in subcutaneous tissue. Very concentrated solutions are instilled in the reservoir and infused at extremely slow rates. Antineoplastic agents and insulin may be administered by this type of pump.

Of the many types of features available in ICDs today, several are worth mentioning. *Macrorate pumps* are capable of delivering 1 to 999 ml/hr, in 1-ml increments. *Microrate pumps,* which are very useful in neonatal intensive care units and for the infusion of critical care drugs in concentrated solutions, are capable of delivering 0.1 to 99.9 ml/hr in increments of 0.1 ml. Both features may be combined in one ICD. *Multiple-solution* or *multiple-channel pumps* allow concurrent administration of two infusion solutions at independent rates. If only a single outflow channel is available, the possibility of incompatibilities must be considered. See the compatibility sections

(Continued)

APPENDIX C
Infusion Control Devices
(*Continued*)

of each monograph for important information regarding potential problems. *Multiple-rate pumps* allow the infusion of one or more solutions at varying rates, permitting ramping (increasing rates) and tapering (decreasing rates) or administration of piggybacks at preselected intervals. Other pumps allow for *weight-based dosing,* whereby the dose may be entered in mcg/kg/min, the patient's weight is entered separately, and the infusion rate appropriate for that patient is calculated and programmed. Among the most novel technologies available is the use of *closed-loop systems.* These ICDs include equipment that is capable of measuring a physiologic parameter (blood pressure, blood sugar) and automatically adjusting the infusion rate (dosage) accordingly.

ICDs are also available with a variety of alarms capable of detecting occlusion, empty fluid containers, completion of infusion, air in the line, and flow rate errors.

Emerging technology in ICDs allows precise administration of medications in a safe and efficient environment. However, their use should not preclude constant vigilance to the IV site itself and the intended therapeutic effect of the drug being administered.

For more detailed information, experts in the clinical setting or the manufacturer should be consulted.

APPENDIX C
Infusion Control Devices

Name (Manufacturer)	Flow Rate/Range	Alarms	Selected Features
Controllers			
Life Care 1050 (Abbott)	Micro: 5–250 ml/hr Macro: 20–400 ml/hr	Dose delivered, empty bag, flow status	Dual-rate automatic piggybacking
Control-A-Flow Regulator (Baxter)	10–250 ml/hr	None	Constant flow rate despite head height, nonelectronic
Volumetric Controller Model 262+ (Ivac)	5–299 ml/hr	Empty bag, occlusion, check flow, closed clamp, infiltrate, low battery	LED display panel, set-up prompts
Rateminder IV (Critikon)	3–500 ml/hr	Occlusion, end of infusion, service check	Cordless, uses any manufacturer's gravity-flow IV set, rate-clip flow regulator
Infusion Pumps/Controllers			
Life Care 5000 "The Plum" (Abbott)	Micro: 0.1–99.9 ml/hr Macro: 1–999 ml/hr	Proximal and distal occlusion, air in line, pressure out of range	Automatic piggybacking, accepts a wide variety of secondary delivery systems
Gemini PC2 (Imed)	Macro: 1–999 ml/hr	Occlusion (patient side or fluid side), close door, check IV set, air in line	Allows delivery of two primary infusion solutions with piggybacking capabilities

(Continued)

APPENDIX C
Infusion Control Devices (*Continued*)

Name (Manufacturer)	Flow Rate/Range	Alarms	Selected Features
Infusion Pumps			
521 Plus Intelligent 522 Plus Intelligent (McGaw)	Macro: 1–999 ml/hr	Air in line, empty container, check IV set, door open, pump on hold, occlusion, completed infusion, repair problem, flow problem	Allows variable delivery modes, has variable pressure settings
Omni-Flow 4000 (Abbott)	Macro: 1.4–800 ml/hr	Cassette unlocked, faulty cassette, air in line, empty container	Can deliver four separate solutions, simultaneously or intermittently at variable rates
Omni-Flow 4000 PLUS (Abbott)	Macro: 1.4–800 ml/hr	Cassette unlocked, faulty cassette, air in line, empty container	Can deliver four separate solutions, simultaneously or intermittently at variable rates, automatic line-purging, computer interface; not intended for use in neonates
The Horizon Modular Infusion System (McGaw)	Micro/macro: 0.1–999 ml/hr	Air in line, door open, container empty, occlusion, set primary or secondary rate of volume, set improperly loaded	Can lock out macro mode for use in pediatrics, tapering capabilities, computer interface; units can be stacked

Device	Rate	Alarms	Features
Sigma 6000 + (Smith and Nephew Sigma Inc)	Micro/macro: 0.1–999 ml/hr	Air in line, occlusion, door open, empty bottle, infusion complete, program complete	Uses standard IV infusion sets, automatic piggybacking
Syringe Pumps			
Bard Mini Infuser System Models 150 XL, 300XL, and 400 (McGaw)	10–120 ml/hr (Bard 400), others are variable	Occlusion, low battery, completed infusion	150 XL uses any 5–60 ml syringe, 300 ml syringe, 300 ml syringe; 150 XL is battery-operated
360 Infuser (Becton Dickinson)	1.5–360 ml/hr	Occlusion, end of infusion, low battery, syringe displacement	Can deliver at various rates or time periods; can be battery-operated
Patient-controlled Analgesia (PCA) Pumps			
Life Care PCA Plus II 4100 Infusor (Abbott)	0.1–200 mg/hr	Check vial, syringe, or injection; check 4-hr limit, door open, occlusion, low battery, reset	Uses prefilled syringes, provides continuous administration plus bolus doses, logs patient requests for breakthrough; patient is limited to 4-hr access; can be battery-operated
CADD-PCA Ambulatory Infusion Pump Model 5800 (Pharmacia Deltec)	Bolus 0–99 mg/hr (0–20 ml/hr) Infusion 0–99 mg/hr (0–6 ml/hr)	Low battery, low or empty reservoir, infusion complete, improper delivery	Doses can be programmed in mg or ml; records doses delivered or attempted; can be battery-operated
Epidural Narcotic Infusion Devices			
Pain Management Provider (Abbott)	0.1–25 ml/hr in 0.1-ml increments		Can be programmed in ml/hr, mg/hr, or mcg/hr; accepts concentrations from 0.1–100 mg/ml or 0.1–100 mcg/ml

APPENDIX D
Food and Drug Administration (FDA) Pregnancy Categories

Category A

No risk to the fetus in the first trimester has been demonstrated by adequate, well-controlled studies. In addition, there does not appear to be risk in the second or third trimester.

Category B

Studies in animals may or may not show risk. If risk has been shown in animals, no risk has been shown in human studies. If risk has not been seen in animals, there are insufficient data in pregnant women.

Category C

Adverse effects have been demonstrated in animal studies, but there are insufficient data for studies in pregnant women. In some clinical situations, the benefits from the use of the drug could outweigh its potential risks.

Category D

Based on information collected in clinical investigations or postmarketing surveillance, human fetal risk has been demonstrated. In specific selected clinical situations, the benefits from the use of the drug could outweigh its potential risks.

Category X

Human fetal risk has been documented clearly. Possible risks to the fetus outweigh potential benefits to pregnant women. Avoid use during pregnancy.

APPENDIX E
Formulas and Nomograms Helpful for Calculating Doses

RATIO AND PROPORTION

A ratio is the same as a fraction and can be expressed as a fraction ($\frac{1}{2}$) or in the algebraic form ($1:2$). This relationship is stated as *one is to two*.

A proportion is an equation of equal fractions or ratios.

$$\frac{1}{2} = \frac{4}{8}$$

To calculate doses, begin each proportion with the two known values, for example 15 grains = 1 gram (known equivalent) or 10 milligrams = 2 milliliters (dosage available) on one side of the equation. Next, make certain that the units of measure on the opposite side of the equation are the same as the units of the known values and are placed on the same level of the equation.

Problem A: $\dfrac{15\,gr}{1\,g} = \dfrac{10\,gr}{x\,g}$

Problem B: $\dfrac{10\,mg}{2\,ml} = \dfrac{5\,mg}{x\,ml}$

Once the proportion is set up correctly, cross-multiply the opposing values of the proportion.

Problem A: $\dfrac{15\,gr}{1\,g} \times \dfrac{10\,gr}{x\,g}$

$$15x = 10$$

Problem B: $\dfrac{10\,mg}{2\,ml} \times \dfrac{5\,mg}{x\,ml}$

$$10x = 10$$

Next, divide each side of the equation by the number with the *x* to determine the answer. Then, add the unit of measure corresponding to *x* in the original equation.

(Continued)

APPENDIX E
Formulas and Nomograms Helpful for Calculating Doses (*Continued*)

Problem A:
$$\frac{15x}{15} = \frac{10}{15}$$

$$x = \frac{2}{3} \text{ or } 0.6 \text{ g}$$

Problem B:
$$\frac{10x}{10} = \frac{10}{10}$$

$$x = 1 \text{ ml}$$

CALCULATION OF IV DRIP RATE
To calculate the drip rate for an intravenous infusion, three values are needed:

I. The amount of solution and corresponding time for infusion. May be ordered as:

1000 ml over 8 hr

or

125 ml/hr

II. The equivalent in time to convert hours to minutes.

1 hr = 60 min

III. The drop factor or number of drops that equal 1 ml of fluid. (This information can be found on the IV tubing box.)

10 gtt = 1 ml

Set up the problem by placing each of the three values in a proportion.

$$\frac{125 \text{ ml}}{1 \text{ hr}} \times \frac{1 \text{ hr}}{60 \text{ min}} \times \frac{10 \text{ gtt}}{1 \text{ ml}}$$

Numbers and units of measure can be canceled out from the upper and lower levels of this equation.

The numbers cancel, leaving:

$$\frac{125\ ml}{1\ hr} \times \frac{1\ hr}{\underset{6}{\cancel{60}}\ min} \times \frac{\overset{1}{\cancel{10}}\ gtt}{1\ ml}$$

The units cancel, leaving:

$$\frac{125\ \cancel{ml}}{1\ \cancel{hr}} \times \frac{1\ \cancel{hr}}{6\ min} \times \frac{1\ gtt}{1\ \cancel{ml}}$$

Next, multiply each level across and divide the numerator by the denominator for the answer.

$$\frac{125\ ml}{1\ hr} \times \frac{1\ hr}{6\ min} \times \frac{1\ gtt}{1\ ml} = \frac{125\ gtt}{6\ min}$$

$$125 \div 6 = 20.8\ or\ 21\ gtt/min$$

CALCULATION OF CREATININE CLEARANCE

To calculate creatinine clearance (Ccr) in adults from serum creatinine:

Male: $Ccr = \dfrac{\text{weight (kg)} \times (140 - \text{age})}{72 \times \text{serum creatinine (mg/dl)}}$

Female: $Ccr = 0.85 \times \text{calculation for males}$

CALCULATION OF IDEAL BODY WEIGHT

To estimate ideal body weight (kg) in adults:

Male = 50 kg + 2.3 kg (each inch >5 ft)
Female = 45.5 kg + 2.3 kg (each inch >5 ft)

To estimate ideal body weight in children:

IBW (kg) = $2.396e^{0.01863\ (ht\ in\ cm)}$
or use the nomogram on page 1062.

(Continued)

APPENDIX E
Formulas and Nomograms Helpful for Calculating Doses (*Continued*)

NOMOGRAM FOR ESTIMATING IDEAL BODY MASS IN CHILDREN*

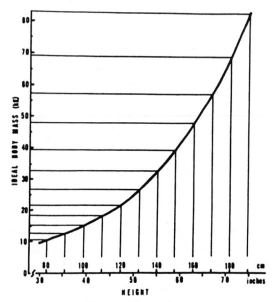

IBM (kg) = 2.396 $e^{0.01863(\text{ht in cm})}$

CALCULATION OF BODY SURFACE AREA
To calculate body surface area (BSA) in adults and children:

1) *Dubois method:*

SA (cm^2) = wt (kg)$^{0.425}$ × ht (cm)$^{0.725}$ × 71.84

SA (m^2) = K × $\sqrt[3]{\text{wt}^2\ (\text{kg})}$ (common K value 0.1 for toddlers, 0.103 for neonates)

2) *Simplified method:*

BSA (m^2) = $\sqrt{\dfrac{\text{ht (cm)} \times \text{wt (kg)}}{3600}}$

---

*From Traub, SL and Kichen, L: Estimating ideal body mass in children. Am J Hosp Pharm 1983; 40:107–110, with permission.

NOMOGRAM FOR ESTIMATING BODY SURFACE AREA IN CHILDREN

For pediatric patients of average size, body surface area may be estimated with the scale on the left. Match weight to corresponding surface area. For other pediatric patients, use the scale on the right. Lay a straightedge on the correct height and weight points for your patient, and observe the point where it intersects on the surface area scale at center

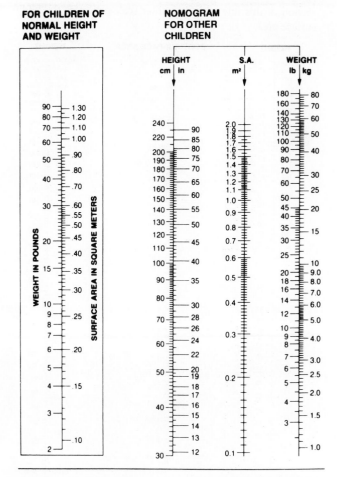

FOR CHILDREN OF NORMAL HEIGHT AND WEIGHT

NOMOGRAM FOR OTHER CHILDREN

From Nelson Text Book of Pediatrics, ed 14. WB Saunders, Philadelphia, 1992, with permission.

APPENDIX E
Formulas and Nomograms Helpful for Calculating Doses (*Continued*)

NOMOGRAM FOR ESTIMATING
BODY SURFACE AREA IN ADULTS
Use a straightedge to connect the patient's height in the left-hand column to weight in the right-hand column. The intersection of this line with the center scale estimates the body surface area.

HEIGHT	BODY SURFACE AREA	WEIGHT
cm 200 — 79 inch	2.80 m²	kg 150 — 330 lb
78		145 — 320
195 — 77	2.70	140 — 310
76	2.60	135 — 300
190 — 75		130 — 290
74	2.50	280
185 — 73	2.40	125 — 270
72		120 — 260
180 — 71	2.30	115 — 250
70		
175 — 69	2.20	110 — 240
68		105 — 230
170 — 67	2.10	100 — 220
66		
165 — 65	2.00	95 — 210
64	1.95	90 — 200
160 — 63	1.90	
62	1.85	85 — 190
155 — 61	1.80	
60	1.75	80 — 180
150 — 59	1.70	75 — 170
58	1.65	— 160
145 — 57	1.60	70 — 150
56	1.55	
140 — 55	1.50	65 — 140
54	1.45	
135 — 53	1.40	60 — 130
52		
130 — 51	1.35	55 — 120
50	1.30	
125 — 49	1.25	50 — 110
48	1.20	— 105
120 — 47	1.15	45 — 100
46	1.10	— 95
115 — 45		40 — 90
44	1.05	— 85
110 — 43	1.00	— 80
42		35 — 75
105 — 41	0.95	— 70
40	0.90	
cm 100 — 39 in	0.86 m²	kg 30 — 66 lb

From Lenter, C (ed): Geigy Scientific Tables, ed 8. CIBA-GEIGY, Basle, Switzerland, with permission.

APPENDIX F
Recommendations for the Safe Handling of Cytotoxic (Antineoplastic) Drugs*

Introduction

Cytotoxic drugs are toxic compounds and are known to have carcinogenic, mutagenic, and/or teratogenic potential. With direct contact they may cause irritation to the skin, eyes, and mucous membranes, and ulceration and necrosis of tissue. The toxicity of cytotoxic drugs dictates that the exposure of health-care personnel to these drugs should be minimized. At the same time, the requirement for maintenance of aseptic conditions must be satisfied.

Potential Routes of Exposure

The following information reviews the routes through which exposure may occur and presents recommendations for the safe handling of parenteral cytotoxic drugs by pharmacists, nurses, physicians, and other personnel who participate in the preparation and administration of these drugs to patients. These guidelines apply in any setting where cytotoxic drugs are prepared—including pharmacies, nursing units, clinics, physicians' offices, and the home health-care environment. The primary routes of exposure during the preparation and administration phases are through the inhalation of aerosolized drug or by direct skin contact.

During drug preparation, a variety of manipulations are performed that may result in aerosol generation, spraying, and splattering. Examples of these manipulations include: the withdrawal of needles from drug vials; the use of syringes and needles or filter straws for drug transfer; the opening of ampules; and the expulsion of air from the syringe when measuring the precise volume of a drug. Pharmaceutical practice calls for the use of aseptic techniques and a sterile environment. Many pharmacies provide this sterile environment by using a horizontal laminar flow work bench. However, while

(Continued)

---

*Produced by the NIH Division of Safety and the NIH Clinical Center Pharmacy Department and Cancer Nursing Service. NIH Publication No. 92-2621.

APPENDIX F
Recommendations for the Safe Handling of Cytotoxic (Antineoplastic) Drugs (*Continued*)

this type of unit provides product protection, it may expose the operator and the other room occupants to aerosols generated during drug preparation procedures. Therefore, a Class II laminar flow (vertical) biological safety cabinet that provides both product and operator protection is needed for the preparation of cytotoxic drugs. This is accomplished by filtering incoming and exhaust air through a high-efficiency particulate air (HEPA) filter. It should be noted that the filters are not effective for volatile materials because they do not capture vapors and gases. Personnel should be familiar with the capabilities, limitations, and proper utilization of the biological safety cabinet selected.

During administration, clearing air from a syringe or infusion line and leakage at tubing, syringe, or stopcock connections should be avoided to prevent opportunities for accidental skin contact and aerosol generation. Dispose of syringes and unclipped needles into a leakproof and puncture-resistant container.

The disposal of cytotoxic drugs and trace contaminated materials (e.g., gloves, gowns, needles, syringes, vials) presents a possible source of exposure to pharmacists, nurses, and physicians as well as to ancillary personnel, especially the housekeeping staff. Excreta from patients receiving cytotoxic drug therapy may contain high concentrations of the drug. All personnel should be aware of this source of potential exposure and should take appropriate precautions as established by your hospital or clinic to avoid accidental contact.

The potential risks to pharmacists, nurses, and physicians from repeated contact with parenteral cytotoxic drugs can be effectively controlled by using a combination of specific containment equipment and certain work techniques, which are described in the recommendations sections. For the most part, the techniques are merely an extension of good work practices by health-care and ancillary personnel, and similar in principle and practice to *Universal Precautions*. These may be supplemented as deemed appropriate for the work being performed. By using these precautions, personnel are better able to minimize possible exposure to cytotoxic drugs.

≋ RECOMMENDED PRACTICES FOR PERSONNEL PREPARING CYTOTOXIC DRUGS

Professionally accepted standards concerning the aseptic preparation of parenteral products should be followed. Only properly trained personnel should handle cytotoxic drugs.

Training sessions should be offered to new professionals as well as to technical and housekeeping personnel who may come in contact with these drugs. Safe handling should be the focus of such training.

Part 1

All procedures involved in the preparation of cytotoxic drugs should be performed in a Class II, Type A or Type B laminar flow biological safety cabinet. The cabinet exhaust should be discharged to the outdoors in order to eliminate the exposure of personnel to drugs that may volatilize after retention on filters of the cabinet. The **cabinet of choice** is a **Class II, Type B** that discharges exhaust to the outdoors and can be obtained with a bag-in/bag-out filter to protect the personnel servicing the cabinet and to facilitate disposal.

Part 2

Alternatively, a **Class II, Type A** cabinet can be equipped with a canopy or thimble unit that exhausts to the outdoors. For detailed information about the design, capabilities, and limitations of various types of biological safety cabinets, refer to the National Sanitation Foundation Standard 49.

The work surface of the safety cabinet should be covered with plastic-backed absorbent paper. This will reduce the potential for dispersion of droplets and spills and facilitate cleanup. This paper should be changed after any overt spill and at the end of each work shift.

Personnel preparing the drugs should wear unpowdered latex surgical gloves and a disposable gown with elastic or knit cuffs. Gloves should be changed regularly and immediately if torn or punctured. Protective clothing should not be worn outside of the drug preparation area. Overtly contami-
(Continued)

APPENDIX F
Recommendations for the Safe Handling of Cytotoxic (Antineoplastic) Drugs (*Continued*)

nated gowns require immediate removal and replacement. In case of skin contact with any cytotoxic drug, thoroughly wash the affected area with soap and water. However, do not abrade the skin by using a scrub brush. Flush the affected eye(s), while holding back the eyelid(s), with copious amounts of water for at least 15 minutes. Then seek medical evaluation by a physician.

Vials containing drugs requiring reconstitution should be vented to reduce the internal pressure with a venting device using a 0.22-micron hydrophobic filter or other appropriate means such as a chemotherapy dispensing pin. This reduces the probability of spraying and spillage.

If a chemotherapy dispensing pin is not used, a sterile alcohol pad should be carefully placed around the needle and vial top during withdrawal from the septum.

The external surfaces contaminated with a drug should be wiped clean with an alcohol pad prior to transfer or transport.

When opening the glass ampule, wrap it and then snap it at the break point using an alcohol pad to reduce the possibility of injury and to contain the aerosol produced. Use a 5-micron filter needle or straw when removing the drug solution.

Syringes and IV bottles containing cytotoxic drugs should be labeled and dated. Before these items leave the preparation area, an additional label reading, "**Caution—Chemotherapy, Dispose of Properly**" is recommended.

After completing the drug preparation process, wipe down the interior of the safety cabinet with water (for injection or irrigation) followed by 70% alcohol using disposable towels. All wastes are considered contaminated and should be disposed of properly.

Contaminated needles and syringes, IV tubing, butterfly clips, etc., should be disposed of intact to prevent aerosol generation and injury. **Do not recap needles.** Place these items in a puncture-resistant container along with any contaminated bottles, vials, gloves, absorbent paper, disposable gowns, gauze, and other waste. The container should then be placed in a box labeled "**Cytotoxic waste only**," sealed, and disposed of according to federal, state, and local requirements. Linen contaminated with drugs, patient excreta, or body fluids should be handled separately.

Hands should be washed between glove changes and after glove removal.

Cytotoxic drugs are categorized as regulated wastes and therefore should be disposed of according to federal, state, and local requirements.

≋ RECOMMENDED PRACTICES FOR PERSONNEL ADMINISTERING PARENTERAL CYTOTOXIC DRUGS

Some cytotoxic drugs are excreted from patients in high concentrations. Personnel should be knowledgeable regarding which drugs fit this description and take care to avoid skin contact and to minimize aerosol generation. When disposing of excreta from patients, all personnel should wear gowns and latex surgical gloves.

A protective outer garment such as a closed-front surgical-type gown with knit cuffs should be worn. Gowns may be of the disposable or washable variety.

Disposable latex surgical gloves should be worn during those procedures where exposure to the drugs may result and when handling patient body fluids or excreta. When bubbles are removed from syringes or IV tubing, an alcohol pad should be placed carefully over the tip of such items in order to collect any of the cytotoxic drugs that may be inadvertently discharged. Discard gloves after each use and wash hands.

Contaminated needles and syringes and IV apparatus should be disposed of intact into a labeled, puncture-resistant container in order to minimize aerosol generation and risk of injury. **Do not recap needles.** The container, as well as other contaminated materials, should be placed in a box labeled "**Cytotoxic waste only**." Linen overtly contaminated with any cytotoxic agent or excreta from a patient within 48 hours following drug administration may be safely handled by using the procedures prescribed for isolation cases. For example, place the contaminated articles in a "yellow" cloth bag

(Continued)

APPENDIX F
Recommendations for the Safe Handling of Cytotoxic (Antineoplastic) Drugs (*Continued*)

lined with a water-soluble plastic bag and then place into the washing machine. Linen without overt contamination can be handled by routine laundering procedures.

In case of skin contact with any cytotoxic drug, thoroughly wash the affected area with soap and water. However, do not abrade the skin by using a scrub brush. Flush the affected eye(s), while holding back the eyelid(s), with copious amounts of water for at least 15 minutes. Then seek medical evaluation by a physician. Always wash hands after removing gloves.

APPENDIX G
Normal Values of Common Laboratory Tests

SERUM TESTS

Hematologic	Male	Female
Hemoglobin	14–18 g/dl	11.5–15.5 g/dl
Hematocrit	39–49%	33–43%
Red blood cells (RBC)	4.3–5.9 million/mm^3	3.5–5 million/mm^3
Leukocytes (WBC)	5,000–10,000/mm^3	
Neutrophils	54–75% (3,000–7,500/mm^3)	
Bands	3–8% (150–700/mm^3)	
Eosinophils	1–4% (50–400/mm^3)	
Basophils	0–1% (25–100/mm^3)	
Monocytes	2–8% (100–500/mm^3)	
Lymphocytes	25–40% (1,500–4,500/mm^3)	
T-lymphocytes	60–80% of lymphocytes	
B-lymphocytes	10–20% of lymphocytes	
Platelets	150,000–450,000/mm^3	
Prothrombin (PT)	9.6–11.8 sec	9.5–11.3 sec
Partial thromboplastin time, activated (aPTT)	25–38 sec	
Bleeding time (Duke)	1–3 min	
" " (Ivy)	3–6 min	
" " (Template)	3–6 min	
Clotting time (Lee-White)	4–8 min	
Fibrinogen	200–400 mg/dl	
Erythrocyte sedimentation rate (ESR)	≤20 mm/hr	≤30 mm/hr

Chemistry	Male	Female
Sodium	135–145 mEq/L	
Potassium	3.5–5.0 mEq/L	
Chloride	95–105 mEq/L	
Bicarbonate (HCO$_3$)	19–25 mEq/L	
Total calcium	9–11 mg/dl or 4.5–5.5 mEq/L	
Ionized calcium	4.2–5.4 mg/dl or 2.1–2.6 mEq/L	
Phosphorus/phosphate	2.5–5 mg/dl	
Magnesium	1.6–2.4 mEq/L	
Glucose	70–110 mg/dl	
Osmolality	280–300 mOsm/kg	
Ammonia (NH$_3$)	10–80 mcg/dl	
Amylase	≤30 U/L	
Creatine phosphokinase, total (CK, CPK)	≤130 U/L	

(Continued)

APPENDIX G
Normal Values of Common Laboratory Tests (*Continued*)

Chemistry	Male	Female
Creatine phosphokinase isoenzymes	CK-MB = ≤5% total CK	
Lactic dehydrogenase (LDH)	50–150 U/L	
Protein: total	6–8 g/dl	
albumin	4–6 g/dl	
globulin	2.3–3.5 g/dl	

Hepatic	Male	Female
SGOT (AST)	≤35 U/L	
SGPT (ALT)	≤35 U/L	
Total bilirubin	0.1–1 mg/dl	
Conjugated bilirubin	0.0–0.2 mg/dl	
Unconjugated (indirect) bilirubin	0.2–0.8 mg/dl	
Alkaline phosphatase	30–120 U/L	

Renal	Male	Female
BUN	6–20 mg/dl	
Creatinine	0.6–1.3 mg/dl	0.5–1.0 mg/dl
Uric acid	2–7 mg/dl	

Lipids	Male	Female
Total cholesterol	400–850 mg/dl	
Desirable	<200 mg/dl	
Borderline high	200–239 mg/dl	
High	>240 mg/dl	
Triglycerides	40–150 mg/dl	
Low-density lipoproteins (LDL)		
Desirable	<130 mg/dl	
Borderline high	130–159 mg/dl	
High	>160 mg/dl	
High-density lipoproteins (HDL)	30–70 mg/dl	

Arterial Blood Gases	Male	Female
pH	7.35–7.45	
pO_2	80–100 mm Hg	
pCO_2	35–45 mm Hg	
O_2 saturation	96–100%	
Base excess	+2–(−2)	
Bicarbonate (HCO_3)	22–26 mEq/L	

URINE TESTS

Urine	Male	Female
pH	4.5–8.0	
Specific gravity	1.010–1.025	

APPENDIX H
Dietary Guidelines for Food Sources

Potassium-Rich Foods

avocados	dried fruits	oranges	spinach
bananas	grapefruit	peaches	sunflower seeds
broccoli	lima beans	potatoes	tomatoes
buttermilk	navy beans	prunes	winter squash
cantaloupe	nuts	rhubarb	

Sodium-Rich Foods

baking mixes (pancakes, muffins)	canned spaghetti sauce	Parmesan cheese
barbecue sauce	cured meats	pickles (dill)
butter/margarine	"fast" foods	potato salad
buttermilk	macaroni and cheese	pretzels, potato chips (salted)
canned chili	microwave dinners	sauerkraut
canned seafood	milk	tomato ketchup
canned soups	onion soup mix (dried)	TV dinners

Calcium-Rich Foods

beans	cream soups	oysters
blackberries	dates	rhubarb
bok choy	figs	salmon
broccoli	milk and dairy products	sardines
cauliflower	molasses (blackstrap)	spinach
clams	oranges	tofu

Vitamin K–Rich Foods

asparagus	cauliflower	liver	rice
beans	cheeses	milk	spinach
broccoli	collards	mustard greens	turnips
brussels sprouts	fish	pork	yogurt
cabbage	lettuce		

Low-Sodium Foods

baked or broiled poultry	grits (not instant)	puffed wheat and rice
canned pumpkin	honey	red kidney and lima beans
cooked turnips	jams and jellies	sherbet
egg yolks	lean meats	unsalted nuts
fresh vegetables	low-calorie mayonnaise	whiskey
fruit	macaroons	
	potatoes	

Foods That Acidify Urine

cheeses	fish	meats	poultry
cranberries	grains (breads and cereals)	plums	prunes
eggs			

Foods That Alkalinize Urine

all fruits except cranberries, prunes, plums   all vegetables   milk

Foods Containing Tyramine

aged cheeses	figs
avocados	Italian flat beans
bananas	liver
beer	meat tenderizer
bouillon	mixed Chinese vegetables
caviar	over-ripe fruit
broad (fava) beans	red and white wine
caffeine-containing beverages	sherry
canned meat	smoked or pickled fish
chocolate	soy sauce
eggplant	yeasts
fermented sausage (bologna, salami, pepperoni, summer)	yogurt

Iron-Rich Foods

cereals	dried fruit	lean red meats
dried beans and peas	leafy green vegetables	organ meats

Vitamin D–Rich Foods

breads	fish	fortified milk
cereals	fish liver oils	

APPENDIX I
Recommended Dietary Allowances (RDAs)[a]

Age (years) and Sex Group	WEIGHT[b] kg	WEIGHT[b] lb	HEIGHT[b] cm	HEIGHT[b] in.	Protein gm	FAT-SOLUBLE VITAMINS Vitamin A μg RE[c]	Vitamin D μg[d]	Vitamin E mg α-TE[e]	Vitamin K μg
Infants									
0.0–0.5	6	13	60	24	13	375	7.5	3	5
0.5–1.0	9	20	71	28	14	375	10	4	10
Children									
1–3	13	29	90	35	16	400	10	6	15
4–6	20	44	112	44	24	500	10	7	20
7–10	28	62	132	52	28	700	10	7	30
Males									
11–14	45	99	157	62	45	1,000	10	10	45
15–18	66	145	176	69	59	1,000	10	10	65
19–24	72	160	177	70	58	1,000	10	10	70
25–50	79	174	176	70	63	1,000	5	10	80
51+	77	170	173	68	63	1,000	5	10	80

Females									
11–14	46	101	157	62	46	800	10	8	45
15–18	55	120	163	64	44	800	10	8	55
19–24	58	128	164	65	46	800	10	8	60
25–50	63	138	163	64	50	800	5	8	65
51+	65	143	160	63	50	800	5	8	65
Pregnant					60	800	10	10	65
Lactating									
1st 6 mo					65	1,300	10	12	65
2nd 6 mo					62	1,200	10	11	65

(Continued)

APPENDIX I
Recommended Dietary Allowances (RDAs)^a (Continued)

Recommended Dietary Allowances (RDAs)—continued

Age (years) and Sex Group	WATER-SOLUBLE VITAMINS							MINERALS						
	Vitamin C	Thiamin	Riboflavin	Niacin	Vitamin B$_6$	Folate	Vitamin B$_{12}$	Calcium	Phosphorus	Magnesium	Iron	Zinc	Iodine	Selenium
	mg	mg	mg	mg NE^f	mg	µg	µg	mg	mg	mg	mg	mg	µg	µg
Infants														
0.0–0.5	30	0.3	0.4	5	0.3	25	0.3	400	300	40	6	5	40	10
0.5–1.0	35	0.4	0.5	6	0.6	35	0.5	600	500	60	10	5	50	15
Children														
1–3	40	0.7	0.8	9	1.0	50	0.7	800	800	80	10	10	70	20
4–6	45	0.9	1.1	12	1.1	75	1.0	800	800	120	10	10	90	20
7–10	45	1.0	1.2	13	1.4	100	1.4	800	800	170	10	10	120	30
Males														
11–14	50	1.3	1.5	17	1.7	150	2.0	1,200	1,200	270	12	15	150	40
15–18	60	1.5	1.8	20	2.0	200	2.0	1,200	1,200	400	12	15	150	50
19–24	60	1.5	1.7	19	2.0	200	2.0	1,200	1,200	350	10	15	150	70

25–50	60	1.5	1.7	19	2.0	200	2.0	800	800	350	10	15	150	70
51+	60	1.2	1.4	15	2.0	200	2.0	800	800	350	10	15	150	70
Females													
11–14	50	1.1	1.3	15	1.4	150	2.0	1,200	1,200	280	15	12	150	45
15–18	60	1.1	1.3	15	1.5	180	2.0	1,200	1,200	300	15	12	150	50
19–24	60	1.1	1.3	15	1.6	180	2.0	1,200	1,200	280	15	12	150	55
25–50	60	1.1	1.3	15	1.6	180	2.0	800	800	280	15	12	150	55
51+	60	1.0	1.2	13	1.6	180	2.0	800	800	280	10	12	150	55
Pregnant	70	1.5	1.6	17	2.2	400	2.2	1,200	1,200	320	30	15	175	65
Lactating													
1st 6 mo	95	1.6	1.8	20	2.1	280	2.6	1,200	1,200	355	15	19	200	75
2nd 6 mo	90	1.6	1.7	20	2.1	260	2.6	1,200	1,200	340	15	16	200	75

[a]The allowances, expressed as average daily intakes over time, are intended to provide for individual variations among most normal persons as they live in the United States under usual environmental stresses. Diets should be based on a variety of common foods in order to provide other nutrients for which human requirements have been less well defined.

[b]Weights and heights of Reference Adults are actual medians for the U.S. population of the designated age, as reported by NHANES II. The median weights and heights of those under 19 years of age were taken from Hamill, P.V.V., Drizd, T.A., Johnson, C.L., Reed, R.B., Roche, A.F., and Moore, W.M.: Physical growth. National Center for Health Statistics Percentiles. Am J Clin Nutr 32:607, 1979. The use of these figures does not imply that the height-to-weight ratios are ideal.

[c]Retinol equivalents. 1 retinol equivalent = 1 μg retinol or 6 μg β-carotene.

[d]As cholecalciferol. 10 μg cholecalciferol = 400 IU of vitamin D.

[e]α-Tocopherol equivalents. 1 mg d-α tocopherol = 1 α-TE.

[f]NE (niacin equivalent) is equal to 1 mg of niacin or 60 mg of dietary tryptophan.

Adapted from National Academy of Sciences, 1989 with permission. From Food and Nutrition Board, National Academy of Sciences—National Research Council (Revised, 1989) (designed for the maintenance of good nutrition of practically all healthy people in the United States).

APPENDIX J
Electrolyte Equivalents and Caloric Values of Commonly Used Large-Volume Parenterals

	mEq/L							
	Na	K	Ca	Mg	Cl	Acetate	Lactate	CALORIES/L
Solution								
D5W	—	—	—	—	—	—	—	170
D10W	—	—	—	—	—	—	—	340
0.9% NaCl	154	—	—	—	154	—	—	—
D5/0.9% NaCl	154	—	—	—	154	—	—	170
D5/0.45% NaCl	77	—	—	—	77	—	—	170
D5/0.2% NaCl	38.5	—	—	—	38.5	—	—	170
D5/LR	130	4	3	—	109	—	28	170–180
D5/Ringer's	147.5	4	4.5	—	156	—	—	170
LR	130	4	3	—	109	—	28	9
Ringer's Injection	147	4	4.5	—	156	—	—	—

D5W = 5% dextrose in water.
D10W = 10% dextrose in water.
0.9% NaCl = 0.9% sodium chloride = normal saline.
D5/0.9% NaCl = 5% dextrose in water with 0.9% sodium chloride
  = D5 with normal saline.
D5/0.45% NaCl = 5% dextrose in water with 0.45% sodium chloride
  = D5 with half normal saline.
D5/0.2% NaCl = 5% dextrose in water with 0.2% sodium chloride
  = D5 with quarter normal saline.
D5/LR = 5% dextrose in water with lactated Ringer's solution.
D5/Ringer's = 5% dextrose in water with Ringer's solution.
LR = lactated Ringer's solution.

APPENDIX K
Endocarditis Prophylaxis Guidelines

TABLE 1.—RECOMMENDED STANDARD PROPHYLACTIC REGIMEN FOR DENTAL, ORAL, OR UPPER RESPIRATORY TRACT PROCEDURES IN PATIENTS WHO ARE AT RISK*

Drug	Dosing Regiment†
STANDARD REGIMEN	
Amoxicillin	3.0 g orally 1 hr before procedure; then 1.5 g 6 hr after initial dose
AMOXICILLIN/PENICILLIN-ALLERGIC PATIENTS	
Erythromycin *or*	Erythromycin ethylsuccinate, 800 mg, or erythromycin stearate, 1.0 g, orally 2 hr before procedure; then half the dose 6 hr after initial dose
Clindamycin	300 mg orally 1 hr before procedure and 150 mg 6 hr after initial dose

*Includes those with prosthetic heart valves and other high-risk patients.
†Initial pediatric doses are as follows: amoxicillin, 50 mg/kg; erythromycin ethylsuccinate or erythromycin stearate, 20 mg/kg; and clindamycin, 10 mg/kg. Follow-up doses should be one half the initial dose. **Total pediatric dose should not exceed total adult dose**. The following weight ranges may also be used for the initial pediatric dose of amoxicillin: <15 kg, 750 mg; 15 to 30 kg, 1500 mg; and >30 kg, 3000 mg (full adult dose).

TABLE 2.—ALTERNATE PROPHYLACTIC REGIMENS FOR DENTAL, ORAL, OR UPPER RESPIRATORY TRACT PROCEDURES IN PATIENTS WHO ARE AT RISK

Drug	Dosing Regimen*
PATIENTS UNABLE TO TAKE ORAL MEDICATIONS	
Ampicillin	Intravenous or intramuscular administration of ampicillin, 2.0 g, 30 min before procedure; then intravenous or intramuscular administration of ampicillin, 1.0 g, or oral administration of amoxicillin, 1.5 g, 6 hr after initial dose

(Continued)

APPENDIX K
Endocarditis Prophylaxis Guidelines (*Continued*)

TABLE 2.—*Continued*

Drug	Dosing Regimen*
AMPICILLIN/AMOXICILLIN/PENICILLIN-ALLERGIC PATIENTS UNABLE TO TAKE ORAL MEDICATIONS	
Clindamycin	Intravenous administration of 300 mg 30 min before procedure and an intravenous or oral administration of 150 mg 6 hr after initial dose
PATIENTS CONSIDERED HIGH RISK AND NOT CANDIDATES FOR STANDARD REGIMEN	
Ampicillin, gentamicin, and amoxicillin	Intravenous or intramuscular administration of ampicillin, 2.0 g, plus gentamicin, 1.5 mg/kg (not to exceed 80 mg), 30 min before procedure; followed by amoxicillin, 1.5 g, orally 6 hr after initial dose; alternatively, the parenteral regimen may be repeated 8 hr after initial dose
AMPICILLIN/AMOXICILLIN/PENICILLIN-ALLERGIC PATIENTS CONSIDERED HIGH RISK	
Vancomycin	Intravenous administration of 1.0 g over 1 hr, starting 1 hr before procedure; no repeated dose necessary

*Initial pediatric doses are as follows: ampicillin, 50 mg/kg; clindamycin, 10 mg/kg; gentamicin, 2.0 mg/kg; and vancomycin, 20 mg/kg. Follow-up doses should be one half the initial dose. **Total pediatric dose should not exceed total adult dose.** No initial dose is recommended in this table for amoxicillin (25 mg/kg is the follow-up dose).

TABLE 3.—REGIMENS FOR GENITOURINARY/ GASTROINTESTINAL PROCEDURES

Drug	Dosage Regimen*
STANDARD REGIMEN	
Ampicillin, gentamicin, and amoxicillin	Intravenous or intramuscular administration of ampicillin, 2.0 g, plus gentamicin, 1.5 mg/kg (not to exceed 80 mg), 30 min before procedure; followed by amoxicillin, 1.5 g, orally 6 hr after initial dose; alternatively, the parenteral regimen may be repeated once 8 hr after initial dose
AMPICILLIN/AMOXICILLIN/PENICILLIN-ALLERGIC PATIENT REGIMEN	
Vancomycin and gentamicin	Intravenous administration of vancomycin, 1.0 g, over 1 hr plus intravenous or intramuscular administration of gentamicin, 1.5 mg/kg (not to exceed 80 mg), 1 hr before procedure; may be repeated once 8 hr after initial dose
ALTERNATE LOW-RISK PATIENT REGIMEN	
Amoxicillin	3.0 g orally 1 hr before procedure; then, 1.5 g 6 hr after initial dose

*Initial pediatric doses are as follows: ampicillin, 50 mg/kg; amoxicillin, 50 mg/kg; gentamicin, 2.0 mg/kg; and vancomycin, 20 mg/kg. Follow-up doses should be half the initial dose. **Total pediatric dose should not exceed total adult dose.**

Adapted from Dajani, AS, et al: Prevention of bacterial endocarditis: recommendations by the American Heart Association. JAMA 1990; 264:2919–2922, with permission.

APPENDIX L
Intravenous Drug Update

Generic name (Brand Name)	Classification	Indication(s)	Dosage	FDA/Market Status
abciximab (ReoPro)	Platelet aggregation inhibitor	Prevention of myocardial ischemia following PCTA in patients at high risk for reclosure	0.25 mg/kg 10–60 min prior to PCTA followed by infusion at 10 mcg/min for 12 hr	Approved 12/94
alteplase (Activase)	Thrombolytic	Management of myocardial infarction	Adults >67 kg: 15 mg bolus, then 50 mg over 30 min, then 35 mg over next 60 min Adults ≤67 kg: 15 mg bolus, then 0.75 mg/kg over 30 min (not to exceed 50 mg), then 0.5 mg/kg over next 60 min (not to exceed 35 mg)	Approved by FDA 3/95 (new method of administration—"front loading")
amiodarone (Cordarone IV)	Antiarrhythmic	Management of acute life-threatening ventricular arrhythmias unresponsive to conventional therapy	Adults: 5–10 mg/kg bolus over 30 min, followed by continuous infusion at 10–20 mg/kg/day; may change to oral therapy after 3–5 days	FDA approval pending*
dexrazoxane (Zinecard)	Cardioprotective agent	Decreases incidence and severity of cardiomyopathy from doxorubicin therapy	Adults: 10 mg/m² dexrazoxane for each 1 mg/m² doxorubicin	Available 9/94

imiglucerase (Cerezyme)	Enzyme replacement	Treatment of symptomatic Type I Gaucher's disease	Adults and children: 60 units/kg q 2 wk (range 2.5 units/kg 3 times weekly–60 units/kg q 1–4 wk)	Approved 3/94; will replace alglucerase
nalmefine hydrochloride (Revex)	Opioid antagonist	Reversal of opioid effects and management of opioid overdosage	Adults: *Reversal of postoperative opioid depression*—0.25 mcg/kg, then 0.25 mcg/kg incremental doses q 2–5 min until desired reversal is obtained (not to exceed 1 mcg/kg cumulative dose); *known or suspected opioid overdosage (patients not physically dependent on opioids)*—0.5 mg/70 kg, may be followed by 1 mg/70 kg 2–5 min later (not to exceed 1.5 mg/70 kg total); *known or suspected opioid overdosage (dependence is suspected)*—0.1 mg/70 kg is challenge dose; if there is no evidence of withdrawal after 2 min, recommended dose should be administered	Marketed 6/95
Rho(D) immune globulin IV (WinRho SD)	Immune globulin	Suppression of sensitization of Rh-negative pregnant women and management of ITP	Adults: *Suppression of Rh isoimmunization*—1500 IU (300 mg) at 28 wk gestation; if given earlier repeat q 12 wk. *Within 72 hr of abortion or amniocentesis at >34 wk*—600 IU (120 mg). *ITP*—250 IU (50 mg)/kg (decrease dose if Hgb<10g/dl), 125–300 IU (25–60 mcg)/kg doses may be repeated as needed	Approved 3/95

(Continued)

APPENDIX L
Intravenous Drug Update
(Continued)

Generic name (Brand Name)	Classification	Indication(s)	Dosage	FDA/Market Status
warfarin (Coumadin)	Anticoagulant	Prevention and treatment of thromboembolic phenomena	Depends on coagulation studies	Marketed 6/95

PCTA = percutaneous transluminal angioplasty

ITP = idiopathic thrombocytopenic purpura

*Not yet approved; information from P and T Quik, Micromedex Inc. Vol. 85. December 1994. Content based on medical literature and product information available at that time.

BIBLIOGRAPHY

Acute Pain Management Guideline Panel: Acute Pain Management in Adults: Operative Procedures. Quick Reference Guide for Clinicians. Agency for Health Care Policy and Research, Public Health Service, US Department of Health and Human Services, Rockville, MD, 1992. AHCPR Pub. No. 92–0019.

American Hospital Formulary Service: Drug Information 95. American Society of Hospital Pharmacists, Bethesda, 1995.

American Pain Society: Principles of Analgesic Use in the Treatment of Acute Pain and Cancer Pain, ed 3. American Pain Society, Skokie, IL, 1992.

Cancer Chemotherapy Guidelines. Recommendations for the Management of Vesicant Extravasation, Hypersensitivity, and Anaphylaxis. Oncology Nursing Society, Pittsburgh, PA, 1992.

Deglin, JH and Vallerand, AH: Davis's Drug Guide for Nurses, ed 4. FA Davis, Philadelphia, 1995.

Facts and Comparisons. JB Lippincott, Philadelphia, 1995.

Koda-Kimble, MA, Young, LY, Kradjian, WA, and Guglielmo, BJ: Handbook of Applied Therapeutics, ed. 2. Applied Therapeutics, Vancouver, WA, 1992.

Koda-Kimble, MA and Young, LY (eds): Applied Therapeutics: The Clinical Use of Drugs, ed 5. Applied Therapeutics, Vancouver, WA, 1992.

Lindley, CM and Deloatch, KH: Infusion Technology Manual: A Self-Instructional Approach. American Society of Hospital Pharmacists, Bethesda, MD, 1993.

Lutz, CA and Przytulski, KR: Nutrition and Diet Therapy. FA Davis, Philadelphia, 1994.

Phelps, SJ and Cochran, EB: Guidelines for Administration of Intravenous Medications to Pediatric Patients, ed. 4. American Society of Hospital Pharmacists, 1993.

Physician's Desk Reference (PDR). Medical Economics Company, Oradell, NJ, 1995.

Semla, TP, Beizer, J, and Higbee, MD: Geriatric Dosage Handbook. Lexi-Comp, Cleveland, 1993.

Trissel, LA. Handbook on Injectable Drugs, ed 8. American Society of Hospital Pharmacists, Bethesda, 1994.

USP Dispensing Information (USP-DI) Drug Information for the Health Care Professional Volume 1. United States Pharmacopeial Convention, Rockville, MD, 1995.

Watson, J and Jaffe, MS: Nurse's Manual of Laboratory and Diagnostic Tests, ed 2. FA Davis, Philadelphia, 1995.

Index

Note: Entries for **generic** names appear in **boldface** type; trade names appear in regular type.